Diabetic Retinopathy

David J. Browning
Editor

Diabetic Retinopathy

Evidence-Based Management

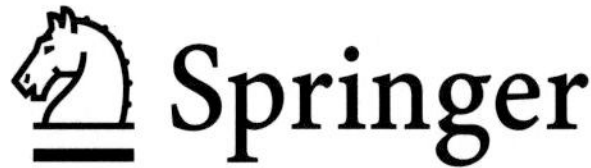

Editor
David J. Browning
Charlotte Eye Ear Nose and Throat
Associates
6035 Fairview Road
Charlotte NC 28210
USA
djbrowning@carolina.rr.com
dbrowning@ceenta.com

ISBN 978-0-387-85899-9 e-ISBN 978-0-387-85900-2
DOI 10.1007/978-0-387-85900-2
Springer New York Dordrecht Heidelberg London

Library of Congress Control Number: 2010920155

Illustrations by Alice Y. Chen (Figures 1.3, 1.4, 1.5, 1.14, 2.1, 2.2, 2.3, 2.4, 2.5, 2.6, 7.3, 7.6, 7.7, 7.9, 7.14, 9.13, 9.21, 9.22, 9.23, 9.24, 9.25, 9.26, 9.27, 9.28, 9.29, 11.1, 11.4, 11.14, 16.6, 16.9). www.aliceychen.com

Printed on acid-free paper

Springer is part of Springer Science+Business Media (www.springer.com)

To my parents,

Warren J. Browning
and
Mary T. Browning

Preface

The goal of this book is to provide a resource for physicians interested in learning the biological basis, clinical manifestations, and current treatment approaches to diabetic eye disease. Diabetes and diabetic eye disease are rapidly increasing in prevalence around the world. Our understanding of the mechanisms that underlie diabetes and our ability to ameliorate ocular complications are advancing at a similarly rapid pace. The disciplines contributing to progress range widely and include biochemistry, physiology, molecular biology, epidemiology, clinical medicine, public policy, economics, and ethics. Although most of the targeted clinical audience for the book will have been exposed to all of the required basic sciences in the past, we have attempted to provide more than allusions to needed concepts at key junctures. For example, Chapter 2 reviews the ideas and vocabulary of molecular and clinical genetics needed for a proper understanding of the subsequent material.

Some redundancy will be found in the text for two reasons. First, we expect users to read the book piecemeal, often stimulated by a clinical encounter of the day. For such users, limited coverage of the pertinent physiology of diabetic macular edema within the chapter dedicated to that topic (Chapter 7) makes pedagogical sense. In such cases, if time and interest permit, the comprehensive coverage provided in the Chapter 1 awaits. Second, redundancy aids understanding when the respective authors approach a topic with differences in framing and explanation.

The book has also been designed to provide the basis for linear study within the context of a course. Subsequent chapters build on antecedent ones. For example, to grasp the rationale for treatment of proliferative diabetic retinopathy (Chapter 9), one must understand its pathophysiology (Chapter 1) and how diabetic retinopathy severity has come to be defined (Chapter 5). Likewise, the significance and conundrums of diabetic macular ischemia (Chapter 8) are best understood after mastering the basis and limitations of ancillary studies (Chapter 6).

Chapters 11, 12, and 13 cover important, and somewhat autonomous, topics involving the effects of diabetes mellitus on the cornea, iris and angle, and optic nerve. Any clinician who cares for patients with diabetic retinopathy will need to be familiar with these concomitant manifestations of diabetic eye disease. More than once as a fellow debriding the corneal epithelium during a vitrectomy have I heard George Blankenship lament, "Doctor, if you're not careful, you'll turn this retina fellowship of yours into a cornea fellowship!" Common pathophysiological themes tie many of the ocular manifestations of diabetes together.

The Chapters 14 and 15 broaden the landscape of consideration from the lab and ophthalmic lane to the community and society. Systems of health-care delivery and their financial incentives influence outcomes in diabetic retinopathy as surely as a patient's blood pressure and glycosylated hemoglobin. We have made an effort to provide specific clinical examples of these effects drawn from practice to ground the discussion.

The last Chapter 16 synthesizes the principles introduced in the earlier chapters in 14 teaching vignettes. Although the Diabetic Retinopathy Study, the Diabetic Retinopathy Vitrectomy Study, the Early Treatment Diabetic Retinopathy Study (ETDRS), and the contemporary clinical trials of the Diabetic Retinopathy Clinical Research Network often provide a foundation of reliable evidence upon which the clinician can base clinical decision making, the complexity of real cases just as often undercuts the extrapolation of classic studies to practice. To cite one example of many, how should one manage clinically significant macular edema in an 80-year-old, when the ETDRS excluded patients older than age 70? Moreover, as level I evidence always, and increasingly, lags behind the development of diagnostic tests and promising treatments for diabetic retinopathy, the importance of experience, informed opinion based on wide reading, and clinical consensus remains as critical as ever in 2010. Chapter 16 was written in this spirit. The cases were circulated among the coauthors who commented independently on them. The coauthor assigned to discuss the case then compiled the independent responses, went back to the literature, and wrote a considered commentary. We hope that you will find these balanced and supported by the evidence marshaled.

We encourage feedback. Your comments, suggestions, and ideas for cases to include in future editions will help us to improve the book.

Charlotte, North Carolina David J. Browning

Acknowledgments

The coauthors thank Catherine Paduani for her excellent editorial skills and friendly, efficient assistance throughout the preparation of the book. We also thank Alice Y. Chen, medical artist, for contributing her impressive talents and for her collaborative spirit.

Scott Pautler thanks Steven M. Cohen, MD for providing the fundus photograph of a combined traction-rhegmatogenous retinal detachment (Fig. 9.14), E. F. Bakke, MD for providing the photograph of iris vascular tufts from his chapter (Fig. 9.5), Curtis Margo, MD for his assistance regarding the histopathology section of Chapter 8 and Donald G. Puro, MDPhD for reviewing the basic science section of Chapter 9. He especially thanks his wife, Carol Pautler, for her sacrifices, patience, and understanding throughout the work.

The editor thanks the coauthors, an inquisitive and stimulating group of experts, for their energy and dedication to the goals we set. He is indebted to Cameron Black, Stephen Clark, Samuel Browning, Clare Browning, and David Manderfield for bibliographic assistance; Michael D. McOwen, Jennifer M. Ballard, Lorraine C. Clark, Uma Balasubramanian, Donna Jo McClain, and Pearl A. Leotaud for their talents and assistance in ophthalmic imaging studies used for illustrations; and Scott Sutherland MD and Scott Jaben MD for their helpful comments on Chapter 10. To his wife, Clare Browning, his thanks for her support, encouragement, and good humor throughout.

Contents

Contributors

Abdhish R. Bhavsar, MD Clinical Research, Retina Center; University of Minnesota; Posterior Segment Research, Phillips Eye Institute, Minneapolis, MN 55404, USA bhavs001@umn.edu

David J. Browning MD, PhD Charlotte Eye Ear Nose & Throat Associates, Charlotte, NC 28210, USA dbrowning@ceenta.com

Geoffrey G. Emerson, MD, PhD Retina Center, Minneapolis, MN 55404, USA geoffrey_emerson@yahoo.com

M. Vaughn Emerson, MD Phillips Eye Institute, Retina Center, Minneapolis, MN 55404, USA drv@retinadocs.com

Saiyid Akbar Hasan, Department of Ophthalmology, Mayo Clinic, Jacksonville, FL 32082, USA hasan.saiyid@mayo.edu

Scott E. Pautler, MD, FACS Department of Ophthalmology, University of South Florida, University Community Hospital, Tampa, FL 33607, USA pautlers@aol.com

Michael H. Rotberg, MD Charlotte Eye Ear Nose & Throat Associates, Charlotte, NC 28210, USA mrotberg@ceenta.com

Kent W. Small, MD Macula and Retina Institute, Cedars-Sinai Medical Center, Los Angeles, CA 90048, USA kentsmall@hotmail.com

Michael W. Stewart, MD Department of Ophthalmology, Mayo School of Medicine, Jacksonville, FL 32082, USA stewart.michael@mayo.edu

David G. Telander, MD, PhD University of California Davis Medical Center, Sacramento, CA 95817, USA dgtelander@ucdavis.edu

Keye Wong, MD University of South Florida, Sarasota, FL 34242, USA iskeye@yahoo.com

Chapter 1
Pathophysiology of Diabetic Retinopathy

Michael W. Stewart

1.1 Retinal Anatomy

1.1.1 History

The retina was first described by Herophilus of Chalcedon around 300 BC. It was named by Rufos of Ephesus (c. 110 AD) and appeared to early anatomists as a surrounding net which supported the vitreous. Though Galen noted structural similarities to the brain, he was unable to provide further understanding regarding its function. It was Kepler who first suggested that the retina served as the eye's primary photoreceptor tissue. By using alcohol fixation, Treviranus (1835) performed the first detailed microscopic retinal studies. Only with the subsequent development of electron microscopy, trypsin digest, clinical fluorescein angiography, and optical coherence tomography have scientists been able to understand the retina's cellular connections, ultrastructure, and retinal vasculature, as well as correlate anatomical and clinical findings.[1]

1.1.2 Anatomy

The retina is a translucent tissue lining the inside posterior 2/3 of the eye, extending from the macula to the ora serrata.[2] It is attached firmly at the disc and ora and is contiguous with the axons of the optic nerve and the nonpigmented epithelium of the pars plana (see Fig. 1.1). Externally, there exist weak attachments to the retinal pigment epithelium via interdigitation between the RPE cells and photoreceptor outer segments. There are firm internal attachments to the vitreous at the optic nerve, macula, retinal vessels, and vitreous base.

The central 5–6 mm is referred to as the retina centralis, an area with more than 1 layer of ganglion cells. The clinical macula, also called the macula lutea owing to xanthophyll in ganglion and bipolar cells, is the central 1.5 mm and is bounded by the termination of the retinal vessels.[3] The central 0.35 mm depression is called the fovea by clinicians and the foveola by anatomists; its photoreceptor layer is entirely composed of cones. The center of foveal depression – the clivus – is located 3.4 mm temporal and 0.8 mm inferior to the center of the optic disc (see Fig. 1.2).

Beyond the macula, the retina spreads peripherally past the vortex veins to the ora serrata. The average equatorial diameter is approximately 24.06–24.08 mm, thereby giving a theoretical retinal area of 1,206 mm.[1,3] The peripheral termination of the retina is at the ora serrata. This lies between 5.73 mm (nasally) and 6.52 mm (temporally) posterior to Schwalbe's line. The ora is defined by protruding anterior retinal extensions (teeth) separated by ciliary epithelium indentations (ora bays) from the pars plana. The strong adhesion of the vitreous to the peripheral retina and pars plana, the vitreous base, extends 1–2 mm anterior to the ora and 1.8–3 mm posterior to the ora bays.[4]

A cross section through the retina just outside the area centralis shows nine layers (internal–external) (see Fig. 1.3): nerve fiber layer, ganglion cell layer, inner plexiform layer, inner nuclear layer, outer

M.W. Stewart (✉)
Department of Ophthalmology, Mayo School of Medicine, Jacksonville, FL 32082, USA
e-mail: stewart.michael@mayo.edu

D.J. Browning (ed.), *Diabetic Retinopathy*, DOI 10.1007/978-0-387-85900-2_1,

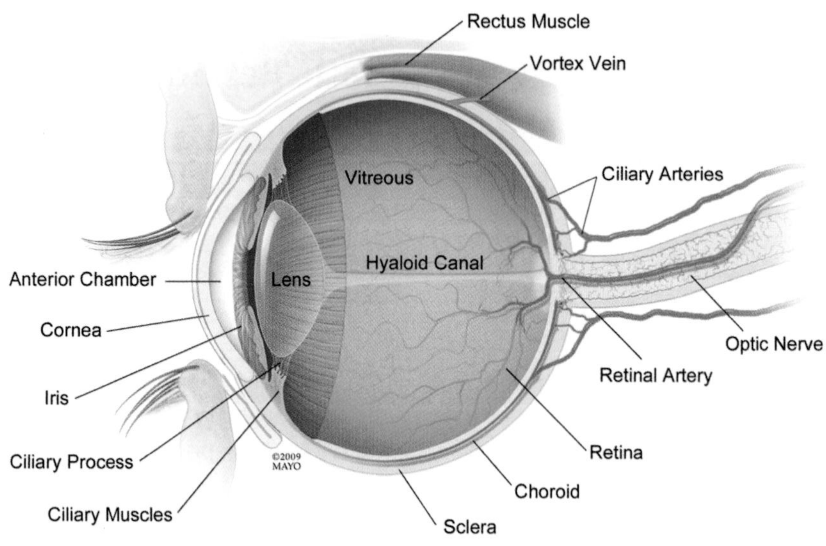

Fig. 1.1 This artistic rendition of the eye shows the retina (*yellow* in cross section) emanating from the optic nerve at the *right*, lining the inside surface of the choroid (*red* and *blue*), and terminating at the ora serrata

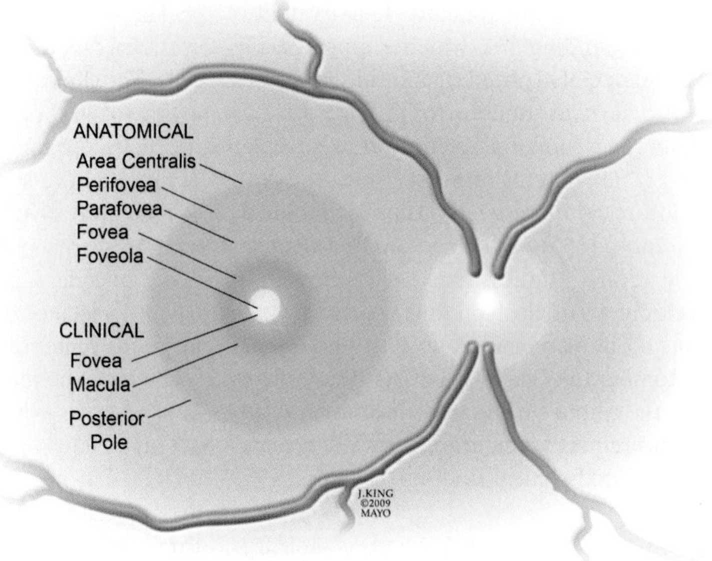

Fig. 1.2 The anatomic classification of areas of the posterior pole is contrasted with the clinical classification

plexiform layer, outer nuclear layer, external limiting membrane, rod and cone inner and outer segments, and retinal pigment epithelium. The retina is thickest around the disc and tapers to 0.18 mm at the equator and 0.11 mm at the ora since the density of all neural elements decreases peripherally.

The layered pattern of the retina enables the conversion of photic energy into neuronal signals. The outer segments of rods and cones convert light energy into a membrane depolarization; in the outer plexiform layer, axons of photoreceptor cells synapse with dendrites of bipolar cells (first-order neurons) and the processes of horizontal cells (integrating neuronal cells); bipolar cells synapse in the inner plexiform layer with dendrites of ganglion cells (second-order neurons) and amacrine cells (provide crosswiring); ganglion cell axons comprise the nerve fiber layer and optic nerve until synapsing

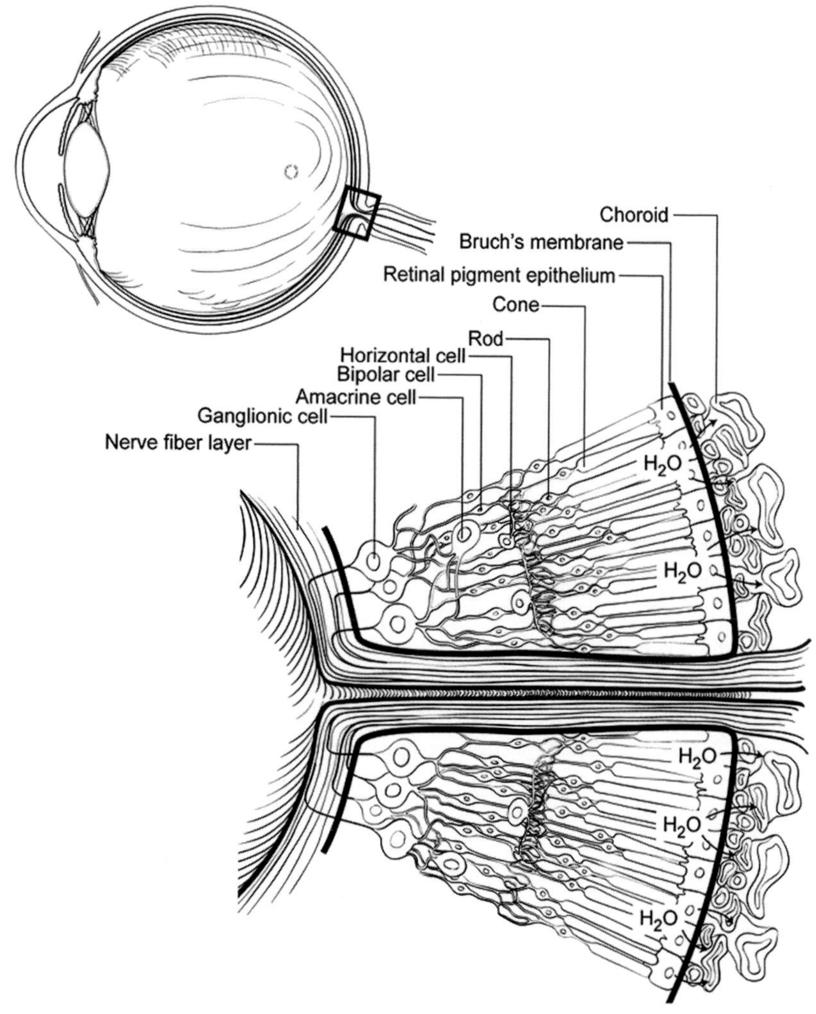

Fig. 1.3 This artistic rendition of the peripapillary retina shows the cellular layers from internal (*left side* of the drawing) to external (*right side* of the drawing). Not labeled are the inner plexiform layer (between the ganglion cell layer and the amacrine/bipolar/horizontal cell layer) and the outer plexiform layer (between the amacrine/bipolar/horizontal cell layer and the rod/cone cell layer). Active transport of water across the retinal pigment epithelium maintains retinal deturgescence

with third-order neurons in the lateral geniculate body. Axons of these cells radiate to the occipital cortex.

The central 0.4 mm zone of the macula is capillary-free, obtaining its nutrients from the choriocapillaris.[5] The foveal center (foveola) is 0.35 mm in diameter and free of rods and blue cones. Long and slender red and green cones are aligned perpendicular to the surface, thereby allowing the greatest light sensitivity. The inner foveal retina lacks the inner nuclear layer, inner plexiform layer, ganglion cell layer, and nerve fiber layer, which minimizes light scatter; it is composed of only Muller's cell processes. The external plexiform layer has an unusual configuration: its axons turn at a right angle, assuming a course parallel with the retina surface. After a short course parallel to the retina surface (while forming Henle's layer), the axons go perpendicular to synapse with dendrites of overlying bipolar cells; this occurs outside the central 0.2 mm diameter of the foveola. Xanthophyll – lutein throughout the posterior pole, zeathanthin mostly in the foveal region – is found in bipolar and ganglion cells and gives the retina its characteristic yellow color. These pigments function to decrease chromatic aberration, absorb potentially toxic blue light, and scavenge free radicals.[6]

The parafovea is a 0.5 mm ring of retina that surrounds the fovea. This region is characterized by a large accumulation of ganglion and inner nuclear cells with a thickened Henle's layer. The density of cones is lower than within the fovea, and rods are beginning to be found. The nerve fiber layer is thickest in the papillomacular bundle.

What is Henle's layer? The outer nuclear layer (ONL), composed of the cell bodies of the rods and cones, has nearly uniform thickness throughout the entire retina. Within the macula, however, the oblique axons displace the cones' cell bodies from their synaptic pedicles in the outer plexiform layer (OPL). These oblique axons with accompanying Muller cell processes form Henle's layer, which is absent in the peripheral retina.

The perifovea is the outermost ring of the area centralis. It comprises the ring from 1.25 to 2.75 mm from the foveal center, defines the periphery of the macula (5.5 mm diameter), and corresponds to a visual field of 18.57°. The perifovea begins where the ganglion cell layer has four nuclei and ends where it thins to a single layer.

How does a 5.5-mm diameter macula perceive a visual field of 18°? Geometrically, an object creates an inverted image which falls upon the concave retina. An image that spans the 5.5 mm curvilinear macula would create a larger image if it were flat on a plane tangent to the posterior pole of the eye. The size of this "straightened" image can be calculated as follows:

The average eye has a diameter of 24.07 mm, creating a radius of 12.035 mm. The angle subtended by a circular segment 5.5 mm in length is (see Fig. 1.4):

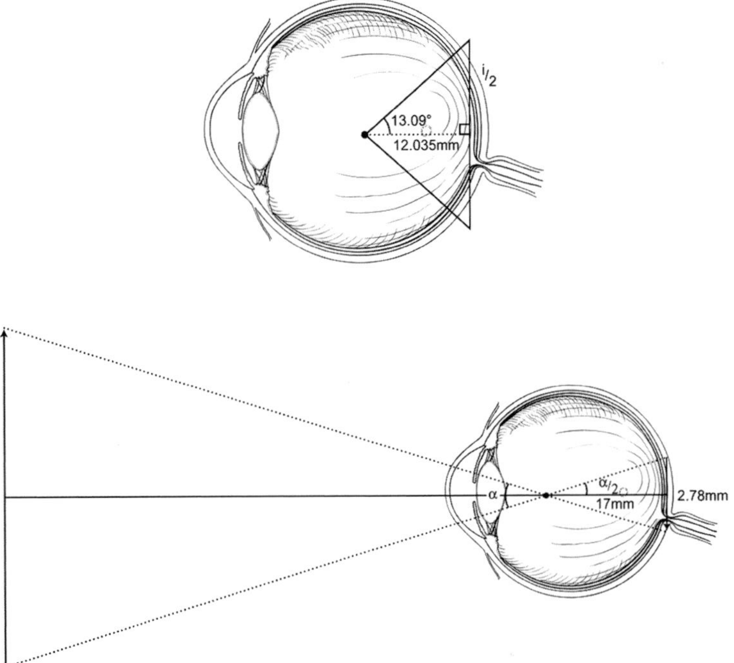

Fig. 1.4 The *top eye* shows the arc subtended by the "straightened" image covering the entire macula; the *bottom eye* shows the object that would create the macular image. Note that the eye's nodal point is situated 17 mm in front of the retina

$$360°(5.5/\text{circumference of eye}) = 26.18°.$$

One-half the straightened image height ($i/2$) can be calculated by

$$\tan(13.09) = (^{i}/_{2})/12.035 \text{ leading to the image height of } i = 2^{*}12.035^{*}\tan(13.09) = 5.56\,\text{mm}.$$

The simplified version of the eye is that of a single lens of 17 mm in front of the retina (the eye's nodal point). Ray tracing shows the relationship between object and image in Fig. 1.2. One-half the angle ($^{\alpha}/_{2}$) subtended by the image from the eyes nodal point can be calculated by

$$\tan(^{\alpha}/_{2}) = 2.78/17,$$

where

$$\alpha = 2 \text{ arc } \tan(2.78/17) = 18.57°.$$

The ora serrata – named for its marginal notches – forms the peripheral edge of the retina as the junction between the multilayered optical retina and the monolayered, nonpigmented epithelium of the ciliary body. The anatomic characteristics of this region are due to its thinness, avascularity, and close relationship to the vitreous base and zonular fibers. The vitreous base normally extends from 2 to 4 mm posterior to the ora. The vitreous cortex collagen fibrils insert into the internal limiting membrane of the retina. Vitreoretinal adhesion is particularly strong along the posterior margin of the vitreous base, making this a common site for retinal tears. As the retina approaches the ora there is gradual loss of the nerve fiber layer, ganglion cell layer, and plexiform layers. These layers are replaced with neuroglia and Muller's cells, which serve as structural support for the entire retina. Both the ILM, into which vitreous base inserts, and the ELM, which continues between the pigmented and nonpigmented layers of pars plana, are thickened.

1.1.3 Microanatomy of the Retina Neurons

The cells within the retina fall into one of three groups: neuronal, glial, and vascular. The neural cells give the retina its primary function: converting light energy into electrical signals. This is accomplished through intricate interaction between the three types of neural cells: photoreceptors, interneurons, and ganglion cells. The photoreceptor cells, the rods and cones, are the primary neurons in the visual pathway. The dense packing of the photoreceptors, combined with their precise axial arrangement, provides for detection of individual photons and the accurate construction of an image. Any change from this axial arrangement causes alteration in vision: micropsia if the cells are abnormally separated, such as with subretinal fluid; metamorphopsia if the alignment is lacking; loss of acuity if the axial alignment is sufficiently disturbed so that the photoreceptor is no longer axial to the inciting light.

The cone cells are comprised of four portions: inner segments, outer segments containing the visual pigment, a perikaryal region containing the cell nucleus, and a synaptic terminal. The light-absorbing visual pigment in rods, rhodopsin, is composed of the light-sensitive chromophore retinal, which is attached to the protein opsin.[7] This is most sensitive to light with a wavelength of 500 nm. The three different types of cones each contains one light-sensitive pigment, resulting in three different spectral sensitivities. The blue, green, and yellow cone pigments are maximally absorbent at 450, 530, and 565 nm, respectively.

The photoreceptor outer segments have two important connections: to the inner segments (cell bodies of the photoreceptors) and to the extracellular matrix, which separates it from the retinal pigment epithelium. The matrix is synthesized by both the photoreceptors and RPE.[8] The acid mucopolysaccharides of the matrix are likely synthesized in the photoreceptor inner segments; disturbances of this would result in separation of photoreceptors from RPE, such as in an exudative retinal detachment. The nuclei of the cones form the outer nuclear layer and lie 3–4 μm internal to the outer limiting membrane. The photoreceptors form junctions with interneurons and Muller cells; the plasma membrane of each photoreceptor and Muller cell is differentiated into a dense band known as the outer limiting membrane. Rods and cones do not contact each other; they are insulated from each other by the Muller cells. The Muller cells contact each other in zonulae adherentes, which are thought to form a diffusion barrier between the intercellular space of the inner retina and the extracellular matrix between the photoreceptor outer segments and the pigment epithelium.

The outer plexiform layer lies between the inner and outer nuclear layers. The synaptic zone, with numerous intercellular junctions and synapses between neural and glial processes, creates the middle limiting membrane. This resembles the outer limiting membrane and may act as a partial barrier to diffusion of fluid and larger molecules. Exudates, hemorrhages, and cysts may be prevented from spreading through the entire retina.

The inner plexiform layer is located between the ganglion and inner nuclear cell layers. In addition to Muller cell branches and retinal blood vessels, it contains synaptic processes of the bipolar, ganglion, and amacrine cells. There are an enormous number of synapses within the inner plexiform layer – 2.9 million dyads (a dyad is a synaptic pair) per square millimeter.[9] Each dyad consists of a bipolar cell making contact with two processes: one from a ganglion cell and the other from an amacrine cell.

The ganglion cell bodies form a distinct layer between the inner plexiform layer and the nerve fiber layer. Through much of the retina there is 1 ganglion cell for every 100 rods and 4–6 cones; however, in the macula the ganglion cell-to-photoreceptor ratio is higher, creating a smaller receptor field for each ganglion cell and, therefore, greater image resolution. Though there are no ganglion cells at the foveal center, the ganglion cells are so densely packed within the macula that there may be two or more for every cone.[10] There are two major groups of ganglion cells: midget and diffuse. The midget ganglion cells cover small areas ($<10\ \mu m^2$) and synapse with only one midget bipolar cell, though each midget bipolar cell may synapse with numerous ganglion cells. On the other hand are the diffuse ganglion cells, also referred to as large and polysynaptic. The ganglion cells' dendrites synapse with retinal bipolar and amacrine cells and the axons synapse with cells in the lateral geniculate body.

The ganglion cell axons course through the inner retina toward the optic nerve forming the nerve fiber layer. They remain unmyelinated until they reach the lamina cribrosa. Axons are in direct contact with each other without interposed glial cells, except for interdigitating Muller cell processes. The axons assume a generally radial course toward the optic nerve except for those immediately temporal to the disc, which form the papillomacular bundle. Since these axons are the first to develop, they form the center of the optic nerve. As axons converge at the optic nerves, the nerve fiber layer becomes thickest; it is thinnest over the macula and far periphery. As is true with all neurons, the axons cannot survive when detached from the cell bodies.[11] Both proximal and distal degenerations are seen after acute retinal or optic nerve ischemia; funduscopically, this can be seen as cotton wool spots or optic disc edema. Though long believed to represent focal infarctions of the retinal nerve fiber layer, cotton wool spots may actually be boundary sentinels of inner retinal ischemia.[12] Following axonal degeneration, defects in the nerve fiber layer can be seen on OCT or funduscopy.

Muller cells form tight junctions with other Muller cells and neural cells. In the outer retina a continuous row of zonulae adherentes forms the outer limiting membrane, a barrier to metabolite movement into and out of the retina.[13] Muller cells constitute the majority of retinal glial cells but the astrocytes are more widely distributed between blood vessels and neurons.

1.1.4 Intercellular Spaces

Neural cells within the retina lie 10–20 μm apart, similar to spacing found in the brain. The intercellular spaces are filled with low-density material that does not limit the diffusion of even large proteins.[14] Large molecules move freely through the retina until reaching the external limiting membrane; intercellular spaces outside the ELM constitute the subretinal space – referred to as the interphotoreceptor matrix – comprising glycosaminoglycans, glycoproteins, and filamentous structures.[15] The most common interreceptor matrix protein is interstitial retinal-binding protein (IRBP), synthesized and secreted by rod photoreceptor cells. It binds all-*trans* retinal and 11-*cis* retinal. Little is known about other matrix proteins.

1.1.5 Internal Limiting Membrane

The ILM is the retina's only true basement membrane. The outer portion consists of the basement membrane of the Muller cells, whereas the inner portion is formed by vitreous fibrils and mucopolysaccharides. It consists of laminin, BM proteoglycans, fibronectin, and collagen.[16] The ILM is 2,000 nm thick over the macula but only 20 nm over the fovea, since the density of Muller cells decreases.[17] Muller cell processes form a continuous but uneven border of attachment with the ILM. The exact nature of the vitreous attachment to the ILM is not known.

1.1.6 Circulation

The retina has the highest oxygen demand of any tissue in the body and relies on two circulations to meet this: the inner 2/3 of the retina relies on the retinal vasculature and the outer 1/3 relies on the choroidal circulation. The choroidal circulation has a high and variable flow rate, transferring molecules easily with the surrounding tissues, whereas the retinal circulation provides a lower, more constant flow with a high rate of oxygen extraction.[18] The central retinal artery supplies the entire circulatory supply for the inner 2/3 of the retina, except for areas served by cilioretinal arteries, which are seen in 20% of eyes.

1.1.7 Arteries

The central retinal artery penetrates the optic nerve about 10 mm posterior to the globe. Its histological structure resembles that of other comparable sized arteries: a luminal diameter of 200 μm, a wall thickness of 35 μm, a single layer of endothelial cells, a subendothelial elastica, an internal elastic lamina, a medium of smooth muscle, and an external elastic lamina that merges with the adventitia. Degenerative diseases that affect muscular arteries, such as atherosclerosis and giant cell arteritis, also affect the intraneural retinal artery. The arteries within the retina are spared from giant cell arteritis because they lack an internal elastic lamina. Atherosclerosis, with its subendothelial plaque formation and hyperplasia of the intimal and endothelial layers, can affect any portion of the retinal artery. When the artery enters the eye, the elastic lamina is lost but the muscularis is unusually prominent.

The retinal circulation is autoregulated by tissue oxygen concentration, metabolic by-products, and intraocular and systemic blood pressures.[19] It is unclear whether the retinal arteries are innervated by sympathetic or parasympathetic nerves but studies suggest that adrenergic-binding sites exist and that retinal blood flow can be altered by adrenergic agonists and antagonists.[20,21] After entering the eye the retinal artery divides into superior and inferior branches, then to smaller branches with either dichotomous (equal-sized bifurcation) or side-arm branching. In smaller branches of the artery, the muscular layer thins from seven cell layers at the disc to two layers at the equator and the luminal diameter thins from 120 μm at the disc to 8–15 μm at the equator. The endothelial cells contain tight junctions that prevent the passage of large molecules into or out of the vascular lumens[22]; therefore, transfer of materials is limited to diffusion and endothelial pinocytosis. The arteries lie in the nerve fiber layer or ganglion cell layer, with only the smaller arterioles descending into the inner plexiform layer to supply capillaries.[23] There exist strong connections between the arteries and cortical collagen in the ILM. Traction on the ILM can cause elevation of the retinal arteries without deeper retina traction. The arteries generally lie superficial to the veins but may lie as deep as the inner nuclear layer at A–V crossing sites. Muller cell and astrocyte processes surround the vessels, insulating them from surrounding retinal neural tissue.

1.1.8 Veins

The wall of the central retinal vein consists of a layer of endothelial cells, subendothelial connective tissue, a medium consisting mostly of elastic fibers, a few smooth muscle cells, and a thin connective tissue adventitia. It is separated from the surrounding neural tissue by Muller cell and astrocyte processes. The lumen decreases in size from 150 μm at the disc to 20 μm at the equator and smooth muscle cells are lost and replaced by pericytes. This allows the venous diameter to change according to the transluminal pressure differential. In patients with diabetes or carotid artery disease, the veins become sausage shaped in response to sluggish flow. Though the central vein is the only outlet for the retinal circulation, potential anastomoses exist between the retinal and choroidal circulations at the disc. They may become manifest in cases of central retinal vein occlusion or compressive lesions of the optic nerve.

1.1.9 Capillaries

Capillaries are distributed throughout the retina except in the foveal avascular zone, the retina adjacent to major arteries and veins, and the far peripheral retina. The capillary network originates from the arterioles in the ganglion cell layer and spreads through the inner nuclear cell layer, but there are no vessels in the outer plexiform and outer nuclear layers. Capillary vessels are distributed in a bilayer schema: a superficial network in the ganglion and nerve fiber cell layers, and a deeper layer in the inner nuclear layer. Vessels range from 5 to 10 μm in diameter. The volume of the outer vascular network is relatively constant, whereas the volume of the inner network varies with the thickness of the nerve fiber layer. Though the perifoveal region has only one capillary layer, up to four different capillary layers are found in the peripapillary region. Peripapillary capillaries drain directly into venules lying on the optic nerve.[24] Within 2 disc diameters of the nerve, these capillaries have long, straight, or slightly curved paths with minimal anastomoses. This unique anatomy makes the capillaries susceptible to elevated IOP and changes in retinal perfusion pressure. This has been used to explain arcuate scotomas in glaucoma, peripapillary flame-shaped hemorrhages in papilledema and hypertension, and cotton wool spots in disorders causing retinal ischemia.

The capillary wall consists of endothelial cells, pericytes, and a basement membrane. The narrow vascular lumen – 3.5–6 μm – coupled with the thin endothelial cell bodies causes nuclei to bulge inward. This requires passing erythrocytes to distort and mold. The endothelial cells are connected by tight junctions that form the blood–retinal barrier.[22] Pinocytic vesicles provide the mechanism for transfer of metabolites from the circulation to the retina. Diseases such as diabetes that disrupt the endothelium also disrupt the blood–retina barrier, causing leakage of protein and lipid into the retina. The leakage is potentially reversible through endothelial cell mitosis and the formation of new tight junctions.[25] The capillary pericytes lie within the endothelial basement membrane. In vivo contraction of mammalian pericytes has not been demonstrated, but pericytes contain contractile proteins and contract in vitro when exposed to endothelin,[26] thromboxane A_2,[27] and angiotensin II.[28] Loss of pericytes, as seen in ischemic retinopathies such as diabetes mellitus, results in weakening of the capillary walls and the formation of microaneurysms.[29]

1.2 Hemodynamics, Macular Edema, and Starling's Law

Movement both into and out of the body's capillaries, including those of the retina, is dependent upon hydrostatic and oncotic pressures. The formation and resorption of macular edema can thus accurately be described by Starling's law (see Fig. 1.5).

The four primary Starling's forces are as follows:

1. Hydrostatic pressure within the capillary lumen (P_c)
2. Hydrostatic pressure within the retinal interstitium (P_i)

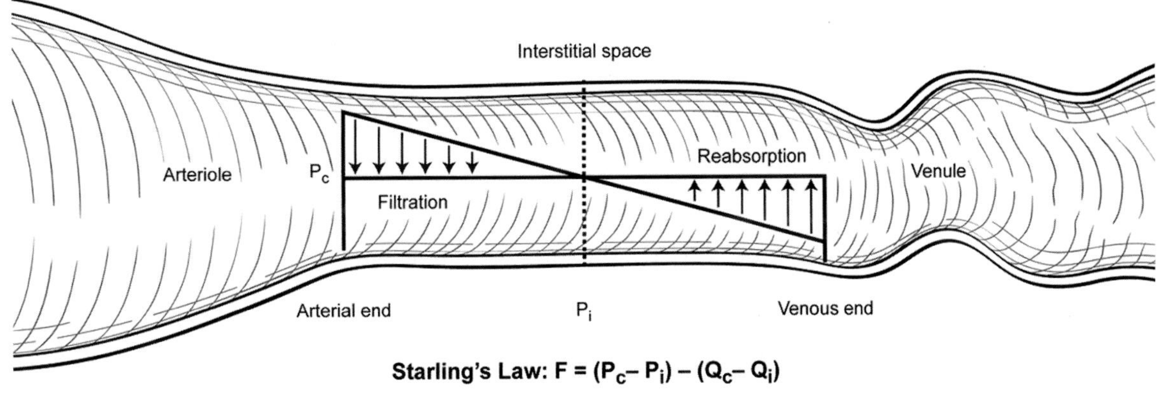

Fig. 1.5 Under physiological circumstances, the drop in transluminal hydrostatic pressure over the length of the capillary causes fluid filtration out of the first half of the capillaries and resorption into the second half. Perturbations in the Starling's equilibrium, by changes in either hydrostatic or oncotic pressures, will result in a horizontal shift of the graph's equilibrium point (P_i)

3. Capillary oncotic pressure (Q_c)
4. Interstitial oncotic pressure (Q_i)

Capillary hydrostatic pressure is determined by systemic blood pressure, whereas tissue hydrostatic pressure is approximately the same as intraocular pressure. Most of the capillary oncotic pressure is created by albumin, whereas, with healthy vascular endothelium, tissue oncotic pressure is determined by interstitial proteins. The net force pushing fluid out of capillaries is the difference between hydrostatic pressures and oncotic pressures and can be represented by the following equation:

$$F = (P_c - P_i) - (Q_c - Q_i),$$

where F is the resultant force determining fluid movement. If F is positive, fluid moves out of the capillary into the interstitium thereby forming tissue edema. However, if F is negative then the net movement of fluid is out of the tissue and into the capillary. At equilibrium,

$$F = 0 = \Delta P - \Delta Q,$$

where there is no net movement of fluid across the capillary walls.

Edema can be defined as the abnormal swelling of soft tissues – in this case the retinal interstitium. Edema can be cytotoxic, where the fluid accumulates within cells, or vasogenic, where fluid accumulates within the interstitial spaces. Cytotoxic edema occurs with severe ischemia, such as following central retinal artery occlusions. Starling's law applies to vasogenic edema, the most common form of edema in retinal vasculopathies such as diabetic macular edema and retinal vein occlusions.

Retinal edema occurs when the net hydrostatic force (forcing fluid into the interstitium) exceeds the net oncotic force (drawing fluid into the capillary lumen) across capillary walls. This is usually due to an increase in transluminal hydrostatic pressure, as occurs with systemic hypertension or ocular hypotony, or due to a decrease in transluminal oncotic pressure, as occurs with increased interstitial proteins due to breakdown of the blood–retinal barrier or with a decrease in plasma proteins as seen with liver disease or protein-wasting nephropathies.

Hydrostatic pressure in the capillaries and venules is dependent upon the arterial blood pressure and the pressure fall through the arterioles. Systemic arterial hypertension increases capillary hydrostatic pressure and aggravates the severity of diabetic macular edema. Patients with diabetic macular edema should undergo a thorough blood pressure assessment and, if systemic hypertension is discovered, appropriate treatment should be initiated. Reduction of systemic blood pressure can result in the improvement of diabetic macular edema.[30,31]

Poiseuille's law describes flow within a tube, where the resistance to flow is inversely related to the radius of the lumen raised to the fourth power. Under hypoxic conditions such as diabetic retinopathy, retinal arterioles dilate, decreasing resistance, resulting in an increase in hydrostatic pressure in the retinal capillaries.[32–34] Retinal blood vessels have been observed to progressively dilate as diabetic macular edema forms.[35]

Less commonly, macular edema is seen in the presence of ocular hypotony. Since tissue hydrostatic pressure equals intraocular pressure, hypotonous eyes develop macular edema due to a widened hydrostatic pressure gradient. Edema may improve if intraocular pressure rises.[36] Interstitial hydrostatic pressure also decreases, with accompanying macular edema or subretinal fluid, when the retina is subjected to vitreous traction.[37]

Oncotic pressure within the capillaries decreases with hypoalbuminemia. This is most commonly seen in patients with the nephrotic syndrome, protein-deficiency malnutrition, or severe liver disease. Oncotic pressure changes commonly accompany the formation of diabetic macular edema. Breakdown of the blood–retinal barrier (BRB) allows albumin to leak into the interstitial spaces, thereby raising tissue oncotic pressure. This draws fluid out of capillaries, across the vascular endothelium, resulting in macular edema. There is a strong correlation between increased VEGF levels, breakdown of the BRB, and macular edema.[38] Endothelial damage, such as that seen with diabetic retinopathy and vein occlusions, compromises the intercellular tight junctions as well as the integrity of the barrier function of the cell membranes. This increased vascular porosity leads to oncotic pressure shifts and interstitial macular edema.

1.3 Biochemical Basis for Diabetic Retinopathy

Diabetes causes similar microvascular abnormalities in the retinal vasculature, renal glomeruli, and vasa vasorum. In the early stages of diabetes, chronic hyperglycemia results in blood flow alterations and increased vascular permeability. This is characterized by decreased activity of vasodilators such as nitric oxide and coexisting increased activity of vasoconstrictors such as angiotensin II and endothelin-1 with the release of vasopermeability augmenting cytokines such as VEGF. Resultant extracellular matrix abnormalities, both qualitative and quantitative, contribute to irreversible increases in vascular permeability. Microvascular cell loss occurs due to programmed cell death, the overproduction of extracellular matrix proteins and the deposition of periodic acid-Schiff-positive proteins induced by growth factors such as TGF-β, all of which subsequently lead to progressive capillary occlusion. Hyperglycemia decreases the production of endothelial and neuronal cell trophic factors leading to edema, ischemia, and hypoxia-driven neovascularization.[39] Atherosclerosis in nondiabetic patients begins with endothelial dysfunction[40] whereas in diabetics this seems to involve insulin resistance due to hyperglycemia.[41]

Four hypotheses have previously been advanced to explain the mechanism of hyperglycemia-induced microvascular damage. These are

1. Increased polyol pathway flux
2. Advanced glycation end products (AGEs)
3. Activation of protein kinase C (PKC)
4. Increased hexosamine pathway flux.

Specific inhibitors of aldose reductase, AGE formation, PKC activation, and the hexosamine pathway each prevent various diabetes-induced abnormalities, but no apparent common element was noted until the recent discovery that each causes overproduction of superoxide by the mitochondrial electron-transport chain[39] (Fig. 1.6). It has been noted that both diabetes and hyperglycemia increase oxidative stress.[42]

To understand how hyperglycemia leads to an increase in reactive oxygen species (ROS) one must look at changes in the electron-transport chain within the mitochondria (see Fig. 1.6). Hyperglycemia, by causing overproduction of electron donors (NADH and $FADH_2$) by the tricarboxylic acid (TCA) cycle,[43] increases the proton gradient across the inner mitochondrial membrane. This prolongs the lifespan of electron-transport intermediates, such as ubisemiquinone, above a threshold

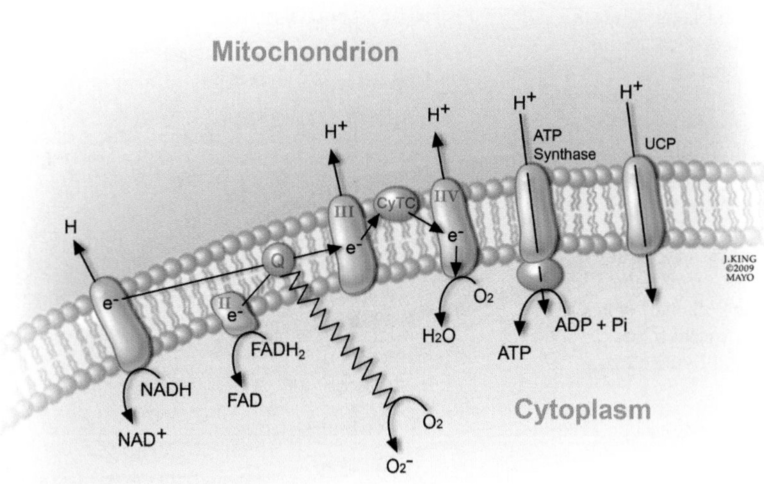

Fig. 1.6 The hyperglycemia-driven production of electron donors ($FADH_2$ and NADH) creates a proton gradient across the mitochondrial membrane, inhibiting electron transport at complex III. This prolongs the half-life of coenzyme Q, thereby leading to the production of superoxide (O_2^-)

value, thereby significantly generating superoxide (Fig. 1.6). Two regulatory enzymes can be exploited to uncouple hyperglycemia-induced production of ROS. Upregulation of manganese superoxide dismutase (MnSOD) eliminates reactive oxygen species production; excess uncoupling protein-1 (UCP-1) eliminated the protein electrochemical gradient.[44] Furthermore, overexpression of either MnSOD or UCP-1 prevented PKC activation, activation of the hexosamine pathway, AGE formation, and an increase in polyol pathway flux. This evidence strongly supports the belief that excessive superoxide is central to the unified theory of diabetic retinopathy.

Other experimental evidence links hyperglycemia, ROS, and the four above-mentioned biochemical pathways (see Fig. 1.7). Hyperglycemia-induced increase in ROS decreases glyceraldehyde 3-phosphate dehydrogenase (GAPDH) activity and, therefore, causes an increase in upstream glycolytic metabolites. This leads to an increase in the polyol pathway flux. Methylglyoxal-derived AGE, the most common AGE resulting from hyperglycemia, probably results from increased triose phosphate levels. Triose phosphate levels rise with GAPDH inhibition by ROS.[45] ROS-induced decreases in GAPDH activity causes a buildup of fructose-6-phosphate, the primary substrate for the hexosamine pathway. Inhibition of GAPDH leads to elevated dihydroxyacetone phosphate levels, leading to increased DAG concentrations and activation of PKC.

Several experimental models have shown that the elevated MnSOD or UCP-1 activity prevents hyperglycemia-induced complications. Overexpression of either protein prevents monocyte adhesion to aortic endothelial cells,[39] the hyperglycemia-induced decrease in eNOS activity,[43] and collagen-induced platelet aggregation and activation.[46] Increased MnSOD activity prevents an increase in collagen synthesis[47] and decreases programmed cell death induced by hyperglycemia.

Since considerable clinical research effort continues to focus on decreasing diabetic complications by minimizing changes in the four-affected pathways, further discussion of the pertinent biochemistry is warranted.

1.3.1 Increased Polyol Pathway Flux

Aldose reductase, the first enzyme in the polyol pathway, has a low affinity for glucose at normal concentrations. In hyperglycemia, however, the

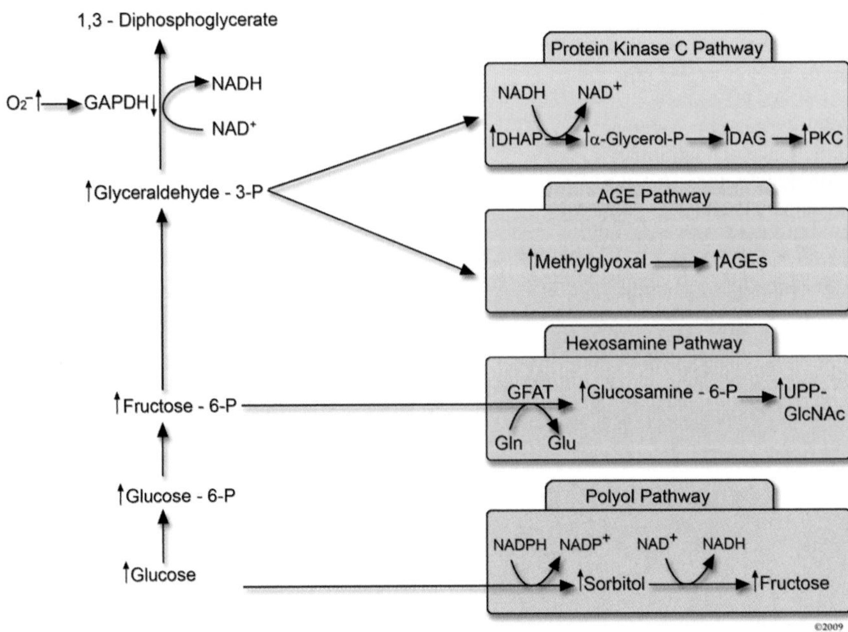

Fig. 1.7 This schematic shows the mechanism by which superoxide production in the mitochondria activates the four biochemical pathways that lead to diabetic retinopathy. Hyperglycemia-induced superoxide (O_2^-) production inhibits GAPDH, causing an accumulation of upstream metabolites. These are diverted into the four alternative metabolic pathways, each of which leads to vascular and interstitial tissue damage

elevated glucose levels result in increased conversion into sorbitol with associated decreases in NADPH. Sorbitol is then oxidized to fructose with NADH reconstitution (Fig. 1.7). It has been proposed that sorbitol oxygenation increases the NADH/NAD+ ratio in the cytosol, thereby inhibiting activity of glyceraldehyde-3-aldehyde dehydrogenase (GAPDH). This leads to increasing concentrations of triose phosphate,[48] which increases the formation of methylglyoxal – a precursor of AGEs – and diacylglycerol, thus activating PKC. Reduction of glucose to sorbitol consumes NADPH; since NADPH is required for regeneration of reduced glutathione, this could exacerbate oxidative stress. Attempts to inhibit the polyol pathway in vivo have yielded mixed results. A 5-year study in diabetic dogs prevented diabetic neuropathy but failed to prevent retinopathy.[49] Zenarestat, an aldose reductase inhibitor, demonstrated a positive effect on diabetic neuropathy in humans.[50]

1.3.2 Advanced Glycation End Products (AGEs)

Intracellular hyperglycemia is the inciting event for the formation of AGEs, which are found in increased concentrations in diabetic retinal blood vessels[51] and glomeruli.[52] They arise from the intracellular auto-oxidation of glucose to glyoxal, the decomposition of the Amadori product (glucose-derived 1 amino-1-deoxyfructose lysine adducts) to 3-deoxyglucosone, and the fragmentation of glyceraldehyde-3-phosphate and dihydroxyacetone phosphate to methylglyoxal, all of which react with amino groups of intracellular and extracellular proteins to form AGEs (see Fig. 1.8).[53–55] The AGE inhibitor aminoguanidine partially prevented microvascular damage in animal models[56] and lowered urinary protein and slowed progression of retinopathy in humans.[57]

The production of intracellular AGE precursors damages target cells by modifying proteins and altering their function. This changes extracellular matrix components and integrins and modifies plasma proteins that bind to AGE receptors. The end result is receptor-mediated production of reactive oxygen species.

AGE formation alters the properties of several extracellular matrix proteins. Crosslinking by AGEs induces an expansion of the molecular packing of type I collagen, thereby altering the function of vessels.[58] AGEs alter type IV collagen from basement membranes.[59] AGE formation on laminin causes decreased polymer self-assembly, decreased binding to type IV collagen, and decreased binding to heparin sulfate proteoglycan.[60]

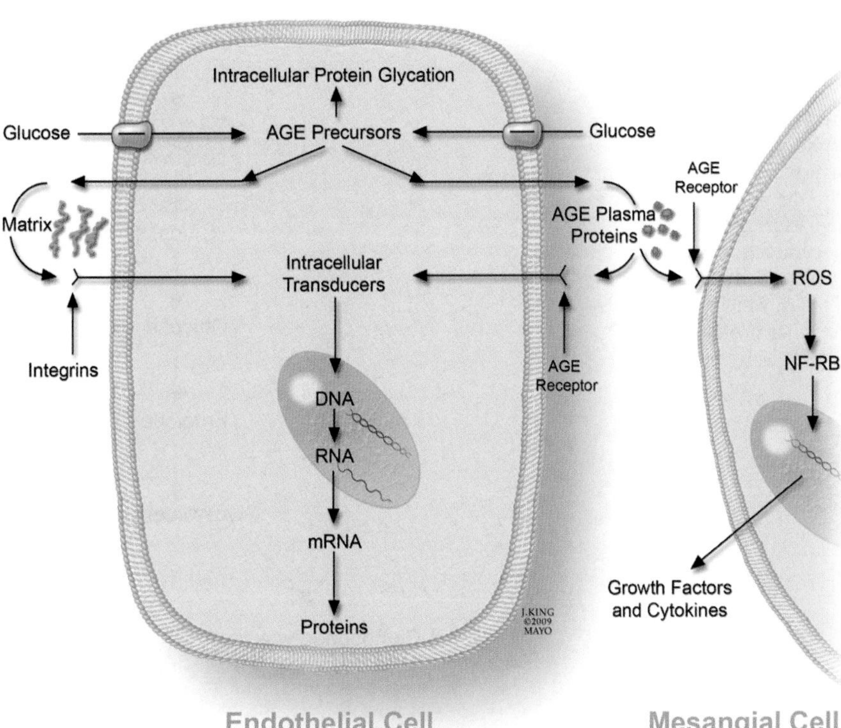

Fig. 1.8 Hyperglycemia leads to the intraocular production of advanced glycation end product (AGE) precursors. These lead to modification matrix proteins and integrins and promote the synthesis of growth factors and cytokines including VEGF

AGE formation on extracellular matrix interferes with matrix–cell interactions. Modification of type IV collagen-binding domains decreases endothelial cell adhesion. Modification of a 6-amino acid growth-promoting sequence in the A chain of laminin reduces neurite outgrowth.[61]

Several cell-associated-binding proteins for AGEs have been identified: OST-48, 80K-H, galectin-3, macrophage scavenger receptor type II, and RAGE. They mediate the long-term effects of AGEs on macrophages, glomerular mesangial cells, and vascular endothelial cells. Their effects include the expression of cytokines and growth factors (interleukin-1, insulin-like growth factor I, tumor necrosis factor-α, TGF-β, macrophage colony-stimulating factor, granulocyte–macrophage colony-stimulating factor, and platelet-derived growth factor) by macrophages and mesangial cells, and the expression of pro-coagulatory and pro-inflammatory molecules (thrombomodulin, tissue factor, and VCAM-1) by endothelial cells. The binding of ligands to endothelial AGE receptors mediates the capillary wall hyperpermeability induced by VEGF.[62] Blockage of RAGE suppressed macrovascular disease in an atherosclerosis-prone type 1 diabetic mouse model. RAGE blockade also inhibited the development of diabetic nephropathy and periodontal disease.

1.3.3 Activation of Protein Kinase C (PKC)

Protein kinase C is a family of at least 11 isoforms, 9 of which are activated by the lipid second messenger diacylglycerol (DAG). Intracellular hyperglycemia increases DAG in both the retina and renal glomeruli by increasing synthesis from dihydroxyacetone phosphate (see Fig. 1.9).[63] This, in turn, activates PKC in vascular cells, retina, and glomeruli. Hyperglycemia also activates PKC isoforms indirectly through ligation of AGE receptors[64] and via increased activity of the polyol pathway.[65] Activation of PKC-β isoforms mediates retinal and renal blood flow abnormalities by depressing nitric oxide production and increasing endothelin-1

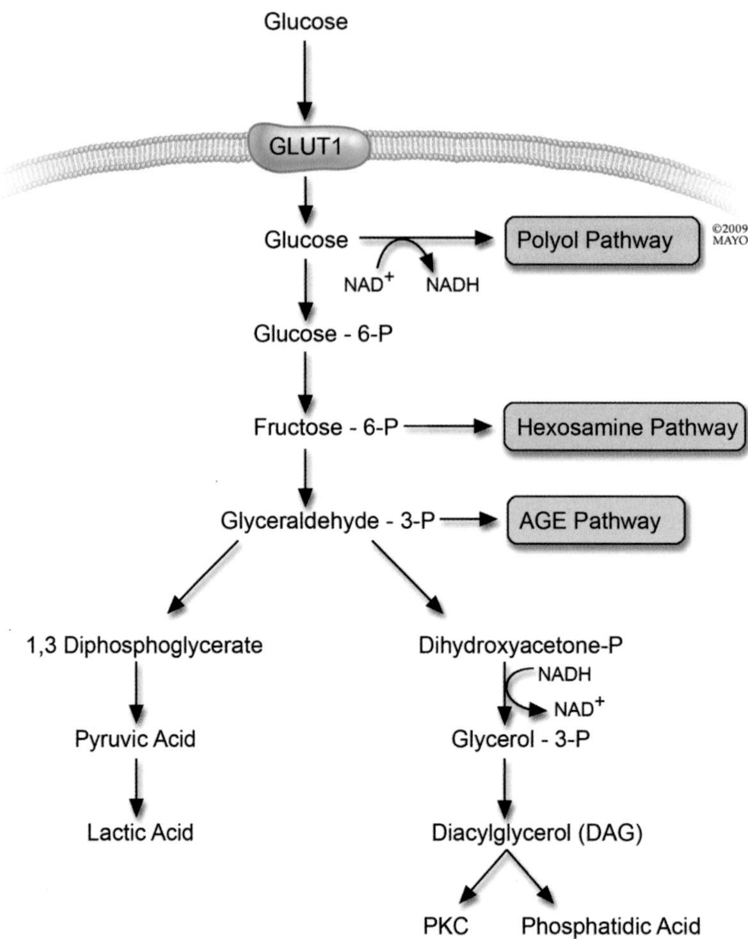

Fig. 1.9 Hyperglycemia-induced superoxide production prevents the normal conversion of glyceraldehyde-3-P into 1,3 diphosphoglycerate. This diverts upstream metabolites into the polyol, hexosamine, and AGE pathways. Excess glyceraldehyde-3-P is converted into diacylglycerol (DAG), which subsequently activates protein kinase C (PKC)

activity.[66] Hyperglycemic activation of PKC induces expression of VEGF in smooth muscle cells.[67]

PKC activation contributes to increased matrix protein accumulation via several mechanisms. PKC induces the expression of TGF-β1, fibronectin, and type IV collagen, which is mediated through the inhibition of nitric oxide production.[68] PKC causes an overexpression of the fibrinolytic inhibitor PAI-1 and activates NF-kB in endothelial and vascular smooth muscle cells.[69,70] PKC regulates and activates various membrane-associated NADP(H)-dependent oxidases.

Treatment with a PKC-β-specific inhibitor reduced PKC activity in the retina and renal glomeruli of diabetic animals, reversed diabetes-induced increases in retinal mean circulation time, normalized glomerular filtration rate, and corrected urinary albumin excretion.[71]

1.3.4 Increased Hexosamine Pathway Flux

Excess activation of the hexosamine pathway causes changes in gene activation, which are known to lead to vascular endothelial dysfunction and other changes consistent with those seen in diabetic retinopathy. Excess intracellular glucose in the form of fructose-6-phosphate is diverted from glycolysis to provide substrates for reactions requiring UDP-*N*-acetylglucosamine (see Fig. 1.10). End products of these diverted reactions include proteoglycans and O-linked glycoproteins. Though the mechanism by which increased flux through the hexosamine pathway mediates hyperglycemia-induced increases in gene transcription is not certain, covalent modification of the transcription factor Sp1 by *N*-acetylglucosamine (G1cNAc) might explain the link between activation of the hexosamine pathway

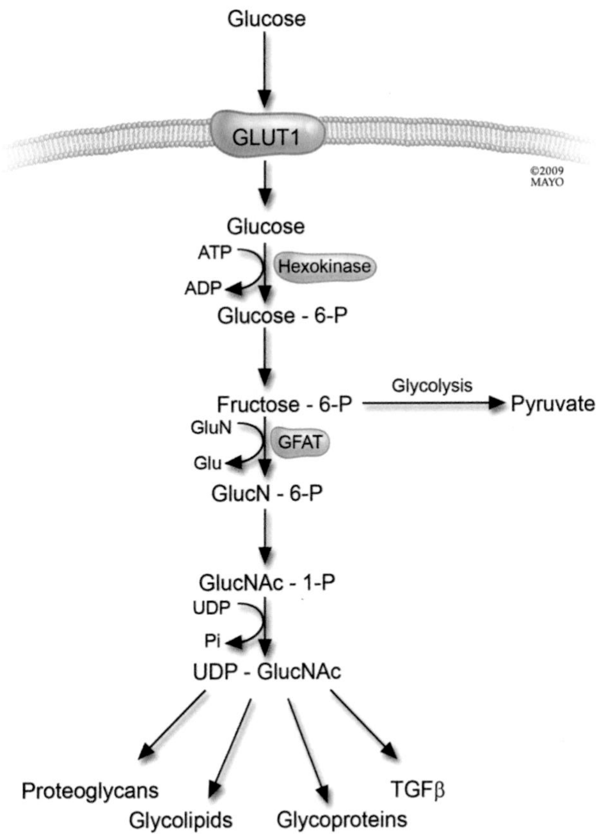

Fig. 1.10 The hexosamine pathway produces glucosamine-6-P by diverting excess fructose-6-P from glycolysis. This leads to the synthesis of glycolipids, glycoproteins, proteoglycans, and TGF-β

and hyperglycemia-induced changes in transcription of the gene for PAI-1. The glycosylated form of Spl promotes significantly more transcription activity than the deglycosylated form. Furthermore, glycosylation of Spl is associated with correspondingly less phosphorylation of Spl, suggesting that the two activities compete for the same binding site and may represent a more generalized mechanism for regulating glucose-responsive gene transcription.[72]

In addition to transcription factors, several nuclear and cytoplasmic proteins are either glycosylated by O-linked GlcNAc or competitively phosphorylated. For example, PKC isoforms are activated by glucosamine without membrane translocation. Hyperglycemia is shown to increase hexosamine pathway activity by 2.4× in aortic endothelial cells, resulting in a 1.7× increase in Spl O-linked GlcNAc. Hyperglycemia caused a 3.8× increase in expression of an 85-base pair DNA region responsible for PAI-1 promotion.

Our current understanding of retinal biochemistry identifies a series of pathways, with positive and negative feedback loops and several shared substrates and enzymes. This allows for considerable and complicated cross-over reactions among pathways suggesting that successful inhibition of any single pathway will likely result in an incomplete clinical response. If the unified theory of diabetic retinopathy – hyperglycemic production of reactive oxygen species – is correct, then research aimed at limiting ROS may yield the most effective therapies.

1.4 Macular Edema

Retinal nutrition is supplied by two circulations: the choriocapillaris which nourishes the outer third of the retina and the two layers (superficial plexus in the axon and ganglion cell layers, deep plexus in the inner nuclear layer) of the retinal capillary circulation. Two distinct types of diabetic maculopathy are seen: ischemic maculopathy due to capillary dropout and macular edema due to exudation from retinal capillaries and/or choriocapillaris.

The exact location of macular edema – extracellular or intracellular – is not well established, as studies point to both locations. Histological studies of enucleated eyes with diabetes and tumors have found swelling and degeneration of Muller, bipolar, ganglion and photoreceptor cells,[73] and extracellular cystic spaces.[74] Though both angiographic ischemia and macular edema may coexist, their effects on visual acuity appear to be independent. Arend et al.[75] found no correlation between blood flow and macular edema, thereby concluding that inner retinal ischemia does not cause macular edema. Retinal thickening appears to correlate with blood–retinal barrier breakdown; however, ischemia was not correlated with macular thickening, thereby suggesting that the major cause of retinal thickening was extracellular expansion.[76] The conclusion of these studies is that although ischemia may lead to a small amount of intracellular swelling, the major contribution to macular edema is extracellular fluid accumulation.[77]

In the absence of retinopathy, diabetes, in various studies, has been shown to increase or decrease retinal blood flow. However, once retinopathy is established, retinal blood flow increases.[78] It is believed that autoregulatory function is lost and both arterioles and venules are noted to dilate and elongate. This leads to decreased arteriole resistance with decreased pressure loss across the length of the arteriole. This would increase effective intraluminal pressure in the retinal capillaries, which according to Starling's law, would lead to fluid passage into the extracellular space. The concomitant release of vasoactive cytokines, such as VEGF, from endothelial cells, neuroglia, and activated leukocytes, creates breakdown of the blood–retinal barrier via several mechanisms, leading to albumin movement into the interstitium.

The choroidal circulation is found to be decreased in diabetic patients.[79] Bulk flow to the choroid is relatively unchanged in diabetics but indocyanine green angiography shows areas of focal choroidal nonperfusion in eyes with diabetic pigment epitheliopathy. Sometimes significant leakage across the pigment epithelium occurs in eyes with only minimal retinopathy.[80] Both intrachoroidal neovascularization and choriocapillaris occlusion occur more commonly in diabetics. Both of these processes likely result from the same inciting events (basement membrane degeneration, angiogenesis) that lead to diabetic retinopathy.[81]

Autoregulation in diabetes

Since the autonomic nervous system terminates at the lamina cribrosa, regulation of retinal blood vessels is mediated by local factors such as endothelin-1, angiotensin II, hyperoxia, CO_2, nitric oxide (NO), and adenosine. Several investigators have uncovered evidence of autoregulatory loss of the retinal vasculature in diabetic patients. Lanigan[82] noted that patients with mild diabetic retinopathy and microalbuminuria had decreased constriction of retinal arterioles and venules associated with sustained handgrip contraction. Inhibitors of NO synthetase cause less pulsation of retinal vessels in diabetic patients than controls suggesting that diabetics have less NO synthetase or their vessels are less sensitive to NO.[83]

Prior to the accumulation of edema, vitreous fluorophotometry has shown breakdown of the blood–retinal barrier. This probably represents early gap junction protein loss allowing molecules smaller than albumin to pass out of the capillary lumen. Other patients may have retinal pigment epitheliopathy as the first manifestation of diabetic retinopathy.[80] RPE dysfunction is probably underappreciated since the development of overlying retinal vascular disease would mask this on fluorescein angiography.

Is the RPE partly to blame for diabetic macular edema?

In addition to commonly seen VEGF-A isoforms, eyes with diabetic macular edema have elevated levels of another of the VEGF family of molecules, placental growth factor (PLGF).[84] These isoforms react with VEGFR-1 but not VEGFR-2.[85] VEGF-induced RPE hyperpermeability has been found to occur only through VEGFR-1.[86] PLGF has been shown to be upregulated under hypoxic conditions as seen in diabetic eye disease. Finally, breakdown of the RPE barrier has been noted in streptozotocin-induced diabetic rats.[87]

Histopathological studies have shown that cystoid macular edema develops in two retinal layers: the inner nuclear layer and the outer plexiform layer.[88] However, large amounts of fluid can spill over into the outer nuclear layer. Both histological studies and OCT examination have suggested the presence of multiple cysts; however, further analysis shows that fluid exists in large cavities spanned by Muller cells.

Fluid leakage from the capillaries of the inner retina is limited by the inner and outer plexiform layers, leading to fluid accumulation within the inner nuclear layer. Fluid accumulation within the inner nuclear layer displaces tissue in the plexiform layers, increasing tissue density leading to a relative barrier to further spread of the edema. Breakdown of the outer blood–retinal barrier often causes fluid to accumulate between the outer plexiform layer and the outer limiting membrane. As demonstrated in horseradish peroxidase studies in diabetic rats,[89] other eyes with intact outer limiting membranes will develop limited exudative retinal detachments with fluid accumulation between the retinal pigment epithelium and photoreceptor outer segments.

1.4.1 Blood–Retinal Barrier

The retina is subject to two distinct blood–retinal barriers: the inner BRB that consists of the retinal capillary endothelial cells and their tight junctions, and the outer BRB that consists of the retinal pigment epithelium and their tight junctions. The cell membranes of the epithelial and endothelial cells are composed of bilayers with hydrophilic glycerols binding hydrophobic long-chain fatty acid moieties (see Fig. 1.11). Under normal, healthy conditions, the cell membranes allow passage of small hydrophobic molecules, water, and small uncharged polar molecules but form an impenetrable barrier to the passage of ions and larger uncharged polar molecules. Breakdown of the BRB in diabetes may involve the inner BRB, the outer BRB, or both.[80]

The tight junctions form the barrier between adjacent endothelium and epithelium cells. The junctions are composed of numerous intercellular proteins, which include occludin, claudin (23 isoforms), 7H6, cingulin, zonula occludens (ZO)-1,2,3, junction adhesion molecule (JAM), membrane-associated guanylate kinases with inverted domain structures (MAGI)-1,2,3, partition defective genes (PAR)3/6, and multi-pdz protein-1 (MUPP1).[90] Some of the proteins have been extensively studied and well characterized. Occludin and the claudins control much of the barrier function (see Fig. 1.12).[91] Occludin is specific to vascular endothelial cells.[92] Loss of occludin in diabetic rats coincides with increased blood–retinal permeability to albumin (m.w. 66 kDa) but not rhodamine-dextran (m.w. 10 kDa), perhaps due to barrier changes, not in pore size, but in hydrophobicity. Claudin-5 prevents passage of small (<0.8 kDa) molecules across the blood–brain barrier[93] and probably serves the same purpose in the retina.[94] ZO-1 in retinal capillary endothelial cell tight junctions is believed to coordinate the assembly of junctional complexes from within the cell[95] and is a reliable indicator of tight-junction function.[96] The junctional adhesion molecules (JAM) facilitate interactions between endothelial cells and leukocytes and help with tight-junction assembly.[97] Additionally, junctional proteins may assist with cellular structure. Intracellular, circumferential actin bundles form at sites of occludin-positive cell

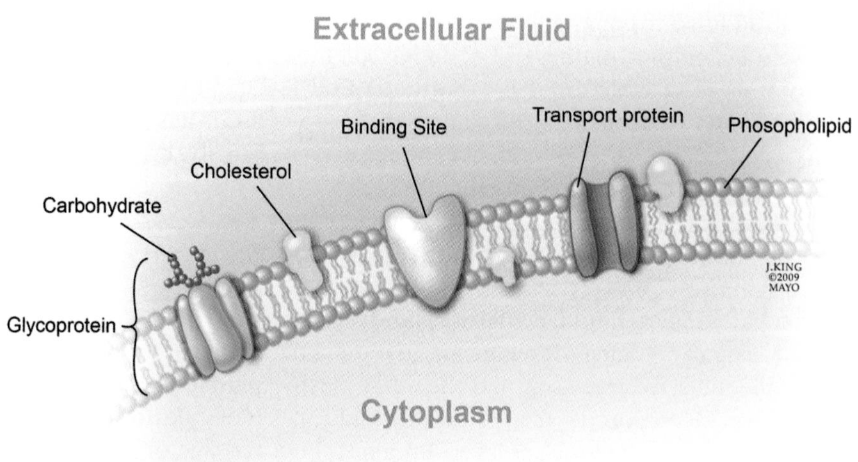

Fig. 1.11 Cell membranes are primarily composed of phospholipids, with hydrophobic lipid tails sandwiched between hydrophilic diglycerides. Situated within the membrane are cholesterol molecules, glycoproteins, various receptor (binding) molecules (e.g., VEGFR-A), and transport channels. Molecular components are not fixed, but float within this "sea" of phospholipids

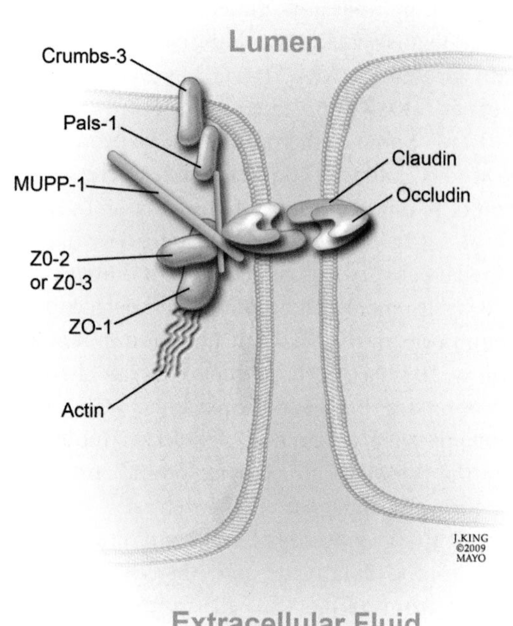

Fig. 1.12 Endothelial cell tight junctions are predominantly composed of claudins and occludin, which span the intercellular space. These are anchored intracellularly by the junctional complex (ZO-1, ZO-2, ZO-3, MUPP-1, Pals-1, and Crumbs-3). Actin binding to the complex, requiring the presence of occludin, provides cellular structure

contact, but actin does not form at areas without occludin.

Transport across the BRB may be either transcellular or paracellular (see Fig. 1.13).[98] Transcellular passage may occur due to changes in the barrier state or pumping capacity of endothelial cells, whereas paracellular passage is due to loss of integrity of the tight junctions. Increased fluorescein levels in the vitreous found by vitreous fluorophotometry precede fluorescein angiographic evidence of diabetic retinopathy in rat and monkey models and humans.[99,100] This suggests that early breakdown of the BRB allows passage of smaller molecules such as fluorescein but still prohibits passage of proteins such as albumin, which are necessary for the formation of macular edema.

VEGF has been shown to break down the BRB by both promoting movement across cells and damaging tight junctions. VEGF injections cause membrane fenestrations in rat and frog endothelial cells but not monkey cells. Transcellular gaps occur with increased frequency and lead to increased hydraulic conductivity. Within 24h after perfusion with VEGF, vesiculovacuolar organelles form a continuous, transcellular chain, separated only by fenestrations, in vascular endothelial cells.[101]

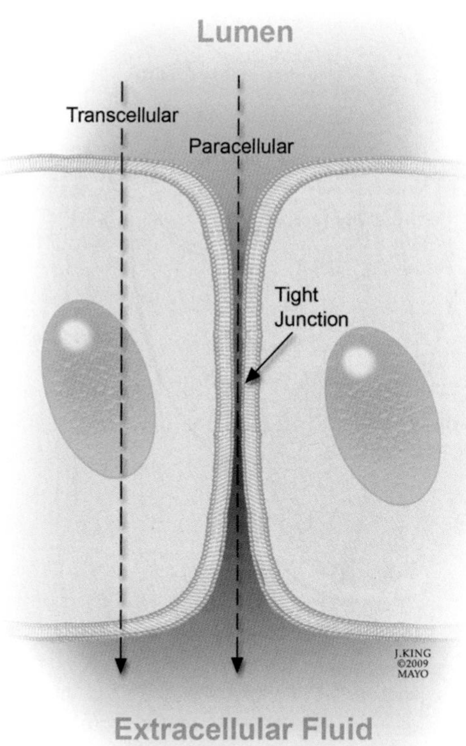

Fig. 1.13 Intravascular fluid may cross the endothelial cell layer through the paracellular space (in the presence of altered tight junctions) or via transcellular transport (membrane fenestrations, transcellular gaps, and vesiculovacuolar organelles)

When exogenous VEGF is administered to eyes affected by diabetes, three changes in the tight junctions have been observed: (1) tight-junction proteins are phosphorylated; (2) existing junctions from the plasma membrane to cell cytoplasm are reorganized; (3) junctional protein levels are decreased.[94]

Diabetes alters the levels of junctional and matrix proteins. The occludin content is decreased in the retinas of diabetic rats. Occludin and ZO-1 levels are decreased in cultured brain endothelial cells treated with VEGF.[102] Retinas of diabetic animals showed increased levels of MMP-2, MMP-9, and MMP-14 mRNA. Hyperglycemia and TGF-β increase levels of MMP-9. Cells treated with MMP-2 and MMP-9 showed gap junction alterations through increased transepithelial electrical resistance and degradation of occludin.[103]

1.4.2 Mechanism of Blood–Retinal Barrier Breakdown

The exact mechanism by which breakdown of the blood–retinal barrier occurs is still being investigated. It could be due to either damage of the junctional complexes between capillary endothelial cells and RPE cells or changes in the cells' membrane state or pumping capacity. Proposed mechanisms for leakage have included fenestration of the endothelial cell cytoplasm, increased transport through vesicles, and increased infolding of the RPE-promoting choroidal to subretinal space transudation.[104] High glucose concentrations have been shown to reduce electrical resistance of cultured capillary endothelial cells and induce breakdown of the blood–retinal barrier mediated by insulin, which does not cross cell membranes. This suggests damage to the intercellular tight junctions.[105] Furthermore, the discovery of vascular endothelial growth factor (VEGF) and other inflammatory cytokines, with their considerable effects on junctional and interstitial proteins, has focused attention on the tight junctions. Cultured astrocytes simultaneously increase both intercellular barrier function and ZO-1 synthesis, suggesting a strong link between the two processes.[106]

Though the precise biochemical pathway leading to breakdown of the blood–retinal barrier is unknown, much recent research has focused on vascular endothelial growth factor (see Fig. 1.14). VEGF molecules fit into a broad group of compounds, which can be divided into several families – A, B, C, D, E, and placental-derived growth factor (PDGF). VEGF molecules stimulate known signaling pathways, including protein kinase C, in endothelial cells.[107,108] Within VEGF family A there are five major molecules and at least three additional minor isoforms.

There are at least four tyrosine kinase VEGF receptors: VEGFR-1, VEGFR-2, VEGFR-3, and neuropilin. VEGFR-3, found primarily in lymphatic cells, does not bind VEGF-A and, therefore, does not affect vascular changes.[109] The role of VEGFR-1 is somewhat controversial; it may function as a decoy receptor or play a role in hematopoiesis, however, it is upregulated in hypoxic conditions via hypoxia-inducible factor (HIF)-1.[110] Furthermore, more recent gene transfer studies

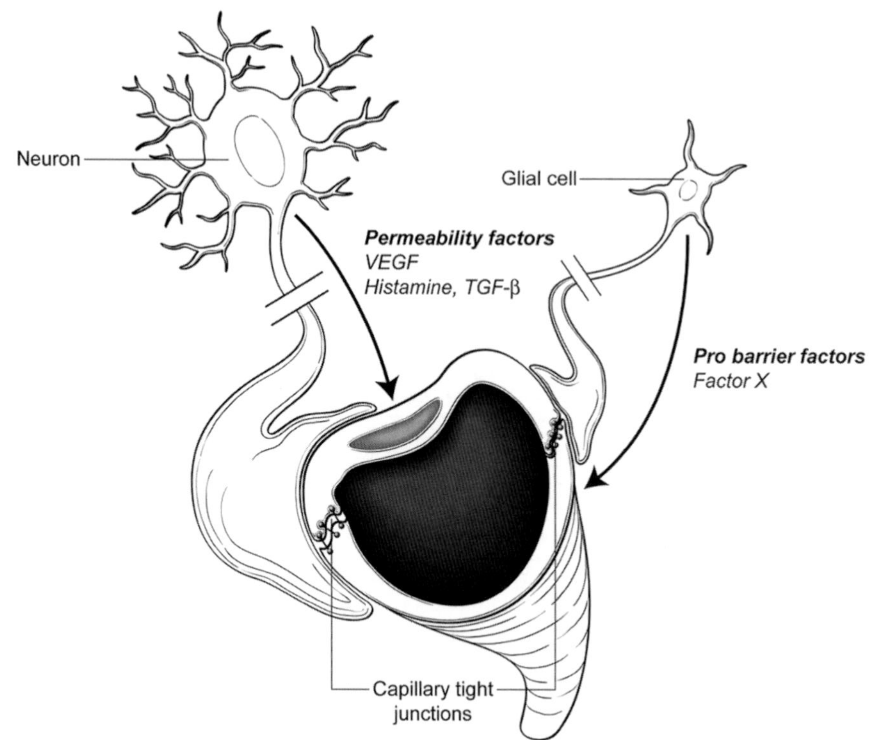

Fig. 1.14 Perturbations in neuroglia homeostasis lead to the release of several vasopermeability (VEGF, histamine, and TGF-β) and probarrier factors, which affect the integrity of capillary tight junctions and endothelial membrane integrity

suggest that VEGFR-1 is pivotal in neovascularization. Phosphorylation of VEGFR-2 induces vascular permeability, angiogenic, and mitogenic changes.[111]

Within the eye, VEGF is produced in retinal pigment epithelial, endothelial, glial, pericytes, Muller and ganglion cells, whereas retinal capillary endothelial cells are its primary targets. VEGF is capable of stimulating angiogenesis (through sprouting, intussusceptions, and recruitment of progenitor cells), increasing vascular permeability and vasodilation, preventing endothelial apoptosis, and recruiting inflammatory cells (see Fig. 1.15).

Physiological angiogenesis is accompanied by very little vascular leakage.[112,113] Pathological angiogenesis, however, has characteristic vascular leakage, as demonstrated by both India ink[114] and tracer studies.[115] In mouse models of experimental neovascularization exogenous administration of a VEGF trap decreased neovascularization by 66%[116] and transfer of VEGFR-1 genes decreased neovascularization by 53–86%.[117,118] These data suggest that VEGF is of critical importance in the development of neovascularization. Though VEGF is sufficient to produce neovascularization from the deep retinal circulation it is insufficient to cause neovascularization on the retinal surface[119] or within the choroid.[120] VEGF is sufficient to cause leakage from normal blood vessels as shown in animal studies following implantation of sustained release devices[121] or intravitreal injections.[116] Though hundreds of papers have been published regarding the effect of VEGF on vascular permeability there have been very few in vitro studies. Notable findings include the ability of VEGF to increase hydraulic conductivity,[122] to increase diffusive permeability to albumin[123] but to have no effect on the oncotic reflection coefficient (the probability that a molecule will bounce off a pore rather than go through it) to albumin.[124] In fact, hydraulic conductivity (a measure of the ease by which fluid moves through a lumen) and compliance (the inverse of stiffness) may be stimulated separately, suggesting that permeability and angiogenesis may be stimulated or inhibited separately.

Nonhypoxic physiological angiogenesis can occur as a result of sheer stress in muscles and under hormonal control in female reproduction. Alternatively, VEGF-induced angiogenesis can occur in conditions characterized by physiological

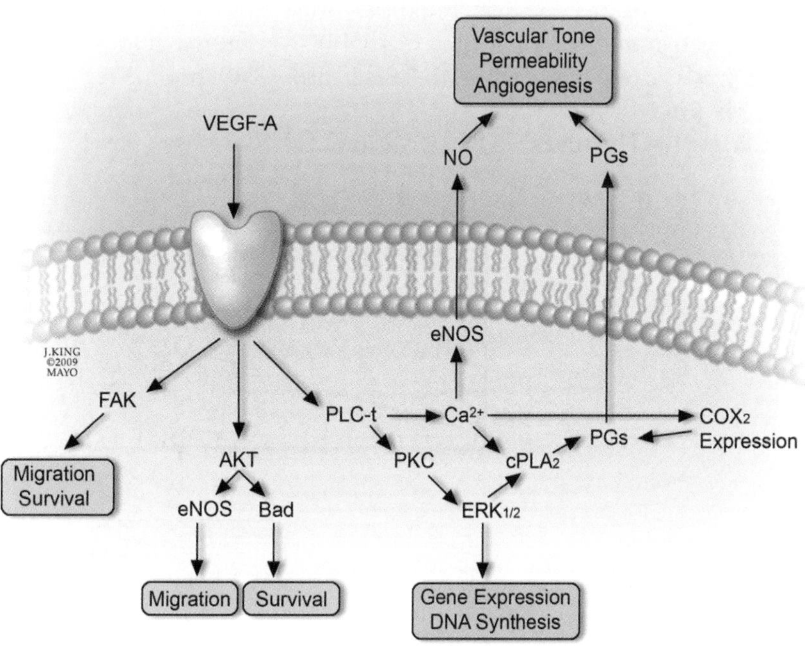

Fig. 1.15 Extracellular vascular endothelial growth factor A (VEGF-A) binds to a transmembrane receptor molecule (VEGFR, a tyrosine kinase) resulting in gene expression and protein synthesis. This leads to cell migration and survival. Through the activation of nitric oxide synthetase and prostaglandin synthesis, vascular tone and permeability are affected and angiogenesis may occur

hypoxia: exercise-induced, in the corpus luteum, and in the endometrium. VEGF release leads to increased vascular permeability through several mechanisms. First, it stimulates inositol triphosphate (IP_3), which leads to intracellular calcium release thereby increasing nitrous oxide and cyclic GMP levels. This causes relaxation of vascular smooth muscle. Vascular permeability, angiogenesis, vessel diameter, and blood flow have been shown to be proportional to nitrous oxide synthetase levels.[125] Second, it stimulates DAG production, which increases cellular permeability directly through DAG-sensitive Ca^{2+} channels. Third, the stimulation of DAG causes PKC (protein kinase C) activation.

In addition to its effects on vascular endothelium, VEGF has been shown to protect against apoptosis. It serves as a survival factor for endothelial cells both in vitro and in vivo. VEGF prevents endothelial apoptosis induced by serum starvation by blocking the phosphatidylinositol 3-kinase/V-akt murine thymoma viral oncogene homolog (PI3 kinase/Akt) pathway possibly through induction of the antiapoptotic proteins Bcl-2, A1, XIAP, and survivin.

VEGF promotes inflammation by inducing ICAM-1 (intercellular adhesion molecule) synthesis and causing leukocyte adhesion.[126] Adherent leukocytes then amplify the effects of VEGF by producing their own.[127] This leads to narrowing of vascular lumens, thereby causing nonperfusion downstream from areas of leukocyte adhesion and leading to loss of occludin and ZO-1 from tight junctions.[128] The loss of these junctional proteins causes breakdown of the blood–retinal barrier.[129]

Intravitreal VEGF levels correlate with the severity of diabetic retinopathy – higher in PDR than BDR.[130] Even within the population of DME patients, aqueous VEGF levels are closely correlated with severity of DME.[131]

VEGF expression is upregulated by numerous growth factors, including TGF-α, TGF-β, epidermal growth factor, IGF-I, FGF, PDGF, and also by inflammatory cytokines, including IL-1-α and IL-8. One of the most important stimulants is hypoxia; VEGF mRNA expression is induced by low tissue O_2 tension. Similarities exist between the hypoxic regulation of VEGF and erythropoietin. A 28-base sequence has been identified in the promoter of the human VEGF gene, which has similar binding characteristics as HIF-1α, a key mediator of hypoxic responses.[132] HIF-1α is a key transcriptional regulator of the hypoxic response, often referred to as the "master switch" (see Fig. 1.16).

In the presence of oxygen, free HIF-1α is hydroxylated, via propyl hydroxylase. The von Hippel–Lindau factor (pVHL) then binds to hydroxylated HIF-1α at the ODD (oxygen-dependent domain) region. The pVHL/HIF-1α complex is then degraded by intracellular proteasomes.[133] Low tissue oxygen tension, however, prevents hydroxylation of HIF-1α at a proline residue,[134] thereby stabilizing HIF-1$^{\alpha}$, which stimulates VEGF synthesis. Hypoxia increases levels of HIF-1α subunits both by

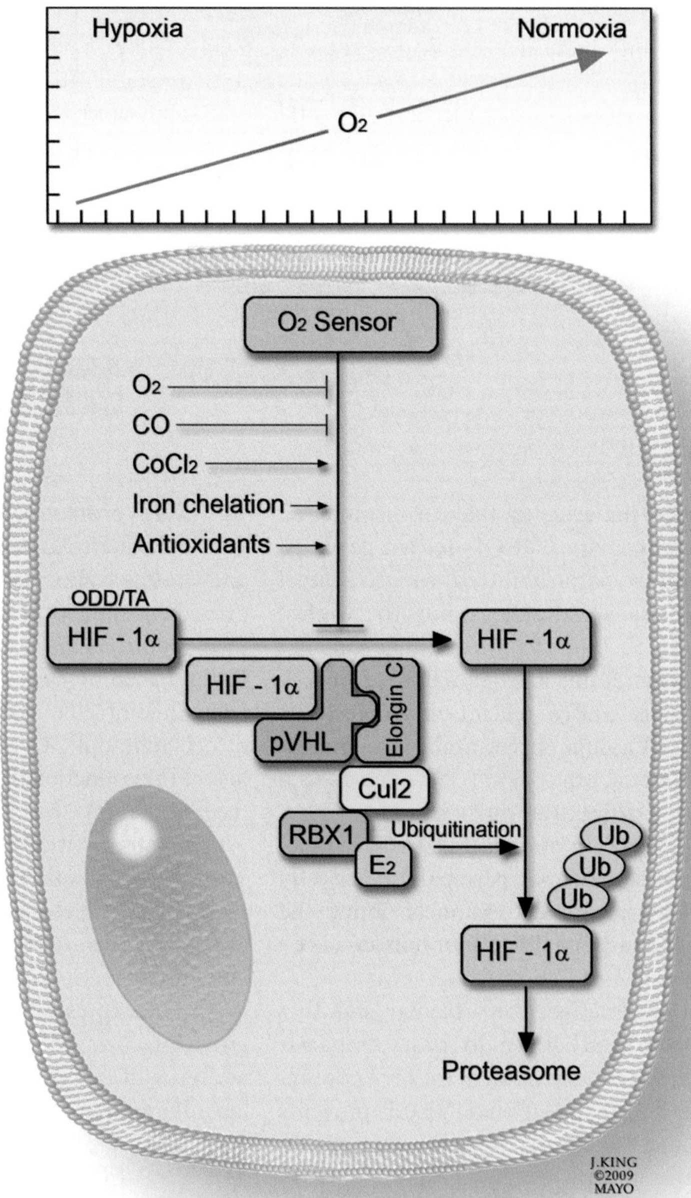

Fig. 1.16 Hypoxia-inducible factor 1α (HIF-1α) is produced within the cell cytoplasm. Under conditions of normal oxygen tension, HIF-1α binds to a molecular complex, which includes the von Hippel–Lindau factor, allowing ubiquination and subsequent degradation by proteosomes. Hypoxic conditions stabilize HIF-1α resulting in VEGF synthesis. Since iron is necessary for HIF-1α function, chelators will mimic hypoxia

stabilizing the protein[135] and by allowing HIF-1α mRNA accumulation.[136] Stabilization of HIF-1α during hypoxia requires an intact mitochondrial electron-transport chain to generate reactive oxygen species (ROS). It is the concentration of ROS that is believed to constitute the cell's oxygen sensor.[137] Low intracellular oxygen tension, indirectly represented by high levels of ROS, limits a cell's ability to hydroxylate HIF-1α. This triggers the hypoxia-induced cascade of protein synthesis, which includes inflammatory cytokines such as VEGF and TNF-α.

In addition to ROS, other molecules affect the stability of HIF-1α. HIF-1α is stabilized by growth factors and cytokines such as IGF-1, 2, and AGEs. Insulin-induced VEGF expression accompanied by elevated HIF-1α may explain why very tight glucose control worsens retinopathy.[138] HIF-1α requires several cofactors: 2-oxoglutarate, vitamin C, and iron. This explains why iron chelators, such as deferoxamine, mimic hypoxia. Several biochemical opportunities exist for HIF-1α modulation, including phosphatidylinositol 3-kinase inhibitors, mitogen-activated protein kinase inhibitors (MAPK), prolyl-4-hydroxylase domain activators, microtubule-disrupting agents, cyclo-oxygenase-2 (COX-2) inhibitors, heat-shock protein inhibitors, and antisense therapy. Breakthroughs in treating ischemic retinal disease may follow new cancer therapies (e.g., topotecan, camptothecin analogs).[139]

Protein kinase C (PKC) is a family of related enzymes, which function as signaling components for several growth factors, hormones, neurotransmitters, and cytokines. The protein kinase C pathway is stimulated by the presence of diacylglycerol. Activated PKC may increase vascular permeability via two mechanisms: the activation of endothelial cell contraction through phosphorylation of the cytoskeletal proteins caldesmon and vimentin[140]; and the activation of serine/threonine phosphatases or the inactivation of kinases both of which lead to dephosphorylation of the tight-junction proteins occludin and the claudins.[141] PKC contributes to increased matrix protein accumulation – a hallmark of diabetic retinopathy – by inhibiting NO synthesis, leading to increased TGF-β1, fibronectin, and type IV collagen.[142]

Several studies have shown how activated PKC may contribute to BRB breakdown. Exogenous VEGF causes BRB breakdown in nondiabetic rats, a process that is blocked by PKC inhibitors.[143] Also, the intravitreal injection of PKC can induce BRB breakdown in nondiabetics. PKC inhibitors prevent hyperglycemia-induced VEGF production.[144] In advanced diabetic retinopathy, PKC may mediate VEGF's action, thereby creating a reinforcing cycle. Hyperglycemia may worsen existing retinopathy by inducing vascular endothelial growth factor synthesis via PKC activation and also by p42/p44 MAPK synthesis. Both of these pathways are independent of HIF-1α stabilization.[138]

Maintenance of normal retinal vasculature requires a balance of angiogenic factors, such as VEGF, and inhibitors, such as angiostatin and pigment epithelium-derived factor (PEDF).[145] PEDF is secreted by Mueller and endothelial cells. Decreased PEDF levels are found in the vitreous of eyes with BDR; PEDF levels rise to normal after PRP for PDR. PEDF is known to have anti-inflammatory and anti-permeability properties.[146] PEDF balances the vasculopathic effects of VEGF through several mechanisms. PEDF inhibits VEGF expression by decreasing HIF levels via MAPK-mediated activation and stimulates endogenous PEDF production.[147] PEDF competes with VRGF for binding to VEGFR-2.

Patients with rheumatoid arthritis are known to have less severe diabetic retinopathy, prompting speculation that the anti-inflammatory medications they take antagonize the effects of vasoactive cytokines. Though these drugs may combat the effects of VEGF, they do not decrease VEGF levels. Aspirin and TNF-α inhibitors decrease ICAM-1 levels and leukocyte adhesion by decreasing nitrous oxide synthetase expression. Aspirin decreases the expression of integrins that bind to ICAM-1 (LFA-1 [CD11a/CD18] and Mac-1 [CD11b/CD18]).

1.4.3 Renin–Angiotensin System

The renin–angiotensin system (RAS) modulates a diverse group of biological functions.[148] The major active product of the system, angiotensin II (ANG II), is converted from angiotensin I by angiotensin-converting enzyme (ACE) (see Fig. 1.17). ANG II influences vasoconstriction, electrolyte homeostasis, modulation of drinking behavior, and stimulation of

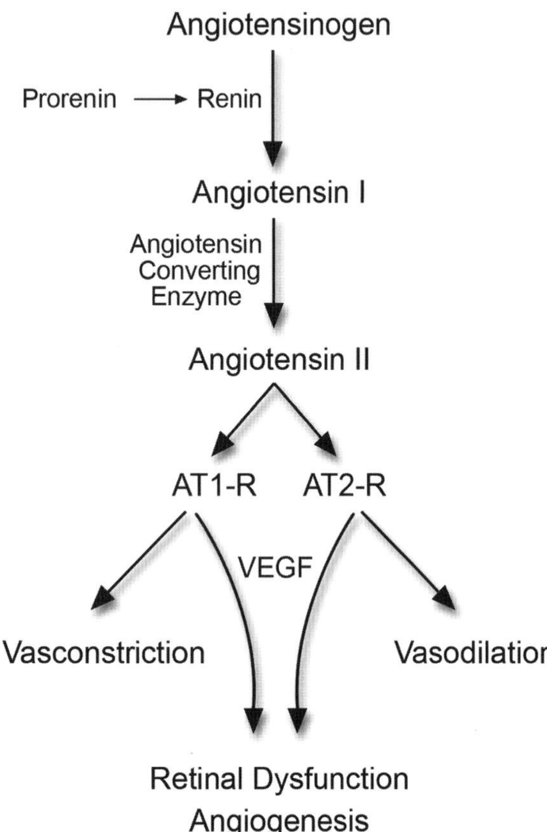

Fig. 1.17 Renin activation followed by the action of angiotensin-converting enzyme (ACE) converts angiotensinogen into angiotensin II. By binding to either of its two receptors, angiotensin II promotes vasoconstriction or vasodilation, in addition to stimulating VEGF production, which leads to vascular permeability changes and angiogenesis

pituitary hormone release.[149–151] As a growth factor, ANG II promotes differentiation, apoptosis, and the deposition of extracellular matrix.[152–155] Angiotensin receptors are located in endothelial cells, glia, and neurons,[156] suggesting that ANG II may regulate functions within these cells.

Angiotensin has significant effects on vascular smooth muscle cells, including cell growth, proliferation, and the deposition of extracellular matrix proteins.[157] These are mediated by factors such as TGF-β1, PDGF, VEGF, insulin-like growth factor, and connective tissue growth factor.[158] Though the ANG II effects on pericytes are less well studied, it does induce pericyte uncoupling and migration.[159]

The pro-angiogenic effect of ANG II in mammalian retinas with oxygen-induced retinopathy is mediated by VEGF.[160] Pharmacological blockade of the RAS decreases angiogenesis by downregulating VEGF and VEGFR2.

The ACE inhibitor captopril prevents degeneration of retinal capillaries; the angiotensin receptor antagonist losartan inhibits leukostasis in streptozotocin-induced rats and vascular cell adhesion molecule-1 (VCAM) expression in human endothelial cells.[161] ACE inhibition prevents the retinal overexpression of VEGF in experimental diabetes.[162] Furthermore, ACE inhibition prevents diabetic retinopathy progression in normotensive type I diabetic patients.[163]

Elevated angiotensin II levels correlate with vitreous VEGF levels in patients with diabetic macular edema.[164] Experimental evidence suggests that this may be mediated through the AT1–R/NF-κB pathway,[165] creating new target sites for the prevention of diabetic retinopathy.

1.5 Development of Proliferative Diabetic Retinopathy

Apoptosis of retinal vascular cells and formation of pericyte ghosts lead to acellular capillaries, hypoxia due to retinal nonperfusion, and subsequent proliferative retinopathy.[166,167] Diabetes-induced TNF-α is an important cause of microvascular cell loss. FOXO1, a forkhead transcription factor that regulates cell death, is stimulated by TNF-α. Inhibition of FOXO1 by RNAi reduces cell apoptosis and microvascular cell death both in vitro and in vivo in type 1 and type 2 diabetic rats.

Hyperglycemia increases FOXO1 protein and RNA levels in retinal capillary endothelial cells. These factors dramatically elevate the levels of genes that modulate endothelial cell behavior, including angiogenesis and vascular remodeling.

The resultant occlusion of retinal capillaries leads to patchy nonperfusion with subsequent hypoxia of the inner 2/3 of the retina. Stabilization of the hypoxia-inducible factor (HIF-1α) results in VEGF production. Intravitreous VEGF levels are higher in PDR than BDR[168] and are temporally related to the development of neovascularization.[169]

In addition to VEGF other growth factors such as insulin-like growth factor I (IGF-1), hepatocyte growth factor (HGF), basic fibroblast growth factor (b-FGF), platelet-derived growth factor (PDGF), pro-inflammatory cytokines, and angiopoietins are involved in the pathogenesis of PDR. Also found within the retina and vitreous are antiangiogenic factors such as pigment epithelium-derived factor (PEDF), transforming growth factor beta (TGF-β), thrombospondin (TSP), and somatostatin. It is postulated that neovascularization results from an imbalance of angiogenic and antiangiogenic factors.[170]

1.6 Summary of Key Points

- As predicted by Starling's law, changes in hydrostatic and oncotic pressures affecting the retinal capillaries (e.g., systemic hypertension, renal failure, hypoalbuminemia) worsen diabetic retinal edema.
- Hyperglycemia-driven activation of four biochemical pathways (increased polyol pathway flux, protein kinase C activation, advanced glycation end products, increased hexosamine pathway flux) explains many of the changes leading to diabetic retinopathy.
- The unified theory of diabetic retinopathy states that the intraocular formation of reactive oxygen species (ROS) fuels the subsequent pathological, biochemical changes.
- Blood–retinal barrier breakdown can be due to either tight-junction damage or transcellular alterations.
- Loss of pericytes, with compensatory synthesis and deposition of extracellular proteins, characterizes early diabetic retinopathy.
- Proliferative diabetic retinopathy may be associated with an imbalance of angiogenic and antiangiogenic factors; however, elevated VEGF levels correlate strongly with the development of neovascularization.

1.7 Future Directions

1. Improved understanding of the biochemical composition and pathological changes of tight junctions will identify new therapeutic targets to prevent blood–retinal barrier breakdown.
2. Research into the pathogenesis and treatment of other chorioretinal vascular diseases will allow the adaptation of new therapies to diabetic retinopathy, as has already occurred with corticosteroids and anti-VEGF agents.
3. Further refinement of the unified theory of diabetic retinopathy will identify pivotal substrates and enzymes, thereby allowing drug development to prevent the onset and progression of retinopathy.
4. Recent drug trials targeting the four individual biochemical pathways have yielded disappointing results. Future studies will learn from oncology's multidrug strategy by simultaneously targeting several biochemical pathways.

References

1. Sigelman J, Ozanics V. Retina. In *Duane's Foundations of Clinical Ophthalmology*. Philadelphia: Lippincott; 1990.
2. Hogan MJ, Alvarado JA, Weddell JE. The retina. In *Histology of the Human Eye*. Philadelphia: WB Saunders; 1971:393–522.
3. Zinn KM, Marmor MF, eds. *The Retinal Pigment Epithelium*. Cambridge, MA: Harvard University Press; 1979.
4. Pfeffer BA. Improved methodology for cell culture of human and monkey retinal pigment epithelium. *Prog Retinal Res*. 1991;10:251.
5. Feeney-Burns L, Burns RP, Gao C-L. Age-related macular changes in humans over 90 years old. *Am J Ophthalmol*. 1990;109:265–278.
6. Handelman GJ, Snodderly DM, Krinsky NI, et al. Biological control of primate macular pigment – biochemical and densitometric studies. *Invest Ophthalmol Vis Sci*. 1991;32:257–267.
7. Wald G, Brown PK. Human rhodopsin. *Science*. 1958;127:222–226.
8. Adler AJ, Severin KM. Proteins of the bovine interphotoreceptor matrix – tissues of origin. *Exp Eye Res*. 1981;2: 755–769.
9. Dowling JE, Boycott BB. Organization of the primate retina – electron microscopy. *Proc R Soc Ser B*. 1966;166: 80–111.
10. Curcio CA, Allen KA. Topography of ganglion cells in human retina. *J Comp Neurol*. 1990;300:5–25.
11. Pollock SC, Miller NR. The retinal nerve fiber layer. *Int Ophthalmol Clin*. 1986;26:201–221.
12. McLeod D. Why cotton wool spots should not be regarded as retinal nerve fiber layer infarcts. *Br J Ophthalmol*. 2005;89:229–237.
13. Ogden TE. The glia of the retina. In: Ryan SJ, Ogden TE, eds. *Retina*, Vol. 1. St. Louis: CV Mosby; 1989:53–56.
14. Smelser GK, Ishikawa T, Pei YF. Electron microscopic studies of intra-retinal spaces – diffusion of particulate

materials. In Rohen JW, ed. *Structure of the Eye, II Symp*. Stuttgart: Schattauer-Verlag; 1965:109–121.
15. Hewitt AT, Adler R. The retinal pigment epithelium and interphotoreceptor matrix – structure and specialized functions. In: Ryan SJ, Ogden TE, eds. *Retina*, Vol. 1. St. Louis: CV Mosby; 1989:57–64.
16. Jerdan JA, Kao L, Glaser BM. The inner limiting membrane: a modified basement membrane? *Invest Ophthalmol Vis Sci (suppl)*. 1986;27:230a.
17. Yamada E. Some structural features of the fovea centralis in the human retina. *Arch Ophthalmol*. 1969;82: 151–159.
18. Archer D, Krill AE, Newell FW. Fluorescein studies of normal choroidal circulation. *Am J Ophthalmol*. 1970;69: 543–554.
19. Ernest JT. Macrocirculation and microcirculation of the retina. In: Ryan SJ, Ogden TE, eds. *Retina*, Vol. 1. St. Louis: CV Mosby; 1989:65–66.
20. Ferrari-Dileo G, Davis EB, Anderson DR. Response of retinal vasculature to phenylephrine. *Invest Ophthalmol Vis Sci*. 1990;30:1181–1182.
21. Shin DH, Tsai CS, Parrow KA, et al. Vasoconstrictive effect of topical timolol on human retinal arteries. *Graefes Arch Clin Exp Ophthalmol*. 1991;229:298–299.
22. Shakib M, Cunha-Vaz JG. Studies on the permeability of the blood–retinal barrier. IV. Junctional complexes of the retinal vessels and their role in the permeability of the blood–retinal barrier. *Exp Eye Res*. 1966;5: 229–234.
23. Hogan MJ, Feeney L. Ultrastructure of the retinal vessels. Part 1. The larger vessels. *J Ultrastruct Res*. 1963;9:10–28.
24. Henkind P. New observations on the radial peripapillary capillaries. *Invest Ophthalmol*. 1967;6:103.
25. Wise GN, Dollery CT, Henkind P. *The Retinal Circulation*. New York: Harper & Row; 1971.
26. Chakravarthy U, Gardiner TA, Anderson P, et al. The effect of endothelin I on the retinal microvascular pericyte. *Microvasc Res*. 1992;43:241–254.
27. Dodge AB, Hechtman HB, Shepro D. Microvascular endothelial-derived autacoids regulate pericyte contractility. *Cell Motil Cytoskel*. 1991;18:180–188.
28. Matsugi T, Chen Q, Anderson DR. Contractile responses of cultured bovine retinal pericytes to angiotensin II. *Arch Ophthalmol*. 1997;115:1281–1285.
29. Cogan DG, Toussaint D, Kuwabara T. Retinal vascular patterns. Part IV. Diabetic retinopathy. *Arch Ophthalmol*. 1961;66:366–378.
30. Matthews DR, Stratton IM, Aldington SJ, et al. Risks of progression of retinopathy and vision loss related to tight blood pressure control in type 2 diabetes mellitus: UKPDS 69. *Arch Ophthalmol*. 2004;122:1631–1640.
31. Stratton IM, Kohner EM, Aldington SJ, et al. UKPDS 50: risk factors for incidence and progression of retinopathy in Type II diabetes over 6 years from diagnosis. *Diabetologia*. 2001;44:156–163.
32. Stefannson E, Landers MB 3rd, Wolbarsht ML. Increased retinal oxygen supply following pan-retinal photocoagulation and vitrectomy and lensectomy. *Trans Am Ophthalmol Soc*. 1981;79:307–334.
33. Stefansson E. The therapeutic effects of retinal laser treatment and vitrectomy. A theory based on oxygen and vascular physiology. *Acta Ophthalmol Scand*. 2001; 79:435–440.
34. Stefansson E. Ocular oxygenation and the treatment of diabetic retinopathy. *Surv Ophthalmol*. 2006;51: 364–380.
35. Kristinsson JK, Gottfredsdotter MS, Stefannson E. Retinal vessel dilatation and elongation precedes diabetic macular oedema. *Br J Ophthalmol*. 1997;81:274–278.
36. Kokame GT, de Leon MD, Tanji T. Serous retinal detachment and cystoid macular edema in hypotony maculopathy. *Am J Ophthalmol*. 2001;131:384–386.
37. Lewis H, Abrams GW, Blumenkranz MS, Campo RV. Vitrectomy for diabetic macular traction and edema associated with posterior hyaloid traction. *Ophthalmology*. 1992;99:753–759.
38. Patel JI, Tombran-Tink J, Hykin PG, et al. Vitreous and aqueous concentrations of proangiogenic, antiangiogenic factors and other cytokines in diabetic retinopathy patients with macular edema: implications for structural differences in macular profiles. *Exp Eye Res*. 2006;82: 798–806.
39. Brownlee M. Biochemistry and molecular cell biology of diabetic complications. *Nature*. 2001;414:813–820.
40. Lucis AJ. Atherosclerosis. *Nature*. 2000;407:233–241.
41. Hseuh WA, Law RE. Cardiovascular risk continuum: implications of insulin resistance and diabetes. *Am J Med*. 1998;105:4S–14S.
42. Guigliano D, Ceriello A, Paolisso G. Oxidative stress and diabetic vascular complications. *Diabetes Care*. 1996; 19:257–267.
43. Du XL, Edelstein D, Dimmeler S, et al. Hyperglycemia inhibits endothelial nitric oxide synthase activity by post-translational modification at the Akt site. *J Clin Invest*. 2001;108:1341–1348.
44. Giardino I, Edelstein D, Brownlee M. BCL-2 expression or antioxidants prevent hyperglycemia-induced formation of intracellular advanced glycation endproducts in bovine endothelial cells. *J Clin Invest*. 1996; 97:1422–1428.
45. Du XL, Edelstein D, Rossetti L, et al. Hyperglycemia-induced mitochondrial superoxide overproduction activates the hexosamine pathway and induces plasminogen activator inhibitor-1 expression by increasing Spl glycosylation. *Proc Natl Acad Sci USA*. 2000;97: 12222–12226.
46. Yamagishi SI, Edelstein D, Du XL, Brownlee M. Hyperglycemia potentiates collagen-induced platelet activation through mitochondrial superoxide overproduction. *Diabetes*. 2001;50:1491–1494.
47. Craven PA, Phillip SL, Melham MF, et al. Overexpression of Mn^{2+} superoxide dismutase increases in collagen accumulation induced by culture in mesangial cells in high-media glucose. *Metabolism*. 2001;50:1043–1048.
48. Williamson JR, Chang K, Frangos M, et al. Hyperglycemic pseudohypoxia and diabetic complications. *Diabetes*. 1993;42:801–813.
49. Engerman RL, Kern TX, Larson ME. Nerve conduction and aldose reductase inhibition during 5 years of diabetes or galactosaemia in dogs. *Diabetologia*. 1994;37:141–144.
50. Greene DA, Arezzo JC, Brown MB. Effect of aldose reductase inhibition on nerve conduction and morphometry

in diabetic neuropathy. Zenarestat study group. *Neurology*. 1999;53:580–591.
51. Stitt AW, Li YM, Gardiner TA, et al. Advanced glycation end products (AGEs) co-localize with AGE receptors in the retinal vasculature of diabetic and of AGE-infused rats. *Am J Pathol*. 1997;150:523–528.
52. Horie K, Miyata T, Maeda K, et al. Immunohistochemical colocalization of glycoxidation products and lipid peroxidation products in diabetic renal glomerular lesions. Implication for glycoxidative stress in the pathogenesis of diabetic nephropathy. *J Clin Invest*. 1997;100:2995–3004.
53. Degenhardt TP, Thorpe SR, Baynes JW. Chemical modification of proteins by methylglyoxal. *Cell Mol Biol*. 1998;44:1139–1145.
54. Wells-Knecht KJ, Zyzak DV, Litchfield JE, et al. Mechanism of autoxidative glycosylation: identification of glyoxal and arabinose as intermediates in the autoxidative modification of proteins by glucose. *Biochemistry*. 1995;34:3702–3709.
55. Thornalley PJ. The glyoxalase system: new developments towards functional characterization of a metabolic pathway fundamental to biological life. *Biochem J*. 1990;269: 1–11.
56. Soulis-Liparota T, Cooper M, Papazoglou D, et al. Retardation by aminoguanidine of development of albuminuria, mesangial expansion, and tissue fluorescence in streptozocin-induced diabetic rat. *Diabetes*. 1991;40: 1328–1334.
57. Bolton WK, Cattran DC, Williams ME, et al. Randomized trial of an inhibitor of advanced glycation end products in diabetic nephropathy. *Am J Nephrol*. 2004;24: 32–40.
58. Huijberts MSP, Wolffenbuttel BH, Boudier HA, et al. Aminoguanidine treatment increases elasticity and decreases fluid filtration of large arteries from diabetic rats. *J Clin Invest*. 1993;92:1407–1411.
59. Tsilibary EC, Charonis AS, Reger LA, et al. The effect of nonenzymatic glucosylation on the binding of the main noncollagenous NC1 domain to type IV collagen. *J Biol Chem*. 1988;263:4302–4308.
60. Charonis AS, Reger LA, Dege JE, et al. Laminin alterations after in vitro nonenzymatic glucosylation. *Diabetes*. 1990;39:807–814.
61. Federoff HJ, Lawrence D, Brownlee M. Nonenzymatic glycosylation of laminin and the laminin peptide CIKVAVS inhibits neurite outgrowth. *Diabetes*. 1993;42: 590–513.
62. Lu M, Kuroki M, Amano S, et al. Advanced glycation end products increase retinal vascular endothelial growth factor expression. *J Clin Invest*. 1998;101:1219–1224.
63. Koya D, King GL. Protein kinase C activation and the development of diabetic complications. *Diabetes*. 1998;47: 859–866.
64. Portilla D, Dai G, Peters JM, et al. Etomoxir-induced PPARalpha-modulated enzymes protect during acute renal failure. *Am J Physiol Renal Physiol*. 2000;278: F667–F675.
65. Keough RJ, Dunlop ME, Larkins RG. Effect of inhibition of aldose reductase on glucose flux, diacylglycerol formation, protein kinase C, and phospholipase A2 activation. *Metabolism*. 1997;46:41–47.
66. Ishii H, Jirousek MR, Koya D, et al. Amelioration of vascular dysfunctions in diabetic rats by an oral PKC beta inhibitor. *Science*. 1996;272:728–731.
67. Williams B, Gallacher B, Patel H, Orme C. Glucose-induced protein kinase C activation of protein kinase C alpha. *Circ Res*. 1997;46:1497–1503.
68. Craven PA, Studer RK, Felder J, et al. Nitric oxide inhibition of transforming growth factor-beta and collagen synthesis in mesangial cells. *Diabetes*. 1997;46:671–681.
69. Pieper GM, Riaz-ul-Haq J. Activation of nuclear factor-kappaB in cultured endothelial cells by increased glucose concentration: prevention by calphostin C. *Cardiovasc Pharmacol*. 1997;30:528–532.
70. Yerneni KK, Bai W, Khan BV, et al. Hyperglycemia-induced activation of nuclear transcription factor kappaB in vascular smooth muscle cells. *Diabetes*. 1999;48: 855–864.
71. Koya D, Haneda M, Nakagawa H, et al. Amelioration of accelerated diabetic mesangial expansion by treatment with a PKC beta inhibitor in diabetic db/db mice, a rodent model for type 2 diabetes. *FASEB J*. 2000;14:439–447.
72. Hart GW. Dynamic O-linked glycosylation of nuclear and cytoskeletal proteins. *Annu Rev Biochem*. 1997;66: 315–335.
73. Fine BS, Brucker AJ. Macular edema and cystoid macular edema. *Am J Ophthalmol*. 1981;92:466–481.
74. Gass JDM, Anderson DR, Davis EB. A clinical, fluorescein angiographic, and electron microscopic correlation of cystoid macular edema. *Am J Ophthalmol*. 1985; 100:82–86.
75. Arend O, Remky A, Harris A, et al. Macular microcirculation in cystoid maculopathy of diabetic patients [see comments]. *Br J Ophthalmol*. 1995;79:628–632.
76. Smith RT, Lee CM, Charles HC, et al. Quantification of diabetic macular edema. *Arch Ophthalmol*. 1987;105: 218–222.
77. Antcliff RJ, Marshall J. The pathogenesis of edema in diabetic maculopathy. *Semin Ophthalmol*. 1999;14:223–232.
78. Sinclair SH. Macular retinal capillary hemodynamics in diabetic patients. *Ophthalmology*. 1991;98:1580–1586.
79. Langham ME, Grebe R, Hopkins S, et al. Choroidal blood flow in diabetic retinopathy. *Exp Eye Res*. 1991; 52:167–173.
80. Weinberger D, Fink-Cohen S, Gaton DD, et al. Non-retinovascular leakage in diabetic maculopathy. *Br J Ophthalmol*. 1995;79:728–731.
81. Fukushima I, McLeod DS, Lutty GA. Intrachoroidal microvascular abnormality: a previously unrecognized form of choroidal neovascularization. *Am J Ophthalmol*. 1997;124:473–487.
82. Lanigan LP. Impaired autoregulation of the retinal vasculature and microalbuminuria in diabetes mellitus. *Eye*. 1990;4:174–180.
83. Schmetterer L, Salomon A, Rheinberger A, et al. Fundus pulsation measurements in diabetic retinopathy. *Graefe's Arch Clin Exp Ophthalmol*. 1997;235:283–287.
84. Ohno-Matsui K, Yoshida T, Uetama T, et al. Vascular endothelial growth factor upregulates pigment epithelium-derived factor expression via VEGFR-1 in human retinal pigment epithelial cells. *Biochem Biophys Res Commun*. 2003;303:962–967.

85. Christinger HW, Fuh G, de Vos AM, Wiesmann C. The crystal structure of placental growth factor in complex with domain 2 of vascular endothelial growth factor receptor-1. *J Biol Chem*. 2004;279:10382–10388.
86. Miyamoto N, de Kozak Y, Jeanny JC, et al. Placental growth factor-1 and epithelial haemato-retinal barrier breakdown: potential implication in the pathogenesis of diabetic retinopathy. *Diabetologia*. 2007;50: 461–470.
87. Bensaoula T, Ottlecz A. Biochemical and ultrastructural studies in the neural retina and retinal pigment epithelium of STZ-diabetic rats: effect of captopril. *J Ocular Pharmacol Ther*. 2001;17:573–586.
88. Tso MO. Pathology of cystoid macular edema. *Ophthalmology*. 1982;89:902–915.
89. Tso MO. Pathological study of cystoid macular oedema. *Trans OSUK*. 1980;100:408–413.
90. Matter K, Balda MS. Occludin and the functions of tight junctions. *Int Rev Cytol*. 1999;186:117–146.
91. Kiuchi-Saichin Y, Gotoh S, Furuse M, et al. Differential expression patterns of claudins, tight junction membrane proteins, in mouse nephron segments. *J Am Soc Nephrol*. 2002;13:875–886.
92. Antonetti DA, Barber AJ, Khin S, et al. Vascular permeability in experimental diabetes is associated with reduced endothelial occludin content: vascular endothelial growth factor decreases occludin in retinal endothelial cells. Penn State Retina Research Group. *Diabetes*. 1998;47:1953–1959.
93. Nitta T, Hata M, Gotoh S, et al. Size-selective loosening of the blood–brain barrier in claudin-5 deficient mice. *J Cell Biol*. 2003;161:653–660.
94. Felinski EA, Antonetti DA. Glucocorticoid regulation of endothelial cell tight junction gene expression: novel treatments for diabetic retinopathy. *Curr Eye Res*. 2005; 30:949–957.
95. Fanning AS, Ma TY, Anderson JM. Isolation and functional characterization of the actin binding region in the tight junction protein ZO-1. *FASEB J*. 2002;16:1835–1837.
96. Gardner TW, Lieth E, Khin SA, et al. Astrocytes increase barrier properties and ZO-1 expression in retinal vascular endothelial cells. *Invest Ophthalmol Vis Sci*. 1997;38:2423–2427.
97. Ebnet K, Suzuki A, Ohno S, Vestweber D. Junctional adhesion molecules (JAMs): more molecules with dual functions? *J Cell Sci*. 2004;117:19–29.
98. Stevenson BR, Keon BH. The tight junction: morphology to molecules. *Annu Rev Cell Dev Biol*. 1998;14:89–109.
99. Cunha-Vaz J, Faria de Abreu JR, Campos AJ. Early breakdown of the blood–retinal barrier in diabetes. *Br J Ophthalmol*. 1975;59:649–656.
100. Jones CW, Cunha-Vaz J, Zweig KO, Stein M. Kinetic vitreous fluorophotometry in experimental diabetes. *Arch Ophthalmol*. 1979;97:1941–1943.
101. Bates DO, Hillman NJ, Williams B, et al. Regulation of microvascular permeability by vascular endothelial growth factors. *J Anat*. 2002;200:581–597.
102. Wang W, Dentler WL, Borchardt RT. VEGF increases BMED monolayer permeability by affecting occludin expression and tight junction assembly. *Am J Physiol Heart Circ Physiol*. 2001;280:H434–H440.
103. Giebel SJ, Menicucci G, McGuire PG, Das A. Matrix metalloproteinases in early diabetic retinopathy and their role in alteration of the blood–retinal barrier. *Lab Invest*. 2005;85:597–607.
104. Vinores SA, Van Niel E, Swerrdloff IL, et al. Electron microscopic immunocytochemical evidence for the mechanism of blood–retinal barrier breakdown in galactosemic rats and its association with aldose reductase expression and inhibition. *Exp Eye Res*. 1993; 57:723–735.
105. Gillies MC, Su T, Stayl J, et al. Effect of high glucose on permeability on retinal capillary endothelium in vitro. *Invest Ophthalmol Vis Sci*. 1997;38:635–642.
106. Gardner TW, Lieth E, Khin SA, et al. Astrocytes increase barrier properties and ZO-1 expression in retinal vascular endothelial cells. *Invest Ophthalmol Vis Sci*. 1997;38:2423–2427.
107. Xia P, Aiello LP, Ishii H, et al. Characterization of vascular endothelial growth factor's effect on the activation of protein kinase C, its isoforms, and endothelial cell growth. *J Clin Invest*. 1996;98:2018–2026.
108. Zachary I, Gliki G. Signaling transduction mechanisms mediating biological actions of the vascular endothelial growth factor family. *Cardiovasc Res*. 2001;49:568–581.
109. Karkkainan MJ, Makinen T, Alitalo K. Lymphatic endothelium: a new frontier of metastasis research. *Nat Cell Biol*. 2002;4:E2–E5.
110. Gerber HP, Condorelli F, Park J, Ferrara N. Differential transcriptional regulation of the two VEGF receptor genes, Flt-1, but not Flk-a/KDR, is up-regulated by hypoxia. *J Biol Chem*. 1997;272:23659–23667.
111. Ferrara N. Vascular endothelial growth factor: basic science and clinical progress. *Endocrin Rev*. 2004; 25:581–611.
112. Spanel-Borowski K, Mayerhofer A. Formation and regression of capillary sprouts in corpora lutea of immature superstimulated golden hamsters. *Acta Anat (Basel)*. 1987;128:227–235.
113. Dejana E, Spagnuolo R, Bazzoni G. Interendothelial junctions and their role in the control of angiogenesis, vascular permeability and leukocyte transmigration. *Thromb Haemost*. 2001;86:308–315.
114. Abell RG. The permeability of blood capillary sprouts and newly formed blood capillaries as compared to that of older capillaries. *Am J Physiol*. 1946;147:231–241.
115. Schoefl GI. Studies on inflammation. III. Growing capillaries: their structure and permeability. *Virchows Arch Pathol Anat*. 1963;337:97–141.
116. Saishin Y, Saishin Y, Takahashi K, et al. VEGF-TRAP(R1R2) suppresses choroidal neovascularization and VEGF-induced breakdown of the blood–retinal barrier. *J Cell Physiol*. 2003;195:241–248.
117. Gehlbach P, Demetriades AM, Yamamoto S, et al. Periocular gene transfer of sFlt-1 suppresses ocular neovascularization and VEGF-induced breakdown of the blood–retinal barrier. *Hum Gene Ther*. 2003;14:129–141.
118. Bainbridge JW, Mistry A, De Alwis M, et al. Inhibition of retinal neovascularization by gene transfer of soluble VEGF receptor sFlt-1. *Gene Ther*. 2002;9:320–326.

119. Tobe T, Ortega S, Luna JD, et al. Targeted disruption of the FGF2 gene does not prevent choroidal neovascularization in a murine model. *Am J Path.* 1998; 153:1641–1646.
120. Oshima Y, Oshima S, Nambu H, et al. Increased expression of VEGF in retinal pigmented epithelial cells is not sufficient to cause choroidal neovascularization. *J Cell Physiol.* 2004;201:393–400.
121. Ozaki H, Hayashi H, Vinores SA, et al. Intravitreal sustained release of VEGF causes retinal neovascularization in rabbits and breakdown of the blood–retinal barrier in rabbits and primates. *Exp Eye Res.* 1997; 64:505–517.
122. Bates DO, Curry FE. Vascular endothelial growth factor increases hydraulic conductivity of isolated perfused microvessels. *Am J Physiol.* 1996;271:H2520–H2528.
123. Wu HM, Huang Q, Yuan Y, Granger HJ. VEGF induces NO-dependent hyperpermeability in coronary venules. *Am J Physiol.* 1996;271:H2735–H2739.
124. Bates DO. The chronic effect of vascular endothelial growth factor on individually perfused frog mesenteric microvessels. *J Physiol.* 1998;513:225–233.
125. Fukumura D, Gohongi T, Kadambi A, et al. Predominant role of endothelial nitric oxide synthase in vascular endothelial growth factor-induced angiogenesis and vascular permeability. *Proc Natl Acad Sci USA.* 2001;98:2604–2609.
126. Lu M, Perez VL, Ma N, et al. VEGF increases retinal vascular ICAM-1 expression in vivo. *Invest Ophthalmol Vis Sci.* 1999;40:1808–1812.
127. Gaudry M, Bregerie O, Andrieu V, et al. Intracellular pool of vascular endothelial growth factor in human neutrophils. *Blood.* 1997;90:4153–4161.
128. Miyamoto K, Khosrof S, Bursell SE, et al. Prevention of leukostasis and vascular leakage in streptozotocin-induced diabetic retinopathy via intercellular adhesion molecule-1 inhibition. *Proc Natl Acad Sci USA.* 1999; 96:10836–10841.
129. Bolton SJ, Anthony DC, Perry VH. Loss of the tight junction proteins occludin and zonula occludens-1 from cerebral vascular endothelium during neutrophil-induced blood–brain barrier breakdown in vivo. *Neuroscience.* 1998;86:1245–1257.
130. Brooks HL Jr., Caballero S Jr., Newell CK, et al. Vitreous levels of vascular endothelial growth factor and stromal-derived factor 1 in patients with diabetic retinopathy and cystoid macular edema before and after intraocular injection of triamcinolone. *Arch Ophthalmol.* 2004;122:1801–1807.
131. Funatsu H, Yamashita H, Ikeda T, et al. Vitreous levels of interleukin-6 and vascular endothelial growth factor are related to diabetic macular edema. *Ophthalmology.* 2003;110:1690–1696.
132. Semenza G. Signal transduction to hypoxia-inducible factor 1. *Biochem Pharmacol.* 2002;64:993–998.
133. Jaakkola P, Mole DR, Tian YM, et al. Targeting of HIF-alpha to the von Hippel–Lindau ubiquitylation complex by O_2-regulated prolyl hydroxylation. *Science.* 2001;292:468–472.
134. Safran M, Kaelin WG Jr. HIF hydroxylation and the mammalian oxygen-sensing pathway. *J Clin Invest.* 2003; 779–783.
135. Wang GL, Jiang BH, Rue EA, Semenza GL. Hypoxia-inducible factor 1 is a basic-helix-loop-helix-PAS heterodimer regulated by cellular O_2 tension. *Proc Natl Acad Sci.* 1995;92:5510–5514.
136. Weiner CM, Booth G, Semenza GL. In vivo expression of mRNAs encoding hypoxia-inducible factor 1. *Biochem Biophys Res Commun.* 1996;225:485–488.
137. Schroedl C, McClintock DS, Budinger GR, Chandel NS. Hypoxic but not anoxic stabilization of HIF-1alpha requires mitochondrial reactive oxygen species. *Am J Physiol Lung Cell Mol Physiol.* 2002;283: L922–L931.
138. Poulaki V, Qin W, Joussen AM, et al. Acute intensive insulin therapy exacerbates diabetic blood–retinal barrier breakdown via hypoxia-inducible factor-1alpha and VEGF. *J Clin Invest.* 2002;109:805–815.
139. Paul SA, Simons JW, Mabjeesh NJ. HIF at the crossroads between ischemia and carcinogenesis. *J Cell Physiol.* 2004;200:20–30.
140. Stasek JE Jr., Patterson CE, Garcia JG. Protein kinase C phosphorylates caldesmon77 and vimentin and enhances albumin permeability across cultured bovine pulmonary artery endothelial cell monolayers. *J Cell Physiol.* 1992;153:62–75.
141. Clarke H, Marano CW, Peralta Soler A, Mullin JM. Modification of tight junction function by protein kinase C isoforms. *Adv Drug Deliv Rev.* 2000;41:283–301.
142. Studer RK, Craven PA, DeRubertis FR. Role for protein kinase C in the mediation of increased fibronectin accumulation by mesangial cells grown in high-glucose medium. *Diabetes.* 1993;42:118–126.
143. Aiello LP, Bursell SE, Clermont A, et al. Vascular endothelial growth factor-induced retinal permeability is mediated by protein kinase C in vivo and suppressed by an orally effective beta-isoform-selective inhibitor. *Diabetes.* 1997;46:1473–1480.
144. Williams B, Gallacher B, Patel H, Orme C. Glucose-induced protein kinase C activation regulates vascular permeability factor mRNA expression and peptide production by human vascular smooth muscle cells in vitro. *Diabetes.* 1997;46:1497–1503.
145. Miller JW, Adamis AP, Aiello LP. Vascular endothelial growth factor in ocular neovascularization and proliferative diabetic retinopathy. *Diabetes Metab Rev.* 1997;13: 37–50.
146. Liu H, Ren JG, Cooper WL, et al. Identification of the antivasopermeability effect of pigment epithelium-derived factor and its active site. *Proc Natl Acad Sci.* 2004;101:6605–6610.
147. Zhang SX, Wang JJ, Gao G, et al. Pigment epithelium-derived factor downregulates vascular endothelial growth factor (VEGF) expression and inhibits VEGF–VEGF receptor 2 binding in diabetic retinopathy. *J Mol Endocrinol.* 2006;37:1–12.
148. Kim S, Iwao H. Molecular and cellular mechanisms of angiotensin II-mediated cardiovascular and renal diseases. *Pharmacol Rev.* 2000;52:11–34.
149. Aguilera G, Kiss A. Regulation of the hypothalamic–pituitary–adrenal axis and vasopressin secretion. Role of angiotensin II. *Adv Exp Med Biol.* 1996;396: 105–112.

150. Culman J, Hohle S, Qadri F, et al. Angiotensin as neuromodulator/neurotransmitter in central control of body fluid and electrolyte homeostasis. *Clin Exp Hypertens.* 1995;17:281–293.
151. Ito M, Oliverio MI, Mannon PJ, et al. Regulation of blood pressure by the type 1A angiotensin II receptor gene. *Proc Natl Acad Sci USA.* 1995;92:3521–3525.
152. Kato H, Suzuki H, Tajima S, et al. Angiotensin II stimulates collagen synthesis in cultured vascular smooth muscle cells. *J Hypertens.* 1991;9:17–22.
153. Otani A, Takagi H, Oh H, et al. Angiotensin II induces expression of the Tie2 receptor ligand, angiopoietin-2, in bovine retinal endothelial cells. *Diabetes.* 2001;50:867–875.
154. Otani A, Takagi H, Suzuma K, Honda Y. Angiotensin II potentiates endothelial growth factor-induced angiogenic activity in retinal microcapillary endothelial cells. *Circ Res.* 1998;82:619–628.
155. Suzuki Y, Ruiz-Ortega M, Lorenzo O, et al. Inflammation and angiotensin II. *Int J Biochem Cell Biol.* 2003; 35:881–900.
156. Nagai N, Noda K, Urano T, et al. Selective suppression of pathologic, but not physiologic, retinal neovascularization by blocking the angiotensin II type 1 receptor. *Invest Ophthalmol Vis Sci.* 2005;46:1078–1084.
157. Tamura K, Nyui N, Tamura N, et al. Mechanism of angiotensin II-mediated regulation of fibronectin gene in rat vascular smooth muscle cells. *J Biol Chem.* 1998; 273:26487–26496.
158. Wilkinson-Berka J. Angiotensin and diabetic retinopathy. *Int J Biochem Cell Biol.* 2006;38:752–765.
159. Kawamura H, Kobayashi M, Li Q, et al. Effects of angiotensin II on the pericyte-containing microvasculature of the rat retina. *J Physiol.* 2004;561:671–683.
160. Ferrara N. Role of vascular endothelial growth factor in the regulation of angiogenesis. *Kidney Int.* 1999;56:794–814.
161. Zhang J-Z. Captopril inhibits capillary degeneration the early stages of diabetic retinopathy. *Curr Eye Res.* 2007;32:883–889.
162. Gilbert RD, Kelly DJ, Cox AJ, et al. Angiotensin converting enzyme inhibition reduces retinal overexpression of vascular endothelial growth factor and hyperpermeability in experimental diabetes. *Diabetologia.* 2000;43:1360–1367.
163. Chaturvedi N, Sjolie AK, Stephenson JM, et al. Effect of lisinopril on progression of retinopathy in normotensive people with type 1 diabetes. The EUCLID study group. EURODIAB controlled trial of Lisinopril in insulin-dependent diabetes mellitus. *Lancet.* 1998;351:28–31.
164. Funatsu H, Yamashita H, Ikeda T, et al. Angiotensin II and vascular endothelial growth factor in the vitreous fluid of patients with proliferative diabetic retinopathy. *Br J Ophthalmol.* 2002;86:311–315.
165. Nagai N, Izumi-Nagai K, Oike Y, et al. Suppression of diabetes-induced retinal inflammation by blocking the angiotensin II type 1 receptor or its downstream nuclear factor-κB pathway. *Invest Oph Vis Sci.* 2007;48: 4342–4350.
166. Mizutani M, Kern TS, Lorenzi M. Accelerated death of retinal microvascular cells in human and experimental diabetic retinopathy. *J Clin Invest.* 1996;97:2883–2890.
167. Benjamin LE. Glucose, VEGF-A, and diabetic complications. *Am J Pathol.* 2001;158:1181–1184.
168. Aiello L, Avery R, Arrigg P, et al. Vascular endothelial growth factor in ocular fluid of patients with diabetic retinopathy and other retinal disorders. *N Engl J Med.* 1994;331:1480–1487.
169. Adamis AP, Miller JW, Bernal MT, et al. Increased vascular endothelial growth factor levels in the vitreous of eyes with proliferative diabetic retinopathy. *Am J Ophthalmol.* 1994;118:445–450.
170. Simo R, Carrasco E, Garcia-Ramirez M, Hernandez C. Angiogenic and antiangiogenic factors in proliferative diabetic retinopathy. *Curr Diabetes Rev.* 2006;2: 71–98.

Chapter 2
Genetics and Diabetic Retinopathy

David G. Telander, Kent W. Small, and David J. Browning

Diabetic retinopathy (DR) is the leading cause of new cases of blindness for people between 20 and 64 years of age in the United States. While glycemic control is the chief risk factor for development and progression of diabetic retinopathy, there is increasing evidence for heritable risk factors. An increasing number of genetic linkage studies have uncovered the role that several genes have in the development and progression of DR.

Unlike sickle cell anemia or Huntington's disease, diabetes mellitus does not demonstrate a mendelian inheritance pattern. No single gene causes diabetes. Rather, it is a complex genetic disease with interaction among genes and the environment. The alleles, or forms of genes, that are associated with complex genetic diseases such as diabetes are often common variants. Rather than being causative, these alleles contribute to the risk of disease expression affecting severity and age of onset.[1] Diabetic retinopathy can be considered as a complex trait as well and may have a constellation of susceptibility and protective genes distinct from those associated with diabetes mellitus. There are many levels to the complexity of the interaction of these genes and gene products. For example, hemoglobin A1c (HbA1c) levels have a genetically determined component in type 1 diabetes that is independent of blood glucose level and are in turn associated with rates of progression of retinopathy.[2]

Non-genetic risk factors for diabetic retinopathy are well known, including duration of diabetes, glycemic control, and hypertension; however, the genetic risk factors for development and progression of diabetic retinopathy are only beginning to be understood.[3,4] A greater than expected prevalence of diabetic retinopathy exists in siblings with diabetic retinopathy than in non-siblings.[5] Differences in frequency of the disease among different ethnicities and populations also suggest a genetic component contributing to diabetic retinopathy.[6,7] Differences in relative prevalence of diabetic macular edema (DME) and proliferative diabetic retinopathy (PDR) in different racial groups further suggest that components of diabetic retinopathy have independent genetic susceptibility profiles.[8] Within a given population, the marked variation in onset and severity of retinopathy that cannot be explained by known risk factors indicates genetic susceptibility to DR.[9] For example, in African-American type 1 diabetics, clinical risk factors could account for only 27% of the variance in DR severity.[10] Because of difficulties unraveling the effects of shared environment from shared genes in family studies, these epidemiologic studies provide suggestive evidence only.[7] Nevertheless, such evidence is an important precursor to molecular genetic explorations searching for specific genetic associations.[7]

2.1 Background for Clinical Genetics

This section is a brief review of genetic concepts for understanding the relevant literature and associated terminology. Lack of familiarity of genetic concepts by clinicians has often been identified as an obstacle in progress toward understanding disease pathogenesis.[11] Our intent in this chapter is to help bridge this obstacle.

D.G. Telander (✉)
Davis Medical Center, University of California, Sacramento, CA 95817, USA
e-mail: dgtelander@ucdavis.edu

D.J. Browning (ed.), *Diabetic Retinopathy*, DOI 10.1007/978-0-387-85900-2_2,

Understanding of molecular genetics begins with the study of deoxyribonucleic acid (DNA), a linear polymer comprised of two strands containing sequences of four nitrogen-containing bases – adenine (A), guanine (G), thymine (T), and cytosine (C) (Fig. 2.1).

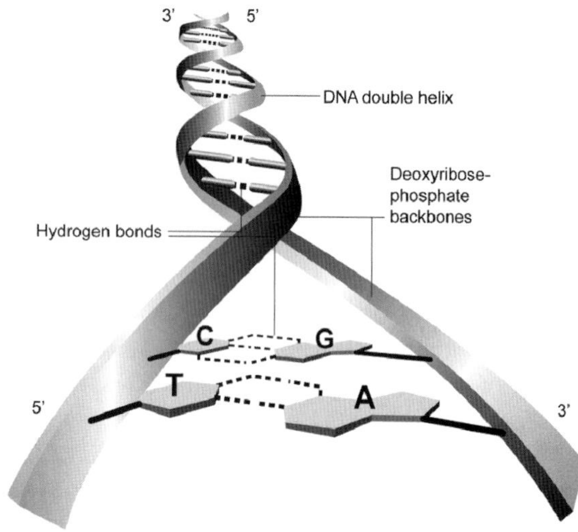

Fig. 2.1 Each strand of DNA consists of a backbone of deoxyribose phosphate sugars with attached purine and pyrimidine bases. The bases show complementarity by forming hydrogen bonds with paired bases in the fellow strand. Adapted with permission from Della[12]

DNA is the template for its own replication. DNA also serves as a template for the creation of ribonucleic acid (RNA) in a process called transcription. This RNA copy of the DNA then in turn serves as the template for synthesis of proteins. In transcription, DNA is always read beginning at the 5′ end and proceeding to the 3′ end. The two strands of a DNA molecule are held together by hydrogen bonds between paired bases. Adenine in one strand always binds to thymine in its fellow strand and likewise for cytosine and guanine. For example, if a section of the sequence of one strand is 5′-ATGAC-3′, then its fellow strand at this locus reads 3′-TACTG-5′. Binding of complementary strands of DNA or between a single strand of DNA and its complementary RNA strand is termed hybridization.[13]

The central dogma of molecular biology states that DNA is transcribed to an RNA which is in turn translated into protein (Fig. 2.2). In the cell nucleus, transcription of DNA occurs first as a messenger RNA precursor (mRNA) that contains the transcript of the protein-coding DNA sequence (exons), the non-protein-coding DNA sequence (introns), and untranslated regions adjacent to the 3′ and 5′ termini. The transcribed introns are spliced out to yield a mature mRNA product (Fig. 2.2). In the cell cytoplasm, mature mRNA is translated as three base segments called codons into amino acids that compose the protein product of the gene.[14] This intricate process of an RNA-guided protein synthesis is called translation.

Humans have 23 pairs of chromosomes, each comprised of DNA and associated proteins. Each chromosome contains many genes, or sequences of DNA that code for proteins, as well as sequences of DNA dedicated to regulatory functions such as initiating transcription or translation. There are 3.3 billion base pairs in the human genome.[1] The latest estimates on the number of genes in the human genome are 20,000–25,000.[15] Ninety-nine percent of the genome does not code for proteins.[16] These noncoding sections of the genome are broken into classes called introns and intergenic DNA. Introns, comprising 24% of the human genome, are segments of DNA adjacent to exons that are initially transcribed into an RNA strand but are then excised from initial RNA transcripts before the final mRNA strand leaves the nucleus for the cytoplasm on the way to protein synthesis (Fig. 2.2). Intergenic DNA, comprising 75% of the genome, remains untranscribed and has unknown function.[16] The remaining 1% of DNA composes the exons that code for proteins.[16,17]

2.2 The Role of Polymorphisms in Genetic Studies

The DNA sequences of any two human beings are 99% identical. The 1% of DNA that differs between any two individuals constitutes the genetic basis of certain diseases. In addition, factors that control the expression of the genes contribute to different phenotypes including disease. The purpose of genetic investigations is to determine which genes contribute to disease. On average, a difference in DNA sequence between two persons is found once per 1,200 base pairs. When a variation of the genetic locus is found in at least 1% of a given human population, the variation is termed as polymorphism.

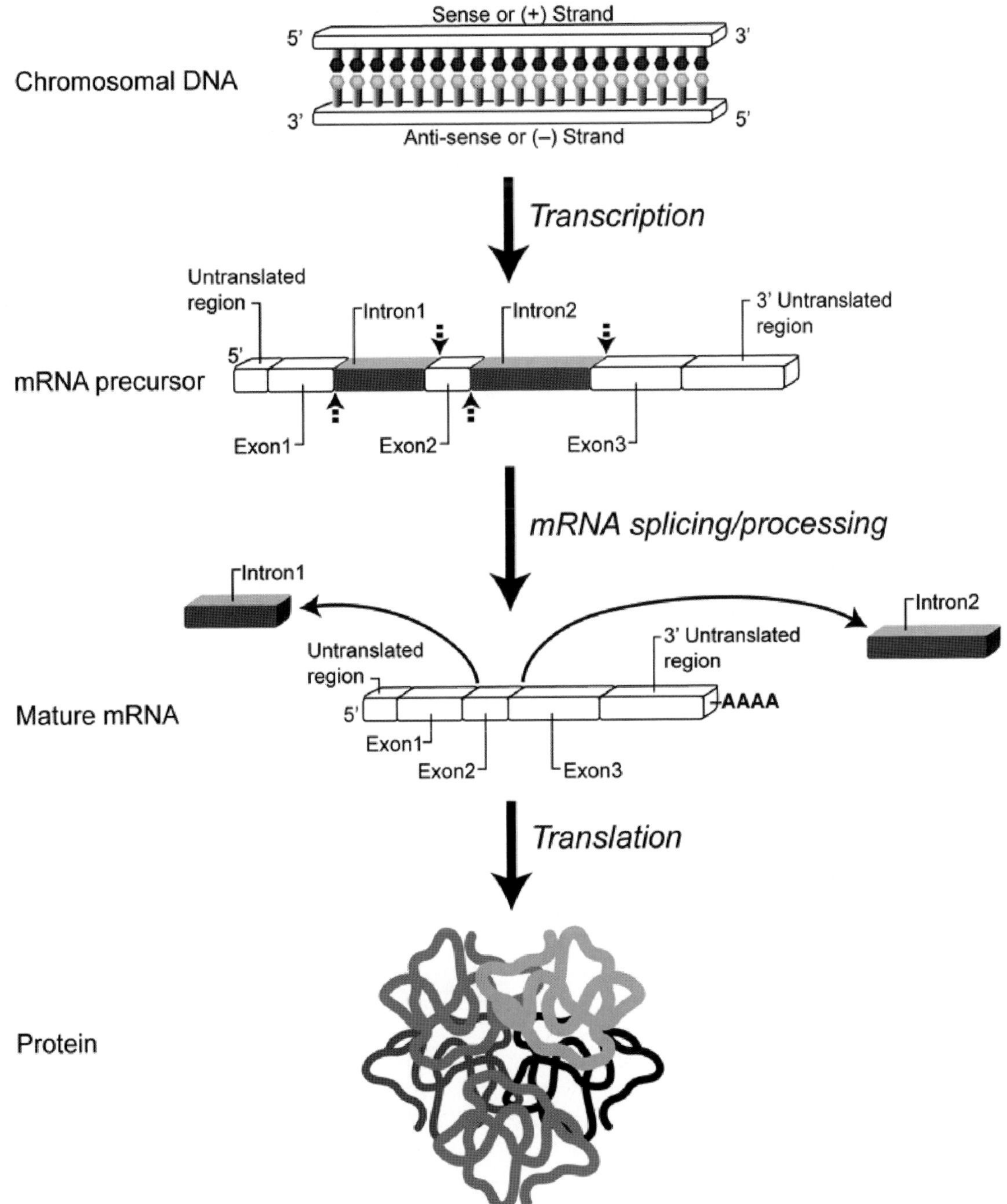

Fig. 2.2 DNA is transcribed into an mRNA precursor which is refined to mature mRNA by the excision of sequences corresponding to introns and transported out of the nucleus into the cytoplasm. Translation of mature mRNA results in a protein product. Adapted with permission from Della[12]

There are several categories of polymorphisms. Single nucleotide polymorphisms (SNPs) are single substitutions of one base for another at a certain position. There are many variations in nomenclature for these, but one common way of naming an SNP is exemplified by c.74C>G. This means that at the level of the coding DNA sequence (indicated by the c. prefix), at position 74, a cytosine is replaced by a guanine. The first letter characterizes the normal base and the second letter following the arrowhead signifies the mutant base. To add to the perplexing nature of the nomenclature, some authors refer to mutations not at the level of the coding DNA, but rather at the level of the altered amino acid sequence in the protein product of the mutant gene. In using this nomenclature, the convention is to list the normal amino acid first followed by the codon number in the sequence of the protein followed by the mutant amino acid. Thus, for example, Ala276-Glu means that at codon 276 one finds glutamine replacing the normally expected alanine.[18]

Another important class of polymorphisms is that of short tandem repeats (STRs) or microsatellites. These are strings of repetitive base pair sequences that vary in length between persons. Thus the alleles are variations in the number of repeats. For example, at a given location, one might find that one person shows CACA [or $(CA)_2$], the next CACACA [or$(CA)_3$], the next CACACACA [or $(CA)_4$], and so on. Nucleotides are repeated in tandem a number of times. SNPs and STRs are scattered at different locations across the human genome, and encyclopedias of such polymorphisms have been compiled. They provide a fine toothed comb such that any part of the human genome can be probed by selecting an SNP or STR located nearby in the genetic map.

Yet another type of polymorphism, more often used in older genetic association studies, is the restriction fragment length polymorphism. Enzymes called restriction endonucleases cleave DNA at sites where certain DNA sequences are detected. There are many restriction endonucleases (Fig. 2.3). By analyzing the length of fragments of

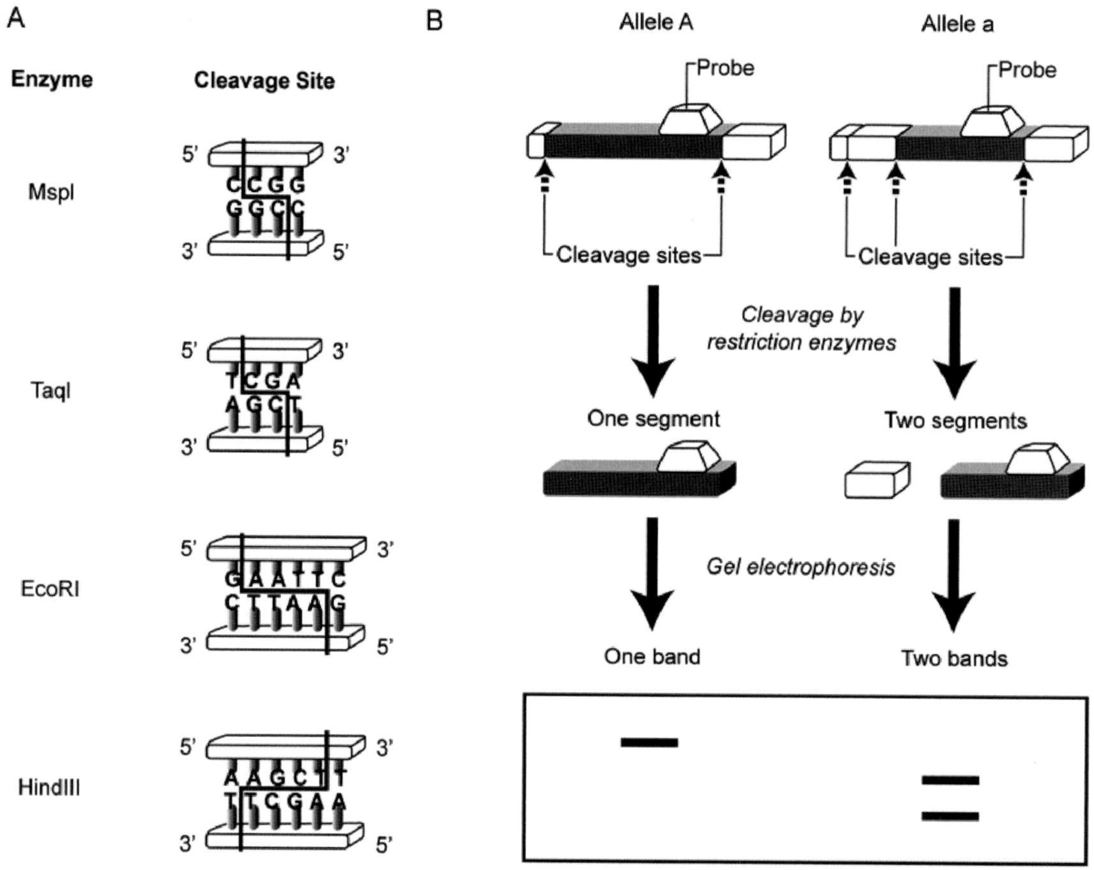

Fig. 2.3 (**a**) Restriction enzymes cleave DNA at specific sites. There are many restriction enzymes. Four (MspI, TaqI, EcoRI, and HindIII) are illustrated here as well as the loci cleaved by them. (**b**) The result of applying a restriction endonuclease to DNA is a set of DNA fragments that can be separated by electrophoresis. The electrophoretic pattern can distinguish different alleles (A and a). Adapted with permission from Musarella[19]

DNA produced by the action of restriction endonucleases, one can deduce the presence or absence of polymorphisms that result in cleavage sites.

Figure 2.4 shows an example of a map of genetic markers, in this case short tandem repeats, corresponding to chromosome 11 and their positional relationship relative to a gene, *PAX6*, that is critical in ocular embryogenesis. From a study of this figure, it will become evident that one can judiciously choose a polymorphism and examine if it is associated with a disease such as diabetic retinopathy. If there is an association between the polymorphism and the disease phenotype, then neighboring genes to this polymorphism may be candidates for investigation regarding pathogenesis of the disease. Neighboring genes become candidates because segments of DNA tend to be inherited together as a unit. Conversely, if one suspects that a certain gene is important in causing a diabetic retinopathy, one could choose to study a polymorphism found in close proximity to that gene based on the genetic map and then look for associations of that polymorphism with presence or absence of the disease. In the case of diabetic retinopathy studies, markers for nonproliferative retinopathy (NPDR), proliferative retinopathy (PDR), diabetic macular edema (DME), or presence of any DR have all been studied. The success of such studies depends critically on how reproducible the classification of patients is with regard to disease status. For example, if patients are misclassified as having PDR, a study may spuriously fail to find an association with a genetic marker. Genes conferring susceptibility for NPDR, PDR, DME, and possibly other diabetic retinopathy phenotypes may be distinct.[6,20]

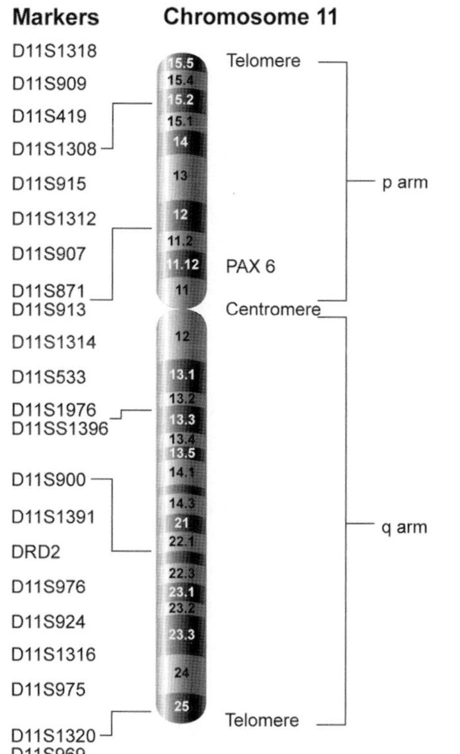

Fig. 2.4 Genetic markers called polymorphisms have been mapped throughout the human genome. In this example, short tandem repeat polymorphisms have been mapped on chromosome 11 and are shown in relation to the position of the PAX6 gene. Adapted with permission from Damji et al.[1]

2.3 Types of Genetic Study Design

One common genetic study design is the case-control format. In such a study, a group of patients with diabetic retinopathy or one of its subtypes and a control group with diabetes but no retinopathy are collected. Information is collected regarding some genetic marker for each person in the population sample. Statistical tests are then performed to examine associations of the genetic marker polymorphisms with presence or absence of the disease state. These may be Chi-square tests, odds ratios, likelihood ratios, or others. In theory, this approach could be used to screen many genetic markers at intervals across the entire genome to test for associations, but several methodological constraints limit such a wide net approach.

The genetic marker may have no causal relationship to diabetic retinopathy, but only manifest linkage with the gene that in fact confers risk. If patients with disease and controls are drawn from genetically different populations, a false-positive association may result. Large numbers of statistical tests performed in genome-wide scans can lead to false-positive associations. In some studies, comparisons of gene frequencies are made between patients with diabetic retinopathy and non-diabetic controls. This can lead to identification of genetic variants associated with vulnerability to diabetes rather than to diabetic retinopathy. To determine genetic variations associated with vulnerability to diabetic retinopathy, it is important to use patients with diabetes but no retinopathy as the control population.[21] The results of this type of genetic association study frequently differ.[22,23] The reasons offered include different ethnic groups studied and different criteria for patient selection such as criteria involving renal function.[24,25] Thus, given the numerous pitfalls and discordant results among studies, it is a general rule that confidence in association studies increases in proportion to the number of studies that replicate a given set of findings. Meta-analyses can be useful in deriving a common thread if one exists in frequently discordant genetic studies.[22]

The Human Genome Project has led to the construction of a genetic map which locates all the known genes and polymorphisms to their particular loci on the 23 pairs of chromosomes (22 pairs of autosomes and 1 pair of sex chromosomes – X and Y). Thus there are 24 genetic submaps, one for each of 22 autosomes and a submap for X and Y. Groups of polymorphisms located on the same chromosomal region tend to be inherited together as a unit and are statistically associated. These are referred to as haplotypes. The HapMap Project is an ongoing international collaboration in which regions of linked polymorphisms are being defined in four international populations.[7] Haplotypes are represented by so-called tag SNPs, which are SNPs that are indicators that an entire ensemble of SNPs is present. The ensemble is the haplotype. The tag SNP is the indicator label for a specific haplotype.

A critical tool in the ability to perform linkage analysis is the polymerase chain reaction. This method of taking a small amount of a specific segment of DNA and generating a large amount of identical DNA provides enough material to be detectable and measurable in order to identify the status of a person with regard to presence or absence of a genetic marker. Thus using PCR, each person in a study can be genotyped for a specific allele. The genotype of the allele can be correlated with disease status to determine associations. In PCR, short synthetic pieces of single-stranded DNA called primers are made which flank a specific small region of DNA of interest in the sample from the person. The double-stranded DNA sample is separated and the primers bind to the region of interest based on their complementary sequences. DNA polymerase and deoxynucleotide triphosphates are then added to the mixture at varying temperatures, resulting in production of new complementary DNA adjacent to the primers at the sequence of interest. Thus two copies of the double-stranded DNA in the region of interest now exist where one had a single copy. The process is repeated many times – 30 times would be typical – producing a billion copies of the DNA sample from a single starter molecule. This larger amount of DNA can then be manipulated, separated, and measured electrophoretically and alleles distinguished. Figure 2.5 illustrates the process of PCR.

Case–control association studies differ from linkage analysis studies, another type of study commonly employed in the investigation of diseases with mendelian inheritance. In a linkage analysis study, a large pedigree with numerous affected members is analyzed using similar molecular genetic techniques. The status of each member of the pedigree with regard to the genetic marker under study is determined. Likewise, the disease status of each member of the family is ascertained. By evaluating the segregation of an allele of the genetic marker with the disease in a pedigree, it is possible to determine the probability that particular alleles are inherited with the disease. Figure 2.6 illustrates the process. To summarize, case–control association analyses examine unrelated population samples. Linkage analyses examine families.

An important method of analysis used in genetics studies of diabetic retinopathy is linkage analysis. In linkage analysis, the expectation is that if an allele makes an important contribution toward disease causation, then the allele should be present in a higher frequency among affected individuals than in the unaffected. Linkage analysis is based on the phenomenon of recombination that occurs during meiosis, or the process of producing sex cells. During meiosis, homologous chromosomes exchange short segments of DNA. The probability that any two small segments of DNA on a chromosome will be separated by this process depends on how far apart they are on the chromosome. The closer the two segments are, the less likely that the segments will be separated by crossing over. Even when there is no known gene directly tied to a disease, this

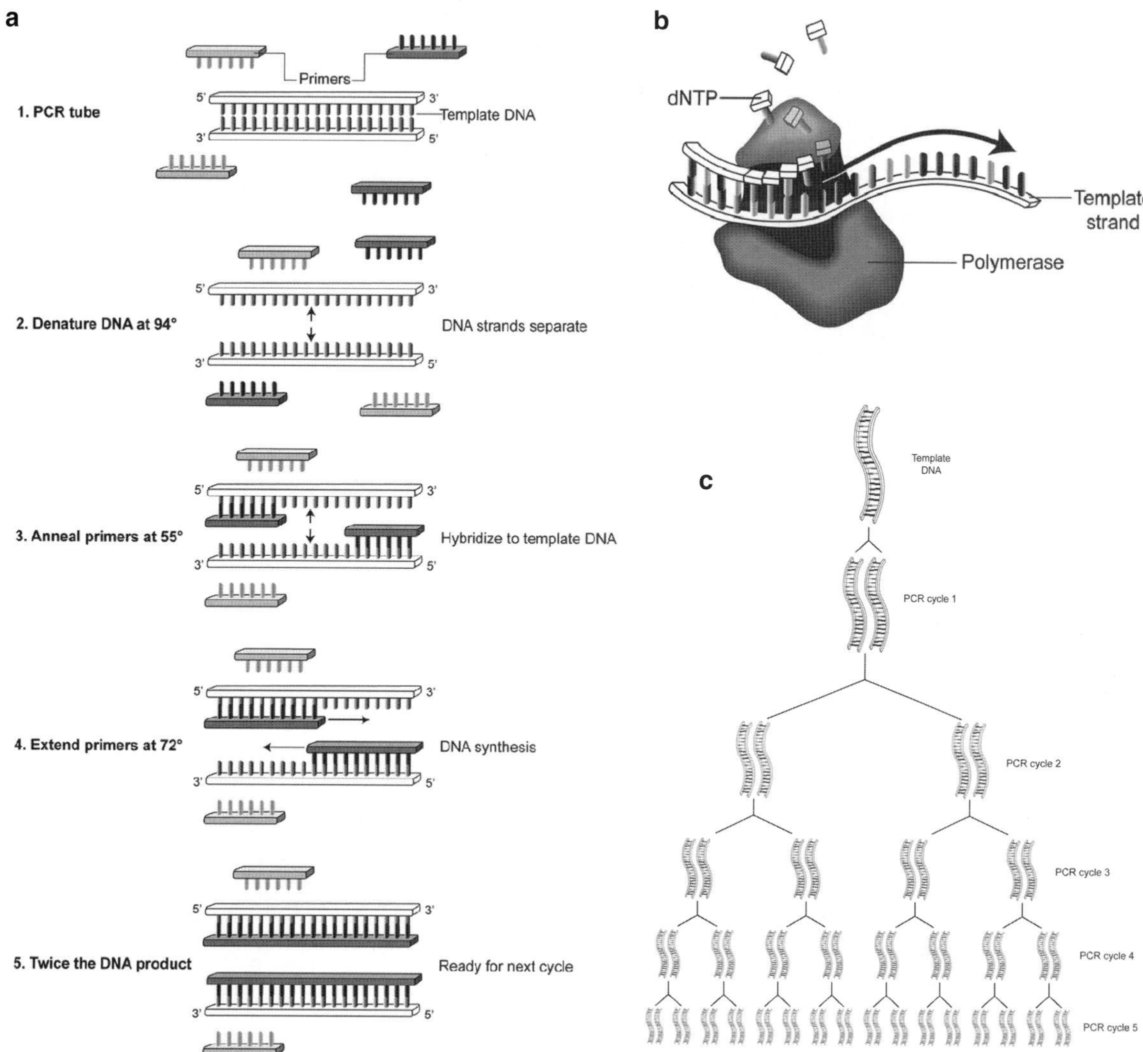

Fig. 2.5 (**a**) Schematic representation of the process of polymerase chain reaction. A double-stranded molecule of DNA called the template from a subject under investigation is broken into two single-stranded components by heating. Primers are specifically synthesized which bind to DNA sequences that flank the region of interest (the region in which one is looking for a particular polymorphism). These primers are added to the mixture and anneal to the complementary sequences in the single separated strands of DNA (hybridization). (**b**) Polymerase enzymes and deoxynucleotide triphosphates (dNTP) are added to the mixture and new DNA is produced starting at the end of the bound primer. Two double-stranded DNA molecules result. The process is repeated many times to produce enough DNA to manipulate electrophoretically. (**c**) Schematic of the exponential amplification of DNA through PCR. After 30 cycles, an initial template molecule of DNA results in 1 billion molecules of identical DNA. Adapted with permission from Della[12] and Dragon[26]

concept is useful. One can quantitate how closely a particular genetic marker is to the presence or absence of the disease by examining large numbers of patients and looking for cosegregation of the genetic marker and the presence or absence of the disease. A metric for quantitating how closely a genetic marker is linked to a disease-causing gene is the LOD score. The LOD score is the logarithm of the odds ratio of linkage of the genetic marker to the disease-causing gene compared to absence of linkage. A LOD score greater than 3 implies an odds ratio exceeding 1000 to 1 in favor of linkage and by convention is taken as evidence of linkage. A LOD score more negative than –2.0 implies odds of 100:1 or

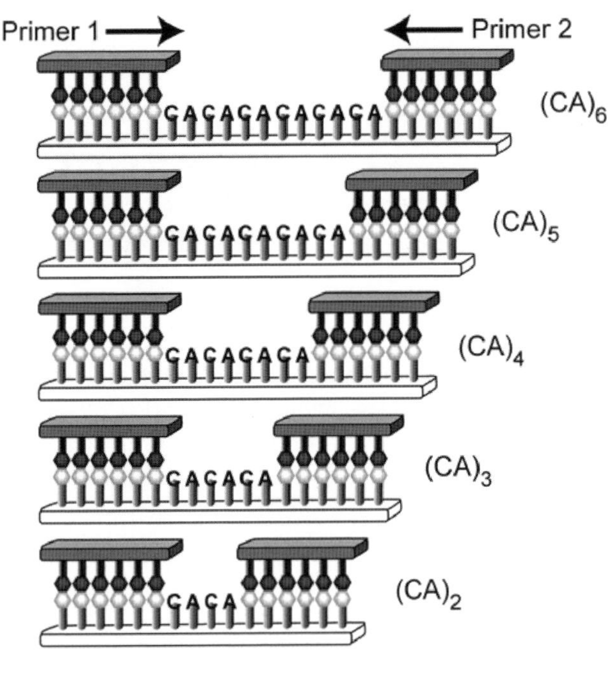

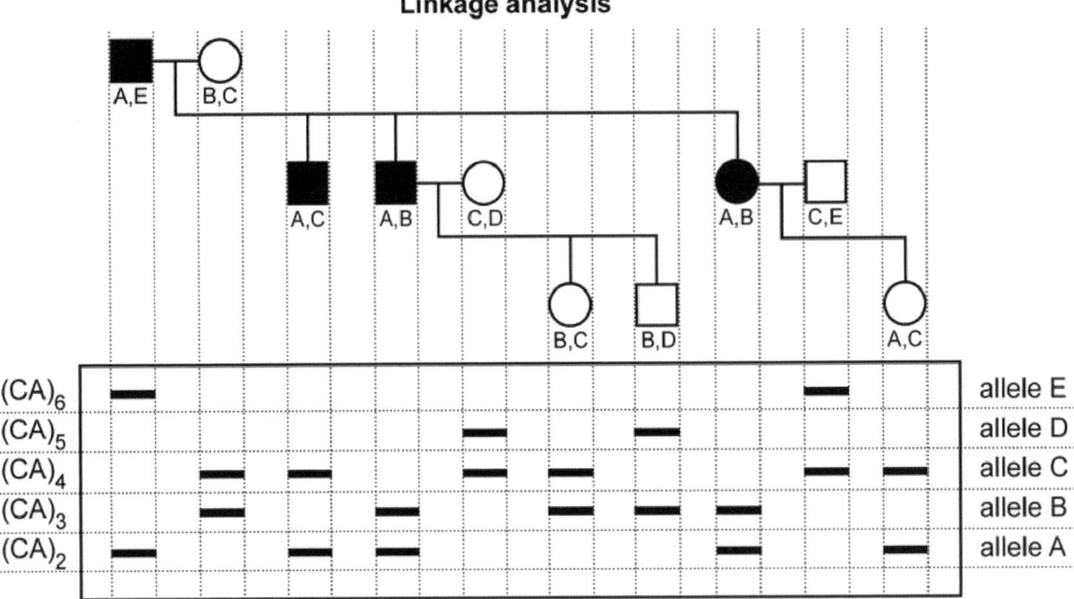

Fig. 2.6 Schematic of the approach to associating polymorphisms with disease. At the top, the DNA of patients is amplified with the polymerase chain reaction to produce enough material to allow the investigator to perform electrophoresis. Electrophoresis allows the investigator to determine which allele a given person in a pedigree possesses, because the number of CA repeats affects the position of the DNA on the electrophoretic gel. Thus any given person can be identified genetically (e.g., a person may have alleles A and B or A and C). Without knowledge of the genetic information, clinicians have independently categorized the patient as having diabetic retinopathy or not. Having diabetic retinopathy is indicated by having the person's symbol filled in the pedigree. In the illustration, an allele A appears to be inherited with the disease because every affected person in the pedigree possesses an allele A and none of the unaffected persons possess it. However, formal analyses need to be performed which take into account other issues such as type of genetic model (parametric, such as autosomal dominant) used or not (non-parametric or model independent) and frequency of all alleles of the marker compared to controls. Adapted with permission from Damji et al.[1]

more that a gene is not linked to the presence of the disease and is taken by convention as evidence that a marker is not linked to the disease. A LOD score between –2.0 and +3.0 is taken as inconclusive.[27]

The LOD Score in Greater Detail

If two genetic markers are unlinked, as for example, would be the case if they were on different chromosomes, then the probability that they will appear in any given gamete from an individual is 0.5. This ceiling fraction arises from the consideration that during meiosis, the probability that the maternal and paternal chromosomes will assort together in the gamete is 1 in 2 (the two possibilities are that they assort together or they do not assort together, and each has equal probability). If the markers lie on the same chromosome, the mechanism that can lead to their separation is recombination caused by crossing over during meiosis. The probability of recombination of two genetic markers increases the farther apart on the chromosome that they are. At a maximum, if the markers are at the extreme opposite ends of the same chromosome, then crossing over could lead to these markers being separated every time meiosis occurred and their being assorted independently into gametes as though they had been on separate chromosomes. Thus the maximum recombination fraction is 0.5. The actual recombination fraction is denoted by the symbol θ, and it will be less than 0.5. The likelihood of recombination fractions of θ and 0.5 are calculated, and a LOD score is defined as $\log_{10}$ (likelihood of observed data if loci are linked at a value of θ/likelihood of observed data if loci are linked at a value of 0.5).

Once linkage of a genetic marker to diabetic retinopathy has been established, candidate genes of interest may be identified using expressed sequence tags. An expressed sequence tag is a short sequence of DNA that is complementary to an expressed mRNA molecule found in the tissue of interest. The expressed mRNA molecule is used to synthesize a complementary DNA molecule of which a fragment is called an expressed sequence tag. Expressed sequence tags are useful in discovering genes and in sequencing genes.[28]

2.4 Studies of the Genetics of Diabetic Retinopathy

2.4.1 *Clinical Studies*

The number of studies exploring possible genetic susceptibility to or protection from diabetic retinopathy is large, and this chapter makes no claim to providing exhaustive coverage of a topic that would require a book unto itself. Rather, our goal is to expose the clinician to an important and expanding field of inquiry in diabetic retinopathy likely to be the source for future breakthroughs in treatment by virtue of illuminating the underlying basic defects. The interested reader is invited to consult comprehensive reviews to explore the topic in greater detail.[6,9]

Heritability for diabetic retinopathy has been reported to be 27% and heritability for PDR has been reported to be 25–52%.[29,30] Among South Asian Indians, the risk of DR is higher in diabetic siblings of probands with DR than in diabetic non-siblings.[4] Some of the differences in epidemiologic aspects of diabetic retinopathy may have a genetic basis, although further study is needed to determine the answer. For example, it has been reported that Hispanic diabetics develop severe DR earlier in their course and progress more rapidly compared with blacks or whites (see Chapter 3).[3] In a twin study, concordance of retinopathy was found in 35 of 37 identical twins concordant for type 2 DM but in only 21 of 31 identical twins concordant for type 1 DM, suggesting a stronger genetic effect in type 2 than in type 1 DM.[5] In the Diabetes Control and Complications Study, there was an increased risk of severe retinopathy among relatives of retinopathy-positive versus retinopathy-negative subjects (odds ratio 3.1, 95% CI 1.2–7.8), suggesting a possible genetic component to retinopathy severity.[31]

In a Mexican-American cohort, more severe diabetic retinopathy in siblings was associated with more severe retinopathy in probands (OR 1.72, 95% CI 1.03–2.88) after accounting for the effects of glycemic control and diabetic duration, but occurrence of diabetic retinopathy showed no such familial aggregation.[32]

2.4.2 Molecular Genetic Studies

Some of the more important candidate genes and associated polymorphisms linked to diabetic retinopathy will be reviewed below. Tables 2.1, 2.2, 2.3, 2.4, 2.5, and 2.6 list selected polymorphisms, genotypes, and haplotypes found to be risk factors, protective factors, or unassociated with different forms of DR. Inspection of the tables will show multiple inconsistencies across studies for such reasons as differences in case definitions, differences in duration of diabetes in the groups studied, in fractions of the two genders, in allele frequencies in the population samples, in methods of detecting DR grading severity of DR, in the recording and statistical handling of possibly confounding risk factors, and in the control groups used.[6,9] For example, the -634C/G polymorphism in the promoter region of the *VEGF gene* has been found to be associated with DR and also to be not associated with DR.[33–35] Many of the listed genetic associations with forms of diabetic retinopathy have not been replicated, and much work remains to be done in diverse human population samples to identify the strong associations from the weak ones and to exclude spurious associations caused by various weaknesses in study designs.[9] The tables we have included are rapidly changing and will be outdated within a short time as further genetic studies of greater statistical power and higher design quality are executed and published.

2.4.3 EPO Promoter

PDR has been found to have 80–90% concordance rate with end-stage renal disease (ESRD).[36] Several candidate gene single-nucleotide polymorphisms (SNPs) have been found and linkage analysis has suggested a diabetic nephropathy locus on chromosome 3q.[37–39] In addition, several researchers have found a locus at chromosome 7q21 associated with an increased risk of nephropathy in diabetes.[37,40–42] In this region of chromosome 7q21, Zhang and colleagues found that the T allele of an SNP rs1617640 in the promoter of the *EPO gene* was significantly associated with PDR and ESRD.[43] Of note, EPO encodes the protein erythropoietin, which is a potent angiogenic factor expressed in the kidney and retina. This protein has been found in human vitreous in PDR.[44]

2.4.4 Aldose Reductase Gene

Hyperglycemia is clearly linked to the microvascular complications of diabetes, and the conversion of glucose to sorbitol by aldose reductase (ALR2) has been shown to be involved in the pathogenesis (see Chapter 1). ALR2 is found in tissues of the eye including the vascular endothelial and retinal pigment epithelial cells.[45] Altered expression of the *ALR2 gene* may play a role in the pathogenesis of diabetic retinopathy. Genetic studies using restriction fragment length polymorphism (RFLP) analysis have inconsistently shown that aldose reductase is associated with diabetic retinopathy (Tables 2.1 and 2.6). Ko et al. have identified one allele (*Z*–2) of a $(CA)_n$ dinucleotide repeat polymorphic marker at the 5′ end of the *aldose reductase gene* in Chinese type 2 diabetic patients having a strong association with early onset of diabetic retinopathy. In Asian Indians as well, the *Z*–2 allele was found to be associated with any DR, PDR, and DME.[46] In Australian type 1 adolescent diabetics, the ALR promoter -106C allele is associated with DR, as is the *Z*–2 allele.[47]

2.4.5 VEGF Gene

Vascular endothelial growth factor (VEGF) has been found to be the primary stimulus for new blood vessel growth and vascular hyperpermeability in diabetic retinopathy.[48,49] Many clinical studies have demonstrated that VEGF concentrations were markedly elevated in both the vitreous and aqueous fluid of

Table 2.1 Genetic markers associated with any diabetic retinopathy (i.e., risk markers)

Genetic marker	Polymorphism	Type DM, ethnicity, N	Odds ratio (95% CI), sample size	X^2	P	References
VEGF gene	−634CC*	2, Japanese, 268	3.20 (1.45, 7.05)		0.0046	Awata et al.[33]
Promoter region of aldose reductase gene	Genotype for $(CA)_n$ repeat:Z–2/X where X is any allele other than $Z+2$	1, British, 322		17.0	<0.0001	Demaine et al.[75]
Promoter region of aldose reductase gene	Z–2 allele for $(CA)_n$ repeat	2, Asian Indian, 214	2.023 (1.06, 3.85)**		0.029	Kumaramanickavel et al.[46]
Promoter region of aldose reductase gene	Z–4 allele for $(CA)_n$ repeat	T2, Chinese, 384	2.44 (1.20, 4.98)**		<0.05	Lee et al.[76]
Promoter region of aldose reductase gene	Z–2 allele	1, Australian, 164	5.49 (3.39, 8.90)**		<0.0005	Kao et al.[47]
Promoter region of aldose reductase gene	−106CC genotype	1, Australian, 164	2.47 (1.30, 4.67)		0.005	Kao et al.[47]
$(CA)_n$ IGF-1 gene promoter polymorphism	Heterozygosity for the 192 or 194 base pair alleles	2, Dutch, 1,146	1.8 (1.0, 3.2)		0.04	Rietveld et al.[55]
SDH	G-888C	2, Polish, 154	1.73 (1.06, 2.83) for NPDR		<0.05	Szaflik et al.[77]
Mitochondrial DNA haplogroups	Haplogroup T	T2, Austrian,149	3.60 (1.02, 12.68)		0.046#	Kofler et al.[78]
Endothelial nitric oxide synthase gene	Intron 4b/b genotype	T2, West African, 384	2.4 (1.39, 4.09)		0.0013	Chen et al.[66]
eNOS promoter	Haplotypes 112 (Glu298/4b/-786C) and 222 (Asp298/4a/-786C)	2, Tunisian, 383	112 (1.34 [1.03, 1.73]) and 222 (2.55 [1.01, 6.44])		112 ($P=0.027$) and 222 ($P=0.048$)	Ezzidi et al.[79]
Inducible nitric oxide synthase	Pentanucleotide STR upstream of transcription start site (allele 210 bp)	T2, Asian Indian, 199	2.03 (0.96, 4.35)		0.044	Kumaramanickavel et al.[80]
Receptor for AGE gene promoter region	-429C allele	2, Caucasian, 215	2.33 (1.30, 4.16)**		0.012	Hudson et al.[81]
Manganese superoxide dismutase gene	VV genotype of theV16A polymorphism	2, Slovenian, 426	2.1 (1.2, 3.4)		0.006	Petrovic et al.[82]
Methylene tetrahydrofolate reductase gene	C677T polymorphism	2, Japanese, 131 with HbA1c≥6.5%	5.33 (1.50,19.0) for NPDR		<0.05	Maeda et al.[74]

*At position 634 relative to the transcription start of the VEGF gene, C is present on both alleles.
#When subjected to a Bonferroni correction, the statistical significance vanished.
**Not given in paper; calculated by DJB from data in the paper.

Table 2.2 Genetic markers associated with diabetic macular edema (i.e., risk markers)

Genetic marker	Polymorphism	Type DM, ethnicity, *N*	Odds ratio (95% CI), sample size	X^2	*P*	References
VEGF gene	C-634G*	2, Japanese, 378	1.81 (1.01, 3.26)		0.047	Awata et al.[83]
Endothelial nitric oxide synthase gene	Intron 4a allele	2, Japanese, 226		NG	0.006	Awata et al.[84]
Endothelial nitric oxide synthase gene	T-786C polymorphism (-786C allele)	2, Japanese, 226		NG	0.029	Awata et al.[84]

*At position 634 relative to the transcription start of the VEGF gene, G is present on one allele and C is present on the other. NG = not given.

Table 2.3 Genetic markers associated with severe nonproliferative or proliferative diabetic retinopathy (i.e., risk markers)

Genetic marker	Polymorphism/genotype/haplotype	Type DM, ethnicity, *N*	Odds ratio (95% CI) or Chi-square statistics	*P*	References
VEGF gene	c.-160CC* genotype	1 and 2, British, 106	10.5 (2.3, 47.7)	0.0003	Churchill et al.[85]
VEGF gene	c.-152AA genotype	1 and 2, British, 106	3.5 (1.5, 7.7)	0.0022	Churchill et al.[85]
VEGF gene	c.-116AA genotype	1 and 2, British, 106	7.9 (3.1, 19.9)	<0.0001	Churchill et al.[85]
VEGF gene	c.-406C allele	1 and 2, British,267	2.5 (1.20, 5.23)	0.027	Ray et al.[51]
VEGF gene	-160C/-152A/-116A haplotype	1 and 2, British, 106	3.34 (1.89, 5.91)	0.0001695	Churchill et al.[85]
VEGF gene	-460C/-417T/-172C/-165C/-160C/-152A/-141A/-116A/+405C haplotype	1 and 2, British, 106	29.9 (3.91, 229)	1.62×10^{-5}	Churchill et al.[85]
VEGF gene	c.-634CC	2, Caucasian, 501	1.85 (1.2, 2.8)	0.04	Errera et al.[34**]
VEGF gene	Homozygosity for rs833070	1, Japanese, 175	1.67 (1.01, 2.54)	0.047	Nakanishi and Watanabe[86]
VEGF gene	Homozygosity for rs2146323	1, Japanese, 175	1.67 (1.01, 2.74)	0.047	Nakanishi and Watanabe[86]
Promoter region of VEGF gene	-2578 A/A genotype	2, Japanese, 469	7.7 (1.8, 30.9)	0.002	Nakamura et al.[52]
Promoter region of the erythropoietin gene	Homozygous for T allele of an SNP rs1617640	1 and 2, US Caucasian, 613	2.01 (1.23,3.29)	0.036	Tong et al.[43]
TNF beta gene	Allele 8 (111 base pair)	2, Asian Indian,207	NG	0.003	Kumaramanickavel et al.[93]
PPARG gene	-2819G allele	2, Italian, 112 females	2.30 (1.09–4.83)	0.02	Costa et al.[87]
ICAM-1 gene	EE genotype of K469E	2, Slovenian, 426	2.0; 95% confidence interval [CI] = 1.1–3.5	0.013	Petrovic et al.[82]
Basic fibroblast growth factor (bFGF) gene	-553T/A	2, Slovenian, 206	2.0, 95% confidence interval = 1.0–3.9	0.03	Petrovič et al.[88]
Solute carrier family 2, member 1	rs841846	1, African American, 437	LR	0.000160	Roy et al.[10]

Table 2.3 (continued)

Genetic marker	Polymorphism/genotype/ haplotype	Type DM, ethnicity, *N*	Odds ratio (95% CI) or Chi-square statistics	*P*	References
Major histo compatibility complex, class 1, B	rs2523608	1, African American, 437	LR	0.00599	Roy et al.[10]
Major histo compatibility complex, DQA1 locus	*0201/0302 genotype	1, Swedish, 56	$X^2 = 15$	0.01	Agardh et al.[56]
FMS-like tyrosine kinase 1	rs622227	1, African American, 437	LR	0.00735	Roy et al.[10]
Angiotensin convertin enzyme insertion/ deletion polymorphism	DD genotype	2, Tunisian, 230	3.516	0.001	Feghhi et al.[70]

*At position 160 relative to the transcription start of the VEGF gene, C is present on both alleles.
**Other studies in other populations have not confirmed this association.[33,89]
LR = logistic regression was used rather than odds ratios. NG = not given in the paper.

Table 2.4 Genetic markers associated with sight-threatening retinopathy (diabetic macular edema or proliferative diabetic retinopathy)

Genetic marker	Polymorphism	Type DM, ethnicity, *N*	Odds ratio (95% CI), sample size	*P*	References
AGER gene polymorphism	c.-374A	1, Scandinavian, 742; 2, Scandinavian, 2957	1.65 (1.11–2.45); 2957 DR, 206 NDC	0.01	Lindholm et al.[90]
Polymorphism for $(CA)_n$ repeat in promoter region of aldose reductase gene	*Z*–2 allele	2, Asian Indian, 214	NG	0.004	Kumaramanickavel et al.[46]

C = Caucasian; NDC = non-diabetic controls; NG = not given in the paper.

Table 2.5 Genetic markers associated with diabetes without retinopathy (i.e., protective markers)

Genetic marker	Polymorphism	Type DM, ethnicity, *N*	Odds ratio (95% CI), sample size	X^2	*P*	References
VEGF genotype	c.-160CT*	1 and 2, British, 106	8.63 (1.96, 37.95)		0.0008	Churchill et al.[85]
	c.-152AG	1 and 2, British, 106	1.87 (1.04, 3.35)		0.0353	Churchill et al.[85]
	c.-116AG	1 and 2, British, 106	4.8 (2.6, 8.8)		<0.0001	Churchill et al.[85]
VEGF gene haplotype associations	-160T/-152G/-116G	1 and 2, British, 106	12.5 (1.61, 100)		0.006181	Churchill et al.[85]
	-460C/-417T/-172C/-165C/-160C/-152A/-141A/-116G/+405G	1 and 2, British, 106	20 (2.86, 100)		0.000373	Churchill et al.[85]
Genotype for $(CA)_n$ repeat in promoter region of aldose reductase gene	*Z*+2/Y where Y is any allele other than *Z*–2	1, Caucasian, 229		30.1	<0.00001	Demaine et al.[75] (see also[91,92]

Table 2.5 (continued)

Genetic marker	Polymorphism	Type DM, ethnicity, *N*	Odds ratio (95% CI), sample size	X^2	*P*	References
EDN1 Lys198Asn polymorphism	EDN1 Asn/Asn	2, Chinese, 343	0.19 (0.07, 0.53), 216 DR, 127 DM controls		0.002	Li et al.[21]
Endothelial nitric oxide (eNOS) gene promoter	(haplotype 122 (Glu298/4a/-786C)]	2, Tunisian, 383	0.51 (0.30, 0.88)		*P*=0.015	Ezzidi et al.[79]
TNF-β gene	STR upstream of promoter region: allele 4 (103 base pair) with (GT)9 repeat	2, Asian Indians, 207	0.236 (0.087, 0.638)**		0.002	Kumaramanickavel et al.[93]
SUMO4 gene	M55V	1, Caucasian, 223	0.37, (0.32, 0.43)		0.004	Rudofsky et al. [94]
Plasminogen activator inhibitor 1 gene	5G/5G genotype	2, Pima Indians, 171		8.22	0.016	Nagi et al.[95]
Receptor for AGE gene	GS genotype for the Gly82Ser polymorphism in exon 3 (Ser 82 allele)	2, Asian Indians, 200	0.34 (0.136, 0.863)**		0.03	Kumaramanickavel et al.[64]

*At position 160 relative to the transcription start of the VEGF gene, C is present on one allele and T on the other allele.
**Not given in paper; calculated by DJB from data in the paper.

Table 2.6 Negative studies looking for associations with various forms of diabetic retinopathy

Genetic marker	Specific polymorphisms (P) and haplotypes (H)	Type DM, ethnicity, *N*	Type retinopathy	References
MMP-2 gene	-168G/T, -735 C/T, -790T/G, -1306C/T, and -1575G/A	2, Czech, 490	PDR	Beranek et al.[96]
MMP-9 gene	-1562C/T, R279Q	2, Czech, 490	PDR	Beranek et al.[96]
IL-6 gene promoter	-174G>C variant	1 and 2, German, 733	Any DR	Rudofsky et al. [97]
Promoter region of VEGF gene	-634C/G polymorphism	2, Japanese, 469	PDR	Nakamura et al.[52]
Promoter region of VEGF gene	-634C/G polymorphism	2, Asian Indian, 208	Any DR	Uthra et al.[35]
Promoter region of VEGF gene	-634C/G polymorphism	2, Slovenian, 555	PDR	Petrovic et al.[98]
Tumor necrosis factor gene	rs1800629, rs1041981, and rs2857713 polymorphisms	2, Chinese, 194	Any DR	Wang et al.[99]
Endothelial nitric oxide synthase gene	G894T polymorphism	2, West African, 384	Any DR	Chen et al.[66]
Endothelial nitric oxide synthase gene	Intron 4a/b polymorphism	2, Japanese, 215	Any DR	Neugebauer et al.[100]
Receptor for AGE gene	Gly82Ser polymorphism in exon 3 (Ser 82 allele)	2, Chinese, 156	Any DR	Liu and Xiang[63]
Receptor for AGE gene promoter region	-429T/C polymorphism	2, Caucasian, 215	Any DR	Hudson et al.[101]
Angiotensin II type 1 receptor gene	A1166C polymorphism	2, Chinese, 827	Any DR	Thomas et al.[102]
Angiotensin I-converting enzyme gene	287 base pair Alu-repetitive sequence in intron 16 insertion/deletion polymorphism	1 and 2, diverse, 2010	Any DR	Fujisawa et al.[68]
Hereditary hemochromatosis gene	C282Y polymorphism	2, Australian,1245	Any DR	Davis et al.[103]

patients with proliferative diabetic retinopathy compared with samples from patients without diabetes and with nonproliferative diabetic retinopathy.[50]

Polymorphisms in the VEGF regulatory regions seem to be significant. In British Caucasians with either type 1 or type 2 diabetes, the VEGF -460C allele increases the risk of proliferative diabetic retinopathy (Table 2.3).[51] In Japanese type 2 diabetics, the C-634G polymorphism in the 5′-untranslated region of the *VEGF gene* was associated with presence of any diabetic retinopathy, and subjects who were homozygous for the C-634C allele had higher fasting serum VEGF levels than those with other genotypes.[33] The association was not found when PDR rather than any DR was the phenotype examined.[52] In Brazilians of European descent, homozygosity for the C-634C allele increases the risk of PDR, but the same result was not found in British Caucasians.[34,51] For PDR in a Japanese population with type 2 diabetes, the -2578C/A polymorphism in the promoter region of the *VEGF gene* was informative. The A/A genotype was associated with higher risk for PDR.[52]

Besides determining genetic markers for increased or decreased risk of diabetic retinopathy, we would be interested to know how such genetic variations confer these properties. With respect to the *VEGF gene*, some information is known. VEGF has a number of isoforms. In the eye, the VEGF-165 isoform seems to be the most important one, which in turn is found in a and b subtypes. $VEGF_{165}a$ is pro-angiogenic, whereas $VEGF_{165}b$ is anti-angiogenic. $VEGF_{165}b$ is the predominant form in the healthy vitreous. Diabetes results in an increase in insulin-like growth factor which downregulates $VEGF_{165}b$ and thus changes the $VEGF_{165}a$/$VEGF_{165}b$ ratio. Studies have also looked at the vitreous levels of VEGF stratified by genotype.[52]

2.4.6 IGF-1

Insulin-like growth factor 1 (IGF-1) is a known regulator of VEGF expression, and Simo et al. found a significantly higher level of IGF-1 in the vitreous of patients with PDR.[53,54] Therefore polymorphisms in the *IGF-1 gene* have been investigated. In patients with impaired glucose tolerance (IGT) or type 2 diabetes, the presence of a variant *IGF-1 gene* polymorphism was associated with an increased risk of retinopathy. The odds ratio for the risk of retinopathy for variant carriers was 1.8 (95% CI 1.0–3.2, $P = 0.04$).[55]

2.5 Genes in or Near the HLA Locus

The HLA locus found on chromosome 6p21 has been studied for genetic linkage to proliferative retinopathy in both type 1 and type 2 diabetes.[6] HLA alleles DRB1*0301, DQA1*0501, and DQB1*0201 have been reported to be associated with severe retinopathy in patients with type 1 DM.[56] In African-American type 1 diabetics, HLA-B was associated with severe DR and progression of DR.[10] In a subgroup of the Wisconsin Epidemiologic Study of Diabetic Retinopathy, persons with HLA-DR4 who were negative for DR3 were more likely to have PDR than those negative for both antigens (odds ratio 5.43, 95% CI 1.04, 28.3).[57] In a Finnish study of adolescents with type 1 DM, HLA DR1 was associated with presence of any DR.[58] Other studies have not found influence of major histocompatibility complex genes on diabetic retinopathy.[6]

2.6 Receptor for Advanced Glycation End Products (RAGE) Genes

Advanced glycation end products of proteins (AGEs) are produced when proteins are chronically exposed to hyperglycemia and have been found in the plasma and tissues of diabetic patients.[59–61] The main effects caused by AGEs are thought to occur through the RAGE receptor including the development of diabetic retinopathy and other complications. The RAGE gene is located in the HLA region on chromosome 6.[62] Studies have been inconsistent on the association of polymorphisms close to this gene and DR. Numerous studies have found no association in Caucasian and Chinese populations.[9,63] Kumaramnickavel et al. found a negative association in an Asian-Indian population.[64] Hudson, using a different SNP, found a positive association in a Caucasian population.[65]

2.7 Endothelial NOS2 and NOS3 Genes

Nitric oxide (endothelial-derived relaxing factor, *S*-nitrosocysteine) regulates vascular tone and inhibits platelet aggregation and monocyte adhesion to endothelial cells. Its production is under control of the nitric oxide synthases coded by distinct endothelial nitric oxide synthase genes. The *NOS3 gene* is expressed constitutively in retinal vascular endothelium and governs normal dilator tone. The *NOS2A gene* is not normally transcribed, but exposure to certain cytokines can lead to its abnormal expression. Warpeha and colleagues found that NOS3 expression is decreased in hyperglycemia, and that a 14 repeat allele of a pentanucleotide polymorphism in the 5′ untranslated region of the *NOS2A gene* results in peak transcription of NOS2A under hyperglycemic conditions. This polymorphism is associated with absence of retinopathy in British Caucasians, thus appearing to be a protective allele. The 4b/b genotype of the 4a/b polymorphism for NOS3 has been associated with DR in West Africans. No association of the 4a or 4b alleles was found with DR in Japanese type 2 diabetics.[67]

2.8 Renin–Angiotensin System-Associated Genes

A meta-analysis of seven studies exploring a possible association of an insertion–deletion polymorphism of the angiotensin-converting enzyme gene found no association. Based on a pooled sample of 1008 subjects with retinopathy and 1002 without retinopathy, the summary odds ratio for the D allele was 0.91, 95% CI 0.73–1.13.[68] In a review by Uhlmann et al., 13 of 15 studies were negative for any association.[9] Counterexamples exist to the general theme of lack of an association. Three studies of Korean, Japanese, and Iranian type 2 diabetics showed an association of the D allele or genotype with any DR, advanced DR, and PDR, respectively.[24,69,70]

The *angiotensin II (type 1) receptor gene* is located on chromosome 3q2125. Genome-wide association scanning detected a tentative linkage for risk of DR with a site close (~20 cm) to this gene.[71]

2.9 Solute Carrier Family 2 (Facilitated Glucose Transporter), Member 1 Gene (SLC2A1)

GLUT1 is the main glucose transporter across endothelial cells in capillaries of the retina and is also found in retinal glial cells, ganglion cells, and photoreceptors.[10,72,73] Hyperglycemia is the strongest clinical risk factor for prevalence, incidence, and progression of DR, thus the *SLC2A1 gene* on chromosome 1 that codes for GLUT1 is a candidate for influencing DR.[10] In African-American type 1 diabetics, SLC2A1 was significantly associated with severe DR (i.e., severe NPDR or PDR) and with progression of retinopathy.[10] However, three other studies, two in Caucasian populations and one in an Asian population, have not found associations.[6]

2.10 Gene–Environment Interaction

Genetic studies are beginning to uncover examples of interaction of genetic and environmental effects on DR. For example, the -677TT genotype for the *methylenetetrahydrofolate reductase gene* polymorphism has been found to be associated with NPDR in patients with higher HbA1c but not in patients with lower HbA1c. Other examples are certain to follow.[74]

2.11 Potential Value of Identifying Genetic Associations with Diabetic Retinopathy

Screening for diabetic retinopathy is an inefficient but currently necessary endeavor. The early phases of PDR and DME may be asymptomatic, which requires that large numbers of asymptomatic people must be examined with dilated fundoscopy to detect those who possess treatable early forms of these complications. Genetic profiling offers the potential to narrow the group predisposed to these complications and preferentially assign screening resources in these people.[86] Likewise, there are likely to exist protective genetic haplotypes that allow health-care providers to lower vigilance in screening for retinopathy. Genetic profiling, therefore, has the potential to help in the allocation of scarce health-care resources. Of course genetic profiling must be safeguarded to prevent the misuse of the information, which could be employed nefariously to deny persons insurance protection.

2.12 Summary of Key Points

- An understanding of basic clinical genetics is essential for today's ophthalmologists as genetic polymorphisms affect risk for diabetic retinopathy.
- Clinical risk factors explain less than 30% of the variation in diabetic retinopathy prevalence and progression. This, together with familial clustering of diabetic retinopathy, indicates that a genetic component of susceptibility to DR exists. The heritable component is polygenic.
- Many genes have been found to be associated with the development of diabetic retinopathy including *EPO, VEGF, aldose reductase, RAGE, NOS, IGF-1*, and others.
- Certain genetic polymorphisms appear to be protective against the development of diabetic retinopathy such as in the *NOS2A gene.*
- Polymorphisms exist that predispose persons to subtypes of diabetic retinopathy and that affect severity of diabetic retinopathy.
- Knowledge of the effects of key polymorphisms will help us to understand how and why patients develop retinopathy and will guide the discovery of future treatments.

2.13 Future Directions

Genetic analysis of diseases such as diabetic retinopathy is complicated as many different genes and environmental factors affect the development of the disease. Genetic studies of patients with retinopathy can be facilitated when strict criteria are used to select a homogeneous population. When possible, a quantitative trait is preferred and any subjective component should be minimized in defining the cohorts. Recent studies have helped demonstrate which genes are associated with different manifestations of diabetic retinopathy.

The future care of patients with diabetic retinopathy is going to be changed by understanding the genetics that influence disease course. New genetic understanding will help elucidate the molecular pathogenesis of disease, which will define new targets of intervention. Moreover, discovery of genetic markers conferring risk for various types of diabetic retinopathy could allow improved screening of the patients that are most at risk. This would allow early detection of disease and limit vision loss. Conversely, knowledge of protective polymorphisms will allow clinicians to discriminate patients who do not need frequent screening allowing the conservation of resources.[96]

Glossary

Allele a form of a gene; a gene may have many forms

Allelic Heterogeneity different mutations of the same gene causing different diseases, for example, different mutations of the *PAX6 gene* cause aniridia, Peters anomaly, and autosomal dominant keratitis

Codon a three-base segment of DNA that codes for an amino acid

Complex Disease a disease that does not manifest mendelian inheritance

Exon a sequence of DNA that codes for a protein

Expressed Sequence Tag a short sequence of DNA complementary to an expressed RNA molecule

Expressivity variation in a disease pattern (phenotype) in patients with a particular genotype. For example, age at onset and severity would be characteristics in which expressivity is manifested

Gene a segment of DNA that codes for a protein

Genetic Map the order of genes and genetic markers, such as polymorphisms, on the chromosomes

Haplotype a combination of alleles at multiple loci on the same chromosome

Hardy–Weinberg Equilibrium a state in which the gene pool of a population is not changing from generation to generation

Heritability the proportion of phenotypic variation in a population attributable to genetic variation. Heritability estimates the relative contributions of genetic and environmental factors to phenotypic variation. It describes the population, not something about an individual. If the heritability of trait *P* is 0.7, it is incorrect to say the 70% of X comes from genetics and 30% comes from the environment. Rather, 70% of the variation of X comes from variation in genotypes in the population and 30% comes from variation in environmental factors in the population

Heterozygous the situation in which the members of a pair of alleles are different

Homozygous the situation in which both members of a pair of alleles are identical

Intergenic DNA untranscribed DNA of unknown function

Intron a sequence of DNA that does not code for a protein; it is excised from the initial RNA transcript

Linkage cosegregation of a gene or DNA marker with another gene or DNA marker close by

Linkage Disequilibrium nonrandom association of alleles at two or more loci; in general, the closer the two loci on a chromosome, the greater the linkage disequilibrium

Locus the position of a gene or genetic marker on the genetic map

Locus Heterogeneity several different mutations causing a similar phenotype, for example, many different genetic mutations cause retinitis pigmentosa

Meiosis sex cell division which produces daughter cells with half the number of chromosomes as the parent cell. The assortment of chromosomes from parent to daughter cells is random. During meiosis, recombination occurs

Mendelian an adjective that implies that only one gene is involved

Mutation a single-letter change to the DNA sequence. A single-letter change that causes the specified codon to change (i.e., under the mutation specifying the wrong amino acid) is called a missense mutation. One that causes a codon change that leads to a stop codon is called a nonsense mutation. One that causes a codon change that leads a stop codon to become a codon for an amino acid is called a sense mutation. Finally, one that causes a codon change but that does not change the specified amino acid (because there are multiple codons for each amino acid) is called a silent mutation.

Penetrance presence or absence of an effect of a gene. Penetrance is dichotomous. Expressivity is graded. Penetrance is defined as the ratio of the prevalence of the expressed trait to the prevalence of the underlying mutation. A high penetrance, i.e., close to 1, implies that nearly everyone who poses the mutation will express the trait.

Polymerase Chain Reaction (PCR) a technique for amplifying quantities of specific genetic material. Involves three steps repeated 30–40 times. The steps are denaturation of double-stranded DNA by heat, annealing of DNA primers to the DNA sequence of interest, and extension of each annealed primer by DNA polymerase producing a new complementary strand of DNA. One gets geometric expansion of the number of DNA fragments of interest and these can be stained and the products separated by size using polyacrylamide gel electrophoresis.

Polymorphism a variation in DNA sequence found in at least 1% of a given human population.

Odds Ratio a measure of the effect size of possessing one or two copies of an allele. For example, suppose possessing allele X is associated with a probability p of having diabetic retinopathy and possessing allele Y is associated with a probability q of having diabetic retinopathy. The odds of having retinopathy are $p/(1–p)$ and $q/(1–q)$ in the two cases, respectively, and the odds ratio is $p/(1–p)/[q/1–q)]$. An odds ratio greater than 1 implies that having diabetic retinopathy is more likely if one has an allele X than if one has an allele Y. An odds ratio less than 1 implies that having diabetic retinopathy is more likely if one has an allele Y than if one has an allele X.

Proband the first affected family member seeking medical attention for a genetic disorder

Promoter a site in a DNA molecule at which RNA polymerase and transcription factors bind to initiate transcription of mRNA

Short Tandem Repeat (STR) a string of repetitive base pair sequences that vary in length between persons

Single Nucleotide Polymorphism (SNP) a variation in the sequence of nucleotide bases comprising DNA; different authors use different nomenclatures for genetic sequences. Some define the sequences at the genetic level. In these cases the nomenclature appears as c.74C>G, where C and G refer to cytosine and guanine nucleotide bases at position 74 of the gene in question. Others define sequences at the level of the protein product of the gene. In these cases the nomenclature appears as p.Asn56Lys, where Asn and Lys refer to the amino acids asparagine and lysine.[104] On average, the DNA sequences at corresponding positions in any two chromosomes from any two people differ at approximately 1 in a 1,000 base pairs.[105]

Transcription Factor a protein that controls whether genes are transcribed or not. Transcription factors bind to regulatory regions in the genome and help control gene expression.

References

1. Damji KF, Allingham RR. Molecular genetics is revolutionizing our understanding of ophthalmic disease. *Am J Ophthalmol.* 1997;124:530–543.
2. Snieder H, Sawtell PA, Ross L, Walker J, Spector TD, Leslie RDG. HbA1c levels are genetically determined even in type 1 diabetes: evidence from healthy and diabetic twins. *Diabetes.* 2001;50:2858–2863.
3. Hallman DM, Huber JC, Gonzalez VH, Klein BE, Klein R, Hanis CL. Familial aggregation of severity of diabetic retinopathy in Mexican Americans from Starr County, Texas. *Diabetes Care.* 2005;28:1163–1168.
4. Rema M, Saravanan G, Deepa R, Mohan V. Familial clustering of diabetic retinopathy in South Indian type 2 diabetic patients. *Diabet Med.* 2002;19:910–916.
5. Leslie RD, Pyke DA. Diabetic retinopathy in identical twins. *Diabetes.* 1982;31:19–21.
6. Warpeha KM, Chakravarthy U. Molecular genetics of microvascular disease in diabetic retinopathy. *Eye.* 2003; 17:305–311.
7. Iyengar SK. The quest for genes causing complex traits in ocular medicine. Successes, interpretations, and challenges. *Arch Ophthalmol.* 2007;125:11–18.
8. Wolfe JA, Horton MB, McAteer MB, Szuter CF, Clayton T. Race, macular degeneration, and diabetic maculopathy. *Arch Ophthalmol.* 1993;111:1603–1604.
9. Uhlmann K, Kovacs P, Boettcher Y, Hammes HP, Paschke R. Genetics of diabetic retinopathy. *Exp Clin Endocrinol Diabetes.* 2006;114(6):275–294.
10. Roy MS, Hallman DM, Fu YP, Machado M, Hanis CL. Assessment of 193 candidate genes for retinopathy in African Americans with type 1 diabetes. *Arch Ophthalmol.* 2009;127:605–612.
11. Gallie BL. Unexploited potential of molecular technology to unravel the pathogenesis of ocular diseases. *Ophthalmology.* 1988;95:1485–1486.
12. Della NG. Molecular biology in ophthalmology. A review of principles and recent advances. *Arch Ophthalmol.* 1996;114:457–463.
13. Freeman WR, Wiley CA. In situ nucleic acid hybridization. *Surv Ophthalmol.* 1989;34:187–192.
14. Mullen LM, Small KW. Molecular genetic techniques and applications in ophthalmology. *Sem Ophthalmol.* 1995;10:268–278.
15. Human Genome Project. How many genes are in the human genome? http://www.ornl.gov/sci/techresources/Human_Genome/faq/genenumber.shtml . 2008. 12-21-2008.
16. Venter JC, Adams MD, Myers EW, et al. The sequence of the human genome. *Science.* 2001;291:1304–1351.
17. Conneally PM. A first step toward a molecular genetic analysis of amyotrophic lateral sclerosis. *NEJM.* 1991;324:1430–1432.
18. Klintworth GK. Advances in the molecular genetics of corneal dystrophies. *Am J Ophthalmol.* 1999;128: 747–754.
19. Musarella MA. Gene mapping of ocular diseases. *Surv Ophthalmol.* 1992;36:285–312.
20. Cunha-Vaz J. Characterization and relevance of different diabetic retinopathy phenotypes. *Dev Ophthalmol.* 2007;39:13–30.
21. Li H, Louey JWC, Choy KW, Liu DTL, Chan WM, Chan YM, et al. EDN1 Lys198Asn is associated with diabetic retinopathy in type 2 diabetes. *Mol Vis.* 2008;14: 1698–1704.
22. Wiwanitkit V. Angiotensin-converting enzyme gene polymorphism is correlated to diabetic retinopathy: a meta-analysis. *J Diabetes Complicat.* 2008;22:144–146.
23. Szaflik JP, Majsterek I, Kowalski M, Rusin P, Sobczuk A, Borucka AI, et al. Association between sorbitol dehydrogenase gene polymorphisms and type 2 diabetic retinopathy. *Exp Eye Res.* 2008;86: 647–652.
24. Matsumoto A, Iwashima Y, Abiko A, Morikawa A, Sekiguchi M, Eto M, et al. Detection of the association between a deletion polymorphism in the gene encoding angiotensin I-converting enzyme and advanced diabetic retinopathy. *Diabetes Res Clin Pract.* 2000;50:195–202.
25. Szaflik JP, Majsterek I, Kowalski M, Rusin P, Sobczuk A, Borucka AI, et al. Association between sorbitol dehydrogenase gene polymorphisms and type 2 diabetic retinopathy. *Exp Eye Res.* 2008;86:647–652.
26. Dragon EA. Polymerase chain reaction. *Sci Am.* 1998; 279:112.

27. Booth A, Churchill A, Anwar R, Menage M, Markham A. The genetics of primary open angle glaucoma. *Br J Ophthalmol.* 1997;81:409–414.
28. Wiggs JL. The human genome project and eye disease. Clinical implications. *Arch Ophthalmol.* 2001;119: 1710–1711.
29. Arar NH, Freedman BI, Adler SG, Iyengar SK, Chew EY, Davis MD, et al. Heritability of the severity of diabetic retinopathy: the FIND-Eye study. *Invest Ophthalmol Vis Sci.* 2008;49:3839–3845.
30. Hietala K, Forsblom C, Summanen P, Groop PH, on behalf of the FinnDiane Study Group. Heritability of proliferative diabetic retinopathy. *Diabetes.* 2008;57: 2176–2180.
31. Diabetes Control and Complications Trial Research Group. Clustering of long-term complications in families with diabetes in the diabetes control and complications trial. *Diabetes.* 1997;46:1829–1839.
32. Hallman DM, Huber JC Jr, Gonzalez VH, Klein BEK, Klein R, Hanis CL. Familial aggregation of severity of diabetic retinopathy in Mexican Americans from Starr County, Texas. *Diabetes Care.* 2005;28:1163–1168.
33. Awata T, Inoue K, Kurihara S, Ohkubo T, Watanabe M, Inukai K, et al. A common polymorphism in the 5'-untranslated region of the VEGF gene is associated with diabetic retinopathy in type 2 diabetes. *Diabetes.* 2002; 51:1635–1639.
34. Errera FIV, Canani LH, Silva ME, Yeh E, Takahashi W, Santos KG, et al. Functional vascular endothelial growth factor -634G>C SNP is associated with proliferative diabetic retinopathy: a case-control study in a Brazilian population of European ancestry. *Diabetes Care.* 2007;30:275–279.
35. Uthra S, Raman R, Mukesh BN, Rajkumar SA, Padmaja KR, Paul PG, et al. Association of VEGF gene polymorphisms with diabetic retinopathy in a south Indian cohort. *Ophthalmology.* 2008;29:11–15.
36. Parving HH, Mauer M, Ritz E. *The Kidney.* Philadelphia: Elsevier; 2004.
37. Iyengar SK, Abboud HE, et al. Genome-wide scans for diabetic nephropathy and albuminuria in multiethnic populations: the family investigation of nephropathy and diabetes (FIND). *Diabetes.* 2007;56:1577–1585.
38. Moczulski DK, Rogus JJ, Antonellas A, Warram JH, Krolewski AS. Major susceptibility locus for nephropathy in type 1 diabetes on chromosome 3q: results of novel discordant sib-pair analysis. *Diabetes.* 1998;47: 1164–1169.
39. Chistiakov DA, Savost'anov KV, Shestakova MV, Chugunova LA, Samkhalova MSh, Dedov II, et al. Confirmation of a susceptibility locus for diabetic nephropathy on chromosome 3q23-q24 by association study in Russian type 1 diabetic patients. *Diabetes Res Clin Pract.* 2004;66:79–86.
40. Kankova K, Stejskalova A, Pacal L, Tschoplova S, Hertlova M, Krusova D, et al. Genetic risk factors for diabetic nephropathy on chromosomes 6p and 7q identified by the set-association approach. *Diabetologia.* 2007;50: 990–999.
41. Placha G, Canani LH, Warram JH, Krolewski AS. Evidence for different susceptibility genes for proteinuria and ESRD in type2 diabetes. *Adv Chronic Kidney Dis.* 2005;12:155–169.
42. Imperatore G, Knowler WC, Nelson RG, Hanson RL. Genetics of diabetic nephropathy in the Pima Indians. *Curr Diabetes Rep.* 2001;1:275–281.
43. Tong Z, Yang Z, Patel S, Chen H, et al. Promoter polymorphism of the erythropoietin gene in severe diabetic eye and kidney complications. *PNAS.* 2008;105: 6998–7003.
44. Watanabe D, Suzuma K, Matsui S, et al. Erythropoietin as a retinal angiogenic factor in proliferative diabetic retinopathy. *N Engl J Med.* 2005;353:782–792.
45. Vinores SA, Van Niel E, Swerdloff JL, Campochiaro PA. Electron microscopic immunocytochemical demonstration of blood-retinal barrier breakdown in human diabetics and its association with aldose reductase in retinal vascular endothelium and retinal pigment epithelium. *Histochem J.* 1993;25:648–663.
46. Kumaramanickavel G, Sripriya S, Ramprasad VL, Upadyay NK, Paul PG, Sharma T. Z-2 aldose reductase allele and diabetic retinopathy in India. *Ophthalmic Genet.* 2003;24:41–48.
47. Kao YL, Donaghue K, Chan A, Knight J, Silink M. A novel polymorphism in the aldose reductase gene promoter region is strongly associated with diabetic retinopathy in adolescents with type 1 diabetes. *Diabetes.* 1999;48:1338–1340.
48. Aiello LP, Northrup JM, Keyt BA, Takagi H, Iwamoto MA. Hypoxic Regulation of Vascular Endothelial Growth Factor in Retinal Cells. *Arch Ophthalmol.* 1995;113:1538–1544.
49. Aiello LP, Bursell SE, Clermont A, Duh E, Ishii H, Takagi C, et al. Vascular endothelial growth factor-induced retinal permeability is mediated by protein kinase C in vivo and suppressed by an orally effective B-isoform-selective inhibitor. *Diabetes.* 1997;46:1473–1480.
50. Aiello LP, Avery RL, Arrigg PG, Keyt BA, Jampel HD, Shah ST, et al. Vascular endothelial growth factor in ocular fluid of patients with diabetic retinopathy and other retinal disorders. *N Engl J Med.* 1994;331:1480–1487.
51. Ray D, Mishra M, Ralph S, Read I, Davies R, Brenchley P. Association of the VEGF gene with proliferative diabetic retinopathy but not proteinuria in diabetes. *Diabetes.* 2004;53:861–864.
52. Nakamura S, Iwasaki N, Funatsu H, Kitano S, Iwamoto Y. Impact of variants in the VEGF gene on progression of proliferative diabetic retinopathy. *Graefes Arch Clin Exp Ophthalmol.* 2009;247:21–26.
53. Pouvlaki V, Joussen AM, Mitsiades N, Mitsiades CS, Iliaki EF, Adamis AP. Insulin-like growth factor-I plays a pathogenetic role in diabetic retinopathy. *Am J Pathol.* 2004;165:457–469.
54. Simo R, Hernandez C, Segura RM, Garcia-Arumi J, Sararois L, Burgos R, et al. Free insulin-like growth factor 1 in the vitreous fluid of diabetic patients with proliferative diabetic retinopathy: a case control study. *Clin Sci.* 2003;104:223–230.
55. Rietveld I, Ikram MK, Vingerling JR, Hofman A, Pols HAP, Lamberts SWJ, et al. An IGF-I gene polymorphism modifies the risk of diabetic retinopathy. *Diabetes.* 2006;55:2387–2391.

56. Agardh D, Gaur LK, Agardh E, Landin-Olsson M, Agardh CD, Lernmark A. HLA-DQB1*0201/0302 is associated with severe retinopathy in patients with severe IDDM. *Ophthalmologica*. 1996;39:1313–1317.
57. Cruickshanks KJ, Vadheim CM, Moss SE, Roth MP, Riley WJ, Maclaren NK, et al. Genetic marker associations with proliferative retinopathy in persons diagnosed with diabetes before 30 years of age. *Diabetes*. 1992;41: 879–885.
58. Falck AA, Knip JM, Ilonen JS, Laatikainen LT. Genetic markers in early diabetic retinopathy of adolescents with type 1 diabetes. *J Diabetes Complicat*. 1997;11:203–207.
59. Brownlee M, Cerami A, Vlassara H. Advanced glycosylation end products in tissue and the biochemical basis of diabetic complications. *N Engl J Med*. 1988;318: 1315–1320.
60. Brownlee M. Glycation and diabetic complications. *Diabetes*. 1994;43:836–841.
61. Brownlee M. The pathobiology of diabetic complications: a unifying mechanism. *Diabetes*. 2005;54: 1615–1625.
62. Hudson BI, Stickland MH, Futers TS, Grant PJ. Effects of novel polymorphisms in the RAGE gene on transcriptional regulation and their association with diabetic retinopathy. *Diabetes*. 2001;50:1505–1511.
63. Liu L, Xiang K. RAGE Gly82Ser polymorphism in diabetic microangiopathy. *Diabetes Care*. 1999;22:646.
64. Kumaramanickavel G, Ramprasad VL, Sripriya S, Upadyay NK, Paul PG, Sharma T. Association of Gly82Ser polymorphism in the RAGE gene with diabetic retinopathy in type II diabetic Asian Indian patients. *J Diabetes Complicat*. 2002;16:391–394.
65. Hudson BI, Stickland MH, Futers TS, Grant PJ. Effects of novel polymorphisms in the RAGE gene on transcriptional regulation and their association with diabetic retinopathy. *Diabetes*. 2001;50:1505–1511.
66. Chen Y, Huang H, Zhou J, et al. Polymorphism of the endothelial nitric oxide synthase gene is associated with diabetic retinopathy in a cohort of West Africans. *Mol Vis*. 2007;13:2142–2147.
67. Neugebauer S, Baba T, Watanabe T. Association of the nitric oxide synthase gene polymorphism with an increased risk for progression to diabetic nephropathy in type 2 diabetes. *Diabetes*. 2000;49:500–503.
68. Fujisawa T, Ikegami H, Kawaguchi Y, Hamada Y, Ueda H, Shintani M, et al. Meta-analysis of association of insertion/deletion polymorphism of angiotensin I-converting enzyme gene with diabetic retinopathy. *Diabetologia*. 1998;41:47–53.
69. Ha SK, Park HC, Park HS, Kang BS, Lee TH, Hwang HJ, et al. ACE gene polymorphism and progression of diabetic nephropathy in Korean type 2 diabetic patients: effect of ACE gene DD on the progression of diabetic nephropathy. *Am J Kidney Dis*. 2003;41:943–949.
70. Feghhi M, Nikzamir A, Esteghamati A, Farahi F, Nakhjavani M, Rashidi A. The relationship between angiotensin-converting enzyme insertion/deletion polymorphism and proliferative retinopathy in type 2 diabetes. *Diabetes Res Clin Pract*. 2008;81:e1–e4.
71. Imperatore G, Hanson RL, Pettitt DJ, Kobes S, Bennett PH, Knowler WC. Sib-pair linkage analysis for susceptibility genes for microvascular complications among Pima Indians with type 2 diabetes. Pima Diabetes Genes Group. *Diabetes*. 1998;47:821–830.
72. Fernandes R, Suzuki Ki, Kumagai AK. Inner blood-retinal barrier GLUT1 in long-term diabetic rats: an immunogold electron microscopic study. *Invest Ophthalmol Vis Sci*. 2003;44:3150–3154.
73. Kumagai AK, Glasgow BJ, Pardridge WM. GLUT1 glucose transporter expression in the diabetic and nondiabetic human eye. *Invest Ophthalmol Vis Sci*. 1994;35: 2887–2894.
74. Maeda M, Yamamoto I, Fukuda M, Motomura T, Nishida M, Nonen S, et al. MTHFR gene polymorphism is susceptible to diabetic retinopathy but not to diabetic nephropathy in Japanese type 2 diabetic patients. *J Diabetes Complicat*. 2008;22:119–125.
75. Demaine A, Cross D, Millward A. Polymorphisms of the Aldose reductase gene and susceptibility to retinopathy in type 1 diabetes mellitus. *Invest Ophthalmol Vis Sci*. 2000;41:4064–4068.
76. Lee SC, Wang Y, Ko GT, Critchley JA, Ng MC, Tong PC, et al. Association of retinopathy with a microsatellite at 5' end of the aldose reductase gene in Chinese patients with late onset type 2 diabetes. *Opthalmic Genet*. 2001; 22:63–67.
77. Szaflik JP, Majsterek I, Kowalski M, Rusin P, Sobczuk A, Borucka AI, et al. Association between sorbitol dehydrogenase gene polymorphisms and type 2 diabetic retinopathy. *Exp Eye Res*. 2008;86:647–652.
78. Kofler B, Mueller E, Eder W, Stanger O, Maier R, Weger M, et al. Mitochondrial DNA haplogroup T is associated with coronary artery disease and diabetic retinopathy: a case control study. *BMC Medical Genetics*. 2009;10:35.
79. Ezzidi I, Mtiraoui N, Mohamed MBH, Mahjoub T, Kacem M, Almawi WY. Endothelial nitric oxide synthase Glu298Asp, 4b/a, and T-786C polymorphisms in type 2 diabetic retinopathy. *Clin Endocrinol*. 2008;68: 542–546.
80. Kumaramanickavel G, Sripriya S, Vellanki RN, Upadyay NK, Bedrinath SS, Rajendran V, et al. Inducible nitric oxide synthase gene and diabetic retinopathy in Asian Indian patients. *Clin Genet*. 2002;61:344–348.
81. Hudson BI, Stickland MH, Futers TS, Grant PJ. Effects of novel polymorphisms in the RAGE gene on transcriptional regulation and their association with diabetic retinopathy. *Diabetes*. 2001;50:1505–1511.
82. Petrovic MG, Cilensek I, Petrovic D. Manganese superoxide dismutase gene polymorphism (V16A) is associated with diabetic retinopathy in Slovene (Caucasians) type 2 diabetes patients. *Dis Markers*. 2008;24: 59–64.
83. Awata T, Kurihara S, Takata N, Neda T, Iizuka H, Ohkubo T, et al. Functional VEGF C-634G polymorphism is associated with development of diabetic macular edema and correlated with macular retinal thickness in type 2 diabetes. *Biochem Biophys Res Commun*. 2005; 333:679–685.
84. Awata T, Neda T, Iizuka H, Kurihara S, Ohkubo T, Takata N, et al. Endothelial nitric oxide synthase gene is associated with diabetic macular edema in type 2 diabetes. *Diabetes Care*. 2004;27:2184–2190.

85. Churchill AJ, Carter JG, Ramsden C, Turner SJ, Yeung A, Brenchley PEC, et al. VEGF polymorphisms are associated with severity of diabetic retinopathy. *Invest Ophthalmol Vis Sci*. 2008;49:3611–3616.
86. Nakanishi K, Watanabe C. Single nucleotide polymorphisms of vascular endothelial growth factor gene intron 2 are markers for early progression of diabetic retinopathy in Japanese with type 1 diabetes. *Clin Chim Acta*. 2009;402:171–175.
87. Costa V, Casamassimi A, Esposito K, Villani A, Capone M, Iannella R, et al. Characterization of a novel polymorphism in PPARG regulatory region associated with type 2 diabetes and diabetic retinopathy in Italy. *J Biomed Biotechnol*. 2009; doi:10.1155/2009/126917.
88. Petrovic MG, Krkovic M, Osredkar J, Hawlina M, Petrovic D. Polymorphisms in the promoter region of the basic fibroblast growth factor gene and proliferative diabetic retinopathy in Caucasians with type 2 diabetes. *Clin Exp Ophthalmol*. 2008;36:168–172.
89. Petrovic MG, Korosec P, Kosnik M, Osredkar J, Hawlina M, Peterlin B, et al. Local and genetic determinants of vascular endothelial growth factor expression in advanced proliferative diabetic retinopathy. *Mol Vis*. 2008;14:1382–1387.
90. Lindholm E, Bakhtadze E, Cilio C, Agardh E, Groop L, Agardh CD. Association between LTA, TNF, and AGER polymorphisms and late diabetic complications. *PLoS ONE*. 2008;3:1–6.
91. Ko BC, Lam KS, Wat NM, Chung SS. An (A-C)n dinucleotide repeat polymorphic marker at the 5' end of the aldose reductase gene is associated with early-onset diabetic retinopathy in NIDDM patients. *Diabetes*. 1995; 44:727–732.
92. Ichikawa F, Yamada K, Ishiyama-Shigemoto S, Yuan X, Nonaka K. Association of an (A-C)n dinucleotide repeat polymorphic marker at the 5'-region of the aldose reductase gene with retinopathy but not with nephropathy or neuropathy in Japanese patients with type 2 diabetes mellitus. *Diabet Med*. 1999;16:744–748.
93. Kumaramanickavel G, Sripriya S, Vellanki RN, Upadyay NK, Badrinath SS, Arokiasamy T, et al. Tumor necrosis factor allelic polymorphism with diabetic retinopathy in India. *Diabetes Res Clin Pract*. 2001;54:89–94.
94. Rudofsky G Jr, Schlotterer A, Humpert PM, Tafel J, Morcos M, Nawroth PP, et al. M55V polymorphism in the SUMO4 gene is associated with reduced prevalence of diabetic retinopathy in patients with type 1 diabetes. *Exp Clin Endocrinol Diabetes*. 2008;116:14–17.
95. Nagi DK, McCormack LJ, Mohamed-Ali V, Yudkin JS, Knowler WC, Grant PJ. Diabetic retinopathy, promoter (4G/5G) polymorphism of PAI-1 gene, and PAI-1 activity in Pima Indians with type 2 diabetes. *Diabetes Care*. 1997;20:1304–1309.
96. Beranek M, Kolar P, Tschoplova S, Kankova K, Vasku A. Genetic variations and plasma levels of gelatinase A (matirx metalloproteinase-2) and gelatinase B (matrix metalloproteinase-9) in proliferative diabetic retinopathy. *Mol Vis*. 2008;14:1114–1121.
97. Rudofsky G Jr, Schlotterer A, Reismann P, Engel J, Grafe IA, Tafel J, et al. The -174G>C IL-6 gene promoter polymorphism and diabetic microvascular complications. *Horm Metab Res*. 2009;41:308–313.
98. Petrovic MG, Korosec P, Kosnik M, Osredkar J, Hawlina M, Peterlin B, et al. Local and genetic determinants of vascular endothelial growth factor expression in advanced proliferative diabetic retinopathy. *Mol Vis*. 2008;14:1382–1387.
99. Wang N, Huang K, Zou H, Shi Y, Zhu J, Tang W, et al. No association found between the promoter variants of TNF-alpha and diabetic retinopathy in Chinese patients with type 2 diabetes. *Curr Eye Res*. 2008; 33:377–383.
100. Neugebauer S, Baba T, Watanabe T. Association of the nitric oxide synthase gene polymorphism with an increased risk for progression to diabetic nephropathy in type 2 diabetes. *Diabetes*. 2000;49:500–503.
101. Hudson BI, Stickland MH, Futers TS, Grant PJ. Effects of novel polymorphisms in the RAGE gene on transcriptional regulation and their association with diabetic retinopathy. *Diabetes*. 2001;50:1505–1511.
102. Thomas GN, Critchley JAJH, Tomlinson B, Yeung VTF, Lam D, Cockram CS, et al. Renin-angiotensin system gene polymorphisms and retinopathy in chinese patients with type 2 diabetes. *Diabetes Care*. 2003;26: 1643–1644.
103. Davis TME, Beilby J, Davis WA, Olnyk JK, Jeffrey GP, Rossi E, et al. Prevalence, characteristics, and prognostic significance of the HFE gene mutations in type 2 diabetes. The Fremantle diabetes study. *Diabetes Care*. 2008;31:1795–1801.
104. den Dunnen JT, Antonarakis SE. Recommendations for the description of sequence variants. *Hum Mutat*. 2008;15:7–12.
105. Hartl DL, Jones EW. Gene linkage and genetic mapping. *Essential Genetics. A Genomics Perspective*. Sudbury: Jones and Bartlett; 2002:121–165.

Chapter 3
Epidemiology of Diabetic Retinopathy

Abdhish R. Bhavsar, Geoffrey G. Emerson, M. Vaughn Emerson, and David J. Browning

3.1 Introduction and Definitions

Epidemiology is the study of factors that determine the occurrence and distribution of disease in a population. In studying the epidemiology of diabetic retinopathy (DR), the literature is large and can be difficult for the clinician to mentally organize. To help in this regard, we note that reports generally display information in grids that are multidimensional. These dimensions can be categorized as follows:

- Outcome variables – indices of visual loss or improvement
- Prevalence and incidence rates
- Risk factors for outcome variables
- Types of diabetes
- Populations sampled
- Eras of sampling

In any single report, it is typical that only a slice of information through this multidimensional epidemiologic study space is reported. In this chapter, we will attempt to provide a broad view of the many dimensions of the topic. For a more detailed study of parts of the topic, the interested reader can pursue the cited references.

The outcome variables reported typically are presence of any DR, presence of proliferative diabetic retinopathy (PDR), presence of diabetic macular edema (DME), and measures of vision loss. There are many other outcome variables, and their meanings often differ slightly among studies, but the most common ones found in the literature are defined as follows:

Presence of Diabetic Retinopathy – the presence of a threshold level of fundus change indicating that the eye has diabetic retinopathy (DR). This threshold level varies among studies. Examples include the presence of a certain number of microaneurysms detected in a specified region of the fundus or the presence of any characteristic lesion of diabetic retinopathy.[1] The Eye Diseases Prevalence Research Group classified presence of DR as mild, moderate, or severe DR, diabetic macular edema, or any combination of these.[2]

Progression of Diabetic Retinopathy – there are a number of diabetic retinopathy severity scales, the best known being the Early Treatment Diabetic Retinopathy Study (ETDRS) classification system and its modifications. Progression means that the level of retinopathy severity has increased on such a scale by a threshold amount, often two steps (e.g., the Wisconsin Epidemiologic Study of Diabetic Retinopathy [WESDR]) or three steps (e.g., the Diabetes Control and Complications Trial [DCCT]).[3,4]

Progression to Proliferative Diabetic Retinopathy – this variable applies to an incidence study and refers to those participants without PDR at the baseline examination who had PDR at the follow-up examination.[5]

Presence of Diabetic Macular Edema or Clinically Significant Macular Edema – DME is the presence of macular thickening within a certain distance from the center of the macula, often

A.R. Bhavsar (✉)
Clinical Research, Retina Center, University of Minnesota, Posterior Segment Research, Phillips Eye Institute, Minneapolis, MN 55404, USA
e-mail: bhavs001@umn.edu

D.J. Browning (ed.), *Diabetic Retinopathy*, DOI 10.1007/978-0-387-85900-2_3,

two disk diameters, as determined by stereoscopic fundus photographs grading. Clinically significant macular edema (CSME) is thickening at or within 500 μm of the center of the macula, presence of lipid with adjacent thickening within 500 μm of the center of the macula, or presence of thickening of at least one disk area in extent, any part of which comes to within one disk diameter of the center of the macula.[6]

Requirement for Laser Photocoagulation – sight-threatening DR due to DME and PDR is treated with laser photocoagulation. This outcome variable therefore is a practical index of progression to a clinically important level of retinopathy. In the United Kingdom Prospective Diabetic Retinopathy Study (UKPDS), 78% of laser treatment was for DME and 22% was for PDR.[7]

Moderate Visual Loss – on the ETDRS visual acuity chart, a loss of visual acuity of three lines or 15 letters; a synonymous term is doubling of the visual angle.

Visual Impairment – best corrected visual acuity in the better seeing eye worse than 20/40.[8]

Moderate Visual Impairment – best corrected visual acuity in the better seeing eye worse than 20/40 but better than 20/200[9]; some studies use different cutpoints for the definition.[5]

Severe Visual Impairment – best corrected visual acuity in the better seeing eye of 20/200 or worse.[9]

Severe Visual Loss – on the ETDRS visual acuity chart, severe visual loss refers to visual acuity of ≤5/200 on two consecutive visits separated by 4 months or more.

Blindness – legal blindness, synonymously termed blindness, means that the visual acuity has dropped to the level of 20/200 or worse.[10] Some studies use a 20/400 threshold for the definition.[11]

Vision Threatening Retinopathy – presence of severe nonproliferative diabetic retinopathy (NPDR), PDR, or clinically significant macular edema (CSME).[1,2]

Epidemiologic studies report prevalence rates, incidence rates, or both. These are measures of frequency of disease at a single time or over time. The definitions of these terms are often confused.

Prevalence – the number of cases of the disease divided by the population at a specified time, expressed as a percentage.[12] A prevalence study is sometimes called a cross-sectional study.[13]

Incidence – the number of new cases that arise during a time divided by the population at risk but disease-free at the beginning of that time.[12]

Prevalence studies are easier to perform than incidence studies because data are collected once rather than twice. Although simpler to perform, they have the drawback that the temporal sequence of the associations cannot be determined.[14] Incidence studies can determine temporal relationships, but have the problem of nonparticipation in the follow-up examination which can potentially bias the data.[5] If the incidence study collects data at widely separated times, the problem of spontaneous onset and resolution of the condition can arise, leading to underestimation of annual incidence. For example, WESDR collected data at 4- and 10-year intervals and arrived at annual incidences of DME smaller than studies with annual data collection.[13]

Epidemiologic results for DR are often presented with reference to the type of diabetes mellitus. There are always two and sometimes three types. All studies distinguish types 1 and 2 diabetes mellitus. In WESDR, the type 1 group is called *younger onset* diabetes, referring to patients with disease onset at less than 30 years of age.[5] WESDR uses the term *older onset, not taking insulin* to refer to some of the patients with type 2 diabetes mellitus.[5] In the WESDR, a third group is defined as *older onset, taking insulin*; this is a mixed group containing patients with types 1 and 2 diabetes mellitus.[5] The unique WESDR nomenclature is important to keep in mind because of the large number of published WESDR reports.

Many variables have been explored in the search for risk and protective associations with aspects of diabetic retinopathy. The risk and protective factors may be different for prevalence rates and incidence rates.[13] For example, male sex was a risk factor for prevalence of CSME but not for incidence of CSME in WESDR.[15,16] The following demographic variables have been found to be informative – type of diabetes, requirement for insulin, duration of diabetes, age at baseline examination, ethnicity, and inconsistently gender. Systemic variables found to be important include the quality of glycemic control, quality of control of any concomitant arterial hypertension and dyslipidemia, effects of certain types of medications, certain genotypes, and era of therapy. There are a few ocular factors of importance, such as level of retinopathy at baseline and presence of modifying concomitant ocular conditions such as glaucoma or optic atrophy. In the present chapter, we will review the effects of demographic factors on the clinically important indices of diabetic retinopathy. The effect of systemic and ocular variables will be discussed in Chapter 4. Genetic variables important for risk and protection are reviewed in Chapter 2.

The last two dimensions considered in many epidemiologic studies characterize the different populations studied and the different eras for which studies have been done. These are important because populations across the world differ and management of diabetes and diabetic retinopathy changes over time. As an example of the former, an estimated 50% of Pima Indians have diabetes, compared to 6.2% of adult Chinese in Taiwan. As an example of the latter, the prevalence rates for diabetic retinopathy among US Whites in 1980–1982 reported in WESDR are higher than in more recent reports, probably reflecting tighter glycemic control over the past 25 years.

Quantifying Risk

The terms odds ratio, relative risk, and hazard ratio are frequently encountered in the epidemiologic literature and may be unclear to clinicians. We will review their definitions.

Odds Ratio – the ratio of the odds of an event occurring in one group to the odds of it occurring in a second group. In the context of this chapter, an example might be the ratio of the odds of a two-step progression of retinopathy in persons with body mass index < 25 to those with body mass index ≥ 25. The odds of an event occurring is the probability of the event occurring divided by the probability of the event not occurring. Thus, if p_1 and p_2 are the probabilities of an event occurring in groups 1 and 2, respectively, the odds are $p_1/(1-p_1)$ and $p_2/(1-p_2)$, respectively, and the odds ratio is $[p_1/(1-p_1)]/[p_2/(1-p_2)]$. When p_1 and p_2 are less than 0.2, the odds ratio is a good estimator of the relative risk.[17]

Relative Risk – if two groups 1 and 2 are defined, and 1 is considered the reference group, then one can define the absolute risks (probabilities) of an outcome for the groups, r_1 and r_2. The relative risk of 2 compared to 1 is r_2/r_1.[17] In the context of this chapter, for example, if the risk of losing three lines of vision over 3 years with untreated DME is 0.24 and the risk with focal/grid laser is 0.12, then the relative risk with focal/grid laser treatment is 0.5 (=0.12/0.24).

Hazard Ratio – in survival analysis, a measure of the effect of a variable on the risk of an event. A hazard ratio of 1 implies no effect of the variable. A hazard ratio of 2 implies that presence of the variable confers twice the risk of an event occurring compared to absence of the variable.[18]

Comparison of epidemiologic studies is difficult. Methodologies differ among studies, such as the criteria for diagnosing diabetes, the tests for ascertaining diabetic retinopathy, and the formats for reporting data.[8] Populations may differ in levels of interacting variables, such as blood pressure, glycosylated hemoglobin, and level of serum lipids. In general terms, many epidemiologic studies must be reviewed to look for a consistent pattern of concordance or discordance of risk and protective factors.[1] Moreover, epidemiologic studies are unable to determine causation. Rather, they reveal associations that may be explored in studies aimed at defining causation and effective treatment. Many associations in epidemiologic studies are univariate and vanish when multivariate analyses are carried out.[14]

That is, the predictive power of a variable in a univariate analysis examining prevalence of DR may be accounted for by some other variable. An example of this is the reported higher prevalence of diabetic retinopathy in blacks than in whites, a difference that in some studies vanishes when the effects of glycemic control and blood pressure between these ethnic groups are taken into account.[14]

3.2 Epidemiology of Diabetes Mellitus

Diabetes mellitus is classified into two types – 1 and 2. In type 1, pancreatic beta cells are destroyed through an autoimmune process leading to an absolute insulin deficiency. In type 2, the peripheral tissues exhibit insulin resistance, and a relative rather than absolute secretory defect of the beta cell is present.[19] Types 1 and 2 diabetes comprise variable fractions of diabetes mellitus depending on the country and region, perhaps reflecting a survivorship effect. In population-based studies in rural China and Barbados, type 1 diabetes comprised <1%.[20,21] In contrast, in the United States, type 1 diabetes comprised 11.9% of the participants in WESDR in 1980–1982.[22] Estimates for the prevalence of types 1 and 2 diabetes in persons over the age of 18 in the United States for 2004–2007 are 0.4 and 7.6% of the population, respectively.[23,24] Thus, currently in the United States, approximately 5 and 95% of patients have types 1 and 2 disease, respectively.

In the United States in 2008, it was estimated that 8% of the population, or 24 million persons, had diabetes mellitus. From 1980 to 2006 the number of persons with diabetes in the United States tripled.[24] Similar statistics apply worldwide.[25] The prevalence of diabetes increases with age (Fig. 3.1).[25,26] Continued growth in prevalence of diabetes mellitus in both developed and less developed countries is projected (Fig. 3.2 and Table 3.1).[27] In the United States, it is estimated that 30% of the cases of diabetes mellitus are undiagnosed, and analogous estimates as high as 76% are reported in other countries.[9,19,20,25]

An increasing prevalence of diabetes has been documented widely (example for India in Fig. 3.3) and is projected for all countries, but the increase is expected to be higher in developing countries.[19] The increase in prevalence is associated with changes in diet, exercise, lifestyle, and increased life expectancy.[19,30] Incidence data on diabetes mellitus worldwide are scarce relative to prevalence data.

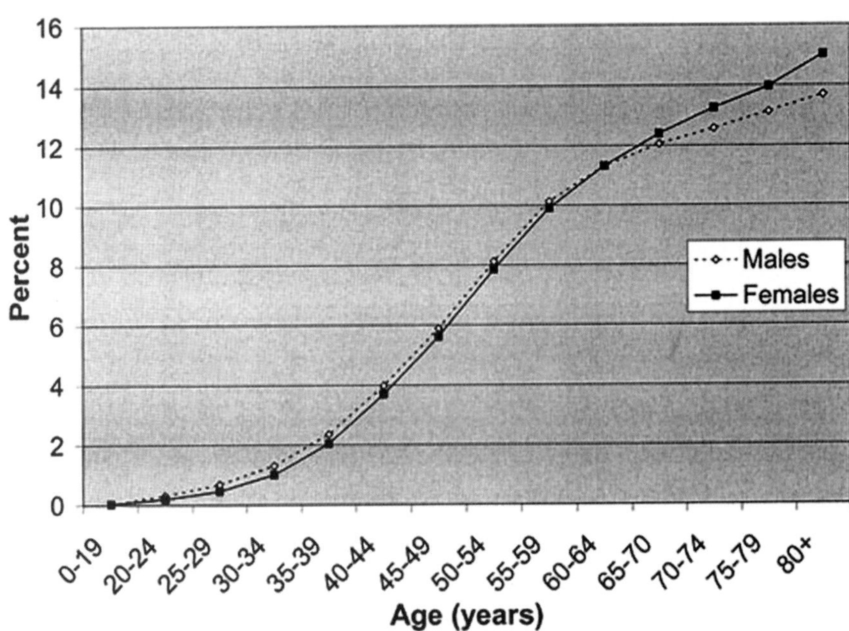

Fig. 3.1 Global gender-specific prevalence of diabetes by age. The *y*-axis is percent of the population having diabetes mellitus. The *x*-axis depicts intervals of age. Reprinted with permission from Wild et al.[27]

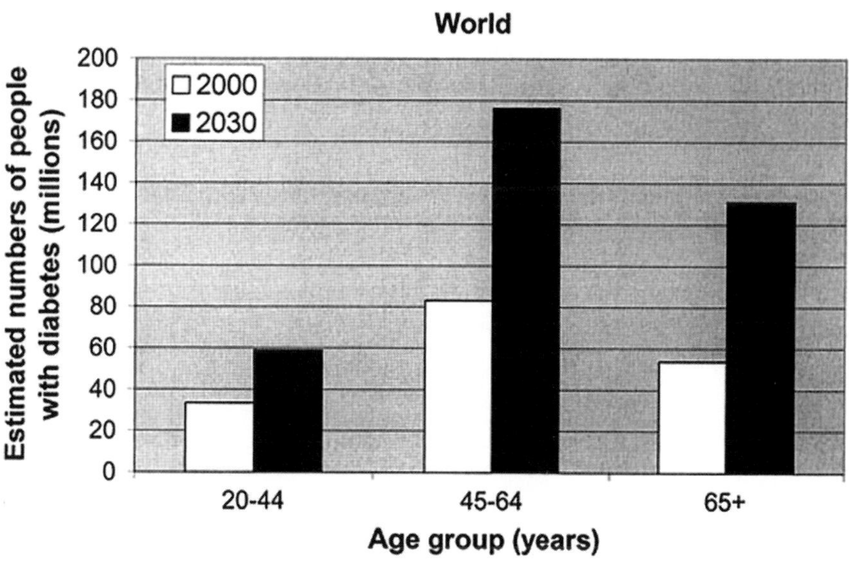

Fig. 3.2 Global estimates of number of persons with diabetes mellitus in 2000 compared with projected numbers for the year 2030 in three age groups. Reprinted with permission from Wild et al.[27]

Table 3.1 Estimated numbers of people with diabetes mellitus in selected countries in 2000 and projections for 2030

	2000		2030	
Ranking	Country	People with diabetes (millions)	Country	People with diabetes (millions)
1	India	31.7	India	79.4
2	China	20.8	China	42.3
3	US	17.7	US	30.3
4	Indonesia	8.4	Indonesia	21.3
5	Japan	6.8	Pakistan	13.9
6	Pakistan	5.2	Brazil	11.3
7	Russian Federation	4.6	Bangladesh	11.1
8	Brazil	4.6	Japan	8.9
9	Italy	4.3	Philippines	7.8
10	Bangladesh	3.2	Egypt	6.7

Reprinted with permission from Wild et al.[27] List of countries with the highest numbers of estimated cases of diabetes for the years 2000 and 2030.

3.3 Factors Influencing the Prevalence of Diabetes Mellitus

Age strongly influences the prevalence of diabetes (Fig. 3.1).[31,34,26] In most studies prevalence increases with age in both genders.[14,21,28,34,37] Not all studies have supported this consensus.[21] The third National Health and Nutrition Examination Study (NHANES III) in the United States showed a peak prevalence for diabetes of 13.2% in those ≥75 years.[28] As a consequence, the prevalence of diabetes is high in residents of nursing and retirement homes.[37,38]

Ethnicity may influence the prevalence of diabetes, although the effects of confounding variables are difficult to unravel. In Indonesia, the prevalence rate of diabetes is lowest (1.7%).[30] In European and in the US white populations, prevalence rates are 2–10%, whereas in Arab, Israeli, Indian, black, and Hispanic American populations, the rates are 14–20%.[21,30] Among Pacific Islanders of Nauru and among Pima Indians in the United States, the prevalence rate is 50%.[30,37] In the United Kingdom, Asian men were shown to have a prevalence four times than that of white men and Asian women were shown to have a prevalence two times than that of white women.[39] In the United States, the NHANES III study demonstrated that non-Hispanic blacks had a 1.6 times higher prevalence of diabetes than non-Hispanic whites and Hispanic Americans had a

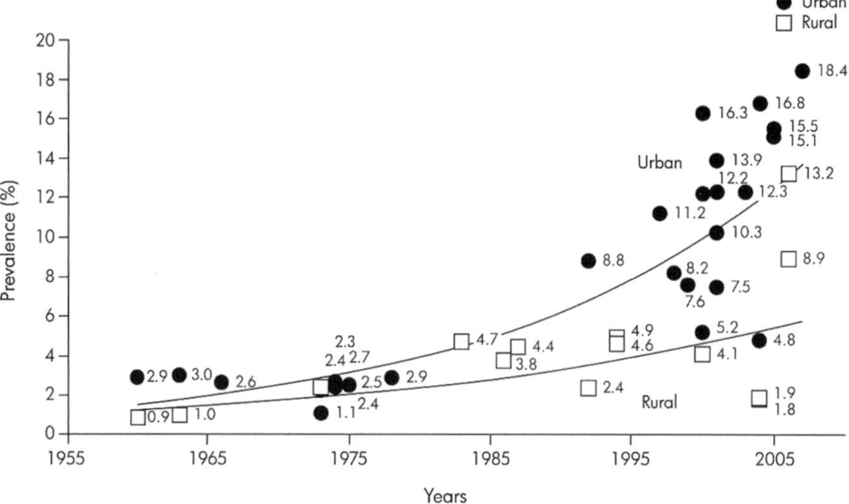

Fig. 3.3 The prevalence of diabetes in India is increasing with time and is increasing more rapidly in urban than in rural areas. A rural–urban gradient in prevalence of diabetes is a consistent finding over time. Reprinted with permission from Gupta and Kumar[30]

1.9 times higher prevalence.[28] The diversity in prevalence rates has been attributed in part to gene–environment interaction. Populations that have been relatively protected from periodic famines (e.g., white Europeans) for 15–20 generations have been hypothesized to have adapted to high-caloric diets and to have low insulin resistance, whereas populations exposed until more recently to regular periodic famines (e.g., Pacific Islanders, Native Americans, Australian Aboriginal peoples, natives of middle eastern desert regions) have retained high insulin resistance and develop DM when exposed to obesogenic environments (Table 3.2).[30,40]

Socioeconomic status has an inconsistent relationship with prevalence of diabetes mellitus. Lower status has been associated with higher diabetes prevalence in some studies and higher status has been associated with higher diabetes prevalence in others.[26,37] The inconsistency does not appear to be haphazard, however. Across the world, as socioeconomic status increases, so does body mass index (BMI), up to approximately 10,000–15,000 international dollars per person gross domestic product.[41] As income rises further, BMI falls. In South Asia, most persons are on the rising limb of this relationship such that rising status correlates with rising obesity and more prevalent diabetes.[30] In contrast, in developed countries most people are on the descending limb of income–BMI relationship such that increasing poverty is associated with obesity and secondarily an increased prevalence of diabetes.

A sedentary lifestyle is associated with a higher prevalence of diabetes. Lifestyle changes that occur when groups move from rural to urban environments has been shown to increase prevalence rates in Native Americans, Australian Aborigines, Polynesian Pacific Islanders, South Asian Indians, and East Indians (Fig. 3.3).[30,37] Urban–rural gradients

Table 3.2 Prevalences of diabetes mellitus by population

Population	Prevalence (%)	Age range (years)	References
Hispanic USA	9.3; 22.9	≥20; ≥40	Harris et al.,[28] Varma et al.[8]
Non-Hispanic white USA	4.8	≥20	Harris et al.[28]
Non-Hispanic black USA	8.2	≥20	Harris et al.[28]
Spain	5–6.8	NG	Mundet et al.[29]
Barbados black	19.4	40–84	Leske et al.[21]
South Asian Indian	10.3*; 28.2	≥20; ≥40	Gupta and Kumar,[30] Raman et al.[31]
Singapore Malay	23.1	40–80	Wong et al.[1]
Australia	7; 9.9	≥49	Cugati et al.[25], Mitchell et al.[32]
Taiwan	4.9; 6.2	≥40;≥30	Chen et al.[33], Chou et al.[34]
China	3.2; 6.9; 12.9	≥20; ≥30; ≥40	Wang et al.,[35,20] Xie et al.[36]

*Median value of 21 epidemiologic studies. NG = not given.
Selected prevalences of diabetes mellitus in various populations.

of diabetes prevalence seem to be diminishing in south Asia over time.[30]

Obesity is an independent risk factor for diabetes, presumably through its effect of increasing insulin resistance of peripheral tissues.[37] In the NHANES III study, increasing obesity was associated with increasing prevalence of diabetes after adjusting for other variables.[42] Central obesity, in particular, is associated with DM. The associations of a high-fat diet and sedentary lifestyle with prevalence of diabetes probably occur through effects on BMI.[37,43]

3.4 Epidemiology of Diabetic Retinopathy

Diabetic retinopathy is the most common microvascular complication of diabetes mellitus and the leading cause of blindness in persons from age 20 to 74 in the United States with 12,000–24,000 new cases of blindness per year.[24,44] Data from WESDR indicate that 1.07 and 1.3% of persons with diabetes develop, respectively, PDR and DME annually, almost all in patients older than 20 years.[5] Based on the estimated US diabetic population over age 20 in 2008 of 14,456,000, an estimated 154,679 new cases of PDR and 187,928 new cases of DME will develop annually. Similar facts and estimates apply to other developed countries.[19] In the United States in the year 2000, the numbers of persons with DR and vision-threatening DR were 4.1 million and 0.9 million, respectively.[2] These numbers are expected to triple by the year 2050 and for those over age of 65 to quadruple.[2] The primary factors responsible include increasing numbers of diabetics, increasing longevity of diabetics, and disproportionate increases in growth rates of Hispanics, in whom prevalence of DR is higher than in non-Hispanic whites and blacks.[2]

The Wisconsin Epidemiologic Study of Diabetes

A disproportionate fraction of the epidemiologic literature of diabetic retinopathy stems from WESDR, thus some background on this study is warranted. Over a 1-year period from 1979 to 1980, diabetic patients were identified from 452 of the 457 primary care practices for diabetics in an 11-county area of Wisconsin.[45,46] After removing patients with incorrect diagnoses, patients who had died or moved, and patients confined to nursing homes, 9,283 patients were identified. Of these, 1,396 were <30 years old at diagnosis and 5,431 were ≥30 years old at diagnosis.[45,46] In the younger onset group, 1,210 were taking insulin and all were examined for the study. From the older onset group, a random sample of 1,370 patients spread over three subgroups stratified by diabetes duration were chosen for study. The older group was further categorized by insulin use or not. Many baseline variables including retinal photography variables were obtained and then the patients were followed over time. The older onset patients were studied over 10 years and the younger onset patients over 25 years. Over 200 reports arising from analyses of this data set have been published, and those results comprise a large portion of the information reviewed in this chapter.[47]

3.5 Diabetes and Visual Loss

Diabetes mellitus is associated with increased levels of all cause visual impairment after adjusting for the effects of age, sex, race, educational level, blood pressure, smoking, and body mass index.[9,48] The relative risk of blindness in persons with diabetes has been reported to be 5.2 times the risk of those without diabetes.[48] The prevalences of visual impairment in adults with and without diabetes vary from 3.8 to 13% and from 1.4 to 2%, respectively.[5,8,9] The prevalence rates of visual impairment by diabetes type from WESDR are shown in Table 3.3. The annual incidence of blindness was 3.3 per 100,000 population.[5]

Incidence rates of loss of vision were obtained in WESDR. Two categories of visual loss examined were doubling of the visual angle and blindness. There were relatively few events for the blindness

Table 3.3 Prevalence of different levels of visual impairment in diabetes mellitus by the visual acuity in the better seeing eye

Group (*N*)	>20/40 (%)	20/40–20/160 (%)	≤20/200 (%)*
Younger onset (996)	91.7	4.7	3.6
Older onset, taking insulin (674)	81.6	15.7	2.7
Older onset, not taking insulin (696)	87.5	10.0	0.3

*Includes patients in whom visual acuity could not be measured.
Adapted with permission from Klein et al.[49] The percentages refer to the number of diabetics of each type (*N*) shown in the *left* column. Younger onset = almost all type 1 diabetes. Older onset, taking insulin = a mixture of patients with type 1 and type 2 diabetes. Older onset, not taking insulin = type 2 diabetes.

outcome and many for the doubling of visual angle outcome, thus for statistical reasons associations between risk factors and outcomes were explored for doubling of the visual angle and not for blindness. The most important results are presented in Tables 3.4 and 3.5. The incidence rates for vision loss are higher for the older onset groups than for the younger onset group. The risk factor analysis is complicated as Table 3.5 illustrates. The most salient point is that increasing age is a risk factor for visual loss in all types of diabetes. In a separate study of African Americans with type 1 diabetes, 6-year incidence rates for doubling of the visual angle and blindness were 13.5 and 0.6%, respectively; increased age was the only demographic risk factor for visual loss.[50]

WESDR provides information of a population that is predominantly white. In black type 1 diabetics, similar data have been reported. The 6-year incidences of doubling of visual angle and blindness were 9.8 and 0.6%, respectively.[50] The risk factors were similar as well, with older age at baseline the strongest demographic predictive variable.[50]

3.6 Prevalence and Incidence of Diabetic Retinopathy

Estimates of the prevalence of diabetic retinopathy need to be understood within the context that retinopathy indistinguishable from diabetic retinopathy occurs in a proportion of persons who have no diabetes mellitus under various definitions of the term. Associations with such fundus changes include hypertension, serum glucose levels within the normal range, BMI, and aging. Estimates of the proportions of persons with this status range from 0.6 to 9.8% depending on methods of retinopathy detection (higher with photographs than clinical examination).[21,51–53] Five- and ten-year incidences of retinopathy in persons without diabetes have been reported to be 6.0–10% and 6.5% in independent studies, respectively.[53–55]

Some studies do not distinguish DR by diabetes type. In a population-based study of this type in adults over the age of 49 from Australia, prevalence and 5-year incidence of any DR were reported to be 35.3 and 22.2%, respectively.[53] In this study, duration of DM was the only demographic baseline factor associated with risk for retinopathy progression.[53] In the Barbados Eye Study of blacks aged 40–84, the prevalence and 4-year incidence of any DR were 28.5 and 30.1%, respectively.[21,56] There were no important demographic risk factors associated with incidence of retinopathy.[56]

Table 3.4 Incidence of vision loss outcomes in WESDR

	Doubling of visual angle		Blindness	
Type of diabetes	10-year incidence, % (*N*)	14-year incidence, % (*N*)	10-year incidence, % (*N*)	14-year incidence, % (*N*)
Younger onset	9.2 (880)	14.2 (880)	1.8 (868)	2.4 (868)
Older onset, taking insulin	32.8 (472)		4.0 (465)	
Older onset, not taking insulin	21.4 (494)		4.8 (490)	

All data from Moss et al.[22,44] Data for visual impairment are similar to data for doubling of visual angle for each group. Too many patients in the older onset groups had died by the 14-year follow-up study, thus only data for the younger onset group were reported.

Table 3.5 Demographic risk factors for doubling of visual angle from diabetic retinopathy in WESDR

Association with doubling of visual angle	Younger onset	Older onset, taking insulin	Older onset, not taking insulin
Increasing age	X	X	X
Increasing duration of diabetes	X	X	
Women		X	X

All data from Moss et al.[22] Data for visual impairment are similar to data for doubling of visual angle for each group. Empty cells mean no association was found on univariate analysis. A *black* X means that an association was found on univariate analysis. A *red* X means that the association persisted in a multivariate analysis. The analyses at 10 and 14 years were similar in results, but in the few cases where they differed, the 14 year results are shown.

3.7 By Diabetes Type

At the time of diagnosis of diabetes, the prevalence of retinopathy is lower in type I than in type 2 diabetes. Prevalence rates of 0–3% and 6.7–38% have been reported at diagnosis in types 1 and 2 diabetes, respectively.[19,58] The same is true at other times after diagnosis of diabetes. When prevalence is recorded without regard for duration of diabetes, prevalence ranges from 38.3 to 82% and from 16.4 to 39% for types 1 and 2 diabetes, respectively.[23,32,45,46,58] In the WESDR scheme of diabetes categorization, prevalence rates of any retinopathy were 71, 70, and 39% for the younger onset, older onset taking insulin, and older onset not taking insulin groups, respectively.[45,46]After adjusting for duration of diabetes, the differences in prevalence rates were no longer statistically significant between types 1 and 2 DM.[8]

In WESDR, for the older onset diabetics, 10-year follow-up data were available, but not 25-year follow-up data, because too many of the patients had died over a 25-year period of follow-up. On the other hand, 25-year follow-up data were available for the younger onset diabetics. Data on 10-year incidence rates of any DR, two-step progression of DR, and two-step improvement of DR are shown in Table 3.6. The incidence rates are higher in the younger onset group for any DR and two-step progression and lower for two-step improvement. In the younger onset group, the prevalence and incidence of DR had decreased in those with more recently diagnosed diabetes, suggesting that change in diabetic management over the years is having a beneficial effect with respect to retinopathy.[59] Studies that use less sensitive methods of retinopathy detection (such as ophthalmoscopic examination) than seven-field fundus photography report lower 10-year incidence rates of any DR than WESDR. For example, a Spanish study reported 10-year incidence rates of any retinopathy in a mixed type diabetic population of 13.8%.[29]

The reported 25-year cumulative risk of DR in persons with type 1 diabetes ranges from 89.1 to 97% in different series.[11,59] In WESDR in persons with younger onset diabetes, the 25-year cumulative rate of two-step progression of DR was 83% (95% CI 80–86%). Multivariate analyses showed that male sex and greater body mass index (BMI) were associated with ≥two-step progression of DR severity.[59]

3.8 By Insulin Use

Among older onset diabetics, both prevalence and incidence of retinopathy depend on use of insulin or not. In WESDR at baseline, the prevalence of any DR at baseline was 70 and 39% in those patients taking and not taking insulin, respectively.[46] WESDR

Table 3.6 Ten-year incidence of any retinopathy, progression of retinopathy, and improvement of retinopathy

Study	10-year incidence of any retinopathy (%)	10-year two-step progression (%)	10-year two-step improvement (%)
Younger onset diabetes	89.3	75.8	9.8
Older onset, insulin using diabetes	79.2	68.7	21.1
Older onset, non-insulin using diabetes	66.9	52.9	26.0

Data from Klein et al.[10]

reported higher 4- and 10-year cumulative incidences of retinopathy in older diabetics taking insulin compared to older diabetics not taking insulin.[10]

Some studies do not classify patients as older onset or younger onset diabetes mellitus or type 1 or 2 DM, but do classify patients as insulin using and non-insulin using. The prevalence of DR is higher in patients using insulin with a 5.79 times higher risk of having retinopathy compared to patients not using insulin.[31,26] This association is considered to arise from the greater severity of diabetes and poorer glycemic control in those individuals taking insulin.[26,46]

3.9 By Age

The prevalence of DR generally increases with age, although nonlinearly, but in some populations decreases in late life, presumably because many patients with diabetes die early, the *survivor effect*.[8,26,20,25,31,46,58,60] However, among Barbados blacks and mixed race persons, prevalence of DR does not depend on age (Table 3.7). In younger onset diabetics, the 10-year incidences of any DR, improvement of retinopathy, and progression of retinopathy are roughly constant over the range of age at baseline examination from puberty to age 34 and shows a slight decline for age ≥35.[10] Among older onset diabetics, an inverse relationship exists between age and 10-year incidence of any DR and progression of DR in adults.[10] The 10-year incidences are 1.5–2.0 times greater in those aged 30–44 compared to those older than 75.[10] A direct relationship, however, is found between age and 10-year incidence of improvement of DR.[63] As with the prevalence relationships, the incidence relationships probably manifest the effects of selective survival. The oldest persons at risk of progression are less likely to survive to have their retinopathy progression detected.

3.10 By Duration of Diabetes Mellitus

Prevalence of retinopathy is associated with duration of diabetes mellitus.[25,14,20,26,36,60] Longer duration of diabetes has been associated with increased prevalence of DR and PDR (Tables 3.8 and 3.14).[8,20,31,46,60,33] The prevalence of DR in newly diagnosed diabetics ranges from 6 to 33.5%.[8,20,26] The proportion of persons with DR having more severe forms of retinopathy increases with increasing duration of diabetes.[20,26,31] The relationship of incidence of various aspects of diabetic retinopathy to duration is more complicated, as there are interactions with diabetes type. For younger onset diabetics, longer duration of diabetes is associated with an increasing 10-year incidence of any DR over durations up to 10 years.[10] Likewise, longer duration of diabetes is associated with increasing 10-year incidence of improvement in retinopathy severity.[10] However, the 10-year incidence of progression of retinopathy declined once duration of diabetes reached 20 years.[10] In the older onset diabetics taking insulin, longer duration of diabetes was associated with decreased risk of incidence of any DR and of progression of retinopathy and had no effect on incidence of improvement of retinopathy.[10] In older onset diabetics not taking insulin, duration of diabetes had no effect on incidence of any DR, improvement of DR, or incidence of progression of DR.[10]

Table 3.7 Relationship of prevalence of diabetic retinopathy and age

	Age (years)					
Population	<40	40–49	50–59	60–69	>70	References
South Asian		13.4	20.9	20.5	14.8	Raman et al.[26]
US Latinos		40.7	46.8	48.7	53	Varma et al.[8]
Chinese	29.4	40.0	45.6	48.7	42.1	Wang et al.[20]
Barbados blacks/mixed race		30.3	27.3	26.6	31.7	Leske et al.[21]
United Arab Emirates	15.8	26.8	30.1	27.3		Al-Maskari and El-Sadig[58]
US whites older, taking insulin	36.2	64.6		67.4	51.5	Klein et al.[46]
US whites older, not taking insulin	28.8	30.5		36.5	39.5	Klein et al.[46]

Selected studies providing prevalence rates for DR by age group. Not all studies divide age ranges the same way. When cutpoints for studies differ, the data are placed into the nearest category of this table.

Table 3.8 Prevalence of any diabetic retinopathy (%) by duration of diabetes (years) in selected studies

	Duration of diabetes mellitus				
Population	<5 years	6–10 years	11–15 years	>15 years	References
South Asian	15.5	30	37.3	40.4	Raman et al.[26]
Asian Indian	11.7	27.5	37.6	29.1	Rema et al.[60]
US Latino	27.5	56.1	59.8	79.6	Varma et al.[8]
African American	9.1	30.4		42.2	Varma et al.[8]
African Barbados	11.9	39.9		59.9	Varma et al.[8]
US whites (NHANES III)	12.6	15.6		32.8	Varma et al.[8]
US whites (San Antonio, TX)	29.6	NA		46.7	Varma et al.[8]
US whites, San Luis Valley, CO	34.1	55.1		88.2	Varma et al.[8]
US whites, Beaver Dam, WI	22.9	37.0		49.9	Varma et al.[8]
US mixed race, type 1		~40	~85	~95	Orchard et al.[61]
United Arab Emirates	6.7	16.5	52.2		Al-Maskari and El-Sadig[58]
US whites older, taking insulin	~48	~65	~72	~82	Klein et al.[46]
US whites older, not taking insulin	~25	~47	~52	~55	Klein et al.[46]
US whites younger	~27	~67	~90	~100	Klein et al.[45]

~ = The numbers are estimated from a published graph in the reference. NA = not available. The wide variation may reflect different ratios of types 1 and 2 diabetes, methods of detecting retinopathy, levels of glycemic control, blood pressure, levels of other systemic variables, and differences based on ethnicity. Some studies break the interval 6–15 years into 5-year subintervals as indicated in the table by separate cells for the subintervals.

3.11 By Ethnicity

There is evidence across different studies that the prevalence of diabetic retinopathy among persons with diabetes mellitus varies by ethnicity, although conclusions are tentative because study designs differ (Table 3.9).[26,60] In general terms, South Asian Indians and Singapore Malay populations have had lower reported prevalences than Caucasian populations.[60] Hispanic Caucasian populations have the highest reported prevalences.[8] Prevalence rates of DR at diagnosis of DM seem to vary by ethnicity as well. Reported rates are lower in South Asian Indians (5.1%) and higher in Hispanic whites (20–35%).[8,60]

Prevalence rates for Hispanic whites are inconsistent.[8] The San Luis Valley Diabetes Study showed a lower prevalence of diabetic retinopathy of 42% in Hispanics compared to 54% in non-Hispanic whites.[62] The NHANES III showed a higher prevalence of diabetic retinopathy in Mexican Americans of 33.4% compared to 18.2% in non-Hispanic whites.[63] Reports that Hispanic diabetics have more severe retinopathy than non-Hispanic whites after adjusting for duration of diabetes, age, glycemic control, and blood pressure are balanced by other studies showing no difference in severity by ethnic group after adjusting for tightness of control.[64,65]

Multiple, but not all, studies report that crude prevalence of DR is higher in blacks than in whites.[14,23,45,68,66] In the NHANES III, the prevalence of diabetic retinopathy was higher in non-Hispanic blacks (26.5%) compared with non-Hispanic whites (18.2%).[63] Likewise in the Barbados Eye Study and the ARIC study, the rates of retinopathy were higher in blacks than in whites.[14,21] In NHANES III and the ARIC study, the differences vanished after controlling for other variables suggesting that it is differences in glycemic or blood pressure control and not ethnicity that is responsible for the prevalence differences.[14] The differences did not go away after adjusting for confounders in the Veterans Affairs Diabetes Trial.[64]

It is uncertain whether ethnic differences reflect genetic predisposition to increased or decreased risk of retinopathy or are instead markers of some other important environmental factor. In a multiethnic population in San Francisco, there was no difference in retinopathy prevalence across ethnic groups suggesting that ethnic differences may be eliminated when social factors are eliminated.[70]

Table 3.9 Prevalence of diabetic retinopathy by ethnicity

Population	Type I (%)	Type II (%)	Mixed cohort (%)	References
USA Caucasian	0–84	7–55	37–61.1	Varma et al.,[8] Williams et al.,[19] Raman et al.[26]
USA biracial (blacks, whites)			20.5	Klein et al.[14]
UK Caucasian	33.6–36.7	21–52	16.5–41	Williams et al.,[19] Raman et al.[26]
Australian Caucasian	42	13–59.7	29.1–32.4	Williams et al.,[19] Raman et al.,[26] Mitchell et al.[32]
European Caucasian	16.6–76.5	32.6–61.8	26.2	Williams et al.[19]
Scandinavian Caucasian	10.8–68.3	18.8–65.9	13.8–75.1	Williams et al.[19]
African American	63.9	26.5–31.4	28.5	Williams et al.[19]
Hispanic American		33.4–46.9	48	Varma et al.,[8] Williams et al.[19]
Mexican			50.5	Villalpando et al.[67]
American Indian	19.7–20.9	19–49.3		Williams et al.[19]
West Indies			28.5	Leske et al.,[21] Raman et al.,[26] Leske et al.[56]
South Asian	13.6	6.7–34.1	18.0	Williams et al.,[19] Raman et al.,[31] Rema et al.[60]
Singapore			21.8	Raman et al.[26]
Singapore Malays			35	Williams et al.,[19] Wong et al.[1]
Mauritius			30	Raman et al.[26]
UK South Asian		11.6		Williams et al.[19]
Indian			12–30.1	Raman et al.,[26] Emanuele et al.[64]
Sri Lanka			15%	Raman et al.[26]
Pakistan			15.7%	Raman et al.[26]
Japanese		31.6–38	38	Williams et al.,[19] Raman et al.[26]
Chinese		19–43.1	28–45.2	Williams et al.,[19] Wang et al.,[20] Raman et al.,[26] Xie et al.[36]
African	26–43	30.5–43	12.7–42.4	Williams et al.[19]
South American		45–51.2		Williams et al.[19]
Taiwan		35.0		Chou et al.[34]
United Arab Emirates			19	Al-Maskari and El-Sadig[58]
Iran			36%*	Amini and Parvaresh[68]
North American Indigenous People			25%**	Naqshbandi et al.[69]

*Median prevalence of 11 studies.

**Median prevalence of five studies.

Adapted and expanded from Williams et al.[19] Wide ranges partially reflect variations in factors of importance among the studies such as criteria for diagnosis of diabetes (e.g., self-reported, oral glucose tolerance test, fasting blood glucose with various cutpoints, random blood glucose with various cutpoints, and hemoglobin A1C), duration of diabetes mellitus among studies (generally longer in developed countries), technical components such as number of photographic fields used for detection and staging of retinopathy, and genetic components inherent in ethnic variation.

3.12 Gender

The effect of gender is inconsistent among population-based studies. In one study in a population of Singapore Malays, women have been reported to have higher prevalence of diabetic retinopathy, diabetic macular edema, and vision-threatening retinopathy, but after adjusting for metabolic and socioeconomic variables, the gender differences lose their statistical significance as associations.[1] In independent studies of South Asian Indians and people from the United Arab Emirates, men had a higher prevalence of DR than women.[26,31,58,60] In an Hispanic population from the United States, a predominantly white population from Australia, a white population in the Netherlands, and a rural Chinese population, no gender differences in prevalence of DR or incidence of DR were found (Table 3.10).[8,20,31,52]

Table 3.10 Estimates of prevalence of forms of diabetic retinopathy by gender

Any DR (F%/M%)	DME (F%/M%)	PDR (F%/M%)	References
42.8/22.9	8.4/1.6	6.9/2.0	Wong et al.[1]
44.8/49.6	10.8/9.8	6.4/5.6	Varma et al.[8]
35.5/38	27.9/32.1	3.1/1.3	Chou et al.[34]
46.5/56.5	8.5/10.6	5.4/5.9	Villalpando et al.[67]
14.6/21.3			Rema et al.[60]
14.6/21.1			Raman et al.[31]
45.1/44.4			Wang et al.[20]
13.9/24.7			Al-Maskari and El-Sadig[58]

Data from selected references on the effect of gender on prevalence of DR. F = female, M = male. DR = diabetic retinopathy. DME = diabetic macular edema. PDR = proliferative diabetic retinopathy.

There may be an interaction between the effect of gender and the type of diabetes. In type 1 diabetes, being female has been associated with higher prevalence of retinopathy; however, men had a higher prevalence of more severe retinopathy.[23,45] Similarly, for younger onset diabetes, the 10-year incidence rate of improvement was higher and rate of progression was lower for females than for males.[10] There was no gender difference in 10-year incidence rates of any DR, improvement in DR severity, or progression in DR severity for older onset diabetics taking insulin. Females had a higher 10-year incidence rate of improvement of retinopathy in the older onset, not taking insulin group, but gender did not influence incidence rates for any DR or progression of DR.[10] The WESDR 25-year analysis in this same cohort demonstrated that being male was significantly associated with progression of retinopathy with a hazard ratio of 1.30 (95% CI 1.11–1.54, $p = 0.0002$). Being male was also associated with less improvement in diabetic retinopathy.

3.13 Age at Onset of Diabetes

Diabetic retinopathy is associated with age at onset of diabetes.[36,45,46] In WESDR, the presence of any retinopathy, proliferative retinopathy, and macular edema were most frequently encountered in younger onset individuals diagnosed prior to 30 years of age, while they were least frequently encountered in older onset individuals diagnosed after 30 years of age who did not require insulin.[45,46] Other studies support the conclusion that earlier age of onset of type 2 diabetes is a risk factor for increased prevalence and severity of DR independent of other traditional risk factors.[71]

3.14 Socioeconomic Status and Educational Level

The reported influence of socioeconomic status on prevalence, incidence, and severity of diabetic retinopathy has been inconsistent. Associations between lower socioeconomic status and worse retinopathy have been reported.[72–74] Other studies have not found such associations.[75,26] Lower education has been associated with higher prevalence of DR and lower prevalence of DR.[36,65]

3.15 Family History of Diabetes

No association of family history of diabetes with presence of diabetic retinopathy has been reported across multiple studies.[26,32,61]

3.16 Changes Over Time

Trends over time in diabetic retinopathy endpoints are shown in Table 3.11. Based on Medicare claims data, in elderly persons with diabetes over the period 1994–2004, there are lower rates of prevalence and incidence of NPDR, PDR, and DME within 1

Table 3.11 Estimated annual incidence of vision loss endpoints in patients with diabetes by diabetes type over time

Endpoint	Period	Younger onset (%)	Older onset, taking insulin (%)	Older onset, not taking insulin (%)
Blindness	1980(2)–1984(6)	0.38	0.82	0.67
	1984(6)–1990(2)	0.05	0.14	0.37
	1990(2)–1995(6)	0.18		
Doubling of visual angle	1980(2)–1984(6)	1.51	3.62	1.87
	1984(6)–1990(2)	0.52	3.31	2.50
	1990(2)–1995(6)	0.85		
PDR	1980(2)–1984(6)	2.71	1.98	0.53
	1984(6)–1990(2)	3.97	3.17	1.34
	1990(2)–1994(6)	2.8%		
	1994(6)–2005(7)	1.6%		

Data from WESDR.[59,10]

year after diagnosis and during 6 years of follow-up more recently.[76] In type 1 diabetics in WESDR, the same trend has been noted in incidence of PDR (Table 3.11).[59]Analogous trends have been noted in other studies from Europe and the United States.[57,77] It is possible that these data reflect improvements in primary care of diabetes mellitus over time. Independent population-based studies have not reported decreased rates of blindness due to diabetes during a time when the rates of PDR and DME have been declining.[78,79] The discordance may reflect a lag phase between improvement in management and decline in some but not all ocular late complications.[78]

3.17 Epidemiology of Diabetic Macular Edema (DME)

In WESDR, the prevalence rates of DME in younger onset, older onset taking insulin, and older onset not taking insulin groups were 6, 12, and 4%, respectively.[45,46] The 4-, 10-, and 25-year incidence rates of DME are shown in Table 3.12. Persons taking insulin have higher rates than those not taking insulin. The association between insulin use and higher incidence of DME may reflect the increased severity of diabetes in insulin users rather than a causal relationship between insulin use and DME. The annual incidence rates of DME show a decrease in the most recent period compared to earlier periods. In WESDR, for the periods from 1990–1992 to 1994–1996 and from 1994–1996 to 2005–2007, the annual rates of incidence were 2.3 and 0.9%, respectively.[80] Similarly, in Denmark, the 20-year cumulative incidence of DME in type 1 diabetics decreased from 18.6% in a cohort diagnosed from 1965 to 1969 to 7.4% for the cohort diagnosed from 1979 to 1984, presumably reflecting better glycemic control in the latter era.[81] The annual incidence of DME in studies in which annual examinations were performed is higher, presumably because some eyes develop and then resolve DME and are not counted in study designs such as WESDR without annual examinations. For example, the annual incidence of DME in type 1 diabetics examined annually with diabetes of duration from 10 to 20 years is 6.7%, approximately three times the rate calculated from WESDR data from a similar era.[13]

Studies consistently report that DME depends on duration of diabetes.[80,8,16,20,82] Prevalence rates of DME vary in younger onset diabetics from 0% in patients whose duration of diabetes is less than 5 years to 29% in patients whose duration of diabetes is 20 or more years.[83] In older onset diabetics, the prevalence varies from 3% in patients whose duration of diabetes is less than 5 years to 28% in patients whose duration of diabetes is 20 or more years. Incidence rates also depend on duration of diabetes. Figures 3.4 and 3.5 show the parabolic relationship of 10-year incidence of DME to duration of diabetes in younger onset and older onset diabetes. In younger onset diabetes, the 10-year incidence of DME on average rises from 7% in a newly diagnosed patient to 27% in a patient who has had diabetes for 12 years and thereafter drops.

Table 3.12 Various incidence rates of diabetic macular edema by diabetes type

Diabetes type	4-year incidence (%)	10-year incidence (%)	25-year incidence (%)
Younger onset	8.2	20.1	29
Older onset, taking insulin	8.4	25.4	
Older onset, taking no insulin	2.9	13.9	

Data from Klein et al.[16,80,82] The 25-year incidence is not available for the older onset groups because too many of these persons had died by the 25-year follow-up time.

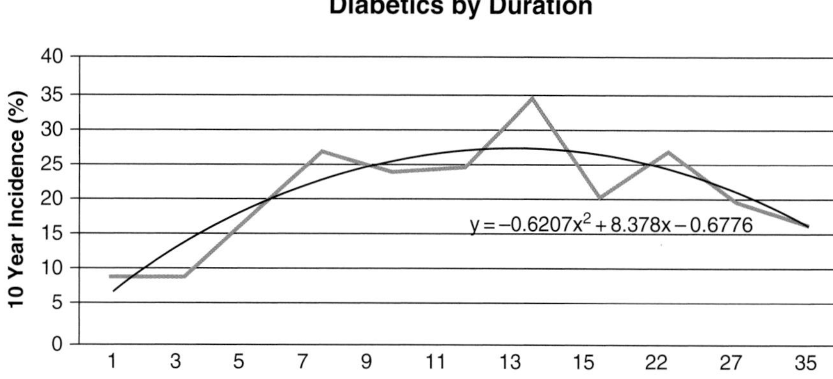

Fig. 3.4 The peak 10-year incidence of DME in younger onset diabetes as assessed from the *fitted curve* would be at approximately 12 years duration. Data from Klein et al.[82]

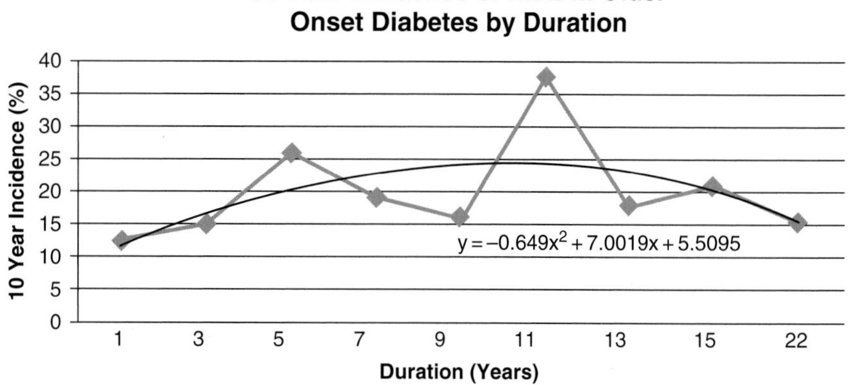

Fig. 3.5 The peak 10-year incidence of DME in older onset diabetes as assessed from the *fitted curve* would be at approximately 10 years duration. Data from Klein et al.[82]

In older onset diabetes, the 10-year incidence of DME on average rises from 12% in a newly diagnosed patient to 25% in a patient who has had diabetes for 10 years and thereafter begins to drop.

Prevalence rates of DME reported for various populations and ethnic groups studied according to diabetes type are shown in Table 3.13. According to the Multiethnic Study of Atherosclerosis (MESA), the prevalence of DME was higher in blacks (11.1%), Hispanics (10.7%), and Chinese (8.9%) than whites (2.7%).[84] In the Atherosclerosis Risk in Communities Study, DME was also more prevalent in blacks than whites.[14] However, race may not be an independent risk factor. When

Table 3.13 Prevalence of diabetic macular edema by type of diabetes and population

Population	Type I (%)	Type II (%)	Mixed cohort (%)	References
USA Caucasian	6	2–4		Williams et al.[19]
USA biracial (blacks, whites)			1.6	Klein et al.[14]
UK Caucasian	2.3–6.4		6.4–6.8	Williams et al.[19]
Australian Caucasian			4.3–10	Williams et al.,[19] Mitchell et al.[32]
European Caucasian		5.4		Williams et al.[19]
Scandinavian Caucasian	16	0.6–26.1	8	Williams et al.[19]
African American		8.6	8.6	Williams et al.,[19] Leske et al.[21]
Hispanic American			10.4	Varma et al.,[8] Williams et al.[19]
South Asian		6.4–13.3		Williams et al.[19]
Indian			1.4	Raman et al.[26]
Chinese		2.7–5.2		Williams et al.,[19] Wang et al.[20]
South American		4.7–6.2		Williams et al.[19]

Wide ranges among studies partially reflect variations in other factors such as duration of diabetes mellitus in addition to ethnic variations.
Adapted and expanded from Williams et al.[19]

adjusted for other baseline variables, ethnicity was not associated with prevalence of vision-threatening retinopathy (primarily DME).[84] The 9-year incidence rate of DME for blacks in the Barbados Eye Study was 8.7%, lower than the 10-year incidence rate of 13.9% reported for the older onset, not taking insulin group in the predominantly white WESDR from an earlier era.[85]

Age at diagnosis influenced incidence of DME in WESDR (Fig. 3.6). The relation of 10-year incidence of DME and age at baseline examination was nonlinear with a peak value at approximately 30 years in younger onset diabetics and at approximately 50 years in older onset diabetics. This relationship did not hold when 25-year incidence of DME was examined with adjustment for other baseline variables.[80]

With control of other baseline variables gender, occupation, income, marital status, educational level, and health insurance status have not been associated with the 25-year incidence of DME in younger onset diabetics.[80,84] The 10-year incidence of DME in both younger onset and older onset diabetics was not associated with gender in WESDR.[82]

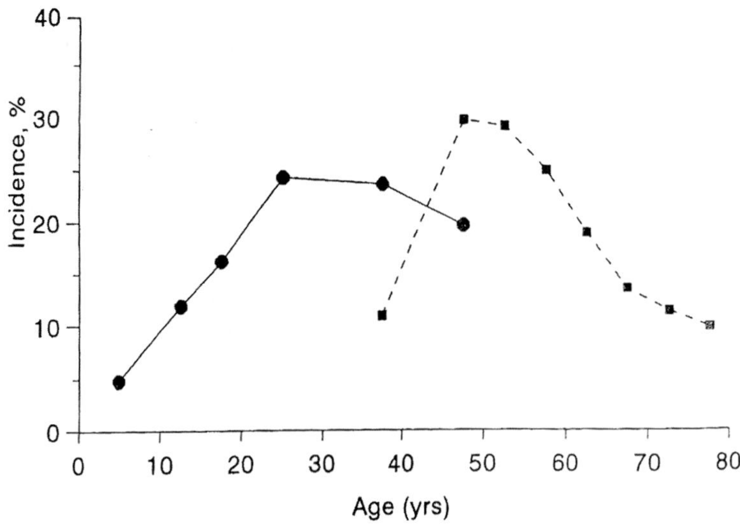

Fig. 3.6 The *solid line* represents data from younger onset diabetics and the *dashed line* from older onset diabetics. Ten year incidence of diabetic macular edema versus age at baseline examination. Reprinted with permission from Klein et al.[82]

3.18 Epidemiology of Proliferative Diabetic Retinopathy (PDR)

In WESDR, the prevalence rates of PDR in younger onset, older onset taking insulin, and older onset not taking insulin groups were 23, 14, and 3%, respectively.[45,46] The 10-year incidence rates of progression to PDR in younger onset, older onset taking insulin, and older onset not taking insulin groups were 29.8, 23.6, and 9.7%, respectively.[10] In an Australian population-based study of adults aged 49 and greater in which type of diabetes was not characterized, the 5-year incidence of PDR was 4.1%.[53] Based on representation in the population, more older onset people develop PDR than do younger onset people, although the risk of developing PDR is higher in younger onset diabetes.[5,46] In type 1 DM, the risk of PDR is nearly zero for the first 10 years of the disease, then rises over 5 years to an roughly stable annual risk for the next 25 years.[86] In 1986, this risk was 30 per 1,000 person-years, but in 2006 this risk was estimated to be lower at 4.5 per 1,000 person-years.[11,86] In type 1 DM, the 20- to 25-year cumulative incidence of PDR seems to be declining over time.[81] Older cohorts had cumulative incidences of 20–40%, but more recent cohorts have rates of 10.9–12.5%.[11,81] These changes may reflect the influence of improved glycemic control and blood pressure in the more recent era.[81]

Duration of DM affects prevalence of PDR with increasing duration associated with higher prevalence rates (Table 3.14). Similarly, duration of diabetes influences 10-year incidence rates of progression to PDR in younger onset diabetics.[10] When duration of diabetes is less than 4 years, the 10-year incidence rate for progression to PDR is approximately 10%.[10] The highest 10-year incidence rate of 49.8% was found in the group with diabetes duration of 10–14 years, and all other groups had rates of 22.9–39.1% with declining rates for the highest values of diabetes duration, probably reflecting the effect of decreasing survival in these subgroups (Fig. 3.7).[10]

Age at baseline examination of diabetes influenced 10-year incidence rates of PDR in the younger onset group of diabetics in WESDR.[10] If age at baseline examination was less than age 10, the 10-year incidence rate for PDR was 0%.[10] If age at baseline examination was in the age range, 10–14, the 10-year incidence rate of PDR was 14.8%.[10] For age at baseline examination above 14 years, the 10-year incidence rates of PDR are roughly equal across a large range of ages (29.0–36.6%).[10]

Younger onset males have a higher prevalence of PDR than younger onset females for unknown reasons.[45] Gender had no influence on the 10-year incidence rate of progression to PDR.[10] The prevalence of PDR varies widely across different ethnic groups (Table 3.15). Reliable patterns are difficult to discern because of the large number of differences in study types and the presence of confounding variables.

3.19 Socioeconomic Impact of Diabetes

Besides the health advantages to the affected patients of proper care of diabetes, there is a socioeconomic aspect to the diagnosis and management of diabetes and its complications. The costs to society of diabetes include direct costs of medical care, costs of disability, lost wages, lost productivity and taxes, and nursing home care. These costs associated with the care of patients with diabetes are disproportionate to the size of the population with

Table 3.14 Prevalence of PDR in selected series by diabetes type and duration of DM

	Duration of diabetes mellitus				
Population/Type	<5 years	6–10 years	11–15 years	>15 years	References
South Asian, mixed type	0.9	1.1	7.9	4.2	Raman et al.[26]
US Latino, mixed type	0.9	5	7.8	18.3	Varma et al.[8]
US whites, younger onset	0	2.3	19.7	52.3	Klein et al.[45]
US whites, older onset, no insulin	~0	~2	~2	~10	Klein et al.[46]
US whites, older onset, on insulin	~3	~10	~10	~20	Klein et al.[46]
US mixed race, type 1	~0	~0	~7	25–80*	Orchard et al.[61]

*The prevalence increases over this range with increasing durations.
Cell entries are in percents. ~ number is estimated from a published graph.

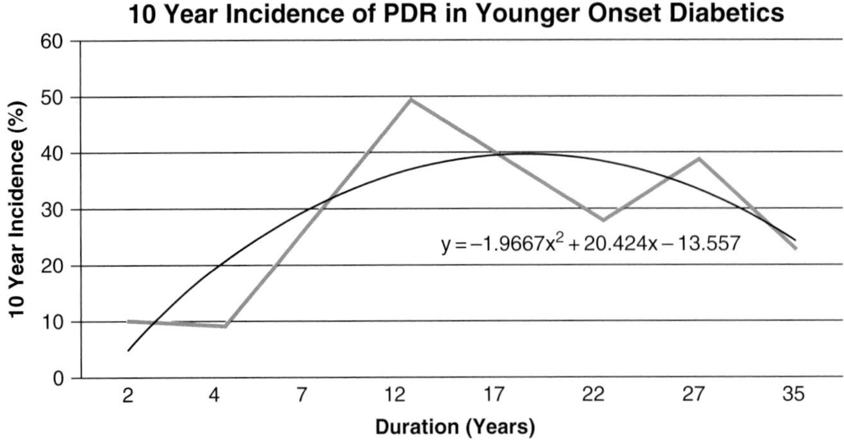

Fig. 3.7 A point estimate duration was chosen from among the categorical duration ranges reported in the data table to allow construction of a graphical approximation in the interests of visualizing the relationship. The *smooth curve* is a parabolic least-squares best-fit line to the data points. The 10-year incidence of PDR peaks for younger onset diabetics with approximately 18 years duration of disease. Data from Klein et al.[10]

Table 3.15 Prevalence of proliferative diabetic retinopathy

Population	Type I (%)	Type II (%)	Mixed cohort (%)	References
USA Caucasian	3.8–25	0.9–5		Williams et al.[19]
USA biracial, blacks and whites			1.8%	Klein et al.[14]
UK Caucasian	1.1–2.0	1.1–4	1.1–8	Williams et al.[19]
Australian Caucasian			1.6–7	Williams et al.,[19] Mitchell et al.[32]
European Caucasian	7.3–17	3.1–15.9	1.8	Williams et al.[19]
Scandinavian Caucasian	2.6–28.4	4.2–14.5	1.7–2.4	Williams et al.[19]
African American	18.9	0.9–1.5	0.9	Williams et al.,[19] Leske et al.[21]
US Hispanic		5.6–6.0	6.1	Varma et al.,[8] Williams et al.[19]
American Indian		5.1–7		Williams et al.[19]
Indian			1.6	Raman et al.[26]
South Asian	1.9	0.7–10.3		Williams et al.[19]
UK South Asian				Williams et al.[19]
Japanese		2.8–10		Williams et al.[19]
Chinese		0.4–12.7	2.2	Williams et al.[19]
African			12.8	Williams et al.[19]
South American		3.4–5.5		Williams et al.[19]

Wide ranges partially reflect variations in factors of importance such as duration of diabetes mellitus among studies in addition to ethnic variations. Adapted and expanded from Williams et al.[19]

diabetes. In the United States in 1992, approximately 3.1% of the population had diabetes but 11.9% of all US health-care expenditures were spent on diabetes. The per capita annual expenditure was $11,000 per person with diabetes and $2,600 per person without diabetes. Half of the diabetes-related expenditures were for the treatment of diabetes and half were for the treatment of chronic complications of diabetes.[87] A decade later, the situation was largely unchanged. In 2002, the per capita expenditure on persons with diabetes was twice that of persons without diabetes. Approximately 20% of all health-care expenditures were for the treatment of diabetes, in spite of having a prevalence of diabetes at less than 5% of the US population.[88] An analogous situation exists in the United Kingdom.[37] Modeling studies of the direct medical costs of managing complications of diabetes suggest estimates of $47,240 per patient over 30 years on average.[89]

3.20 Socioeconomic Impact of Diabetic Retinopathy

Across the world, studies point to an important economic impact of diabetic retinopathy. In the United States, from 1996 to 2000, the total Medicare payments for diabetic retinopathy were $590 million. The Medicare payments per beneficiary per year for the treatment of diabetic retinopathy varied from $1,176 in the first year of diagnosis to $366 in years five and after.[90] In 2004, the total direct medical costs were estimated to be $493 million for diabetic retinopathy, with an average annual total cost per patient with diabetic retinopathy of $629.[91]

In Germany in 2002, the annual costs per patient associated with diabetic retinopathy were estimated to be 1,433 euros. Medical devices and temporary working disability accounted for 58% of the costs. Hospitalization accounted for 10% and visits to ophthalmologists accounted for 9%. Thus, a large portion of the costs were related to productivity losses and a relatively smaller portion of the costs were related to direct ophthalmic care.[92] A similar situation has been reported in Nova Scotia, Canada, where only 13.5% of costs were related to direct care of diabetic retinopathy but 48.2% of the costs associated with diabetic retinopathy were due to lost productivity.[93]

In cost effectiveness studies the emphasis shifts to estimates of costs per person year of vision saved. In a computer model of the costs of type I diabetes, over a period of 60 years in the United States, it was predicted that 72% of persons would develop PDR requiring panretinal photocoagulation and 48% of individuals would develop DME requiring focal laser treatment. The model predicted a cost of $966 per person-year of vision saved from proliferative diabetic retinopathy and a cost of $1118 per person-year of central acuity saved from clinically significant macular edema. Compared to the average cost of $6900 for 1 year of Social Security Disability due to vision loss, the treatment expenses for DR represent a preferable alternative based on economic considerations alone.[94] When a similar model was applied to patients with type II diabetes in the United States based on data from 1990, screening and treatment of diabetic retinopathy would result in annual savings of $472.1 million and 94,304 person-years of sight.[95] Similar conclusions have been reached in cost–benefit analyses done in other countries.[96]

Another method of evaluating the relative value of diagnostic and treatment regimens is to assess their cost per quality-adjusted life year (QALY). In patients with type 2 diabetes, the diagnosis and treatment of diabetic retinopathy ranged from $3198–3849 per QALY compared with no treatment depending on the use of insulin.[97] The World Health Organization has suggested that very cost-effective regimens are those that cost less than the per capita gross domestic product for the country being discussed.[98] For the United States with a 2008 per capita gross domestic product of $43,730, these values are in a range considered highly justifiable.[99]

3.21 Summary of Key Points

- The prevalence of diabetes is increasing worldwide probably as an effect of increased caloric consumption and decreased exercise.
- Diabetes monotonically increases in prevalence with age, but diabetic retinopathy does not. In the oldest subgroups, prevalence of diabetic retinopathy declines, probably as a survivorship effect.
- The prevalence of diabetes among populations varies from 1.7% in Indonesians to 50% in Pima Indians. The factors responsible for the wide range are unclear, but may include genetic factors.
- The order of incidence of doubling of the visual angle from highest to lowest is older onset, insulin taking diabetics>older onset, not taking insulin diabetics>younger onset diabetics. The order of prevalence of moderate visual loss is older onset, insulin taking diabetics > older onset, not taking insulin diabetics > younger onset diabetics.
- The order of incidence of blindness from highest to lowest is older onset, taking insulin diabetics > older onset, not taking insulin diabetics > younger onset diabetics. Because of the effect of duration of disease, the order of prevalence of blindness is younger onset diabetics > older onset taking insulin > older onset not taking insulin.

- The prevalence of blindness and visual impairment is declining over time even as the incidence of diabetic retinopathy has not declined probably reflecting better disease detection, better glycemic control, better blood pressure control, better lipid control, better screening, and advances in treatment of diabetic retinopathy.
- The range of prevalence of various forms of diabetic retinopathy is wide across different populations reflecting the effects of many variables.
- The strongest risk factor association with prevalence of diabetic retinopathy is duration of diabetes.
- Increasing age is a consistent risk factor for doubling of visual angle across all types of diabetes.
- The order of incidence of a two-step progression of retinopathy severity from highest to lowest is younger onset > older onset taking insulin > older onset not taking insulin.
- The order of 10-year incidence of diabetic macular edema is older onset taking insulin > younger onset > older onset not taking insulin.
- The order of 10-year incidence of proliferative diabetic retinopathy is younger onset > older onset taking insulin > older onset not taking insulin.
- The socioeconomic costs of diabetes and diabetic retinopathy are disproportionately high relative to the number of persons with diabetes.
- Diagnosis and treatment of diabetic retinopathy are very cost effective for society apart from the health benefits gained by those affected.

3.22 Future Directions

The biggest epidemiologic challenge for the future is reversing the spread of obesogenic lifestyles. The downstream effects of successful efforts at this level could include lowered incidence of diabetes and diabetic retinopathy, reduced loss of vision, and reduced health-care costs. Unraveling factors responsible for the variations in prevalence of diabetes and diabetic retinopathy across the world will probably require genetic studies at the population level. Targeting health-care resources to the most at risk populations will continue to challenge societies, as those at risk are often economically deprived and have least access to medical care, which tends to follow wealth.

References

1. Wong TY, Cheung N, Tay WT, et al. Prevalence and risk factors for diabetic retinopathy. The Singapore Malay eye study. *Ophthalmology*. 2008;115:1869–1875.
2. Saaddine JB, Honeycutt AA, Narayan KM, et al. Projection of diabetic retinopathy and other major eye diseases among people with diabetes mellitus: United States 2005–2050. *Arch Ophthalmol* 2008;126: 1740–1747.
3. Diabetes Control and Complications Trial Research Group. Progression of retinopathy with intensive versus conventional treatment in the diabetes control and complications trial. *Ophthalmology*. 1995;102:647–661.
4. United Kingdom Prospective Diabetes Study Group. United Kingdom prospective diabetes study 24: a 6-year, randomized, controlled trial comparing sulfonylurea, insulin, and metformin therapy in patients with newly diagnosed type 2 diabetes that could not be controlled with diet therapy. *Ann Intern Med*. 1998;128:165–175.
5. Klein R, Klein BEK, Moss SE. The epidemiology of ocular problems in diabetes mellitus. In: Feman SS, ed. *Ocular Problems in Diabetes Mellitus*. St. Louis: CV Mosby Co; 1989:255–264.
6. Early Treatment Diabetic Retinopathy Study Research Group. Photocoagulation for diabetic macular edema. *Arch Ophthalmol*. 1985;103:1796–1806.
7. UK Prospective Diabetes Study (UKPDS) Group. Intensive blood-glucose control with sulphonylureas or insulin compared with conventional treatment and risk of complications in patients with type 2 diabetes (UKPDS 33). *Lancet*. 1998;352:837–853.
8. Varma R, Torres M, Pena F, et al. Prevalence of diabetic retinopathy in adult Latinos. *Am Acad Ophthalmol*. 2004; 111:1298–1306.
9. Zhang X, Gregg EW, Cheng YJ, et al. Diabetes mellitus and visual impairment. National health and nutrition examination survey, 1999–2004. *Arch Ophthalmol*. 2008; 126:1421–1427.
10. Klein R, Klein B, Moss S, Cruickshanks K. The Wisconsin epidemiologic study of diabetic retinopathy. *Arch Ophthalmol*. 1994;112:1217–1228.
11. Skrivarhaug T, Fosmark DS, Stene LC, et al. Low cumulative incidence of proliferative diabetic retinopathy in childhood-onset type 1 diabetes: a 24 year follow-up study. *Diabetologia*. 2006;49:2281–2290.
12. Jekel JF, Elmore JG, Katz DL. *Epidemiology, Biostatistics, and Preventive Medicine*, 1st ed. Philadelphia: WB Saunders; 1996:216–217.
13. Vitale S, Maguire MG, Murphy RP, et al. Clinically significant macular edema in type I diabetes. *Ophthalmology*. 1995;102:1170–1176.
14. Klein R, Sharrett AR, Klein BEK, et al. The association of atherosclerosis, vascular risk factors, and retinopathy in adults with diabetes. The atherosclerosis risk in communities study. *Ophthalmology*. 2002;109:1225–1234.
15. Klein R, Klein BEK, Moss SE, et al. The Wisconsin epidemiologic study of diabetic retinopathy IV. Diabetic macular edema. *Ophthalmology*. 1984;91: 1464–1474.

16. Klein R, Moss SE, Klein BE, et al. The Wisconsin epidemiologic study of diabetic retinopathy. XI. The incidence of macular edema. *Ophthalmology*. 1989;96:1501–1510.
17. Jaeschke R, Guyatt G, Barratt A, et al. Therapy and understanding the results. Measures of association. In: Guyatt G, Rennie D, eds. *User's Guides to the Medical Literature. A Manual for Evidence-Based Clinical Practice*. Chicago: American Medical Association; 2002:351–368.
18. Kleinbaum DG, Klein M. *Survival Analysis. A self-Learning Text*. 2nd ed. New York: Springer; 2005:32–33.
19. Williams R, Airey M, Baxter H, et al. Epidemiology of diabetic retinopathy and macular edema: a systematic review. *Eye*. 2004;18:963–983.
20. Wang FH, Liang YB, Zhang F, et al. Prevalence of diabetic retinopathy in rural China: the Handan eye study. *Ophthalmology*. 2009;116:461–467.
21. Leske MC, Wu SY, Hyman L, et al. Diabetic retinopathy in a black population-the Barbados eye study. *Ophthalmology*. 1999;106:1893–1899.
22. Moss SE, Klein R, Klein BEK. Ten-year incidence of visual loss in a diabetic population. *Ophthalmology*. 1994; 101:1061–1070.
23. Roy MS, Klein R, O'Colmain BJ, et al. The prevalence of diabetic retinopathy among adult type 1 diabetic persons in the United States. *Arch Ophthalmol*. 2004;122:546–551.
24. National diabetes fact sheet, 2007. http://www.cdc.gov/diabetes/pubs/pdf/ndfs_2007.pdf. Accessed November 30, 2008.
25. Cugati S, Kifley A, Mitchell P, Wang JJ. Temporal trends in the age-specific prevalence of diabetes and diabetic retinopathy in older persons: population-based survey findings. *Diabetes Res Clin Pract*. 2006;74:301–308.
26. Raman R, Rani PK, Rachepalle SR, et al. Prevalence of diabetic retinopathy in India. Sankara Nethralaya diabetic retinopathy epidemiology and molecular genetics study report 2. *Ophthalmology*. 2009;116:311–318.
27. Wild S, Roglic G, Green A, et al. Global prevalence of diabetes: estimates for the year 2000 and projections for 2030. *Diabetes Care*. 2004;27:1047–1053.
28. Harris MI, Flegal KM, Cowie CC, et al. Prevalence of diabetes, impaired fasting glucose, and impaired glucose tolerance in U.S. adults. The Third National Health and Nutrition Examination Survey, 1988–1994. *Diabetes Care*. 1998;21:518–524.
29. Mundet X, Pou A, Piquer N, et al. Prevalence and incidence of chronic complications and mortality in a cohort of type 2 diabetic patients in Spain. *Prim Care Diabetes*. 2008;2:135–140.
30. Gupta R, Kumar P. Global diabetes landscape–type 2 diabetes mellitus in South Asia: epidemiology, risk factors, and control. *Insulin*. 2008;3:78–94.
31. Raman R, Rani PK, Rachepalle SR, et al. Prevalence of diabetic retinopathy in India. Sankara Nethralaya diabetic retinopathy epidemiology and molecular genetics study report 2. *Ophthalmology*. 2008;116:311–318.
32. Mitchell P, Smith W, Wang J, Attebo K. Prevalence of diabetic retinopathy in an older community/the blue mountain eye study. *Ophthalmology*. 1998;105: 406–411.
33. Chen MS, Kao CS, Chang CJ, et al. Prevalence and risk factors of diabetic retinopathy among noninsulin-dependent subjects. *Am J Ophthalmol*. 1992;114:723–730.
34. Chou P, Liao MJ, Kuo HS, et al. A population survey on the prevalence of diabetes in Kin-Hu, Kinmen. *Diabetes Care*. 1994;17:1055–1058.
35. Wang K, Li T, Xiang H. Study on the epidemiological characteristics of diabetes mellitus and IGT in China. *Zhonghua liu xing bing xue za zhi = Zhonghua liuxingbingxue zazhi* 1998;19:282–285.
36. Xie XW, Xu L, Wang YX, Jonas JB. Prevalence and associated factors of diabetic retinopathy. The Beijing eye study 2006. *Graefe's Arch Clin Exp Ophthalmol*. 2008; 246:1519–1526.
37. Gadsby R. Epidemiology of diabetes. *Adv Drug Deliv Rev*. 2002;54:1165–1172.
38. Sinclair AJ, Gadsby R, Penfold S, et al. Prevalence of diabetes in care home residents. *Diabetes Care*. 2001;24: 1066–1068.
39. Simmons D, Williams DRR, Powell MJ. Prevalence of diabetes in a predominantly Asian community: preliminary findings of the Coventry diabetes study. *Br Med J*. 1989;298:18–21.
40. El Haddad O, Saad M. Prevalence and risk factors for diabetic retinopathy among Omani diabetics. *Br J Ophthalmol*. 1998;82:901–906.
41. Ezzati M, Vander Hoorn S, Lawes CMM, et al. Rethinking the "Diseases of Affluence" paradigm: global patterns of nutritional risks in relation to economic development. *PLos Med*. 2005;2:e133.
42. Nguyen NT, Magno CP, Lane KT, et al. Association of hypertension, diabetes, dyslipidemia, and metabolic syndrome with obesity: findings from the National health and nutrition examination survey, 1999 to 2004. *J Am Coll Surg*. 2008;207:928–934.
43. Tuomilehto J, Lindstrom J, Eriksson JG, et al. Prevention of type 2 diabetes mellitus by changes in lifestyle among subjects with impaired glucose tolerance. *N Engl J Med*. 2001;344:1343–1350.
44. Moss SE, Klein R, Klein BEK. The 14-year incidence of visual loss in a diabetic population. *Ophthalmology*. 1998;105:998–1003.
45. Klein R, Klein BEK, Moss SE, et al. The Wisconsin epidemiologic study of diabetic retinopathy. II. Prevalence and risk of diabetic retinopathy when age at diagnosis is less than 30 years. *Arch Ophthalmol*. 1984;102:520–526.
46. Klein R, Klein BEK, Moss SE, et al. The Wisconsin epidemiologic study of diabetic retinopathy. III. Prevalence and risk of retinopathy when age at diagnosis is 30 or more years. *Arch Ophthalmol*. 1984;102:527–532.
47. Varma R. From a population to patients: the Wisconsin epidemiologic study of diabetic retinopathy. *Ophthalmology*. 2008;115:1857–1858.
48. Trautner C, Icks A, Haastert B, et al. Incidence of blindness in relation to diabetes. *Diabetes Care*. 1997;20: 1147–1153.
49. Klein R, Klein BEK, Moss SE. Visual impairment in diabetes. *Ophthalmology*. 1984;91:1–9.
50. Roy MS, Skurnick J. Six-year incidence of visual loss in African Americans with type 1 diabetes mellitus. *Arch Ophthalmol*. 2007;125:1061–1067.
51. Tapp RJ, Shaw JE, Harper CA, et al. The prevalence of and factors associated with diabetic retinopathy in the Australian population. *Diabetes Care*. 2003;26:1731–1737.

52. van Leiden HA, Dekker JM, Moll AC, et al. Risk factors for incident retinopathy in a diabetic and nondiabetic population. The Hoorn study. *Arch Ophthalmol.* 2003; 121:245–251.
53. Cugati S, Cikamatana L, Wang JJ, et al. Five-year incidence and progression of vascular retinopathy in persons without diabetes: the Blue Mountains eye study. *Eye.* 2006;20:1239–1245.
54. Klein R, Klein BE, Moss SE. The relation of systemic hypertension to changes in the retinal vasculature: the Beaver Dam eye study. *Trans Am Ophthalmol Soc.* 1997;95:329–350.
55. Voutilainen-Kaunisto RM, Terasvirta ME, Uusitupa MI, Niskanen LK. Occurrence and predictors of retinopathy and visual acuity in type 2 diabetic patients and control subjects: 10 year follow-up from the diagnosis. *J Diabetes Complicat.* 2001;15:24–33.
56. Leske MC, Wu SY, Hennis A, et al. Incidence of diabetic retinopathy in the Barbados eye studies. *Ophthalmology.* 2003;110:941–947.
57. Porta M, Bandello F. Diabetic retinopathy. A clinical update. *Diabetologia.* 2002;45:1617–1634.
58. Al-Maskari F, El-Sadig M. Prevalence of diabetic retinopathy in the United ARab Emirates: a cross-sectional survey. *BMC Ophthalmol.* 2007;7:11–19.
59. Klein R, Knudtson MD, Lee KE, et al. The Wisconsin epidemiologic study of diabetic retinopathy XXII. The twenty five year progression of retinopathy in persons with type 1 diabetes. *Ophthalmology.* 2008;115:1859–1868.
60. Rema M, Premkumar S, Anitha B, et al. Prevalence of diabetic retinopathy in Urban India: the Chennai urban rural epidemiology study (CURES) eye study, I. *Invest Ophthalmol Vis Sci.* 2005;46:2328–2333.
61. Orchard TJ, Dorman JS, Maser RE, et al. Prevalence of complications in IDDM by sex and duration. Pittsburgh epidemiology of diabetes complications study II. *Diabetes.* 1990;39:1116–1124.
62. Hamman RF, Mayer EJ, Moo-Young GA, et al. Prevalence and risk factors of diabetic retinopathy in non-hispanic whites and Hispanics with NIDDM. *Diabetes.* 1989;38:1231–1237.
63. Harris MI, Klein R, Cowie CC, et al. Is the risk of diabetic retinopathy greater in non-Hispanic blacks and Mexican American than in non-Hispanic whites with type 2 diabetes? A US population study. *Diabetes Care.* 1998;21:1230–1235.
64. Emanuele N, Sacks J, Klein R, et al. Ethnicity, race, and baseline retinopathy correlates in the veterans affairs diabetes trial. *Diabetes Care.* 2005;28:1954–1958.
65. Munoz B, O'Leary M, Fonseca-Baker F, et al. Knowledge of diabetic eye disease and vision care guidelines among Hispanic individuals in Baltimore with and without diabetes. *Arch Ophthalmol.* 2008;126:968–974.
66. Roy MS. Diabetic retinopathy in African Americans with type 1 diabetes-the New Jersey 725 II. Risk factors. *Arch Ophthalmol.* 2000;118:105–115.
67. Villalpando MAEG, Villalpando CG, Perez BA, Stern MP. Diabetic retinopathy in Mexico. Prevalence and clinical characteristics. *Arch Med Res.* 1994;25:355–360.
68. Amini M, Parvaresh E. Prevalence of macro- and microvascular complications among patients with type 2 diabetes in Iran: a systematic review. *Diabetes Res Clin Pract.* 2009;83:18–25.
69. Naqshbandi M, Harris SB, Esler JG, Antwi-Nsiah F. Global complication rates of type 2 diabetes in indigenous peoples: a comprehensive review. *Diabetes Res Clin Pract.* 2008;82:1–17.
70. Lim A, Stewart J, Chui TY, et al. Prevalence and risk factors of diabetic retinopathy in a multi-racial underserved population. *Ophthalmic Epidemiol.* 2008;15: 402–409.
71. Wong J, Molyneaux L, Constantino M, et al. Timing is everything: age of onset influences long-term retinopathy risk in type 2 diabetes, independent of traditional risk factors. *Diabetes Care.* 2008;31:1985–1990.
72. Roy MS, Affouf M. Six-year progression of retinopathy and associated risk factors in African American patients with type 1 diabetes mellitus. *Arch Ophthalmol.* 2006;124: 1297–1306.
73. Bihan H, Laurent S, Sass C, et al. Association among individual deprivation, glycemic control, and diabetes complications: the EPICES score. *Diabetes Care.* 2005; 28:2680–2685.
74. Bachmann MO, Eachus J, Hopper CD, et al. Socioeconomic inequalities in diabetes complications, control, attitudes and health service use: a cross-sectional study. *Diabetic Med.* 2003;20:921–929.
75. Haffner SM, Mitchell BD, Moss SE, et al. Is there an ethnic difference if the effect of risk factors for diabetic retinopathy? *Ann Epidemiol.* 1993;3:2–8.
76. Sloan FA, Belsky D, Ruiz D Jr, Lee P. Changes in incidence of diabetes mellitus-related eye disease among US elderly persons, 1994–2005. *Arch Ophthalmol.* 2008; 126:1548–1553.
77. Brown JB, Pedula KL, Summers KH. Diabetic retinopathy. Contemporary prevalence in a well-controlled population. *Diabetes Care.* 2003;26:2637–2642.
78. Rossing P. The changing epidemiology of diabetic microangiopathy in type 1 diabetes. *Diabetologia.* 2005;48: 1439–1444.
79. Trautner C. Incidence of blindness in southern Gerany between 1990 and 1998. *Diabetologia.* 2001;44: 147–150.
80. Klein R, Knudtson MD, Lee KE, et al. The Wisconsin epidemiologic study of diabetic retinopathy XXIII: the twenty-five year incidence of macular edema in persons with type 1 diabetes. *Ophthalmology.* 2009;116:497–503.
81. Hovind P, Tarnow L, Rossing K, et al. Decreasing incidence of severe diabetic microangiopathy in type 1 diabetes. *Diabetes Care.* 2003;26:1258–1264.
82. Klein R, Klein BE, Moss SE, Cruikshanks KJ. The Wisconsin epidemiologic study of diabetic retinopathy. XV. The long-term incidence of macular edema. *Ophthalmology.* 1995;102:7–16.
83. Klein R, Klein BEK, Moss SE, et al. Diabetic macular edema. *Ophthalmology.* 1984;91:1464–1474.
84. Wong TY, Klein R, Islam FMA, et al. Diabetic retinopathy in a multi-ethnic Cohort in the United States. *Am J Ophthalmol.* 2006;141:446–455.
85. Leske MC, Wu SY, Hennis A, et al. Nine-year incidence of diabetic retinopathy in the Barbados eye studies. *Arch Ophthalmol.* 2006;124:250–255.

86. Krolewski AS, Warram JH, Rand LI, et al. Risk of proliferative diabetic retinopathy in juvenile-onset type 1 diabetes: a 40 year follow-up study. *Diabetes Care.* 1986;9:443–452.
87. Herman WH, Eastman RC. The effects of treatment on the direct costs of diabetes. *Diabetes Care.* 1998;21: C19–C24.
88. Hogan P, Dall T, Nikolov P. Economic costs of diabetes in the US in 2002. *Diabetes Care.* 2003;26:917–932.
89. Caro JJ, Ward AJ, O'Brien JA. Lifetime costs of complications resulting from type 2 diabetes in the U.S. *Diabetes Care.* 2002;25:476–481.
90. Salm M, Belsky D, Sloan FA. Trends in cost of major eye diseases to medicare, 1991–2000. *Am J Ophthalmol.* 2006;142:976–982.
91. Rein DB, Zhang P, Wirth KE, et al. The economic burden of major adult visual disorders in the United States. *Arch Ophthalmol.* 2006;124:1754–1760.
92. Happich M, Reitberger U, Breitscheidel L, et al. The economic burden of diabetic retinopathy in Germany in 2002. *Graefe's Arch Clin Exp Ophthalmol.* 2008;246:151–159.
93. Smith AF. The economic impact of ophthalmic services for persons with diabetes in the Canada province of Nova Scotia: 1993–1996. *Ophthalmic Epidemiol.* 2001;8: 13–25.
94. Javitt JC, Canner JK, Sommer A. Cost effectiveness of current approaches to the control of retinopathy in type 1 diabetes. *Ophthalmology.* 1989;96:255–264.
95. Javitt JC, Aiello LP, Chiang Y, et al. Preventive eye care in people with diabetes is cost-saving to the Federal government. Implications for health-care reform. *Diabetes Care.* 1994;17:909–917.
96. Matz H, Falk M, Gottinger W, Kieselbach G. Cost-benefit analysis of diabetic eye disease. *Ophthalmologica.* 1996;210:348–353.
97. Javitt J, Aiello L. Cost-effectiveness of detecting and treating diabetic retinopathy. *Ann Intern Med.* 1996;124: 164–169.
98. Sarin R. Criteria for deciding cost-effectiveness for expensive new anti-cancer agents. *J Cancer Res Ther.* 2008;4:1–2.
99. The Economist. *Pocket World in Figures.* London: Profile Books Ltd; 2008:236.

Chapter 4
Systemic and Ocular Factors Influencing Diabetic Retinopathy

David J. Browning

4.1 Introduction

Epidemiologic studies have established that certain systemic factors have associations with incidence and progression of diabetic retinopathy (DR). These provide a foundation for treating the manifestations of diabetic retinopathy. Before an ophthalmologist considers using laser treatment, intravitreal injections, and surgery, optimizing the systemic factors that influence diabetic retinopathy is prudent.[1] In general these factors apply to both genders and all races, although the strengths of the associations may vary across subgroups.[2–4] Many more associations are present with univariate testing than with multivariate testing, suggesting that the information carried by these associations may be redundant across more than one factor.[5] For example, hyperglycemia is associated with dyslipidemia. Thus in a study with the goal of determining the importance of dyslipidemia as a predictor of DR, it is important to analyze the data adjusting for baseline glycemic control (HbA1c) to determine if dyslipidemia is independently important as a predictive variable.[6] Accordingly predictive variables found on multivariate testing are more important than those found by univariate testing. In addition, predictive factors are not always the same for different end points. For example, those factors that predict proliferative diabetic retinopathy (PDR), any diabetic retinopathy, and diabetic macular edema (DME) may be different.[6,7]

D.J. Browning (✉)
Charlotte Eye Ear Nose & Throat Associates, Charlotte, NC 28210, USA
e-mail: dbrowning@ceenta.com

In addition to systemic factors, there are ocular factors that have been hypothesized to impact diabetic retinopathy, such as high myopia and pre-existing chorioretinal scarring. Although less important than systemic factors, these have historical significance. It was awareness of the protective effect of pre-existing chorioretinal scarring that led Meyer-Schwickerath to think of purposefully inducing scarring with the xenon photocoagulator in diabetic retinopathy.[8] Socioeconomic factors also have importance and are often overlooked or ignored as inaccessible to change by clinicians. Nevertheless, the effects of these factors are evident in daily practice and therefore they will also be covered in this chapter.

The methods used in determining systemic and ocular associations with DR are the same as those used in epidemiologic studies of demographic variables. The important terms and concepts in these types of studies are defined in Chapter 3 (Epidemiology) and the reader in need of a review is referred there before proceeding further.

4.2 Systemic Factors

4.2.1 Glycemic Control

Glycemic control has a strong influence on many indices of diabetic retinopathy such as prevalence of retinopathy, incidence of retinopathy progression of retinopathy, need for focal and scatter photocoagulation, and loss of visual acuity.[9–18] The influence of glycemic control is apparent in both type 1 and type 2 diabetes. Thresholds for blood glucose used

D.J. Browning (ed.), *Diabetic Retinopathy*, DOI 10.1007/978-0-387-85900-2_4,

in making the diagnosis of diabetes mellitus are chosen, in part, because of the sharp increase in prevalence of retinopathy manifested by patients when glucose rise above these levels.[19] The concept of a laboratory cutpoint for blood glucose normality is vague, however, and 5–9.8% of patients over age 40 in developed countries have typical lesions of diabetic retinopathy even though they do not meet criteria for diabetes.[14,19,20] Retinopathy consistent with diabetic retinopathy can develop in certain patients whose blood glucoses range in the normal range for the population; in adults over the age of 49, the 5-year incidence of such an event is 10%.[17] This may in part reflect increased genetic susceptibility to the effects of hyperglycemia (see Chapter 2). Responsiveness to treatments for manifestations of diabetic retinopathy may also depend on glycemic control. Failure of DME to respond to focal/grid laser photocoagulation has been associated with higher glycosylated hemoglobin.[21]

Diabetic Retinopathy "Without" Diabetes Mellitus

Occasionally a patient will be examined and found to have retinal stigmata of diabetic retinopathy and yet have no evidence of diabetes mellitus. Such an example is shown in Fig. 4.1. This patient had been under regular medical care for years with hypertension and some high normal blood sugars, but no abnormal glycosylated hemoglobins. At the time of these photographs, the glycosylated hemoglobin was 5.5% and there was no other hemoglobinopathy. Communication with the patient's internist revealed that repeated glucose testing over the previous few years had revealed no abnormal values. Such cases may reflect a patient with an unusual susceptibility to development of diabetic retinopathy at blood glucose levels lower than the laboratory cutpoints for population normals. Presumably, the synergistic effect of elevated blood pressure and genetic susceptibility may combine to produce such a picture. It has been shown that in patients without diabetes mellitus according to conventional criteria, the blood glucose is higher in those who have retinal lesions of diabetic retinopathy than in those without such lesions.[22]

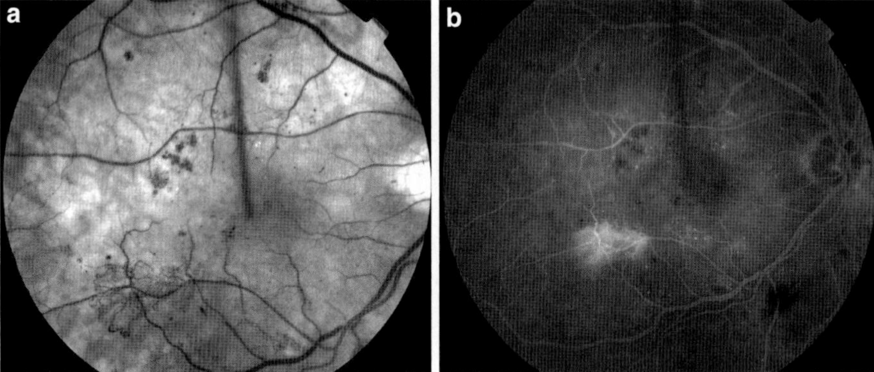

Fig. 4.1 Red-free fundus photograph (**a**) and fluorescein angiogram frame (**b**) of the right eye of a 74-year-old man with no history of diabetes mellitus, a current glycosylated hemoglobin of 5.5% (normal, and indicative of a mean blood glucose of 97 mg/dl), no hemoglobinopathy, and treated hypertension. There are typical lesions of diabetic retinopathy including microaneurysms, lipid exudates, intraretinal microvascular abnormalities, and neovascularization

4.2.1.1 Type 1 Diabetes Mellitus

Epidemiologic studies strongly associate glycemic control with severity of retinopathy in type 1 diabetes mellitus (DM).[16] In multivariate analyses from the Wisconsin Epidemiologic Study of Diabetic Retinopathy (WESDR), the 10-year and 25-year incidences of DME were related to higher baseline glycosylated hemoglobin.[23] The hazard ratio per 1% increase in glycosylated hemoglobin was 1.17 (95% confidence interval [CI] 1.10–1.25, $P < 0.001$).[24] Higher baseline glycosylated hemoglobin was also associated with ≥2-step progression of DR severity.[4] Higher baseline HbA1c was a predictor of progression to PDR in type 1 DM in a Norwegian study and with an increased 6-year incidence of doubling of the visual angle in African Americans with type 1 DM.[25,7]

The Diabetes Control and Complications Trial (DCCT) was a randomized trial that investigated the effect of tight blood glucose control compared to conventional control in patients with type 1 diabetes mellitus ranging in age from 13 to 39 years at the time of enrollment (Table 4.1). There were two cohorts studied. The primary-prevention cohort consisted of 726 patients with no baseline diabetic retinopathy. The secondary-intervention cohort consisted of 715 patients with mild-to–moderate nonproliferative diabetic retinopathy (NPDR) at baseline. The intensive control patients received three to four injections of short-acting insulin per day or subcutaneous insulin infusions. Fingerstick blood glucose checks were done four times daily. The conventional control group received one to two injections of insulin daily and checked blood glucose once daily. Median HbA1cs were 9.1 and 7.3% for the conventional and intensive control groups, respectively, over a mean duration of follow-up of 6.5 years. Over 9 years of follow-up, a 3-step progression of retinopathy on the ETDRS retinopathy severity scale was decreased 76% with tight glucose control.[26,27] For the primary-prevention cohort, the risk of any retinopathy was reduced by 27% over a mean follow-up of 6.5 years (from 90 to 70% for the conventional versus intensive treatment groups).[9] For this cohort, the cumulative 8.5 year rates of 3-step or more retinopathy progression were 54.1 and 11.5% for the conventional and intensive therapy groups, respectively. For the secondary-intervention cohort, the cumulative 8.5 year rates of 3-step or more retinopathy progression were 49.2 and 17.1%, respectively (Fig. 4.2). The beneficial effects became apparent after approximately 2–3 years of therapy and were evident for all levels of baseline retinopathy, but were greatest when intensive therapy was initiated earlier in the course of type 1 diabetes and with less severe levels of baseline retinopathy.[9] The risks of receiving any laser therapy over 9 years of follow-up were 30 and 7.9% for the conventional and intensive treatment groups, respectively ($P = 0.001$).[9]

There was a strong exponential relationship between the risk of retinopathy progression and the duration of follow-up for any given level mean glycosylated hemoglobin during the study (Fig. 4.3). As the mean glycosylated hemoglobin during the study increased, the steepness of the relationship between retinopathy progression risk and duration in the study increased. Thus, risk of retinopathy progression depends on both duration of retinopathy and level of glycemic control.[29] The risk relationships were similar in the primary-prevention and secondary-intervention cohorts. There was no threshold glycosylated hemoglobin value below which further normalization of glucose failed to provide additional benefit.[27,30]

The potential impact that tighter glycemic control could have on ocular and other microvascular complications was shown from modeling of DCCT outcomes and US epidemiologic data regarding type 1 diabetes. Cumulative incidence of PDR and DME would be reduced by approximately one-half and one-third, respectively, with tighter control compared to conventional control.[31] The predicted average number of years free of proliferative retinopathy, DME, and blindness would increase by 14.7, 8.2, and 7.7 years, respectively, if tighter control were achieved.[31]

The Epidemiology of Diabetes Interventions and Complications Study (EDIC) was an extension study involving 1,375 (95%) of the participants in the DCCT study. The goal of this study was to determine the later effects of the interventions tested in the DCCT. Upon advice, most patients in both treatment groups were on an intensive regimen of glucose control for the EDIC study and had convergence of group mean glycosylated hemoglobin values during the course of EDIC (8.07% versus 7.98% overall mean glycosylated hemoglobin values for the former conventional and intensive control groups, respectively, over 10 years follow-up).[32] The benefit from the difference in glycosylated hemoglobin in the former intensively controlled group during the years of the DCCT waned slightly. The cumulative incidence of a 3-step progression of retinopathy was 53% as much in the former intensive control group as in the former conventional control group throughout the 10 years of the EDIC study (Fig. 4.4). Over the first 4 years of EDIC, the risk reduction for 3-step progression of retinopathy was 70%. Over years 4–10

Table 4.1 Diabetes control and complications trial 1983–1993

Major design features
Patients randomized to conventional treatment or intensive treatment group

Conventional treatment group
Insulin injections once or twice a day
Daily self-monitoring of urine or blood glucose
Clinical visits every 3 months
Diet and exercise education

Intensive treatment group
Insulin pump or three or more insulin injections a day
Self-monitoring of blood glucose (SMBG) four or more times a day
Insulin dosage adjusted according to SMBG, diet, and exercise
Diet and exercise plan
Initial hospitalization to implement treatment
Weekly to monthly clinical visits with frequent telephone contact

Randomization
1,441 patients
Primary prevention
Secondary intervention
Conventional versus intensive blood glucose control

End points
Development/progression of diabetic retinopathy (DR)
Neuropathy/nephropathy outcomes

Major eligibility criteria
Type 1 diabetes mellitus (DM)
Age 13–39 years
Absence of hypertension, hypercholesterolemia, and severe diabetic or medical complications

Primary-prevention cohort
Type 1 DM for 1–5 years
No DR on seven-field stereoscopic fundus photography
Urinary albumin secretion – 40 mg/24 h

Primary-prevention major conclusions (mean follow-up 6.5 years)
Intensive blood glucose control
27% reduction in development of DR
78% reduction in 3-step progression of DR

Secondary-intervention cohort
Type 1 DM for 1–15 years
Very mild-to-moderate nonproliferative DR
Urinary albumin secretion – 200 mg/24 h

Secondary-intervention major conclusions (mean follow-up 6.5 years)
Intensive blood glucose control
54% reduction in 3-step progression of DR
47% reduction in proliferative DR and severe levels of nonproliferative DR
56% reduction in photocoagulation
23% reduction in macular edema

Overall major conclusions (mean follow-up 6.5 years)
Intensive blood glucose control
Reduced clinically meaningful retinopathy by 27–76%
Reduced clinically meaningful nephropathy by 34–57%
Reduced clinical risk of other microvascular complications of DM

Reproduced with permission from Aiello[28].

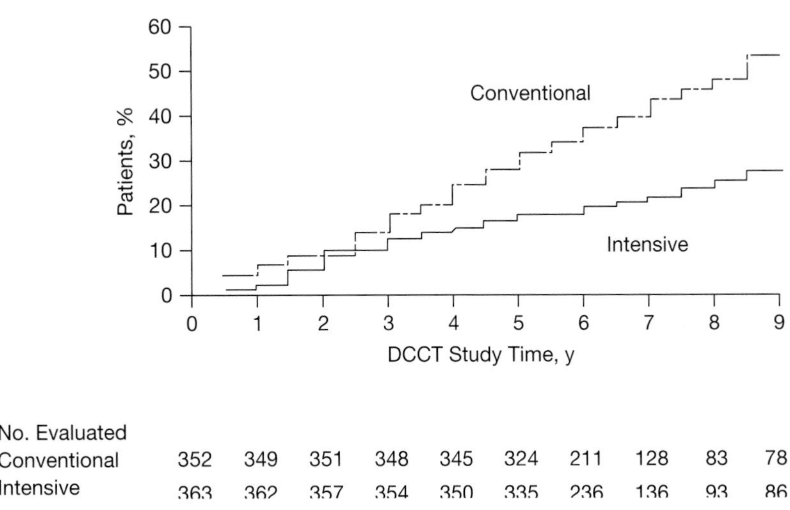

No. Evaluated										
Conventional	352	349	351	348	345	324	211	128	83	78
Intensive	363	362	357	354	350	335	236	136	93	86

Fig. 4.2 The cumulative incidence of a 3-step retinopathy progression on the ETDRS retinopathy severity scale in the DCCT for the conventional and intensive blood glucose control groups for the secondary-intervention cohort (patients with some baseline diabetic retinopathy). The numbers in the table at the bottom refer to participants evaluated in the two groups at each of the time points. Reproduced with permission from DCCT[27]

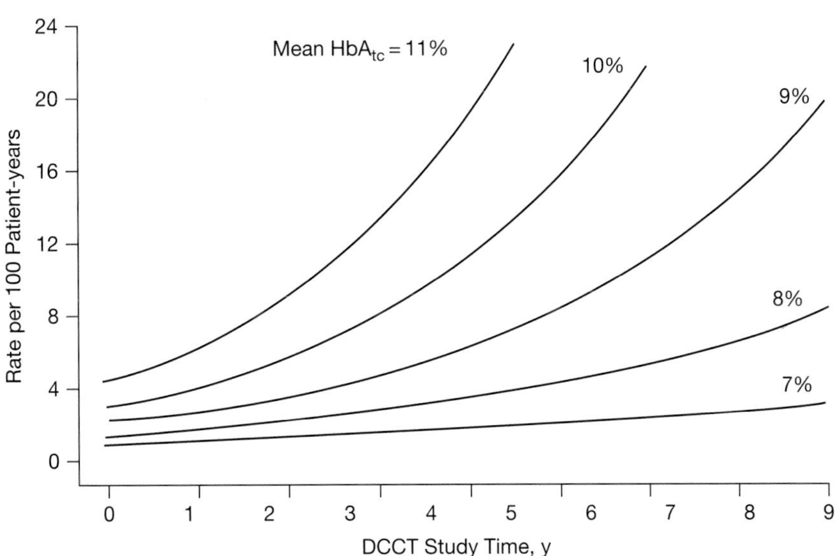

Fig. 4.3 Family of curves representing the relationship of risk of retinopathy progression versus time in the DCCT study for any given mean HbA1c level during the study for the conventional treatment group. The *y*-axis is rate of 3-step progression of retinopathy severity per 100 patient years of follow-up. For any given mean glycosylated hemoglobin level, the relationship of risk of retinopathy progression to duration is exponential. The steepness of the exponential relationship increases as the mean glycosylated hemoglobin increases. A similar family of curves, but much less steep, was found for the intensive treatment group. Reprinted with permission from DCCT[27]

the risk reduction was 38%. Thus, some waning of the protective effect of former intensive glycemic control was noted.[32] Other end points were consonant with the retinopathy progression end point. At 4 years into the EDIC study, laser therapy (either focal or scatter) had been given to 6% of the former conventional control group, but 1% in the former intensive control group ($P = 0.002$).[27]

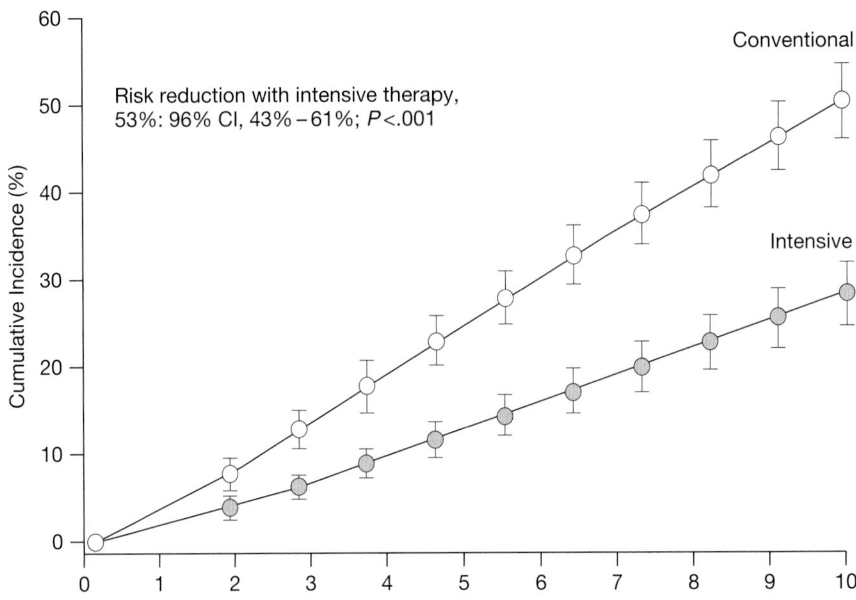

Fig. 4.4 Cumulative incidence of a 3-step progression in retinopathy severity on the ETDRS retinopathy severity scale for the former conventional and former intensive glucose control groups of the DCCT study for 10 years of follow-up during the EDIC study. Reproduced with permission from Diabetes Control and Complications Trial/ Epidemiology of Diabetes Interventions and Complications Research Group[32]

The beneficial effects of intensive glucose control on retinopathy progression do not become apparent for approximately 2–3 years. In fact, there is an early paradoxical early worsening of retinopathy experienced in the first 6 months of intensive retinopathy control.[33] Once the benefits of intensive control accrue, however, they persist even if the intensity of control is relaxed. The relationship of glycemic control to retinopathy, therefore, has a characteristic of momentum and has been termed metabolic memory.[27,32] In the EDIC study, metabolic memory was noted to wane faster in patients with more severe retinopathy at the baseline of the period of intensive control, thus the goal should be to institute intensive control as early in the course of type 1 diabetes as possible.[32] Metabolic memory works in the reverse direction as well. A period of poor glycemic control has adverse effects on retinopathy progression that persist beyond the period of poor control.[32]

The beneficial effects of more intensive glycemic control are not without risks, such as a higher rate of severe hypoglycemia and increased weight gain.[34,35] The two adverse effects may be linked, as subjects on intensive regimens may eat more to prevent hypoglycemia.[35] Behaviors associated with increased risk of hypoglycemic episodes include taking excess insulin, increasing exercise without other adjustments, delaying or missing meals, and drinking alcohol.

4.2.1.2 Type 2 Diabetes Mellitus

As with type 1 diabetes, epidemiologic evidence supports the importance of glycemic control with multiple aspects of diabetic retinopathy in type 2 DM. Increasing HbA1c is associated with higher risk of any DR, PDR, and DME.[15,36,37] Incidence of diabetic retinopathy over 9.4 years of follow-up increased with increasing glycosylated hemoglobin.[19] The odds ratio for the group with the highest tertile of glycosylated hemoglobin was 3.29 (95% CI 1.85–40.60) compared with the lowest tertile.[19] In a cross-sectional study of type 2 diabetics, more severe retinopathy was associated with higher glycosylated hemoglobin.[38]

The United Kingdom Prospective Diabetes Study (UKPDS) was a randomized trial that examined the effect of tight glycemic control in patients with type 2 diabetes mellitus. In this study of 3,867 patients randomized to intensive therapy with a sulfonylurea or insulin at the outset or to conventional therapy based on diet, the intensive glycemic control and conventional glycemic control groups had median glycosylated hemoglobins of 7.0 and 7.9%, respectively, over a median follow-up of 10 years (Table 4.2).[10] Over this interval, the rates of laser photocoagulation and progression of retinopathy were 27% lower in patients with tighter glycemic control compared to those with conventional control

Table 4.2 United Kingdom prospective diabetes study, 1977–1999

Major design features
Randomization
4,209 patients
Primary prevention
Secondary intervention
Conventional versus intensive blood glucose control
End points
Development/progression of diabetic retinopathy (DR)
Neuropathy/nephropathy/cardiovascular outcomes
Patients randomized to conventional treatment or intensive treatment group
Conventional treatment group
Diet control
Followed by sulfonylurea, insulin, metformin
Intensive treatment group
Sulfonylurea
Insulin
Overweight: metformin
Major eligibility criteria
Newly diagnosed type 2 diabetes mellitus
Primary-prevention cohort
Newly diagnosed type 2 diabetes mellitus
No DR on seven-field stereoscopic fundus photography
Secondary-intervention cohort
Newly diagnosed type 2 diabetes mellitus
Very mild-to-moderate nonproliferative DR
Major conclusions (median follow-up, 10.0 years)
Reduced clinically meaningful retinopathy by 27–76%
17% reduction in 2-step progression of DR
29% reduction in need for laser photocoagulation
23% reduction in vitreous hemorrhage
24% reduction in need for cataract extraction
16% reduction in legal blindness
Reduced clinically meaningful nephropathy by 34–57%
Elevated blood pressure is independent risk factor for 2-step progression of DR

Reproduced from Aiello[28].

($P < 0.05$).[10] The relative risk of any retinal photocoagulation (most of which was focal) in the intensive glycemic control group was 0.71 (95% CI 0.53–0.96, $P = 0.0031$).[10] More recently, the Action in Diabetes and Vascular Disease: Preterax and Diamicron Modified Release Controlled Evaluation (ADVANCE) trial randomized 11,140 patients with type 2 DM to intensive or standard glucose control. After a median of 5 years of follow-up the median glycosylated hemoglobins were 6.5 and 7.3% for the intensive and standard control groups, respectively. The rates of new or worsening DR were 6.0 and 6.3%, respectively. The relative risk reduction with intensive treatment was 5% (95% CI 10–18%).[39] In type 2 diabetics, once glycemic control approaches a target glycosylated hemoglobin of 7.0%, the evidence suggests that at least with regard to retinopathy end points, further efforts at intensifying control may produce little benefit.

As with type 1 diabetes, tighter glycemic control in type 2 diabetics carries a risk of hypoglycemic episodes and the gravity of the risk may be greater in type 2 than in type 1 patients.[10,34] The Action to Control Cardiovascular Risk in Diabetes (ACCORD) study was terminated early because of an excess rate of fatal myocardial infarction in the intensive control group (1.41% versus 1.14% per year for the intensive and standard glycemic control groups, respectively).[40] Therefore, less stringent glycosylated hemoglobin goals may be preferable in patients with a history of severe hypoglycemia, limited life expectancy, advanced microvascular or macrovascular complications, or extensive comorbid conditions.[40] Once glycosylated hemoglobin levels reach 7.0%, efforts to tighten glucose control have been successful, and further tightening may be ill advised.[41] Tighter glycemic control requires great effort by patients, and in the large majority of patients for whom intensive control is appropriate, reinforcement and encouragement should be part of the clinical encounter with the ophthalmologist.

4.2.1.3 Rapidity of Improvement in Glycemic Control

In general, improved metabolic control of diabetes mellitus is associated with less rapid progression of retinopathy over extended follow-up periods, however, if metabolic control is greatly improved over a short period, there can be paradoxical worsening in retinopathy thought to be mediated by concomitant increases in insulin-like growth factor 1 (Fig. 4.5).[41–44] In the DCCT, using a variety of definitions of early worsening of retinopathy, intensive glycemic control was associated with early worsening in 13.1% of patients at the 6- or 12-month follow-up visits compared to 7.6% of patients in the conventional treatment group ($P < 0.001$).[42] Despite this early worsening, and despite the fact that such early worsening is associated with higher cumulative incidence in 3-step retinopathy progression at all subsequent follow-up times, the beneficial long-term effects of intensive glycemic control outweigh the negative effects of early worsening, such that intensive control is still recommended. In certain subsets of patients, for example, those approaching proliferative retinopathy with high-risk characteristics, institution of intensive control may be delayed until completion of scatter laser, especially if the baseline glycosylated is high. Although some have intentionally treated individual patients with reversion to poor control because of deterioration of diabetic retinopathy despite laser treatment, this approach is controversial.[41] Accelerated retinopathy with sudden tightening of control has been put forth as an explanation for findings of decreased NPDR but not PDR in some more recent epidemiologic studies compared to WESDR, but this explanation has been discounted.[36] Instead, methodological differences in studies over time have been suggested, including detection bias with nonexamination of patients with less severe disease, as more likely explanations for the apparently paradoxical data.[45]

How Is Early Worsening Defined and Does It Matter?

There are many definitions of early worsening. Early is generally taken to mean sometime between 3 and 12 months after the initiation of tighter glycemic control. Worsening has at least four definitions[42]:

1. Progression of $\geq$3 steps on the ETDRS retinopathy severity scale.
2. Development of cotton wool spots or intraretinal microvascular abnormalities in patients initially free of these lesions.
3. Development of severe nonproliferative retinopathy, proliferative retinopathy, or clinically significant macular edema in eyes initially without these characteristics.
4. When any of the previous three definitions is met at a given visit in the 6- to 12-month time window.

Regardless of the definition used, all analyses from the DCCT point to the same conclusion – that it is the magnitude of the change in HbA1c that occurs rather than the rate of change of the HbA1c that determines risk of early worsening. This result runs counter to many suggestions arising from case series that slower improvement in glycemic control could reduce the incidence of early worsening.[41] To test this hypothesis properly, a randomized clinical trial would need to be performed, which is unlikely to ever occur. Despite the absence of data to support the position, continued advice to slow the rate of improvement in glycemic control is published.[41,42,46]

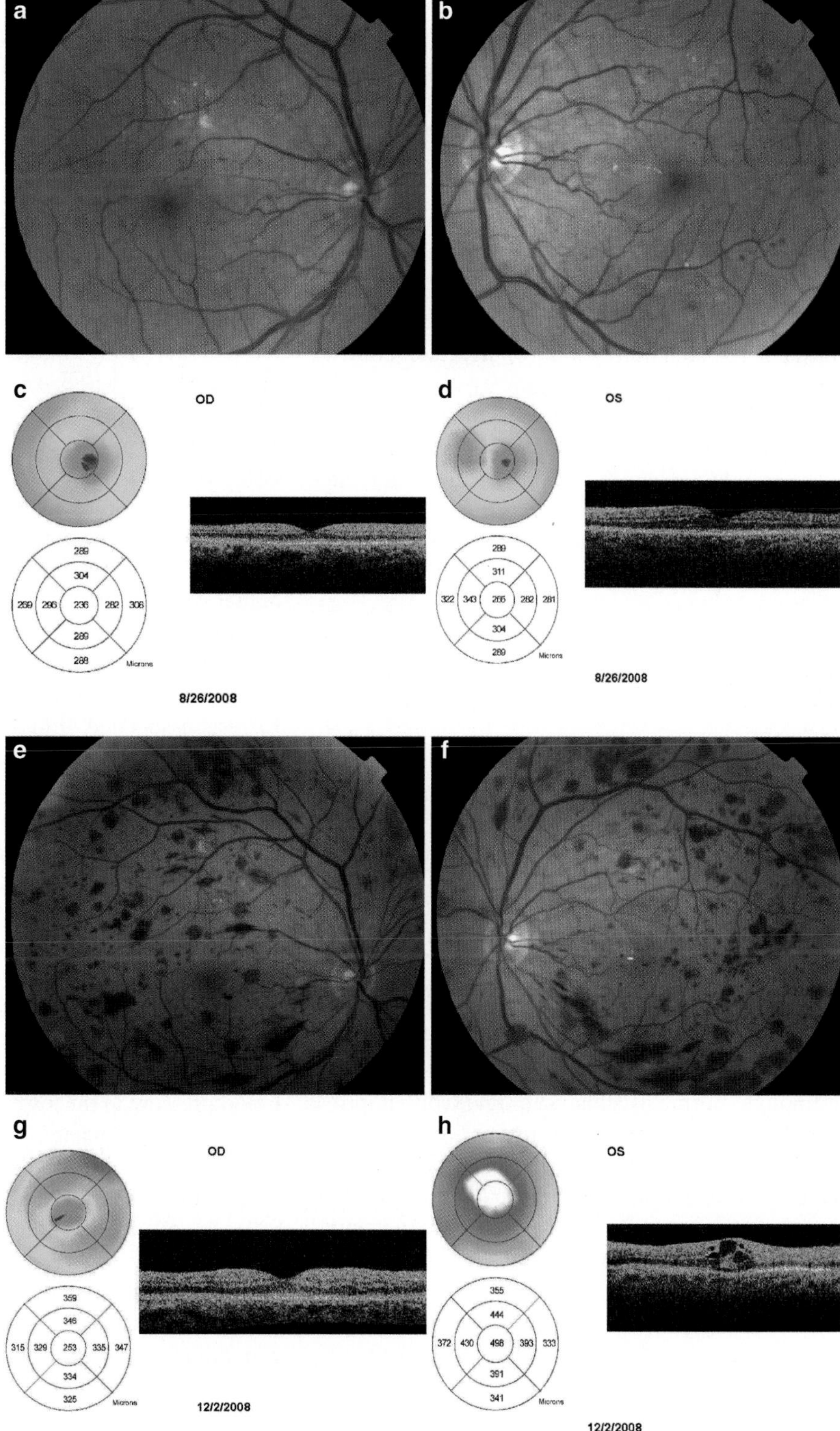

Fig. 4.5 Fundus photographs and OCT images of a 48-year-old patient with 28 years of type 1 diabetes mellitus. When first examined, his best corrected visual acuity was 20/20 in both eyes, subclinical diabetic macular edema was present in the *right fundus* (**a**, **c**), and clinically significant diabetic macular edema was present in the *left fundus* (**b**, **d**). Focal/grid laser photocoagulation was recommended for the left eye, but he desired to try to improve the left eye by working on systemic factors alone. He abruptly and markedly improved his blood glucose and blood pressure and over 4 months lost 20 pounds of body weight. His retinopathy deteriorated bilaterally. His subclinical DME in the right eye evolved to clinically significant macular edema (**e**, **g**) and his clinically significant macular edema in the left eye worsened (**f**, **h**)

In diabetic patients undergoing phacoemulsification cataract extraction with intraocular lens implantation, rapid improvement in glycemic control was associated with a higher rate of progression of diabetic macular edema, and probably should be avoided.[47]

4.2.2 Glycemic Variability

Besides the absolute level of glycemic control, there has been speculation that variability in glycemic control may be a factor in some retinopathy end points.[48] In a study of 100 patients followed for 11 years, the incidence of PDR in type 1 diabetics was not related to glycemic variability as assessed by the standard deviation of the blood glucose concentration.[48]

4.2.3 Insulin Use in Type 2 Diabetes

Type 2 diabetics may be managed with diet alone, with diet plus oral agents, or in more difficult cases with both of these plus insulin. Use of insulin has been associated with an increased prevalence of diabetic retinopathy and incidence of DR.[11–13,36,49,50,18]

4.2.4 Pancreas and Pancreas–Renal Transplantation

Although normoglycemia can markedly improve ophthalmic outcomes when achieved earlier in the course of diabetic retinopathy, most patients who come to isolated pancreas transplantation or combined pancreas–renal transplantation have advanced retinopathy.[51,52] Studies have not shown a difference in change in visual acuity, change in retinopathy severity, or need for laser treatment in patients receiving combined renal–pancreas transplants versus renal transplantation alone or in patients receiving isolated pancreatic transplants.[51–53] Therefore, even if normoglycemia is achieved in such patients, the retinopathy may be too advanced to benefit. The number of patients with milder levels of retinopathy undergoing transplantations is small, however, and it remains a possibility that they will show slower retinopathy progression.

4.2.5 Blood Pressure

Theoretically, blood pressure might be expected to be an important factor in diabetic retinopathy incidence and progression given the impaired autoregulatory capacity of the retinal vasculature in diabetic retinopathy.[54] In such a state, higher blood pressure leads to higher pressure within the retinal capillaries and would be expected to promote macular edema.[55] Indeed, in type 2 diabetic Pima Indians, a strong association of higher blood pressure with development of retinal exudates has been reported.[56] In multivariate analyses in type 1 DM, higher systolic BP was associated with a higher 25-year incidence of DME.[24] The hazard ratio per 10 mmHg increase in baseline systolic BP was 1.15 (95% CI 1.04–1.26, $P = 0.004$).[24] Higher diastolic BP was associated with an increased 10-year incidence of DME in a univariate analysis, but the relationship vanished in multivariate analysis after controlling for other baseline variables.[23]

Although the pathophysiologic pathway between elevated blood pressure and other aspects of DR is less clear, in the Wisconsin Epidemiologic Study of Diabetic Retinopathy, progression to PDR and baseline severity of retinopathy were associated with baseline diastolic blood pressure in type 1 diabetics.[16] The risk of progression to PDR increased from 3 to 20% for those with diastolic blood pressure in the lowest versus highest quartiles at baseline.[57] Epidemiologic evidence exists associating higher systolic blood pressure and prevalence and severity of diabetic retinopathy in both types 1 and 2 DM and seems to be a particular important factor when the glycemic control is poorer (interaction).[14–16,36] Incidence of DR over 9.4 years of follow-up increased in patients with concomitant hypertension.[19] The adjusted odds ratio for the hypertensive group was 2.36 (95% CI 1.02–5.49) for the hypertensive group compared to the nonhypertensive group.[19] In the Barbados Eye Study, the 4-year incidence of DR increased in patients with elevated systolic blood pressure.[18] In a cross-sectional study, severity of retinopathy was associated with higher systolic blood pressure.[38] A diagnosis of hypertension has been associated with an increased prevalence of DR.[36,58] But not all studies have found an association between hypertension and prevalence of diabetic retinopathy, progression of retinopathy, or progression to PDR.[7,50,11,5,38,59,60]

The importance of blood pressure for diabetic retinopathy outcomes has also been noted in randomized controlled trials in both types 1 and 2 diabetics. In the EDIC study involving patients with type 1 diabetes, the risk of further progression of retinopathy increased significantly with higher mean blood pressure at DCCT closeout (11% increase in risk per 5 mmHg increase in mean blood pressure; $P < 0.001$).[32] The UKPDS contained a trial within a trial in which 758 patients with type 2 diabetes mellitus were randomized to tight blood pressure control and 390 patients to less tight blood pressure control.[61] Over a median follow-up of 8.4 years the mean differences in systolic and diastolic blood pressure of the two groups were 10 and 5 mmHg, respectively.[61] The mean HbA1c of the two groups was no different over this time. The group with tight blood pressure control had a 35% reduction in the risk of retinal photocoagulation (78% of which was for DME), a 34% reduction in risk of 2-step progression of retinopathy severity level on graded fundus photographs, a 47% reduction in the risk of losing three or more lines of best corrected visual acuity on the ETDRS chart, and significant reductions in incidence of microaneurysms, hard exudates, and cotton wool spots.[55,61,62] The visual acuity outcome has been attributed primarily to the beneficial effect of tighter blood pressure control on rates of development and progression of diabetic macular edema. No differences in rates of vitreous hemorrhage, blindness, and cataract extraction were detected between groups. Whether the blood pressure was lowered with a beta blocker (atenolol) or an angiotensin-converting enzyme inhibitor (captopril) did not matter.[62,63]

Reduction in blood pressure also appears to be beneficial for type 2 diabetics who do not meet the conventional definition of hypertension – that is, systolic blood pressure >140 mmHg or diastolic blood pressure > 90 mmHg. In a randomized controlled trial comparing antihypertensive treatment with no treatment in normotensive type 2 diabetics, lowering systolic blood pressure by a mean of 9 mmHg and diastolic blood pressure by a mean of 6 mmHg over 5 years led to a reduction in progression of retinopathy from 46 to 34% for the treated versus control groups, respectively ($P = 0.02$).[64] Changes not reaching statistical significance were also noted in number of patients developing retinopathy from no retinopathy and in percentage of patients developing proliferative retinopathy.[64]

Evidence exists for a similar beneficial effect of lower blood pressure and blood pressure reduction in type 1 diabetes, but is not as strong as for type 2 diabetes. In an observational study of younger type 1 diabetics, elevated diastolic blood pressure alone and in combination with elevated systolic blood pressure correlated significantly with more severe retinopathy and was associated with progression of retinopathy.[65] Further relevant evidence on blood pressure reduction in type 1 diabetics is reviewed in the section on drugs affecting the rennin–angiotensin system (see below).

Although clinical blood pressure readings are taken during the day, the possible effects of nocturnal blood pressure are also important. Nocturnal blood pressure is generally lower than daytime blood pressure. A nondipper is defined as a person in whom the nocturnal blood pressure is >0.9 times the daytime blood pressure, whether referring to diastolic or systolic blood pressure. In both types 1 and 2 diabetics who are normotensive and without renal impairment, severity of diabetic retinopathy has been associated with a decreased fall in nocturnal systolic blood pressure and nocturnal mean blood pressure, whereas no associations have been found with daytime blood pressure measurements.[66,67]

Despite the data demonstrating the importance of treating hypertension in patients with diabetic retinopathy, many ophthalmologists do not include blood pressure measurement in their routine care of diabetic patients thereby missing an opportunity to help to preserve sight and prevent cardiovascular adverse outcomes.[68] In one study, only 65% of type 2 diabetic patients requiring focal/grid photocoagulation for DME had blood pressure <140/80 with or without treatment, a level deemed by the British National Institute for Health and Clinical Excellence as suboptimal.[69] As with intensive glycemic control, more intensive antihypertensive therapy requires great effort by the patient. Almost one-third of patients in the UKPDS required three or more drugs to adequately control their blood pressure. Concerns about nocturnal hypotension and possibly related nonarteritic ischemic optic neuropathy have led to recommendations to avoid taking antihypertensive medications before bedtime.[70]

4.2.6 Serum Lipids

Elevated serum lipids have been speculated to cause or exacerbate diabetic retinopathy by several mechanisms. Oxidized low-density lipoprotein cholesterol may be toxic to capillary endothelium and pericytes by stimulating inflammation and release of cytokines.[71] They may increase serum viscosity and affect the fibrinolytic system.[72,73] Observational and epidemiologic studies inconsistently support an association of aspects of diabetic retinopathy with elevated serum lipids.[60,73,74] In a population-based epidemiologic study, univariate analysis showed a significant trend associating an increased severity of diabetic retinopathy and retinal hard lipid exudates with increased cholesterol in persons using insulin regardless of age, but this effect vanished in multivariate analysis.[75] Similarly, multiple logistic regression of NPDR, PDR, and DME against mean total cholesterol showed no association in a multi-ethnic California health maintenance organization.[36] The Veterans Affairs Diabetes Trial found no association of total cholesterol, LDL cholesterol, or HDL cholesterol with baseline retinopathy severity.[38] The Blue Mountains Eye Study found no association of baseline HDL cholesterol, total cholesterol, or triglycerides with progression of retinopathy.[60] A case series found that patients with significant hard lipid exudates had higher levels of serum triglycerides but not cholesterol compared to patients without such exudates.[74] In Korean type 2 diabetics, those with PDR had a higher lipoprotein (a) level than those without PDR after controlling for other factors associated with PDR.[76]

In the ETDRS, increased baseline cholesterol or low-density lipoproteins were associated with a higher frequency of hard exudates that were in turn associated with increased risk of visual loss.[77] Thus, by a chain of reasoning, but not by a direct study result, elevated serum lipid levels are indirectly associated with an increased risk of visual impairment from DME.[71] Multiple reports suggest that lipid-lowering therapy can reduce retinal hard exudates, but effects on visual acuity are inconsistent.[78,79] A diet restricted in animal fat and supplemented with unsaturated fat (corn oil diet) has been shown to reduce the severity of retinal hard lipid exudates. No beneficial effect on visual acuity was noted, although possibly because of the small number of participants.[80] Such diets are associated with reduced serum cholesterol and lipid levels. Oral clofibrate with or without androsterone is effective in reducing the severity of hard exudates in patients with diabetic retinopathy while simultaneously lowering serum cholesterol in patients with elevated baseline cholesterol.[78,81] Treatment did not affect visual acuity nor did it slow progression to proliferative retinopathy.[78,81]

In persons with type 1 diabetes mellitus, severity of retinopathy is positively associated with triglycerides and negatively associated with HDL cholesterol. Using nuclear magnetic resonance analysis of whole serum to determine concentrations of 15 different lipoprotein subclasses by particle size, diabetic retinopathy is negatively associated with VLDL size.[82] In a separate study of type 1 diabetes, high triglycerides and high LDL at baseline were also associated with subsequent progression of retinopathy at 2 years follow-up.[83] In the DCCT, the total-to-HDL cholesterol ratio and the LDL predicted development of CSME and retinal hard exudates after controlling for known confounders.[6] There were no associations of multiple lipid variables and other end points such as PDR and 3-step progression of retinopathy.[6] In EDIC, the 3-step progression of retinopathy was significantly higher in patients with hyperlipidemia at DCCT closeout (70% increase in risk for those with hyperlipidemia versus those without; $P=0.001$).[32] In WESDR among patients with younger onset diabetes, there was no association of baseline serum lipids and DME after controlling for HBA1c and other risk factors.[84] An elevated serum triglyceride level was a predictor of progression to PDR in a study of type 1 DM.[7]

Response of DME to focal/grid laser photocoagulation may depend on levels of various serum lipid fractions. In a retrospective study of 65 eyes of 39 patients with DME with either type 1 or 2 diabetes receiving focal/grid laser treatment, the visual acuity response was better in patients with normal serum triglycerides and HDL cholesterol than in patients with elevated triglycerides and low HDL cholesterol.[85]

Hydroxy-3-methylglutaryl coenzyme A reductase inhibitors (statins) are effective in reducing serum lipids and some evidence suggests that they can improve DME regression rates as an adjunctive therapy with focal/grid photocoagulation.[86,87] In a small clinical trial of patients with diabetic retinopathy and hypercholesterolemia, patients taking simvastatin 20 mg/day had less worsening of visual acuity and fundus fluorescein angiography indices of retinopathy severity than the placebo group after 6 months follow-up.[88] However, in a case–control study of male diabetic patients with newly detected diabetic retinopathy (cases) or not (controls) over a 4-year period, there was no association between statin use and incident diabetic retinopathy.[89]

4.2.7 Anemia

Cases have been published that suggest that anemia can exacerbate development of proliferative diabetic retinopathy and diabetic macular edema.[90–93] Correction of anemia by subcutaneous injections of erythropoietin has been associated with improvement in macular hard exudates and visual acuity, although not with changes in the pattern of fluorescein angiography.[90,91] In population-based studies, however, hematocrit has not been associated with prevalence or severity of diabetic retinopathy.[58]

4.2.8 Nephropathy

Epidemiologic data from WESDR suggested that proteinuria was associated with prevalence of DR and incidence of PDR in younger onset diabetics after controlling for other variables.[94,95] Other independent studies have agreed.[11,59] Proteinuria was an independent risk factor for 25-year incidence but not 10-year incidence of DME in type 1 DM.[23,24] Proteinuria was not associated with 10-year incidence of DME in older onset diabetics in WESDR.[23] Low serum albumin, which may be reflective of diabetic nephropathy, and microalbuminuria have been associated with more severe diabetic retinopathy.[38,58] In black type 1 diabetics, proteinuria was an independent risk factor for 6-year incidence of doubling of the visual angle.[25] Proteinuria was associated with severity of DR at baseline in older onset diabetics and in younger onset diabetics with duration of disease greater than 10 years.[15,16] Proteinuria was also associated with the 20- to 40-year cumulative incidence of PDR in type 1 diabetics.[96] The epidemiologic association of nephropathy and DR is inconsistent, however. In some studies no association has been found.[49,7,5,59]

Diabetes mellitus is one of many causes of the nephrotic syndrome characterized by massive proteinuria, hypoalbuminemia, and decrease in serum osmolarity. This, together with retention of salt and water, can exacerbate DME. Diuresis with furosemide can improve DME in such a situation.[97]

Hemodialysis has been associated with dilation of retinal vessels in patients with end-stage renal disease of varied etiology.[98] Retinal vessel dilation is an effect that in isolation would tend to exacerbate macular edema. The reduction of systemic salt and water associated with hemodialysis is apparently more important than the attendant retinal vascular dilation because hemodialysis in the setting of renal failure can improve or resolve DME.[99] Analogous improvement or sustained improvement initially brought on by hemodialysis has been reported after renal transplantation.[100] Renal transplantation has also been associated with stabilization of diabetic retinopathy.[100]

4.2.9 Pregnancy

Pregnancy can accelerate the course of diabetic retinopathy. Nonproliferative diabetic retinopathy and proliferative retinopathy develop in 18–58 and 5–16% of type 1 diabetic women who become pregnant, respectively.[101] The increased cardiac output, increased plasma volume, increased retinal blood flow, and occasional onset of anemia concomitant with pregnancy can be associated with new onset

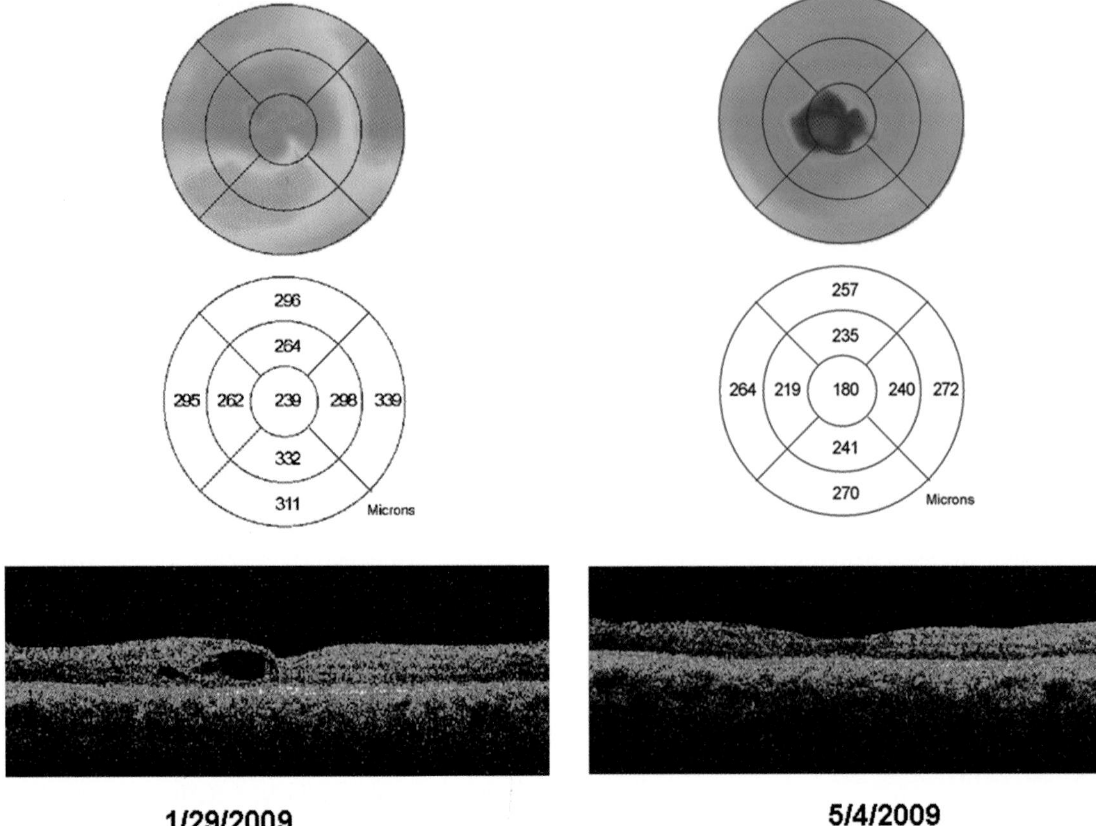

Fig. 4.6 OCTs illustrating the potential exacerbation of DME by pregnancy and the potential spontaneous resolution once delivery occurs. This 37-year-old woman had previously been treated with focal/grid laser photocoagulation for DME of the left eye with resolution. She became pregnant in July of 2008 and over the course of pregnancy experienced recurrent DME (*left panel*) that was observed rather than treated. The corrected visual acuity dropped from 20/25 to 20/32 during the pregnancy. She had an uneventful delivery in April of 2009, and at follow-up in May 2009, the pregnancy associated DME had spontaneously resolved with return of visual acuity to 20/25 (*right panel*)

DME that can resolve spontaneously after delivery (Fig. 4.6).[101,102] Development and progression of capillary nonperfusion is irreversible and can permanently impair visual acuity.[101] The progression of retinopathy during pregnancy is related to baseline retinopathy at conception with faster progression seen in patients with more advanced retinopathy.[103] Poorer glycemic control at conception and faster improvement early in pregnancy are additional risk factors associated with higher risk of progression of retinopathy.[104] There can be spontaneous regression of changes in nonproliferative retinopathy and even proliferative retinopathy after delivery, but if high-risk proliferative retinopathy develops, panretinal laser photocoagulation is indicated rather than observation with anticipation of spontaneous postpartum regression.[105,106] Proliferative diabetic retinopathy can develop rapidly, and more frequent ophthalmoscopic monitoring is required during pregnancy, especially when simultaneous hypertension exacerbates the situation.[101] Panretinal laser photocoagulation should be applied for high-risk PDR and appears as effective as in patients with similar degrees of retinopathy who are not pregnant.[101] Fetal morbidity and loss is higher in patients with proliferative diabetic retinopathy, but an earlier general recommendation that proliferative retinopathy is an indication for therapeutic abortion is now considered unsupported by the improved prognosis for fetal survival and maternal eyesight associated with advances in medical care.[107] The use of intraocular anti-VEGF drugs in the setting of pregnancy has not been reported and is fraught with concerns for adverse side effects for the fetus.

4.2.10 Other Systemic Factors

There are many other systemic factors that have been hypothesized to influence diabetic retinopathy. These factors are generally considered to have lesser impact, and in a number of cases the scant evidence available suggests that they have no impact. The waist-to-hip ratio has been associated with a higher incidence of DR and DME.[19,108] Use of diuretics, lower serum albumin, higher serum von Willebrand factor, and lower plasminogen activator inhibitor level have all been associated with worse DR.[58,38] Less alcohol consumption and hypomagnesemia have been associated with worse DR.[58,109] Lower serum growth hormone has been associated with relative protection from DR.[110] Factors that have not been found to have an association with aspects of diabetic retinopathy include elevated total cholesterol[7,36,58–60,12], HDL-cholesterol[19,58,60,12], LDL cholesterol[61], non-HDL cholesterol[19], lipoprotein (a)[58], serum creatinine[12], frequency of exercise[5], smoking[11,5,7,13,19,49,58,60], use of aspirin[13], hematocrit[58], white blood cell count[58], platelet count[58], use of beta blockers[58], serum fibrinogen[38,60], and diabetic neuropathy[49].

In several cases, the evidence for associations is inconsistent as for example in the case of hyperhomocysteinemia[111,112,113]. Table 4.3 shows selected characteristics inconsistently associated with DR across studies.

4.2.11 Influence on Visual Loss

The influence of systemic factors on visual loss, summarized by the index doubling of the visual angle, is shown in Table 4.4. All of these data derive from

Table 4.3 Inconsistent relationships of various systemic factors to prevalence, incidence, or severity of diabetic retinopathy

Factor	Positive association reported	No association detected
Body mass index	11	12;5;13;19;19;24;50;58;60
Serum triglycerides	38	7;19;59;60
Systolic BP	38;36;58	12
Diastolic BP	12	38;58
Proteinuria (higher prevalence)	11;59	5;7;59
Presence of macrovascular disease	58 (stroke) 38 (amputation)	5, 49;58 (CAD) 11;38 (stroke, CABG) 59
Hyperhomocysteinemia	111	112;113

Factors in the left-hand column have been tested for an association with presence of or severity of diabetic retinopathy. Columns 2 and 3 list studies that report a positive association or lack of an association, respectively. Results of multivariate testing were taken if the univariate and multivariate results were discordant. BP = blood pressure; CAD = coronary artery disease; CABG = coronary artery bypass grafting.

Table 4.4 Influence of Systematic Factors on Doubling of the Visual Angle in Three Types of Diabetes Mellitus

	Younger onset	Older onset, taking insulin	Older onset, not taking insulin
Increasing baseline HbA1C	X	X	(X)
Higher SBP	X	X	
Higher DBP	X		X
Proteinuria	X	X	
Smoking history			X
Smoking pack years	X		X (but in a paradoxical direction)
DME	X	X	X
Retinopathy severity	X	X	X

Data for visual impairment are similar to data for doubling of visual angle for each group. Empty cells mean no association was found on univariate analysis. A black X means that an association was found on univariate analysis. A red X means that the association persisted in a multivariate analysis. The analyses at 10 and 14 years were similar in results, but in the few cases where they differed, the 14-year results are shown. The parenthesis means that the association was present on multivariate analysis only. All data from Moss[114].

WESDR. Less information is available for African Americans with type 1 DM. From the New Jersey 725 study, baseline poor glycemic control and proteinuria were predictors for higher 6-year incidence rates of doubling of the visual angle.[25]

4.3 Effects of Systemic Drugs

4.3.1 Diuretics

In a univariate analysis, the use of diuretics by patients with diabetes was associated with more severe diabetic retinopathy.[58] Furosemide has been associated with improvement in DME in a patient with the nephrotic syndrome.[97] This clinical observation contradicts the implication of an experimental study in monkeys showing inhibition of the retinal pigment epithelial pump by furosemide and was explained by hypothesizing a normalization of vascular oncotic pressure in the patient with nephrotic syndrome.[97,115] History of diuretic use at baseline was not associated with 10-year incidence of DME in WESDR.[23]

4.3.2 Renin–Angiotensin System Drugs

The renin–angiotensin system is a biochemical pathway active within the retina and suspected to be of clinical importance in the regulation of retinovascular tone and inflammatory pathways (see Chapter 1).[116,117] Renin cleaves angiotensinogen to yield angiotensin I, which is in turn cleaved by angiotensin-converting enzyme (ACE) or chymase into angiotensin II. Angiotensin II binds to the angiotensin II receptor (type I) to produce vasoconstriction and activation of nuclear factor-κB. ACE inhibitors and angiotensin receptor (type 1) blockers treat hypertension by inhibiting this pathway, leading to vasodilation.[117] Angiotensin II also promotes angiogenesis and increased vascular permeability, providing a rationale for how ACE inhibitors might beneficially affect DME and progression to PDR.[116]

The clinical effects of drugs designed to act at various points of the RAS pathway have been inconsistent. In a controlled, open label study, the ACE inhibitor lisinopril was effective in reducing DME.[118] An acute decrease in blood pressure associated with a dose of captopril in hypertensive diabetics with nonproliferative retinopathy was not associated with an acute change in the blood–retinal barrier permeability, but over 6 months of captopril therapy the permeability declined.[119,120] In normotensive diabetics treated with captopril for 18 months, the blood–retinal barrier permeability also declined.[121] The EURODIAB Controlled Trial of Lisinopril in Insulin-Dependent Diabetes examined normotensive patients randomized to lisinopril 10–20 mg/day or placebo over 2 years of follow-up. Retinopathy severity was graded from fundus photographs and retinopathy end points were secondary outcomes. The odds ratios for risk of progression by two levels of retinopathy severity was 0.27 (95% CI 0.07–1.99, $P=0.05$) and for progression to PDR was 0.18 (95% CI 0.04–0.82, $P=0.03$).[122] A meta-analysis of four clinical studies of ACE inhibitors on progression of DR led to a conclusion of a suggested beneficial effect.[117]

On the other hand, the ACE inhibitor captopril was no more effective than atenolol in retarding progression of retinopathy in the UKPDS.[61] In a univariate analysis from a separate epidemiologic study, the use of angiotensin-converting enzyme inhibitors by patients with diabetes was associated with more severe, rather than less severe, diabetic retinopathy.[58]

In a trial of candesartan, a blocker of the angiotensin receptor (type 1), in which retinopathy end points were the primary outcomes, results depended on the presence or absence of retinopathy at baseline. Treatment of type 1 diabetic patients without retinopathy at baseline showed a reduction in incidence of 3-step progression of retinopathy at 4.7 years of follow-up.[123] In a parallel study involving patients with baseline diabetic retinopathy and similar follow-up, candesartan did not affect 3-step progression of retinopathy.[123] A phase 2 randomized clinical trial is presently underway comparing the renin inhibitor aliskiren versus amlopidine in patients with hypertension and DME (Novartis protocol SPP100A2244). Further work will be needed to unravel the complicated effects of the RAS pathway on DR.

4.3.3 Aldose Reductase Inhibitors

Aldose reductase inhibitors are hypothesized to be useful in treating diabetic retinopathy based on two mechanisms. First, hyperglycemia can cause increases in intracellular sorbitol mediated by the enzyme aldose reductase. Increased intracellular sorbitol in turn causes cytoplasmic swelling via osmosis. Second, the conversion of glucose to sorbitol catalyzed by aldose reductase requires NADPH as a cofactor. By depleting cellular NADPH supplies, the aldose reductase reaction reduces intracellular defenses against reactive oxygen species. Aldose reductase inhibitors thus act in two ways to mitigate the adverse effects of hyperglycemia.

Two aldose reductase inhibitors have been used clinically in the context of diabetic retinopathy. Sorbinil slightly reduces the rate of new microaneurysm formation. Tolrestat decreases leakage from focal intraretinal lesions on fluorescein angiography. Both effects, however, can be achieved by glucose control itself, and in clinical practice, the minimal beneficial effects and significant side effects of these drugs have prevented their widespread adoption as a method of treating diabetic retinopathy.[55]

4.3.4 Drugs That Target Platelets

Forty-five years ago it was observed that patients with rheumatoid arthritis taking aspirin who also had diabetes seemed to have a lower prevalence of DR than would have been expected, prompting the hypothesis that aspirin might be a medical therapy for DR.[124] The hypothesis is rational because of evidence that capillary microthrombi are important in the pathogenesis of diabetic retinopathy and that hyperglycemia impairs platelet function.[125] Subsequently, anti-platelet aggregation drugs have been studied in clinical trials designed to investigate their effects on diabetic retinopathy.[55]

Aspirin decreases platelet aggregation by inhibiting platelet cyclooxygenase-1. This in turn reduces production of thromboxane A2, a mediator of platelet aggregation. In a clinical trial of aspirin 1 g orally per day compared to placebo, there was a statistically significant but clinically unimpressive decrease in microaneurysm counts associated with aspirin use. The lack of a clinically important effect together with a high incidence of gastrointestinal side effects with this high-dose aspirin therapy has not led to widespread advocacy of aspirin therapy for early diabetic retinopathy, but many patients do take such therapy for cardiovascular indications.[55,126] Worries that aspirin therapy might lead to worse vitreous hemorrhaging in more advanced diabetic retinopathy was one concern studied in the ETDRS. In that study, the risk of vitreous hemorrhage and visual loss in the aspirin group was no higher than in the placebo group. In addition, progression of retinopathy was no different between the aspirin and control groups.[127] Other studies provide supportive evidence of lack of effect of aspirin on time to occurrence or recurrence rates of diabetic vitreous hemorrhage.[128] There is no evidence that aspirin use influences prevalence of DR.[13,23] The 10-year incidence of DME in both younger onset and older onset diabetics was not associated with baseline use of aspirin.[23]

Dipyridamole inhibits platelet aggregation by inhibiting platelet reuptake of adenosine and inhibiting platelet adenosine deaminase, both actions that increase extracellular adenosine concentrations, an anti-platelet aggregation mechanism independent of that of aspirin. A clinical trial comparing combination therapy with aspirin 1 g orally per day and dipyridamole 25 mg orally per day reduced microaneurysm counts compared to placebo and compared to aspirin alone. The effect, although statistically significant, was clinically unimpressive, and such therapy has not been adopted for the treatment of diabetic retinopathy. As with aspirin monotherapy, there are many patients who take such combined therapy for independent cardiovascular indications, and they may be accruing a small benefit with regard to their retinopathy.[55,126]

Ticlopidine is an adenosine diphosphate receptor inhibitor that reduces platelet aggregation. Oral therapy reduced microaneurysm counts but side effects such as thrombotic thrombocytopenic purpura and neutropenia outweighed the retinopathy benefits, and in general it is not used for the treatment of diabetic retinopathy.[55]

In summary, considerable basic science suggests that anti-platelet drugs might have beneficial effects on DR, but no clinical trials have yet proven their importance.[129] It is possible that different dosing regimens or combinations of drugs may realize the promise of this therapeutic avenue.[130]

4.3.5 Statins

Hydroxymethylglutaryl coenzyme A reductase inhibitors (HMGCaA reductase inhibitors, or statins) have been associated with a reduction in recurrence rates of diabetic vitreous hemorrhage and reduction in rates of retinopathy progression in small clinical studies.[88,128] In a case–control chart review, use of statins was not associated with reduced development of diabetic retinopathy.[89] Statins may have beneficial effects on diabetic retinopathy by reduction of serum cholesterol levels, by direct anti-apoptosis effects on retinal endothelial cells, and by protection of the blood–retinal barrier through anti-inflammatory effects.[72,131] Statins may also change the response to focal/grid laser for DME. In a small randomized trial, atorvastatin increased the resolution in macular hard exudates at 18 weeks following laser treatment compared to patients with similar severity of DME not receiving drug.[86]

4.3.6 Protein Kinase C Inhibitors

Protein kinase C β (PKC β) is activated in diabetes with multiple effects linked to development and progression of DR including thickening of basement membranes, increased leukocyte vascular adhesion, increased vascular permeability, and prolongation of retinal circulation time (see Chapter 1).[132,133] Ruboxistaurin is a PKC β inhibitor that has been shown to reduce the progression of DME > 100 μm from the center of the macula to DME <100 μm from the center of the macula in a randomized clinical trial over 3 years.[134] In addition, the drug reduced the frequency of sustained moderate visual acuity loss, the rate of decrease of visual acuity associated with severe DME, and the need for focal/grid laser treatment.[134,135] Ruboxistaurin is in continued phase 3 randomized trials and is not available for clinical use.

4.3.7 Thiazolidinediones (Glitazones)

Thiazolidinediones are oral antidiabetic drugs that bind to peroxisome proliferator–activator receptor gamma and act as insulin sensitizers. They have been found to raise plasma vascular endothelial growth factor and to be associated with peripheral edema in 3–7.5% of patients taking them, especially when used in combination with insulin.[136–138] Retrospective case reports and case series have suggested that use of these drugs may be associated with induction or exacerbation of DME.[139,131,141] Cessation of thiazolidinedione use led to reduction of DME in 73% and resolution of DME in 36% of patient, respectively.[140] A case–control study did not show a higher incidence of DME in diabetics taking thiazolidinediones as might have been expected from the anecdotal reports, but did show a delay in progression of severe NPDR to PDR in patients taking these drugs.[142] A prospective cohort study from a managed care organization with 170,000 diabetic patients showed that thiazolidinedione use was associated with DME with an odds ratio of 2.6 (95% CI 2.4–3.0).[143]

4.3.8 Miscellaneous Drugs

Use of oral hypoglycemic drugs has been associated with an increased 4-year incidence of DR compared to management of diabetes by diet.[18] The atypical antipsychotic drug risperidone has been reported to exacerbate diabetes and has been associated with lipemia retinalis.[144]

4.4 Ocular Factors Influencing Diabetic Retinopathy

Diabetic retinopathy severity is affected by certain ocular factors.[58] In a multivariate model incorporating demographic variables (age, gender, race, duration of diabetes, stroke history, coronary artery disease history, drinking history, smoking history) and systemic variables (fasting blood glucose, diabetes medications, serum lipids, blood pressure, hypertension medication use, diuretic use, and certain laboratory tests), the following ocular variables were associated with increasing severity of DR: smaller retinal arteriole/venule ratio, presence of retinal A/V nicking, and focal arteriolar narrowing.[58] In black type

1 diabetics, greater baseline retinopathy severity is an independent risk factor for 6-year incidence of doubling of the visual angle.[25]

In WESDR, greater baseline retinopathy severity was associated with a higher incidence rate of DME in both younger and older onset diabetics (Figs. 4.7 and 4.8).[23] Other studies have confirmed the association in type 1 diabetics.[24] Using the state of no DR as the reference level, and a modification of the ETDRS adaptation of the modified Airlie House classification of DR (see Chapter 5), the hazard ratios for incidence of DME for retinopathy severity levels 21 (minimal NPDR), 31–37 (mild NPDR), 43–53 (moderate–severe NPDR), and 60+ (PDR) were 1.52, 2.71, 3.26, and 3.40, respectively.[24]

In addition to systemic factors associated with progression of retinopathy, certain ocular factors are predictive. The main ocular factor associated with progression to PDR in type 1 DM is presence of NPDR.[7] In WESDR, multivariate analyses showed that less severe retinopathy at baseline was associated with ≥2-step progression of DR severity.[4]

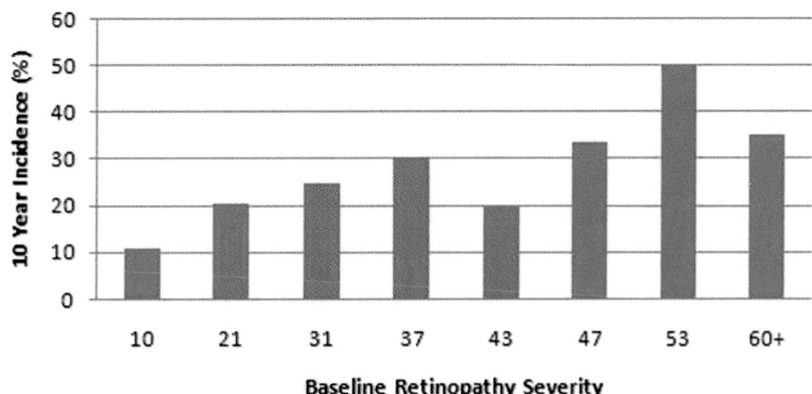

Fig. 4.7 Graph of the 10-year incidence of DME in younger onset diabetics in WESDR by baseline DR severity. Data from Klein et al.[23] The definitions of the retinopathy severity

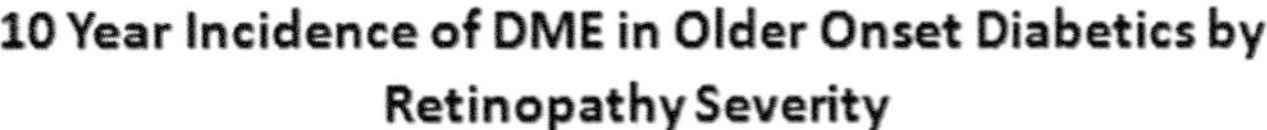

levels follow: 10 = no diabetic retinopathy; 21, 31, 37, 43, 47, and 53 = nonproliferative diabetic retinopathy of increasing severity; and 60+ = proliferative diabetic retinopathy

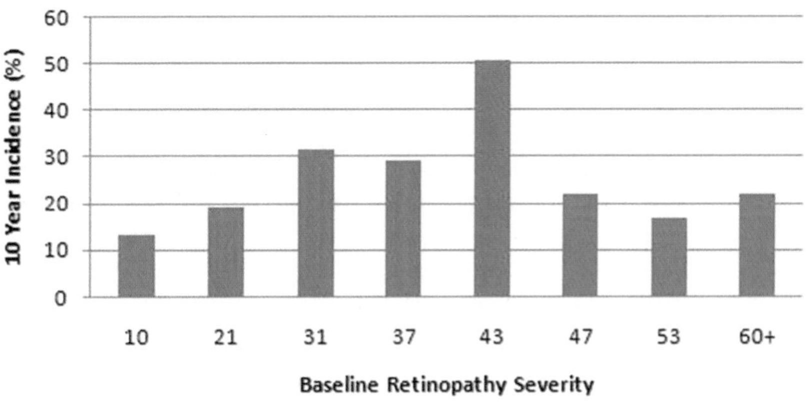

Fig. 4.8 Graph of the 10-year incidence of DME in older onset diabetics regardless of insulin use in WESDR by baseline DR severity. Data from Klein et al.[23] The definitions of the retinopathy severity levels follow: 10 = no diabetic retinopathy; 21, 31, 37, 43, 47, and 53 = nonproliferative diabetic retinopathy of increasing severity; and 60+ = proliferative diabetic retinopathy

Greater baseline severity of diabetic retinopathy was associated with a higher rate of progression to proliferative retinopathy in the ETDRS. Of eyes with levels 35 (mild NPDR), 43, and 47 (moderate NPDR), and 53 (severe NPDR) retinopathy at baseline, 15.2, 21, 27, and 57.8%, respectively, progressed to high-risk proliferative diabetic retinopathy after 5-year follow-up.[145] A similar result was found in the UKPDS in patients with type 2 diabetes. In patients with no retinopathy at baseline, 0.2 and 2.6% required photocoagulation at 3 and 9 years of follow-up, respectively.[146] In patients with microaneurysms or more severe retinopathy in both eyes at baseline, 15.3 and 31.9% required laser photocoagulation at 3 and 9 years, respectively. The commonest indication for laser treatment was diabetic macular edema.[146] In adult patients with type 1 diabetes, there was an association of larger arteriolar and venular caliber with progression of retinopathy severity from mild to severe and with development of proliferative diabetic retinopathy.[147]

Diabetic retinopathy is generally symmetric between the two eyes. The Spearman correlation coefficient between the two eyes for diabetic retinopathy severity at 10-year follow-up in WESDR was 0.90, 0.82, and 0.82 for the younger onset, older onset taking insulin, and older onset not taking insulin groups, respectively.[148] Thus, asymmetry of retinopathy provides clues regarding protective or predisposing ocular risk factors for retinopathy. Some factors associated with protection from PDR are optic atrophy, higher intraocular pressure, unilateral glaucoma, and chorioretinal scarring.[149–152] Bilateral glaucoma has not been found to influence prevalence of DR.[13] Myopia has been inconsistently associated with protection from diabetic retinopathy; higher degrees of myopia seem to provide more protection when an association has been discerned.[13,153] Although ipsilateral carotid occlusive disease was raised as a possible protective factor against development of PDR in a study based on ophthalmodynamometry, a later prospective study using fluorescein angiography to document neovascularization found no association.[154,155] There are also regionally protective factors for diabetic retinopathy within the same eye. For example, diabetic eyes with tilted disk syndrome and inferior staphylomas may have sparing from diabetic retinopathy in the area of the thinner retina inferiorly.[156]

4.5 Diabetic Retinopathy and Associated Comorbidity

Systemic factors influence not only diabetic retinopathy but also aspects of diabetic retinopathy can be warning signs regarding systemic health. In a population-based study of adults aged 40 and above in Beijing, diabetic-like retinopathy was an independent predictor of all cause mortality.[157] In population-based studies from the Australia and the United States, baseline presence of retinopathy was associated with increased mortality from coronary heart disease and cardiovascular disease (coronary heart disease and stroke), respectively.[158,159] Presence of CSME was significantly associated with all cause mortality and ischemic heart disease mortality in patients with type 2 diabetes, but not with type 1 diabetes.[160] In two independent Finnish population-based studies, PDR in type 2 DM was associated with coronary heart disease death.[161,162] In the Atherosclerosis Risk in Communities Study, presence of DR at baseline was associated with a higher rate of congestive heart failure after 9 years of follow-up.[163] Such broad-based evidence across multiple countries suggests that patients with diabetic retinopathy need heightened surveillance for the detection of cardiovascular disease.[160,163] DME may be an indicator of generalized vascular hyperpermeability as reflected in urinary albumin excretion and transcapillary escape of albumin.[164]

4.6 Economic Consequences

Glycemic control has economic consequences. In a modeling study based on existing epidemiologic studies, a change in the average HbA1c level for the population from 7.25 to 9.6 was associated with an increase in 30-year average direct medical cost to manage the diabetic complications from \$35,000 to \$49,000, other variables being held constant.[165] Conversion from conventional to intensive glucose control has been predicted to cost \$19,987 per quality adjusted life year gained, a number well within the range considered to represent a good value.[31,166]

4.7 Summary of Key Points

- Systemic associations with diabetic retinopathy are often overlooked. Their recognition offers approaches to treatment that may help ocular outcomes and other aspects of health as well.
- Retinopathy identical to that associated with diabetes is seen in 5–10% of persons over age 40 who do not have diabetes mellitus as conventionally defined.
- In type 1 diabetes mellitus, there is no glycemic threshold below which further reduction in HbA1c toward normal does not result in further improvement in retinopathy end points, but the risk of hypoglycemia correspondingly goes up as well. A HbA1c goal is therefore an individualized decision for each patient. In general, a goal of 7.0% strikes a balance between benefits and risks.
- Metabolic memory is a term indicating that glycemic control has consequences for retinopathy progression that persist for years. Tight control early in the course of diabetes is thus a goal.
- Rapid improvement in glycemic control can cause short-term worsening of retinopathy, but is still associated with long-term better outcomes than continued conventional control.
- Lowering blood pressure benefits multiple aspects of DR in all subtypes of the disease.
- Awareness of the potential for pregnancy to be associated with rapid progression of DR, of the need for a screening examination early in the course of pregnancy, and of the need for follow-up examinations calibrated according to the severity of retinopathy will prevent unnecessary visual loss.
- Patients with renal insufficiency can manifest DME that is better managed at the systemic level first before considering specific ocular intervention such as laser photocoagulation. Control of blood pressure, systemic fluid retention, and anemia can lead to resolution of edema in such cases.
- Patients with more advanced diabetic retinopathy need systemic monitoring for coronary artery disease and peripheral vascular disease as their risk is higher compared to patients without retinopathy.

4.8 Future Directions

Continuous improvement in glucose monitoring techniques with the possibility of eliminating fingersticks and more widespread use of insulin pumps may help more diabetics achieve intensive glycemic control with beneficial effects on retinopathy and other complications. Improved communication between internists, who manage the important systemic risk factors, and ophthalmologists, who monitor the retinopathy, may be expected in an era of increasing use of the electronic medical record with benefits for outcomes. The relationship of many drugs with potential effects on the retina and the course of DR is largely unexplored and will probably increase in the future. Because of possible interactions of multiple drugs, large databases will be advantageous in such investigations, again aided by the increasing adoption of the electronic medical record.

References

1. Klein R. Is intensive management of blood pressure to prevent visual loss in persons with type 2 diabetes indicated? *Arch Ophthalmol.* 2004;122:1707–1709.
2. Rabb MF, Gagliano DA, Sweeney HE. Diabetic retinopathy in blacks. *Diabetes Care.* 1990;13:1202–1206.
3. Roy MS, Affouf M. Six-year progression of retinopathy and associated risk factors in African American patients with type 1 diabetes mellitus. *Arch Ophthalmol.* 2006;124:1297–1306.
4. Klein R, Knudtson MD, Lee KE, Gangnon R, Klein BEK. The Wisconsin epidemiologic study of diabetic retinopathy XXII. The twenty five year progression of retinopathy in persons with type 1 diabetes. *Ophthalmology.* 2008;115:1859–1868.
5. Chen MS, Kao CS, Chang CJ, Wu TJ, Fu CC, Chen CJ, et al. Prevalence and risk factors of diabetic retinopathy among nonisulin-dependent diabetic subjects. *Am J Ophthalmol.* 1992;114:723–730.
6. Miljanovic B, Glynn RJ, Nathan DM, Manson JE, Schaumberg DA. A prospective study of serum lipids and risk of diabetic macular edema in type 1 diabetes. *Diabetes.* 2004;53:2883–2892.
7. Skrivarhaug T, Fosmark DS, Stene LC, Bangstad HJ, Sandvik L, Hanssen KF, et al. Low cumulative incidence of proliferative diabetic retinopathy in childhood-onset type 1 diabetes: a 24 year follow-up study. *Diabetologia.* 2006;49:2281–2290.
8. Meyer-Schwickerath G, Schott K. Diabetic retinopathy and photocoagulation. *Am J Ophthalmology.* 1968;66: 597–603.

9. Diabetes Control and Complications Trial Research Group. Progression of retinopathy with intensive versus conventional treatment in the diabetes control and complications trial. *Ophthalmology*. 1995;102:647–661.
10. UK Prospective Diabetes Study (UKPDS) Group. Intensive blood-glucose control with sulphonylureas or insulin compared with conventional treatment and risk of complications in patients with type 2 diabetes (UKPDS 33). *Lancet*. 1998;352:837–853.
11. Rema M, Premkumar S, Anitha B, Deepa R, Pradeepa R, Mohan V. Prevalence of diabetic retinopathy in urban India: the Chennai urban rural epidemiology study (CURES) eye study, I. *Invest Ophthalmol Vis Sci*. 2005; 46:2328–2333.
12. Cugati S, Kifley A, Mitchell P, Wang JJ. Temporal trends in the age-specific prevalence of diabetes and diabetic retinopathy in older persons: population-based survey findings. *Diab Res Clin Pract*. 2006;74: 301–308.
13. McKay R, McCarty CA, Taylor HR. Diabetic retinopathy in Victoria, Australia: the visual impairment project. *Br J Ophthalmol*. 2000;84:865–870.
14. Tapp RJ, Shaw JE, Harper CA, de Courten MP, Balkau B, McCarty DJ, et al. The prevalence of and factors associated with diabetic retinoapthy in the Australian population. *Diabetes Care*. 2003;26:1731–1737.
15. Klein R, Klein BEK, Moss SE, et al. The Wisconsin epidemiologic study of diabetic retinopathy. III. Prevalence and risk of retinopathy when age at diagnosis is 30 or more years. *Arch Ophthalmol*. 1984;102:527–532.
16. Klein R, Klein BEK, Moss SE, et al. The Wisconsin epidemiologic study of diabetic retinopathy. II. Prevalence and risk of diabetic retinopathy when age at diagnosis is less than 30 years. *Arch Ophthalmol*. 1984;102: 520–526.
17. Cugati S, Cikamatana L, Wang JJ, Kifley A, Liew G, Mitchell P. Five-year incidence and progression of vascular retinopathy in persons without diabetes: the Blue Mountains eye study. *Eye*. 2006;20:1239–1245.
18. Leske MC, Wu SY, Hennis A, Nemesure B, Hyman L, Schachat A, et al. Incidence of diabetic retinopathy in the Barbados Eye Studies. *Ophthalmology*. 2003;110:941–947.
19. van Leiden HA, Dekker JM, Moll AC, Nijpels G, Heine RJ, Bouter LM, et al. Risk factors for incident retinopathy in a diabetic and nondiabetic population. The Hoorn Study. *Arch Ophthalmol*. 2003;121:245–251.
20. Yu T, Mitchell P, Berry G, Li W, Wang JJ. Retinopathy in older persons without diabetes and its relationship to hypertension. *Arch Ophthalmol*. 1998;116:83–89.
21. Do DV, Shah SM, Sung JU, Haller JA, Nguyen QD. Persistent diabetic macular edema is associated with elevated hemoglobin A1c. *Am J Ophthalmol*. 2005;139: 620–623.
22. Stolk RP, Vingerling JR, de Jong PT, Dielemans I, Hofman A, Lamberts SW, et al. Retinopathy, glucose, and insulin in an elderly population. The Rotterdam Study. *Diabetes*. 1995;44:11–15.
23. Klein R, Klein BE, Moss SE, Cruikshanks KJ. The Wisconsin epidemiologic study of diabetic retinopathy. XV. The long-term incidence of macular edema. *Ophthalmology*. 1995;102:7–16.
24. Klein R, Knudtson MD, Lee KE, Gangnon R, Klein BEK. The Wisconsin epidemiologic study of diabetic retinopathy XXIII: the twenty-five year incidence of macular edema in persons with type 1 diabetes. *Ophthalmology*. 2009;116:497–503.
25. Roy MS, Skurnick J. Six-year incidence of visual loss in African Americans with type 1 diabetes mellitus. *Arch Ophthalmol*. 2007;125:1061–1067.
26. Epidemiology of Diabetes Interventions and Complications (EDIC) Research Group. Epidemiology of Diabetes Interventions and Complications (EDIC); design, implementation, and preliminary results of a long-term follow-up of the Diabetes control and complications trial cohort. *Diabetes Care*. 1999;22:99–111.
27. The Writing Team for the Diabetes Control and Complications Trial/Epidemiology of Siabetes Interventions and Complications Research Group. Effect of intensive therapy on the microvascular complications of type 1 diabetes mellitus. *JAMA*. 2002;287:2563–2569.
28. Aiello LM. Perspectives on diabetic retinopathy. *Am J Ophthalmol*. 2003;136:122–135.
29. The Diabetes Control and Complications Trial Research Group. The relationship of glycemic exposure (HbA1c) to the risk of development and progression of retinopathy in the diabetes control and complications trial. *Diabetes*. 1995;44:968–983.
30. Diabetes Control and Complications Trial Research Group. The absence of a glycemic threshold for the development of long-term complications: the perspective of the diabetes control and complications trial. *Diabetes*. 1996;45:1289–1298.
31. Diabetes Control and Complications Trial Research Group. Lifetime benefits and costs of intensive therapy as practiced in the diabetes control and complications trial. *JAMA*. 1996;276:1409–1415.
32. Diabetes Control and Complications Trial/Epidemiology of Diabetes Interventions and Complications Research Group. Prolonged effect of intensive therapy on the risk of retinopathy complications in patients with type 1 diabetes mellitus: 10 years after the diabetes control and complications trial. *Arch Ophthalmol*. 2008; 126:1707–1715.
33. The Diabetes Control and Complications Trial Research Group. The effect of intensive diabetes treatment on the progression of diabetic retinopathy in insulin-dependent diabetes mellitus. The diabetes control and complications trial. *Arch Ophthalmol*. 1995;113:36–51.
34. The DCCT Research Group. Epidemiology of severe hypoglycemia in the diabetes control and complications trial. *Am J Med*. 1991;90:450–459.
35. Wing RR, Cleary PA, The DCCT Research Group. Weight gain associated with intensive therapy in the diabetes control and complications trial. *Diabetes Care*. 1988;11:567–573.
36. Brown JB, Pedula KL, Summers KH. Diabetic retinopathy. Contemporary prevalence in a well-controlled population. *Diabetes Care*. 2003;26:2637–2642.
37. Kalesnykiene V, Sorri I, Voutilainen R, Uusitupa M, Niskanen L, Uusitalo H. The effect of glycemic control on the quantitative characteristics of retinopathy lesions in patients with type 2 diabetes mellitus: 10 year follow-up study. *Graefe's Arch Clin Exp Ophthalmol*. 2009;247: 335–341.

38. Emanuele N, Sacks J, Klein R, Reda D, Anderson R, Duckworth W, et al. Ethnicity, race, and baseline retinopathy correlates in the veterans affairs diabetes trial. *Diabetes Care*. 2005;28:1954–1958.
39. The ADVANCE Collaborative Group. Intensive blood glucose control and vascular outcomes in patients with type 2 diabetes. *N Engl J Med*. 2008;358:2560–2572.
40. Skyler JS, Bergenstal R, Bonow RO, Buse J, Deedwania P, Gale EAM, et al. Intensive glycemic control and the prevention of cardiovascular events: implications of the ACCORD, ADVANCE, and VA diabetes trials: a position statement of the American Diabetes Association and a scientific statement of the American College of Cardiology Foundation and the American Heart Association. *Diabetes Care*. 2009;32:187–192.
41. Chantelau E, Meyer-Schwickerath R. Reversion of "early worsening" of diabetic retinopathy by deliberate restoration of poor metabolic control. *Ophthalmologica*. 2003;217:373–377.
42. Diabetes Control and Complications Trial Research Group. Early worsening of diabetic retinopathy in the diabetes control and complications trial. *Arch Ophthalmol*. 1998;116:874–886.
43. Chantelau E. Evidence that upregulation of serum IGF-1 concentration can trigger acceleration of diabetic retinopathy. *Br J Ophthalmol*. 1998;82:725–730.
44. Kroc Collaborative Study Group. Blood glucose control and the evolution of diabetic retinopathy and albuminuria. *New Engl J Med*. 1984;311:365–372.
45. Klein R. Has the frequency of proliferative diabetic retinopathy declined in the US? *Diabetes Care*. 2003;26: 2691–2692.
46. Knott RM. Insulin-like growth factor type 1 – friend or foe? *Br J Ophthalmol*. 1998;82:719–721.
47. Suto C, Hori S, Kato S, Muraoka K, Kitano S. Effect of perioperative glycemic control in progression of diabetic retinopathy and maculopathy. *Arch Ophthalmol*. 2008; 124:38–45.
48. Bragd J, Adamson U, Backlund LB, Lins PE, Moberg E, Oskarsson P. Can glycaemic variability, as calculated from blood glucose self-monitoring, predict the development of complications in type 1 diabetes over a decade? *Diabetes Metab*. 2008;34:612–616.
49. Raman R, Rani PK, Rachepalle SR, Gnanamoorthy P, Uthra S, Kumaramanickavel G, et al. Prevalence of diabetic retinopathy in India. Sankara Nethralaya diabetic retinopathy epidemiology and molecular genetics study report 2. *Ophthalmology*. 2009;116:311–318.
50. Narendran V, John RK, Raghuram A, Ravindran RD, Nirmalan PK, Thulasiraj RD. Diabetic retinopathy among self reported diabetics in southern India: a population based assessment. *Br J Ophthalmol*. 2002;86:1014–1018.
51. Ramsay R, Goetz F, Sutherland E, Mauer S, Robison L, Cantrill H, et al. Progression of diabetic retinopathy after pancreas transplantation for insulin-dependent diabetes mellitus. *New Engl J Med*. 1988;318:208–214.
52. Bandello F, Vigano C, Secchi A, Martinenghi S, Di Carlo V, Pozza G, et al. Diabetic retinopathy after successful kidney-pancreas allotransplantation: a survey of 18 patients. *Graefe's Arch Clin Exp Ophthalmol*. 1991; 229:315–318.
53. Friberg TR, Tzakis AG, Carroll PB, Starzl TE. Visual improvement after long-term success of pancreatic transplantation. *Am J Ophthalmol*. 1990;110:564–565.
54. Sinclair SH, Grunwald JE, Riva CE, Braunstein SN, Nichols CW, Schwartz SS. Retinal vascular autoregulation in diabetes mellitus. *Ophthalmology*. 1982;89:748–750.
55. Donaldson M, Dodson PM. Medical treatment and diabetic retinopathy. *Eye*. 2003;17:550–562.
56. Knowler WC, Bennett PH, Ballintine EJ. Increased incidence of retinopathy in diabetics with elevated blood pressure. *N Engl J Med*. 1980;302:645–650.
57. Klein R. Is blood pressure a predictor of the incidence or progression of diabetic retinopathy? *Arch Intern Med*. 1989;149:2427–2432.
58. Klein R, Sharrett AR, Klein BEK, Moss SE, Folsom AR, Wong TY, et al. The association of atherosclerosis, vascular risk factors, and retinopathy in adults with diabetes. The atherosclerosis risk in communities study. *Ophthalmology*. 2002;109:1225–1234.
59. Al-Maskari F, El-Sadig M. Prevalence of diabetic retinopathy in the United Arab Emirates: a cross-sectional survey. *BMC Ophthalmol*. 2007;7:11–19.
60. Cikamatana L, Mitchell P, Rochtchina E, Foran S, Wang JJ. Five-year incidence and progression of diabetic retinopathy in a defined older population: the Blue Mountains eye study. *Eye*. 2007;21:465–471.
61. UK Prospective Diabetes Study Group. Tight blood pressure control and risk of macrovascular and microvascular complications of type 2 diabetes: UKPDS 38. *BMJ*. 1998;317:703–713.
62. UK Prospective Diabetes Study (UKPDS) Group. Risks of progression of retinopathy and vision loss related to tight blood pressure control in type 2 diabetes mellitus. *Arch Ophthalmol*. 2004;122:1631–1640.
63. UK Prospective Diabetes Study Group. Efficacy of atenolol and captopril in reducing risk of macrovascular and microvascular complications in type 2 diabetes: UKPDS 39. *BMJ*. 1998;317:713–720.
64. Schrier RW, Estacio RO, Esler A, Mehler P. Effects of aggressive blood pressure control in normotensive type 2 diabetic patients on albuminuria, retinopathy and strokes. *Kidney Int*. 2002;61:1086–1097.
65. Chase HP, Garg SK, Jackson WE, Thomas MA, Harris S, Marshall G, et al. Blood pressure and retinopathy in type I diabetes. *Ophthalmology*. 1990;97:155–159.
66. Klein R, Moss SE, Sinaiko AR, Zinman B, Gardiner R, Suissa S, et al. The relation of ambulatory blood pressure and pulse rate to retinopathy in type 1 diabetes mellitus the renin-angiotensin system study. *Ophthalmology*. 2006;113:2231–2236.
67. Knudsen ST, Poulsen PL, Hansen KW, Ebbehoj E, Bek T, Mogensen CE. Pulse pressure and diurnal blood pressure variation: association with micro- and macrovascular complications in type 2 diabetes. *Am J Hypertens*. 2002;15:244–250.
68. Al-Husainy S, Farmer J, Gibson JM, Dodson PM. Is measurement of blood pressure worthwhile in the diabetic eye clinic? *Eye*. 2005;19:312–316.
69. Sivaprasad S, Jackson H. Blood pressure control in type II diabetics with diabetic retinopathy. *Eye*. 2007;21: 708–711.

70. Hayreh SS. Role of retinal hypoxia in diabetic macular edema: a new concept. *Graefe's Arch Clin Exp Ophthalmol.* 2008;246:353–361.
71. Cusick M, Chew EY, Chan CC, Kruth HS, Murphy RP, Ferris FL III. Histopathology and regression of retinal hard exudates in diabetic retinopathy after reduction of elevated serum lipid levels. *Ophthalmology.* 2003;110: 2126–2133.
72. Misra A, Vikram NK, Kumar A. Diabetic maculopathy and lipid-lowering therapy. *Eye.* 2004;18:107–108.
73. Chowdhury TA, Hopkins D, Dodson PM, Vafidis GC. The role of serum lipids in exudative diabetic maculopathy: is there a place for lipid lowering therapy? *Eye.* 2002;16:689–693.
74. Brown GC, Ridley M, Haas D, Lucier AC, Sarin LK. Lipemic diabetic retinopathy. *Ophthalmology.* 1984;91: 1490–1495.
75. Klein BEK, Moss SE, Klein R, Surawicz TS. The Wisconsin epidemiologic study of diabetic retinopathy XIII. Relationship of serum cholesterol to retinopathy and hard exudate. *Ophthalmology.* 1991;98: 1261–1265.
76. Kim CH, Park HJ, Park JY, Hong SK, Yoon YH, Lee KU. High serum lipoprotein(a) levels in Korean type 2 diabetic patients with proliferative diabetic retinopathy. *Diabetes Care.* 1998;21:2149–2151.
77. Chew EY, Klein ML, Ferris FL, Remaley NA, Murphy RP, Chantry K, et al. Association of elevated serum lipid levels with retinal hard exudate in diabetic retinopathy-early treatment diabetic retinopathy study (ETDRS) report 22. *Arch Ophthalmol.* 1996;114: 1079–1084.
78. Duncan LJP, Cullen JF, Ireland JF, Nolan J, Clarke BF, Oliver MF. A three-year trial of Atromid therapy in exudative diabetic retinopathy. *Diabetes.* 1968;17:458–467.
79. Gordon B, Chang S, Kavanagh M, Berrocal M, Yannuzzi L, Robertson C, et al. The effects of lipid lowering on diabetic retinopathy. *Am J Ophthalmol.* 1991;112: 385–391.
80. King RC, Dobree JH, Kok D'A, Foulds WS, Dangerfield WG. Exudative diabetic retinopathy. Spontaneous changes and effects of a corn oil diet. *Br J Ophthalmol.* 1963;47:666–672.
81. Harrold BP, Marmion VJ, Gough KR. A double-blind controlled trial of clofibrate in the treatment of diabetic retinopathy. *Diabetes.* 1969;18:285–291.
82. Lyons TJ, Jenkins AJ, Zheng D, Lackland DT, McGee D, Garvey WT, et al. Diabetic retinopathy and serum lipoprotein subclasses in the DCCT/EDIC Cohort. *Invest Ophthalmol Vis Sci.* 2004;45:910–918.
83. Orchard TJ, Dorman JS, Maser RE, Becker DJ, Ellis D, LaPorte RE, et al. Factors associated with avoidance of severe complications after 25 yr of IDDM. Pittsburgh epidemiology of diabetes complications study I. *Diabetes Care.* 1990;13:741–747.
84. Klein BEK, Klein R, Moss SE. Is serum cholesterol associated with progression of diabetic retinopathy or macular edema in persons with younger-onset diabetes of long duration? *Am J Ophthalmol.* 1999;128: 652–654.
85. Kremser BG, Falk M, Kieselbach GF. Influence of serum lipid fractions on the course of diabetic macular edema after photocoagulation. *Ophthalmologica.* 1995; 209:60–63.
86. Gupta A, Gupta V, Thapar S, Bhansali A. Lipid-lowering drug atorvastatin as an adjunct in the management of diabetic macular edema. *Am J Ophthalmol.* 2004;137: 675–682.
87. Gupta A, Gupta V, Dogra MR, Pandav SS. Risk factors influencing the treatment outcome in diabetic macular oedema. *Ind J Ophthalmol.* 1996;44:145–148.
88. Sen K, Misra A, Kumar A, Pandey RM. Simvastatin retards progression of retinopathy in diabetic patients with hypercholesterolemia. *Diabetes Res Clin Pract.* 2002;56:1–11.
89. Zhang J, McGwin G Jr. Association of statin use with the risk of developing diabetic retinopathy. *Arch Ophthalmol.* 2007;125:1096–1099.
90. Berman DH, Friedman EA. Partial absorption of hard exudates in patients with diabetic end-stage renal disease and severe anemia after treatment with erythropoietin. *Retina.* 1994;14:1–5.
91. Friedman EA, Brown CD, Berman DH. Erythropoietin in diabetic macular edema and renal insufficiency. *Am J Kidney Dis.* 1995;26:202–208.
92. Shorb SR. Anemia and diabetic retinopathy. *Am J Ophthalmol.* 1985;100:434–436.
93. Chadha V, Styles C. Progression of diabetic retinopathy following coronary artery bypass graft. *Eye.* 2007;21: 864–865.
94. Cruikshanks KJ, Ritter LL, Klein R, Moss SA. The association of microalbuminuria with diabetic retinopathy. The Wisconsin epidemiologic study of diabetic retinopathy. *Ophthalmology.* 1993;100:862–867.
95. Klein R, Moss SE, Klein BEK. Is gross proteinuria a risk factor for the incidence of proliferative diabetic retinopathy? *Ophthalmology.* 1993;100: 1140–1146.
96. Krolewski AS, Warram JH, Rand LI, Christlieb AR, Busick EJ, Kahn CR. Risk of proliferative diabetic retinopathy in juvenile-onset type 1 diabetes: a 40 year follow-up study. *Diabetes Care.* 1986;9:443–452.
97. Ciardella AP. Partial resolution of diabetic macular edema after systemic treatment with furosemide. *Br J Ophthalmol.* 2004;88:1224–1225.
98. Nagaoka T, Takeyama Y, Kanagawa S, Sakagama K, Mori F, Yoshida A. Effect of hemodialysis on retinal circulation in patients with end stage renal disease. *Br J Ophthalmol.* 2004;88:1026–1029.
99. Perkovich BT, Meyers SM. Systemic factors affecting diabetic macular edema. *Am J Ophthalmol.* 1988;105: 211–212.
100. Ramsay RC, Knobloch WH, Barbosa JJ, Sutherland DE, Kjellstrand CM, Najarain JS, et al. The visual status of diabetic patients after renal transplantation. *Am J Ophthalmol.* 1979;87:305–310.
101. Sinclair S, Nesler C, Foxman B, Nichols C, Gabbe S. Macular edema and pregnancy in insulin-dependent diabetes. *Am J Ophthalmol.* 1984;97:154–167.
102. Loukovaara S, Harju M, Kaaja R, Immonen I. Retinal capillary blood flow in diabetic and nondiabetic women

during pregnancy and postpartum period. *Invest Ophthalmol Vis Sci*. 2003;44:1486–1491.
103. Dibble CM, Kochenour NK, Worley RJ, Tyler FH, Swartz M. Effect of pregnancy on diabetic retinopathy. *Obstet Gynec*. 1982;59:699–704.
104. Chew EY, Mills JL, Metzger BE, Remaley NA, Jovanovic-Peterson L, Knopp RH, et al. Metabolic control and progression of retinopathy. The diabetes in early pregnancy study. National institute of child health and human development diabetes in early pregnancy study. *Diabetes Care*. 1995;18:631–637.
105. Moloney J, Drury M. The effect of pregnancy on the natural course of diabetic retinopathy. *Am J Ophthalmol*. 1982;93:745–756.
106. Chan WC, Lim LT, Quinn MJ, Knox FA, McCance D, Best RM. Management and outcome of sight-threatening diabetic retinopathy in pregnancy. *Eye*. 2004;18: 826–832.
107. Horvat M, Maclean H, Goldberg L, Crock G. Diabetic retinopathy in pregnancy: a 12-year prospective survey. *Br J Ophthalmol*. 1980;64:398–403.
108. Wong TY, Klein R, Islam FMA, Cotch MF, Folsom AR, Klein BEK, et al. Diabetic retinopathy in a multi-ethnic Cohort in the United States. *Am J Ophthalmol*. 2006;141:446–455.
109. McNair P, Christiansen C, Madsbad S, Lauritzen E, Faber O, Binder C, et al. Hypomagnesemia, a risk factor in diabetic retinopathy. *Diabetes*. 1978;27: 1075–1077.
110. Greenwood R, Ireland J, Jones D, Mahler R. Diabetic complications in a patient with coexisting anterior hypopituitarism. *Diabetes*. 1975;24:1027–1031.
111. Golbahar J, Rahimi M, Tabei MB, Aminzadeh MA. Clinical risk factors and association of hyperhomocysteinemia with diabetic retinopathy in Iranian type 2 diabetes patients: a cross-sectional study from Shiraz, Southern Iran. *Diabetes Metab Syndr Clin Res Rev*. 2008;2:192–201.
112. Soedamah-Muthu SS, Chaturvedi N, Teerlink T, Idzior-Walus B, Fuller JH, Stehouwer CDA, et al. Plasma homocysteine and microvascular and macrovascular complications in type 1 diabetes: a cross-sectional nested case-control study. *J Intern Med*. 2005;258: 450–459.
113. Hultberg B, Agardh E, Andersson A, Brattstrom L, Isaksson A, Israelsson B, et al. Increased levels of plasma homocysteine are associated with nephropathy, but not severe retinopathy in type 1 diabetes mellitus. *Scand J Clin Lab Invest*. 1991;51: 277–282.
114. Moss SE, Klein R, Klein BEK. Ten-year incidence of visual loss in a diabetic population. *Ophthalmology*. 1994;101:1061–1070.
115. Tsuboi S, Pederson JE. Experimental retinal detachment XI. Furosemide-inhibitable fluid absorption across retinal pigment epithelium in vivo. *Arch Ophthalmol*. 1986;104:602–603.
116. Nagai N, Izumi-Nagai K, Oike Y, Koto T, Satofuka S, Ozawa Y, et al. Suppression of diabetes-induced retinal inflammation by blocking the angiotensin II type 1 receptor or its downstream nuclear factor-{kappa}B pathway. *Invest Ophthalmol Vis Sci*. 2007;48: 4342–4350.
117. Sjolie AK, Chaturvedi N. The retinal renin-angiotensin system: implications for therapy in diabetic retinopathy. *J Human Hypertens*. 2002;16:S42–S46.
118. Funatsu H, Yamashita H, Shimuzu E, Mimura T, Nakamura S, Hori S. Quantitative measurement of retinal thickness in patients with diabetic macular edema is useful for evaluation of therapeutic agents. *Diabetes Res Clin Pract*. 2004;66:219–227.
119. Engler CB, Parving HH, Methiesen ER, Larsen M, Lund-Andersen H. Blood-retina barrier permeability in diabetes during acute ACE-inhibition. *Acta Ophthalmol*. 1991;69:581–585.
120. Parving HH, Larsen M, Hommel E, Lund-Andersen H. Effect of antihypertensive treatment on blood-retinal barrier permeability to fluorescein in hypertensive Type 1 (insulin-dependent) diabetic patients with background retinopathy. *Diabetologia*. 1989;32:440–444.
121. Larsen M, Hommel E, Parving HH, Lund-Andersen H. Protective effect of captopril on the blood-retina barrier in normotensive insulin-dependent diabetic patients with nephropathy and background retinopathy. *Graefe's Arch Clin Exp Ophthalmol*. 1990;228: 505–509.
122. Sjolie A, Stephenson J, Aldington S, Kohner E, Janka H, Stevens L, et al. Retinopathy and vision loss in insulin-dependent diabetes in Europe: the EURODIAB IDDM complications study. *Ophthalmology*. 1997;104: 252–260.
123. Chaturvedi N, Porta M, Klein R, Orchard T, Fuller J, Parving HH, et al. Effect of candesartan on prevention (DIRECT-Prevent 1) and progression (DIRECT-Protect 1) of retinopathy in type 1 diabetes: randomised, placebo controlled trials. *Lancet*. 2008;372: 1394–1402.
124. Powell EDU, Field RA. Diabetic retinopathy and rheumatoid arthritis. *Lancet*. 1964;2:17–18.
125. Cerbone AM, Macarone-Palmieri N, Saldalamacchia G, Coppola A, Di Minno G, Rivellese AA. Diabetes, vascular complications and antiplatelet therapy: open problems. *Acta Diabetol*. 2008; DOI 10.1007/s00592-008-0079-y.
126. Damad Study Group. Effect of aspirin alone and aspirin plus dipyridamole in early diabetic retinopathy: a multicenter randomized controlled clinical trial. *Diabetes*. 1989;38:491–498.
127. Early Treatment Diabetic Retinopathy Study Research Group. Effects of aspirin treatment on diabetic retinopathy. ETDRS report number 8. *Ophthalmology*. 1991; 98(Suppl):757–765.
128. Banerjee S, Denniston AKO, Gibson JM, Dodson PM. Does cardiovascular therapy affect the onset and recurrence of preretinal and vitreous hemorrhage in diabetic eye disease? *Eye*. 2004;18:821–825.
129. Zheng L, Howell SJ, Hatala DA, Huang K, Kern TS. Salicylate-based anti-inflammatory drugs inhibit the early lesion of diabetic retinopathy. *Diabetes*. 2007;56: 337–345.
130. Kohner EM. Aspirin for diabetic retinopathy. *BMJ*. 2003;327:1060–1061.

131. Li J, Wang JJ, Chen D, Mott R, Yu Q, Ma JX, et al. Systemic administration of HMG-CoA reductase inhibitor protects the blood-retinal barrier and ameliorates retinal inflammation in type 2 diabetes. *Exp Eye Res*. 2009; DOI 10.1016/j.exer.2009.02.013: 1-8.
132. Aiello LP, Bursell SE, Clermont A, Duh E, Ishii H, Takagi C, et al. Vascular endothelial growth factor-induced retinal permeability is mediated by protein kinase C in vivo and suppressed by an Orally effective B-isoform-selective inhibitor. *Diabetes*. 1997;46: 1473–1480.
133. Koya D, King GL. Protein kinase C activation and the development of diabetic complications. *Diabetes*. 1998; 47:859–866.
134. PKC-DRS2 Group. Effect of Ruboxistaurin on visual loss in patients with diabetic retinopathy. *Ophthalmology*. 2006;113:2221–2230.
135. Davis MD, Sheetz MJ, Aiello LP, Milton RC, Danis RP, Zhi X, et al. Effect of ruboxistaurin on the visual acuity decline associated with longstanding diabetic macular edema. *Invest Ophthalmol Vis Sci*. 2009;50: 1–4.
136. Emoto M, Sato AT, Tanabe K, Tanizawa Y, Matsutani A, Oka Y. Troglitazone treatment increases plasma vascular endothelial growth factor in diabetic patients and its mRNA in 3T3-L1 adipocytes. *Diabetes*. 2001;50: 1166–1170.
137. Mudaliar S, Chang AR, Henry RR. Thiazolidinediones, peripheral edema, and type 2 diabetes: incidence, pathophysiology, and clinical implications. *Endocr Pract*. 2003;9:406–416.
138. Hollenberg NK. Considerations for management of fluid dynamic issues associated with thiazolidinediones. *Am J Med*. 2003;115:111S–115S.
139. Oshitari T, Asaumi N, Watanabe M, Kumagai K, Mitamura Y. Severe macular edema induced by pioglitazone in a patient with diabetic retinopathy: a case study. *Vasc Health Risk Manage*. 2008;4: 1137–1140.
140. Ryan EH, Han DP, Ramsay RC, Cantrill HL, Bennett SR, Dev S, et al. Diabetic macular edema associated with glitazone use. *Retina*. 2006; 26:562–570.
141. Colucciello M. Vision loss due to macular edema induced by rosiglitazone treatment of diabetes mellitus. *Arch Ophthalmol*. 2005;123:1273–1275.
142. Shen LQ, Child A, Weber GM, Folkman J, Aiello LP. Rosiglitazone and delayed onset of proliferative diabetic retinopathy. *Arch Ophthalmol*. 2008;126: 793–799.
143. Fong DS, Contreras R. Glitazone use associated with diabetic macular edema. *Am J Ophthalmol*. 2009;147: 583–586.
144. Gopal L, Sunder KS, Rao SK, Soni M, Sharma S, Ramakrishnan S. Hyperlipidemia in a poorly controlled diabetic presenting with lipemic aqueous and lipemia retinalis. *Retina*. 2004;24:312–315.
145. Early Treatment Diabetic Retinopathy Study Research Group. Fundus photographic risk factors for progression of diabetic retinopathy: ETDRS report number 12. *Ophthalmology*. 1991;98:823–833.
146. Kohner EM, Stratton IM, Aldington SJ, Holman RR, Matthews DR, UK Prospective Diabetes Study Group. Relationship between the severity of retinopathy and progression to photocoagulation in patients with type 2 diabetes mellitus in the UKODS (UKPDS 52). *Diabetes Med*. 2001;18: 178–184.
147. Klein R, Klein BE, Moss SE, Wong TY, Hubbard L, Cruikshanks KJ, et al. The relation of retinal vessel caliber to the incidence and progression of diabetic retinopathy. XIX: the Wisconsin epidemiologic study of diabetic retinopathy. *Arch Ophthalmol*. 2004;122: 76–83.
148. Klein R, Klein BEK, Moss SE, Cruikshanks KJ. The Wisconsin epidemiologic study of diabetic retinopathy. XIV. Ten-year incidence and progression of diabetic retinopathy. *Arch Ophthalmol*. 1994;112: 1217–1228.
149. Valone J, McMeel J, Franks E. Unilateral proliferative diabetic retinopathy. *Archives of Ophthalmol*. 1981;99: 1357–1361.
150. Browning D, Flynn H, Blankenship G. Asymmetric retinopathy in patients with diabetes mellitus. *Am J Ophthalmol*. 1988;105:584–589.
151. Madsen P. Ocular findings in 123 patients with proliferative diabetic retinopathy. *Doc Ophthalmol*. 1971;29: 345–349.
152. Mooney A. Diabetic retinopathy – a challenge. *Br J Ophthalmol*. 1963;47:513–520.
153. Jain I, Luthra C, Das T. Diabetic retinopathy and its relation to errors of refraction. *Arch Ophthalmol*. 1967; 77:59–60.
154. Gay A, Rosenbaum A. Retinal artery pressure in asymmetric diabetic retinopathy. *Arch Ophthalmol*. 1966; 75:758–762.
155. Duker J, Brown G, Bosley T, Colt C, Reber R. Asymmetric proliferative diabetic retinopathy and carotid artery disease. *Ophthalmology*. 1990;97:869–874.
156. Malinowski SM, Pulido JS, Flickinger RR. The protective effect of the tilted disk syndrome in diabetic retinopathy. *Arch Ophthalmol*. 1996;114:230–231.
157. Xu L, Wang YX, Wang J, Jonas JJ. Mortality and ocular diseases. The Beijing eye study. *Ophthalmology*. 2009;116:732–738.
158. Wong TY, Klein R, Nieto FJ, Klein BEK, Sharrett AR, Meuer SM, et al. Retinal microvascular abnormalities and 10-year cardiovascular mortality. A population-based case-control study. *Ophthalmology*. 2003;110: 933–940.
159. Liew G, Wong T, Mitchell P, Cheung N, Wang JJ. Retinopathy prevents coronary heart disease mortality. *Heart*. 2008; DOI:10.1136/hrt.2008.146670.
160. Hirai FE, Knudtson MD, Klein BEK, Klein R. Clinically significant macular edema and survival in type 1 and type 2 diabetes. *Am J Ophthalmol*. 2008;145: 700–706.
161. Miettinen H, Haffner SM, Lehto S, Ronnemaa T, Pyorala K, Laakso M. Retinopathy predicts coronary heart disease in NIDDM patients. *Diabetes Care*. 1996;19: 1445–1448.
162. Juutilainen A, Lehto S, Ronnemaa T, Pyorala K, Laakso M. Retinopathy predicts cardiovascular

mortality in type 2 diabetic men and women. *Diabetes Care*. 2007;30:292–299.

163. Cheung N, Wang JJ, Rogers SL, Brancati F, Klein R, Sharrett AR, et al. Diabetic retinopathy and risk of heart failure. *J Am Coll Cardiol*. 2008;51:1573–1578.
164. Knudsen ST, Bek T, Poulsen PL, Hove MN, Rehling M, Mogensen CE. Macular edema reflects generalized vascular hyperpermeability in type 2 diabetic patients with retinopathy. *Diabetes Care*. 2002;25: 2328–2334.
165. Caro JJ, Ward AJ, O'Brien JA. Lifetime costs of complications resulting from type 2 diabetes in the U.S. *Diabetes Care*. 2002;25:476–481.
166. Sarin R. Criteria for deciding cost-effectiveness for expensive new anti-cancer agents. *J Cancer Res Ther*. 2008;4:1–2.

Chapter 5
Defining Diabetic Retinopathy Severity

Keye Wong

The fundus abnormalities seen in diabetic retinopathy can conceptually be split into three categories – those findings resulting from leaking microvasculature (hemorrhages, lipid exudates, retinal edema); those findings resulting from structural damage to the microvasculature wall (microaneurysms); and those findings resulting from ischemia with a subsequent overproduction of vascular growth factors (cottonwool patches, intraretinal microvascular abnormalities [IRMA], preretinal neovascularization, fibrous proliferation, and vitreous hemorrhage). The severity of each of these findings can be classified and quantified based on the degree of retina involvement, e.g., the number of microaneurysms and hemorrhages in each quadrant or photographic field, the area of retina affected by neovascular tissue or IRMA, or the area of macula involved with retinal thickening. Classification schemes are a means to categorize the varying degrees of such findings to facilitate communication. As with all specialized languages, the value of these languages depends upon who is speaking to whom. The ultimate goal of classification schemes is to provide a system to improve patient care. This may be achieved initially by precise communication among researchers to define categories by which the natural history and subsequent response to intervention(s) can be identified. Once these research goals have been achieved these classification schemes should be understandable and reproducible by practicing clinicians. If not, then modification of these classification schemes is desirable to allow clinicians to communicate among themselves and with their patients the expected results of therapies demonstrated to be beneficial in clinical trials. One should realize that the goals of communication between researchers may be different from the goals of communication between clinicians and may likewise be different from the goals of communication between clinician and patient. Evolution of classification schemes is desirable dependent upon who is communicating with whom.

Historically, the initial classification schemes for diabetic retinopathy were developed to facilitate communication among researchers. In 1968 the US Public Health Service held a symposium at the Airlie House in Warrington, PA, to develop a classification system for diabetic retinopathy.[1] The "Airlie House" classification system used five standard photographic fields (field 2 centered on the foveola; fields 4 and 5 just above and below the foveola respectively; fields 1 and 3 just nasal and temporal to the foveola respectively). Fundus lesions (hemorrhages, microaneurysms, lipid, neovascularization, etc.) were classified into one of three categories: absent, mild to moderate, or severe. However, with only three levels of severity graders using the Airlie House classification often found it difficult to reach consensus. This system therefore fell short in its ability to communicate with consistency between researchers. The Airlie House classification scheme did not define enough distinction between "mild to moderate" lesions and "severe" lesions so that most lesions were lumped into the "mild to moderate" category. In the "lumpers" vs. "splitters" distinction, there was not enough "splitting."

The Diabetic Retinopathy Study (DRS) subsequently created the modified Airlie House

K. Wong (✉)
University of South Florida, Sarasota, FL 34242, USA
e-mail: iskeye@yahoo.com

D.J. Browning (ed.), *Diabetic Retinopathy*, DOI 10.1007/978-0-387-85900-2_5,

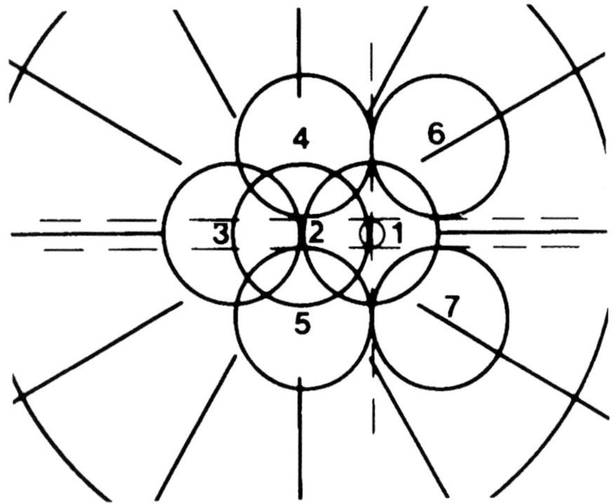

Fig. 5.1 Seven standard fields of the modified Airlie House classification (shown for the *right eye*). Field 1 is centered on the optic disc, field 2 on the macula. Field 3 is temporal to the macula. Fields 4–7 are tangential to the *horizontal lines* passing through the *upper* and *lower poles* of the disc and to a *vertical line* passing through its center. Reproduced from ETDRS Research Group[3]

classification system with a greater degree of "splitting." Two additional photographic fields were analyzed (field 6 superonasal and field 7 inferonasal) to the optic nerve head (see Fig. 5.1).

In addition, more gradations of severity for individual components were added.[2] The primary question asked by the DRS was whether photocoagulation helped to prevent severe visual loss from proliferative diabetic retinopathy. Eligible patients had either proliferative diabetic retinopathy or severe nonproliferative diabetic retinopathy (defined as follows) (see Table 5.1).

Table 5.1 DRS definition of severe nonproliferative diabetic retinopathy

Any three of the following characteristics:
Soft exudates definitely present in ≥ 2 of photographic fields 4–7
IRMA definitely present in ≥ 2 of photographic fields 4–7
Venous beading definitely present in ≥ 2 of photographic fields 4–7
Hemorrhages and/or microaneurysms $\geq$ severe ($\geq$ std photo 2A) in ≥ 1 of photographic fields 4–7
Or
IRMA $\geq$ standard photo 8A in ≥ 2 of photographic fields 4–7 and definitely present in the remaining two fields

IRMA = intraretinal microvascular abnormalities (dilated preexisting vessels or intraretinal new vessels).
Adapted with permission from ETDRS Report No. 12.[4]

One eye received photocoagulation and the other eye received observation only during the study period. The principal outcome measure was visual acuity of <5/200 at two consecutive 4-month intervals (defined as "severe visual loss"). For the targeted study population, the modified Airlie House classification scheme allowed researchers to classify lesions consistently and to demonstrate the benefit of *immediate* scatter laser photocoagulation in patients with "high-risk" proliferative diabetic retinopathy. These "high-risk" characteristics were (1) neovascularization of the disc, (2) neovascularization of the disc > standard photograph 10A (see Fig. 5.2), (3) neovascularization elsewhere, and (4) vitreous hemorrhage (defined as hemorrhage more forward in the vitreous cavity than preretinal hemorrhage – standard photograph 13)[3] (see Fig. 5.3).

However, for patients with lesion characteristics which approached but did not yet reach the definitions of "high-risk" proliferative diabetic retinopathy,

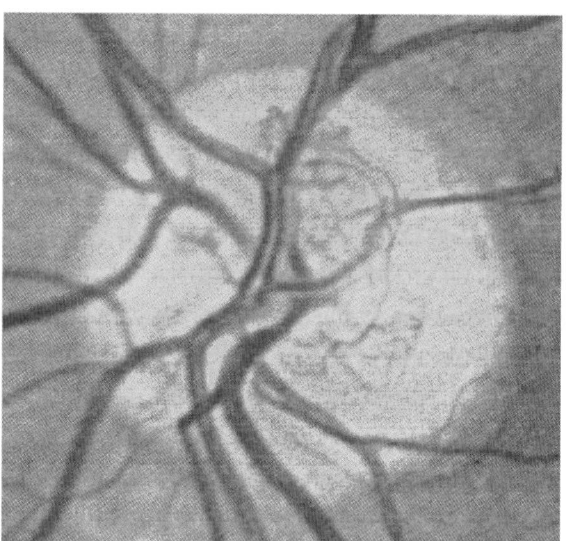

Fig. 5.2 Standard photograph 10A, defining the lower boundary of Grade 3 (moderate) NVD. NVD covers approximately one-third the area of the standard disc (4.7 mm diameter on the original transparency) and about one-fifth the area of this unusually large disc (6.0-mm diameter on the original transparency). The unusual size of this disc was not taken into consideration when it was chosen as a standard, and is disregarded in grading (i.e., the area of the NVD in the photograph being graded is compared with that in the standard, without regard to the size of the discs). Reproduced with permission from the Early Treatment Diabetic Retinopathy Study Research Group

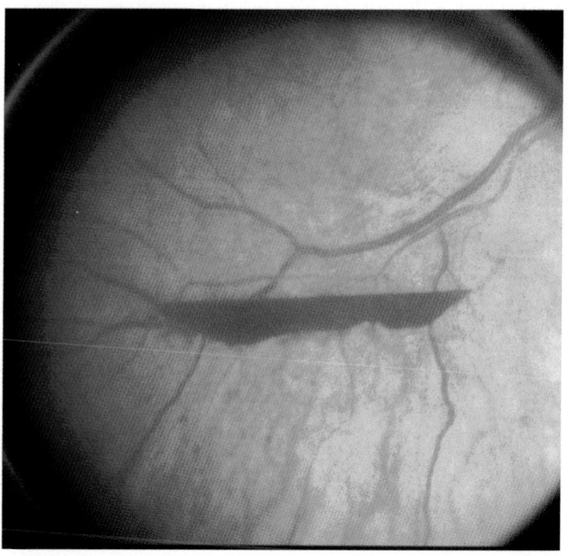

Fig. 5.3 Standard photograph 13, one of two standards used (interchangeably) to define the lower boundary of Grade 3 (moderate) preretinal hemorrhage. Reproduced with permission from the Early Treatment Diabetic Retinopathy Study Research Group

the DRS results were not helpful in determining whether *immediate* photocoagulation was a better treatment strategy as compared to *deferral* of scatter photocoagulation until "high-risk" characteristics developed. The Early Treatment Diabetic Retinopathy Study (ETDRS) therefore was designed to answer whether a strategy of earlier treatment with scatter photocoagulation was beneficial. As in the DRS, the primary end point was the rate of development of visual acuity <5/200 at two consecutive 4-month visits. However, since DRS results had already indicated that eyes with proliferative diabetic retinopathy and high-risk characteristics were at increased risk of "severe visual loss," ETDRS data were also analyzed to determine rates of progression to proliferative diabetic retinopathy.

The ETDRS additionally asked whether laser photocoagulation of diabetic macular edema was helpful. The primary end point for this group of patients with macular edema was the rate of development of loss of 15 or more letters from baseline (defined as "moderate visual loss").

In attempting to answer these two study questions, the classification system of the modified Airlie House system was felt to have not enough detail in the categories of moderate to severe NPDR and the "interim" ETDRS scale was designed. Besides the modified Airlie House lesions of microaneurysms, IRMA, NVE, and fibrous proliferations, the ETDRS asked that photographs be graded additionally for hard exudates, cottonwool patches, arteriovenous nicking, retinal elevation, and vitreous hemorrhage.[3] Venous abnormalities were further subdivided into venous beading, venous narrowing, venous loops, venous sheathing, and perivascular exudate. The grading of each of these 17 factors in multiple stereoscopic fields with several steps of severity presents a rather complicated grading scheme. The ETDRS "interim" scale classification is shown in Table 5.2.

Table 5.2 ETDRS interim scale

Level	Definition
30 A	Venous loops definitely present
30 B	Soft exudates, IRMA, or venous beading questionable
30 C	Hemorrhages present but less than severe in 1–3 fields
30 D	Definite hard exudates
30 E	Hard exudates > moderate in 1 field
41 A	Definite IRMA in 1–3 fields
41 B	Definite soft exudates in 1–3 fields
45 A	Definite soft exudates in 4–5 fields
45 B	Definite IRMA in 4–5 fields or moderately severe IRMA in 1 field
45 C	Definite venous beading in 1 field
45 D	Severe hemorrhages in 1–3 fields
51 A	Severe hemorrhages in 4–5 fields

Reproduced from ETDRS Report No. 12.[4]

Subsequent analysis of ETDRS data validated the prognostic power of this "interim" scale and this interim scale was thereby modified to a "final" scale[4] (see Table 5.3).

One may notice that the numbers used are different between the interim and final scales (see Table 5.4).

In contrast to the numerical severity levels (of use principally to professional graders), the verbal definitions[5] of the ETDRS classification scheme in general are more easily understood (e.g., macular edema, mild NPDR, high-risk PDR) (see Table 5.5).

However, some of the definitions (e.g., clinically significant macular edema, severe NPDR) remain so complex as to make clinical application problematic (as evidenced by the impetus behind the

Table 5.3 ETDRS final scale

Level	Definition
10	Microaneurysms and other characteristics absent
20	Microaneurysms definite, other characteristics absent
35 A	Definite venous loops in 1 field
35 B	Questionable soft exudates, IRMA, or venous beading
35 C	Hemorrhage present
35 D	Definite hemorrhage in 1–5 fields
35 E	Moderately severe hemorrhages in 1 field
35 F	Definite soft exudates in 1 field
43 A	Moderately severe hemorrhages in 4–5 fields or severe hemorrhages in 1 field
43 B	Definite IRMA in 1–3 fields
47 A	Both 43 A and 43 B definitions
47 B	Definite IRMA in 4–5 fields
47 C	Severe hemorrhages in 2–3 fields
47 D	Definite venous beading in 1 field
53 A	≥2 level 47 definitions
53 B	Severe hemorrhages in 4–5 fields
53 C	Moderately severe IRMA in 1 field
53 D	Definite venous beading in 2–3 fields
53 E	2 or more level 53 definitions

Reproduced from ETDRS Report No. 12.[4]

Table 5.4 Comparison of ETDRS interim vs. final scales

Interim scale	Final scale	Severity
30 A		
30 B		
30 C		
30 D		
30 E		
	35 A	Mild NPDR
	35 B	
	35 C	
	35 D	
	35 E	
	35 F	
41 A		
41 B		
	43 A	Moderate NPDR
	43 B	
45 A		
45 B		
45 C		
45 D		
	47 A	Moderately severe NPDR
	47 B	
	47 C	
	47 D	
51 A		
51 B		
51 C		
	53 A	Severe NPDR
	53 B	
	53 C	
	53 D	
	53 E	
55 A		
55 B		
55 C		
55 D		
	61	Mild PDR
	65	Moderate PDR
	71	High-risk PDR

Adapted from ETDRS Report No. 12.[4]

proposed International Clinical Diabetic Retinopathy and Diabetic Macular Edema Severity Scales).

Although complicated the ETDRS severity scale has become the de facto gold standard for grading diabetic retinopathy severity in clinical trials. In the recently described International Classification Scheme (see below) the Global Diabetic Retinopathy Project Group believed that "retina specialists were considered to be familiar with the ETDRS classification system and expected to continue using either it or their personal customized modifications."[6] They are likely making this statement in reference to the verbal definitions as the numerical levels are of value only for communication among researchers or the extremely obsessive–compulsive clinician.

The additional value which the ETDRS classification provides in "splitting" categories can be found in natural history data. Based on a patient's current ETDRS retinopathy level, one can predict the chance of developing high-risk proliferative retinopathy[7] (see Table 5.6).

In retrospect, a careful inspection of this data demonstrates a deficiency of the ETDRS classification scheme, whereas moderate NPDR (level 47) carries an 8.6% 1-year risk of developing high-risk PDR, severe NPDR (level 53e) carries a 45% risk of developing high-risk PDR. Therefore, a jump in a single numerical level of severity (47–53) results in a big jump in risk (8.6–45%). Ideally, the risk of developing high-risk PDR will show a linear change in risk as one progresses along the severity scale.

The demonstration by the ETDRS that a patient's 1- and 3-year risk of progressing to high-risk proliferative retinopathy increases dramatically when that patient's severity level increases from moderate to severe NPDR has led to a concerted effort by the

Table 5.5 ETDRS definitions of commonly used terms

A. Macular edema	Thickening of retina within 1 disc diameter of the center of the macula; and/or hard exudates ≥ standard photograph 3 in a standard 30° photographic field centered on the macula (field 2), with some hard exudates within 1 disc diameter of the center of the macula
B. Clinically significant macular edema	Retinal thickening at or within 500 μm of the center of the macula; and/or hard exudates at or within 500 μm of the center of the macula, if associated with thickening of the adjacent retina; and/or a zone or zones of retinal thickening one disc area in size at least part of which was within 1 disc diameter of the center
C. Mild NPDR	At least one microaneurysm, and definition not met for D, E, F, or G below
D. Moderate NPDR	Hemorrhages and/or microaneurysms ≥ standard photograph 2A, and/or soft exudates, venous beading, or intraretinal microvascular abnormalities definitely present, and definition not met for E, F, or G below
E. Severe NPDR	Soft exudates, venous beading, and intraretinal microvascular abnormalities all definitely present in at least two of fields 4 through 7; or two of the preceding three lesions present in at least two of fields 4 through 7 and hemorrhages and microaneurysms present in these four fields, equaling or exceeding standard photograph 2A in at least one of them; or intraretinal microvascular abnormalities present in each of fields 4 through 7 and equaling or exceeding standard photograph 8A in at least two of them; and definition not met for F or G below
F. Early PDR	New vessels; and definition not met for G below
G. High-risk PDR	New vessels on or within 1 disc diameter of the optic disc (NVD) ≥ standard photograph 10A (about 1/4 to 1/3 disc area), with or without vitreous or preretinal hemorrhage; or vitreous and/or preretinal hemorrhage accompanied by new vessels, either NVD < standard photograph 10A or new vessels elsewhere (NVE) ≥ 1/4 disc area
H. Less severe retinopathy	Mild or moderate nonproliferative retinopathy
I. More severe retinopathy	Severe nonproliferative or early proliferative retinopathy
J. Severe visual loss	Visual acuity < 5/200 at two consecutive follow-up visits (scheduled at 4-month intervals).
K. Moderate visual loss	Loss of 15 or more letters between baseline and follow-up visit, equivalent to doubling of the initial visual angle (i.e., 20/20–20/40 or 20/50–20/100)

Reproduced from ETDRS Report No. 9.[7]

Table 5.6 Risk of developing high-risk proliferative retinopathy in all eyes assigned to deferral by baseline retinopathy severity level

ETDRS retinopathy level	1-year risk of developing HR PDR (%)	3-year risk of developing HR PDR (%)	5-year risk of developing HR PDR (%)
Level ≤ 35	0.8	6.7	15.5
Level 43	3.3	14.2	26.5
Level 47	8.6	24.4	39.4
Level 53a–d	14.6	39.5	56.0
Level 53e	45.0	64.9	71.3
Level 61	21.7	48.6	63.8
Level ≥ 65	45.5	67.2	74.7

Reproduced from ETDRS Report No. 9.[7]

American Academy of Ophthalmology to educate ophthalmologists to attempt differentiate severe NPDR from lesser levels. A simplified technique to identify severe NPDR is the 4:2:1 rule.[8] The 4:2:1 rule classifies severe NPDR as eyes with hemorrhages in four quadrants > standard photograph 2A (see Fig. 5.4); or venous beading in two quadrants > standard photograph 6A (see Fig. 5.5); or IRMA > standard photograph 8A in one quadrant (see Fig. 5.6).

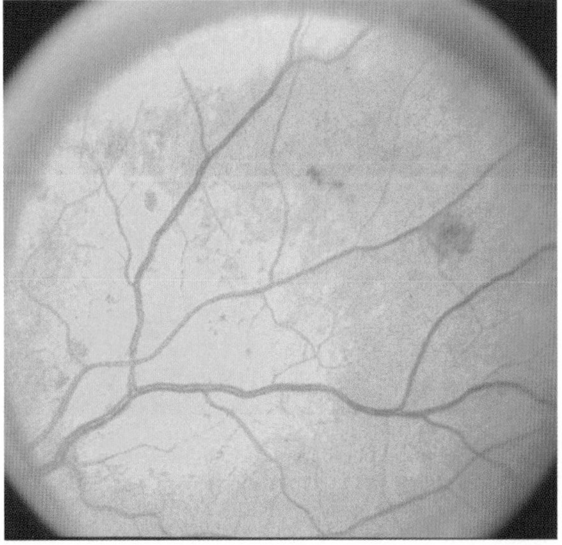

Fig. 5.4 Standard photograph 2A, intermediate standard for hemorrhages/microaneurysms. This is the minimum grade of hemorrhages and microaneurysms necessary for diagnosing severe nonproliferative diabetic retinopathy. Reproduced with permission from the Early Treatment Diabetic Retinopathy Study Research Group

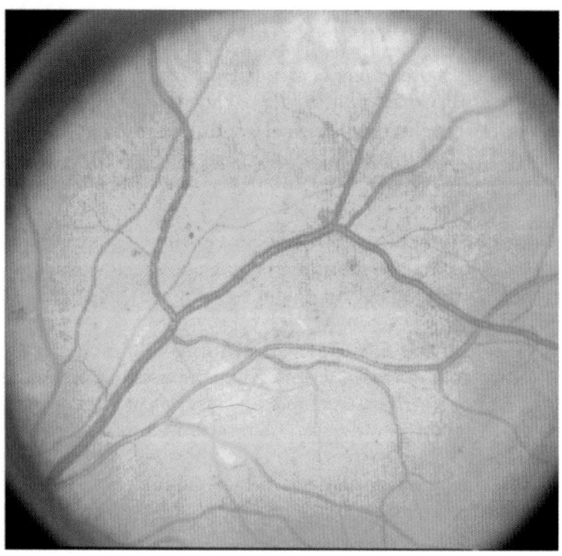

Fig. 5.5 Standard photograph 6A, less severe of two standards for venous beading. Two main branches of the superior temporal vein show beading that is definite, but not severe. Reproduced with permission from the Early Treatment Diabetic Retinopathy Study Research Group

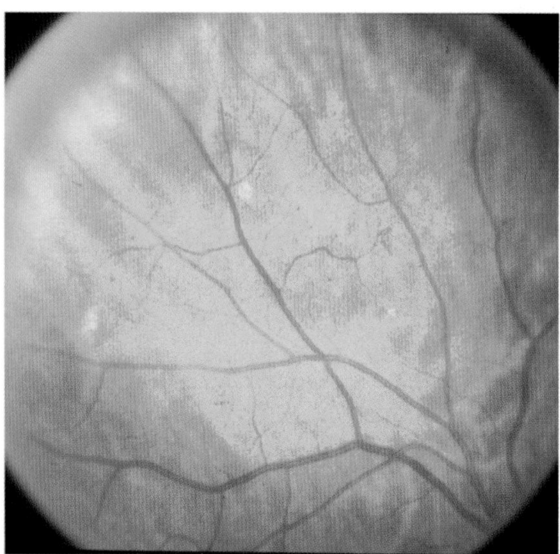

Fig. 5.6 Standard photograph 8A, less severe of two standards for grading soft exudates and IRMA. This is the minimum standard for grading IRMA sufficient to diagnose severe nonproliferative diabetic retinopathy. Reproduced with permission from the Early Treatment Diabetic Retinopathy Study Research Group

One should recognize, however, that the 4:2:1 description of severe NPDR describes a level of disease severity that is less than the DRS definition of severe NPDR (see Table 5.1) and also less than the ETDRS definition of severe NPDR. The ETDRS definition of severe NPDR is characterized by any one of three clinical descriptions.[9] In the *first* description, soft exudates, venous beading, and IRMA *all* have to be present in at least two photographic fields (quadrants). The 4:2:1 rule makes no mention of soft exudates and requires IRMA in only one quadrant. The *second* ETDRS description most closely approximates the 4:2:1 rule with hemorrhages in all four quadrants (but only greater than standard photograph 2A in one of them) *and* also with two of the following three lesions (soft exudates, venous beading, or IRMA) present in two fields. The 4:2:1 rule requires only hemorrhages in four quadrants *or* venous beading in two quadrants *or* IRMA in one quadrant. In contrast, the *second* ETDRS description requires hemorrhages in four quadrants *and* two of the three lesions in *two* quadrants. The *third* ETDRS description of severe NPDR stipulates IRMA in four quadrants with at least two of the quadrants having severity $\geq$ standard photograph 8A. The 4:2:1 rule therefore describes a level of diabetic retinopathy severity which is probably intermediate between the ETDRS definition of moderate and severe NPDR. Although probably reasonable, one must realize that the 4:2:1 rule is an extrapolation but not identical to "severe NPDR" as defined in the ETDRS. The scant evidence available suggests that clinicians are poor at correctly discerning severe NPDR despite the intensive educational efforts toward the goal of accurate diagnosis.[10]

The second question asked by the ETDRS was whether laser photocoagulation of diabetic macular edema was helpful in reducing the rate of moderate visual loss. Enrolled patients could have 20/20 visual acuity in which vision gain was not likely. The ETDRS was conducted in an era prior to optical coherence tomography and defined macular edema and clinically significant macular edema based on examination of stereo fundus photographs. When macular edema was defined as retinal thickening within 1 disc diameter of the center of the macula, protocol laser treatment was not shown to reduce the risk of moderate visual loss within the initial 2 years following treatment (see Fig. 5.7).

When macular edema was more strictly defined to be closer to the fovea (clinically significant

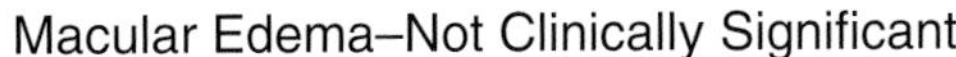

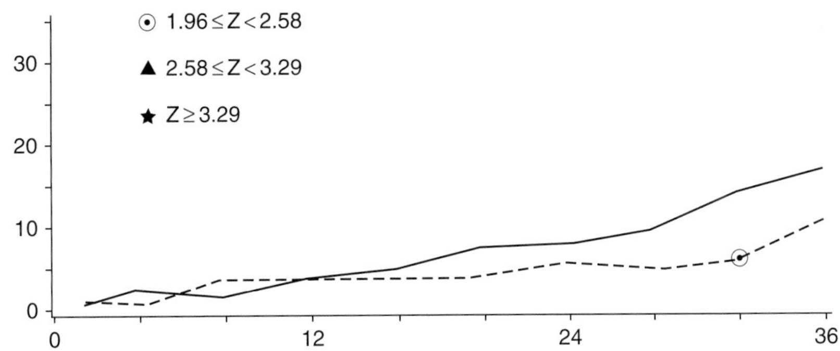

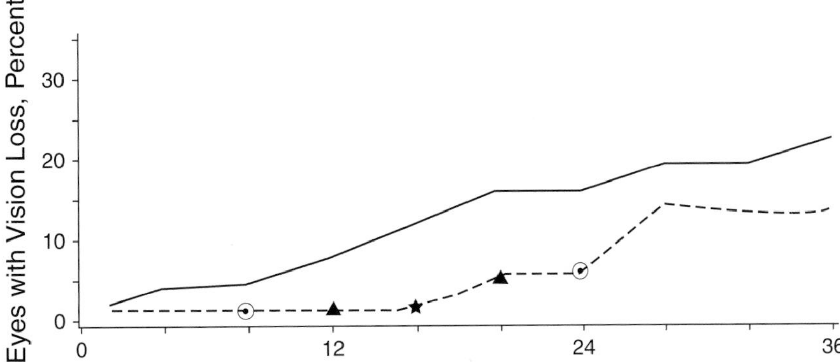

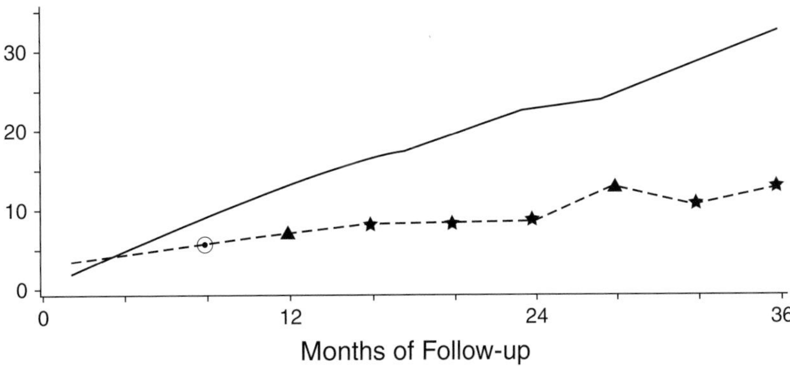

Fig. 5.7 Comparison of percentages of eyes that experienced visual loss of 15 or more letters (equivalent to at least doubling of the initial visual angle) in eyes classified by severity of macular edema in baseline fundus photographs and assigned to either immediate photocoagulation for macular edema (*broken line*) or deferral of photocoagulation unless high-risk characteristics develop (*solid line*). Reproduced with permission from ETDRS Research Group[11]

macular edema), the rate of moderate visual loss was decreased by 50% (24% of untreated eyes compared to about 12% of treated eyes at 3 years).[11] Based on this data, the ETDRS recommended that "eyes with CSME with center involvement should be considered for immediate laser treatment." Since the ETDRS demonstrated that subclassifying diabetic macular edema severity as "clinically significant" or "not clinically significant" resulted in a differential response to laser therapy, it is important for the clinician to recognize this distinction. However, like ETDRS severity levels, the definition of CSME is a research definition initially designed for use by professional graders reviewing stereoscopic fundus photographs. In clinical practice the ability to distinguish "clinically significant macular edema" from "macular edema" may be difficult to reproduce. Furthermore, following laser therapy it may also be difficult to clinically determine improvement or resolution of clinically significant macular edema. In the DRS and ETDRS there was a lack of concordance between the professional graders and clinicians in determining macular edema with the two groups agreeing only 55% of the time on the diagnosis after taking into account the agreement due to chance.[12] This subjective variability in diagnosing CSME may have practical implications in reproducing the beneficial results of laser therapy demonstrated in the ETDRS.

The DRS and the ETDRS demonstrated two thresholds of diabetic retinopathy severity for recommending laser therapy to help prevent vision loss: (1) proliferative diabetic retinopathy with high-risk characteristics and (2) clinically significant macular edema. The Global Diabetic Retinopathy Project Group has attempted to simplify the classification scheme to facilitate early detection of these threshold levels.[6] They have proposed an International Classification Scale to help communication between comprehensive ophthalmologists and primary care physicians to hopefully allow these threshold levels to be detected earlier.

Rather than utilizing 12 levels of severity (level 10–85) with 12 corresponding descriptive terms (mild NPDR, moderate NPDR, moderately severe NPDR, mild PDR, high-risk PDR, etc.), this international panel of experts proposed reducing the number of levels. The distinguishing feature of this classification scheme is an attempt to distinguish patients with severe NPDR or worse from patients with less than severe NPDR. The rationale proposed lies in using the 4:2:1 rule as a simplified method to identify severe NPDR. As previously stated these definitions of severe NPDR approximate each other but are not equivalent.

In reviewing the ETDRS data the Global Diabetic Retinopathy Project Group realized that the presence of IRMA and venous beading was more predictive of the risk of progressing to high-risk PDR, whereas retinal hemorrhages and microaneurysms alone were poorly predictive. For this reason their classification scheme deemphasizes the recognition of hemorrhages and microaneurysms (see Table 5.7).

A separate severity scale was proposed for diabetic macular edema (see Table 5.8).

The global issues prompting a separate severity scale for diabetic macular edema were purported to be the use of direct ophthalmoscopy by primary care physicians to examine the retina. The ETDRS standard of diagnosing "clinically significant macular edema" as the indication to benefit from laser treatment would therefore not be applicable to practitioners untrained in the use of slit lamp biomicroscopy. This proposed International Classification Scheme merits consideration in facilitating communication but has not been validated with regard to its ability to overdiagnose or underdiagnose clinically significant macular edema.

Table 5.7 Proposed International Clinical Diabetic Retinopathy Severity Scale

Proposed disease severity level	Findings observable on dilated ophthalmoscopy
No apparent retinopathy	No abnormalities
Mild NPDR	Microaneurysms only
Moderate NPDR	More than just microaneurysms but less than severe NPDR
Severe NPDR	Any of the following: more than 20 intraretinal hemorrhages in each of four quadrants; definite venous in 2+ quadrants; prominent intraretinal microvascular abnormalities in 1+ quadrant; and no signs of PDR
PDR	One or more of the following: neovascularization, vitreous/preretinal hemorrhage

Reproduced with permission from Wilkinson et al.[6]

Table 5.8 Proposed International Diabetic Macular Edema Severity Scale

Proposed disease severity level	Findings observable on dilated ophthalmoscopy
DME apparently absent	No apparent retinal thickening or hard exudates in posterior pole
DME apparently present	Some apparent retinal thickening or hard exudates in posterior pole
If DME present	Mild DME: Some retinal thickening or hard exudates in posterior pole but distant from the center of the macula
If DME present	Moderate DME: Retinal thickening or hard exudates approaching the center of the macula but not involving the center
If DME present	Severe DME: Retinal thickening or hard exudates involving the center of the macula

Reproduced with permission from Wilkinson et al.[6]

The advent of optical coherence tomogram technology to quantitate retinal thickness along with its universal acceptance has further complicated the issue of classifications schemes to classify diabetic macular edema. CSME as the indication for benefiting from laser therapy is either present or absent. The quantitative analyses provided by OCT allow the possibility of further splitting diabetic macular edema into subclassifications analogous to the progressive splitting of classifications between the Airlie House classification, modified Airlie House classification, and ETDRS classification schemes. It is not unreasonable that varying degrees of diabetic macular edema may respond differently to varying approaches of laser combined with pharmacologic therapy. However, in the absence of studies demonstrating such benefit, the ETDRS currently provides the most complete data set and "clinically significant macular edema" (either present or absent) remains the gold standard classification scheme.

The varying definitions of diabetic "macular edema" and "clinically significant macular edema" lend itself to difficulties in communication among clinicians. Although the ETDRS provided distinctly different definitions to "diabetic macular edema" and "clinically significant macular edema" some clinicians merge the two definitions into an undefined term "clinically significant diabetic macular edema." Further vagaries in undefined terminology are "diffuse" and "focal" diabetic macular edema. The varying definitions for these terms are based on using different modalities (clinical examination, fundus photography, optical coherence tomography, and fluorescein angiography) to describe them. Although commonly used, these terms currently are poorly defined without evidence that additional subclassification of diabetic macular edema into "focal" and "diffuse" changes clinical outcome or treatment decisions.[13]

A DME severity scale using professional grading of the ETDRS stereo photographs has recently been proposed.[14] This scale categorized edema based on the grader-determined area of edema within the macula and also the degree of retinal thickening at the foveal center relative to a reference thickness. The objective of this severity scale was to determine whether splitting macular edema into more levels than "present" or "absent" might be beneficial. Not surprisingly this study did find an association. Greater severity of both diabetic macular edema and edema that had been present for a longer duration was associated with vision loss. Given the ability of OCT to accurately and reproducibly quantify macular thickness, the results of this DME severity scale study imply that accurate subclassification of diabetic macular edema may be helpful.

The beneficial role of fluorescein angiography in classifying diabetic retinopathy severity is unclear. The ETDRS did perform and evaluate fluorescein angiograms in a systematic fashion. It graded the size of the foveal avascular zone (FAZ), FAZ outline, capillary loss, capillary dilatation, focal narrowing, vessel wall staining, severity of leakage, source of leakage, cystoid spaces, and RPE defects.[15] These characteristics were graded typically on a 3- to 5-step scale. Graders varied in their assessment of the degree of severity. With regard to grading severity of features of ischemia, there was complete agreement in grading FAZ size in 74%; complete agreement in grading FAZ outline in 47%; and complete agreement in grading capillary loss in 47%. With regard to fluorescein angiographic signs of leakage there was complete agreement in grading severity of leakage in 63%; complete agreement in grading source of leakage in 60%; and complete agreement in grading cystoid spaces in 92%. It seems that if professional graders disagreed on classifying the severity level of fluorescein angiographic findings 40–50% of the time, consistent and reproducible grading of these lesions by clinicians may be a challenge. Reproducibility of grading fluorescein angiograms in diabetic retinopathy has not improved in the 20 years since the ETDRS, and although their use was employed in the first clinical trial of the Diabetic Retinopathy Clinical Research Network (DRCR.net), these gradings have since been abandoned as insufficiently reproducible and a poor allocation of resources in Network studies.

Besides being difficult to reproduce the gradings, it is not certain that the additional information gained from fluorescein angiographic classification helps in predicting risk of progression or for recommending therapy. In the DRS, the indication for benefiting from laser photocoagulation was the presence of high-risk characteristics detected by fundus photography (and not fluorescein angiography). In the ETDRS, the indication for benefiting from laser photocoagulation was clinically significant macular edema diagnosed clinically and confirmed by professional graders interpreting stereo fundus photography (and not fluorescein angiography). The Global Diabetic Retinopathy Project Group did not include fluorescein angiographic characteristics in their disease severity scales. The 4:2:1 rule does not include fluorescein angiographic findings. Although a greater severity of fluorescein leakage, capillary loss, and arteriolar abnormalities were associated with a greater risk of progression to proliferative retinopathy, the ETDRS did not find this to be of clinical importance because the information available from color photography alone was sufficient to predict progression and to make recommendations for treatment.[16] The information gained from fluorescein angiography may certainly change the extent and pattern of laser application.[17] In the ETDRS, the protocol laser treatment specified a grid pattern of laser to areas of nonperfusion[18] and direct treatment to areas of focal leakage. However, it is possible that modifying the precise treatment parameters of the ETDRS may not adversely affect treatment outcome.[19]

Although the ETDRS utilized fluorescein angiography to direct laser therapy, current clinical practice suggests that fluorescein angiograms are not universally utilized. In a recent study of the DRCR Network utilizing 35 clinical centers across the United States, laser treatment of diabetic macular edema was directed by fluorescein angiography in only 51% of cases.[20] Although this suggests that clinicians believe that laser treatment without fluorescein guidance is effective, to date there is no clinical trial to compare the vision outcomes of laser treatment for diabetic macular edema with and without fluorescein guidance.

Ultrawide field fluorescein angiography systems provide information from the retinal periphery (ischemia and vascular leakage) outside of the area investigated by the standard fields of the ETDRS.[21] Pending the results of clinical trials it is unclear as to whether this additional information will have prognostic value for diabetic patients or will provide information to alter therapy.

5.1 Summary of Key Points

- Terms in *italics* are specific definitions. Understanding these definitions helps foster better communication to improve patient outcomes.
- The *4:2:1 rule* approximates the ETDRS definition of *severe NPDR*.
- Laser therapy of *clinically significant macular edema* reduces the risk of *moderate visual loss*, whereas laser therapy of *macular edema* did not show benefit over 24 months.
- Identification of *high-risk characteristics*of PDR and application of scatter laser photocoagulation lead to a significant reduction in the risk of *severe visual loss*.
- ETDRS severity levels are too complex for clinical use.
- Clinical examination and fundus photography provide sufficient information for classifying diabetic retinopathy. Information from fluorescein angiography may help guide therapy but does not affect classification schemes.

5.2 Future Directions

- Determination of whether additional information from imaging studies (optical coherence tomography and ultrawide field fundus photography/fluorescein angiography) is helpful in subclassifying diabetic retinopathy.
- Determination of whether utilizing the simplified definitions of the "International Clinical Diabetic Retinopathy and Diabetic Macular Edema Disease Severity Scales" alters patient outcomes.
- Determination of whether response to therapeutic interventions for diabetic macular edema or high-risk PDR varies dependent upon baseline hemoglobin A1c or systemic blood pressure control.

5.3 Practice Exercises

Exercise 1 – Does this patient have "severe NPDR"? (see Figs. 5.8–5.14)

Severe NPDR:

ETDRS definition 1: Soft exudates, venous beading, and intraretinal microvascular abnormalities all definitely present in at least two of fields 4 through 7 (Table 5.9).

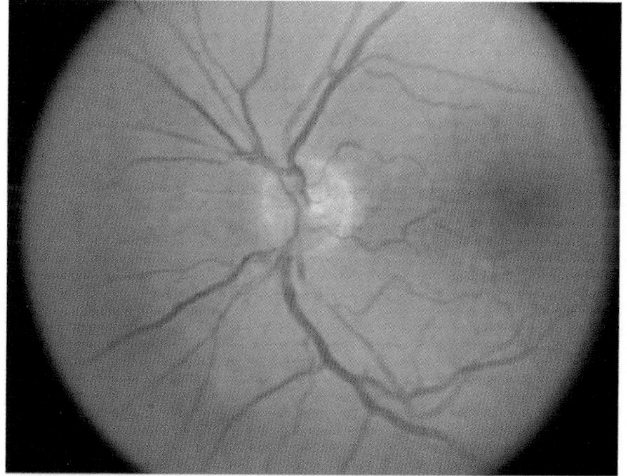

Fig. 5.8 Exercise 1: Field 1

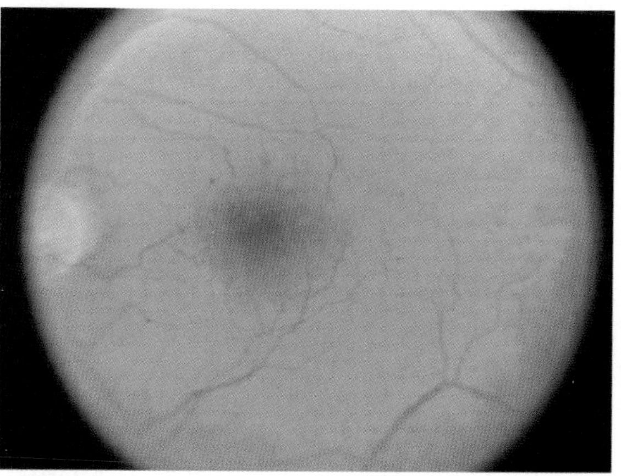

Fig. 5.9 Exercise 1: Field 2

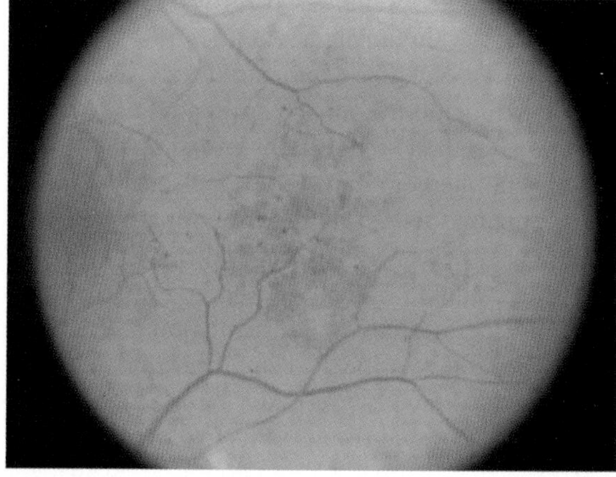

Fig. 5.10 Exercise 1: Field 3

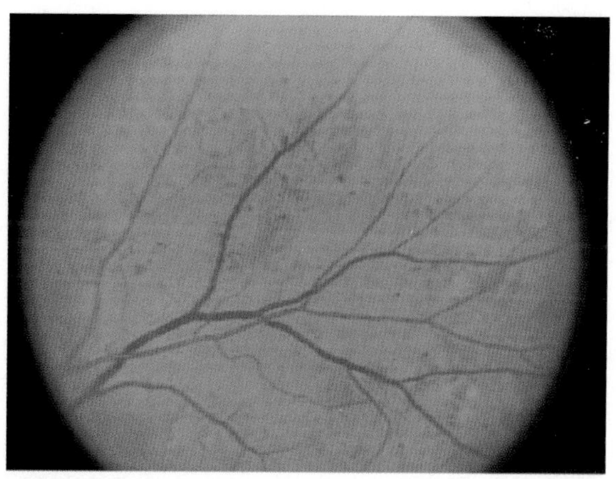

Fig. 5.11 Exercise 1: Field 4

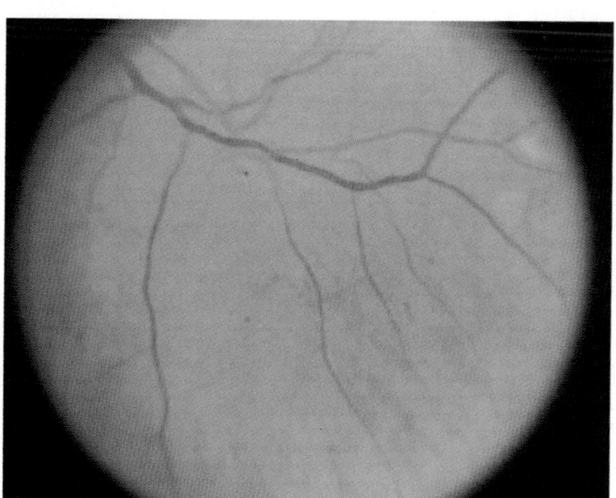

Fig. 5.12 Exercise 1: Field 5

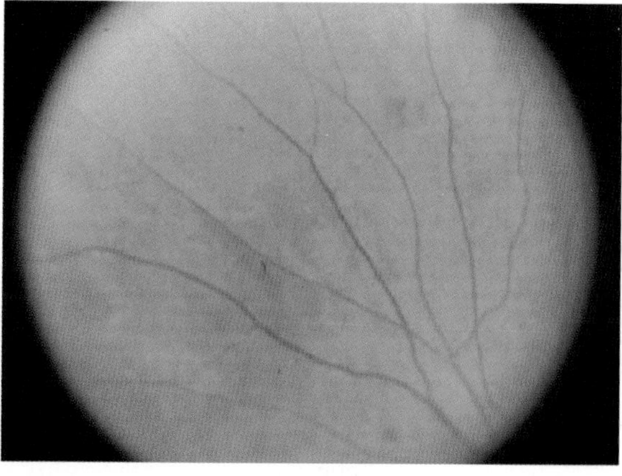

Fig. 5.13 Exercise 1: Field 6

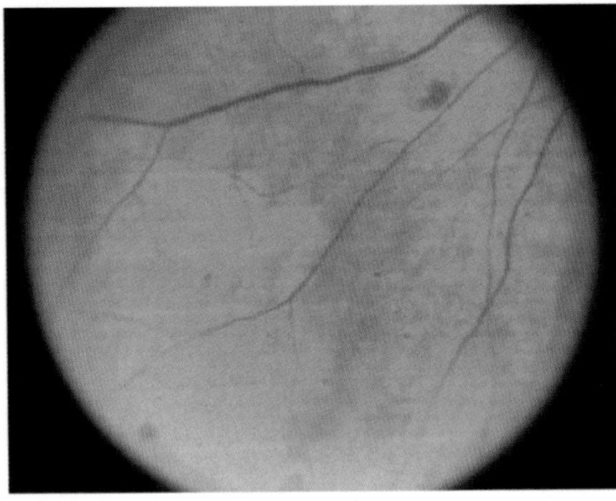

Fig. 5.14 Exercise 1: Field 7

Table 5.9 Table for grading fundus photographs using ETDRS definition 1 in exercise 1

Field	1	2	3	4	5	6	7
SE							
VB							
IRMA							

ETDRS definition 2: Two of the preceding three lesions present in at least two of fields 4 through 7 and hemorrhages and microaneurysms present in these four fields, equaling or exceeding standard photograph 2A in at least one of them (Table 5.10).

Table 5.10 Table for grading fundus photographs using ETDRS definition 2 in exercise 1

Field	1	2	3	4	5	6	7
SE							
VB							
IRMA							

ETDRS definition 3: Intraretinal microvascular abnormalities present in each of fields 4 through 7 and equaling or exceeding standard photograph 8A in at least two of them (Table 5.11).

Table 5.11 Table for grading fundus photographs using ETDRS definition 1 in exercise 1

Field	1	2	3	4	5	6	7
SE							
VB							
IRMA							

DRS definition 1: Any three of the following: Soft exudates definitely present in ≥ 2 of photographic fields 4–7; IRMA definitely present in ≥ 2 of photographic fields 4–7; venous beading ≥ definitely present in ≥ 2 of photographic fields 4–7; hemorrhages/microaneurysms ≥ standard photo 2A in ≥ 1 of photographic fields 4–7 (Table 5.12).

Table 5.12 Table for grading fundus photographs using DRS definition 1 in exercise 1

Field	1	2	3	4	5	6	7
SE							
VB							
IRMA							

4:2:1 rule: four quadrants of > 20 hemorrhages or two quadrants of venous beading or one quadrant of IRMA (Table 5.13).

Table 5.13 Table for grading fundus photographs using 4:2:1 rule in exercise 1

Field	1	2	3	4	5	6	7
SE							
VB							
IRMA							

Exercise 2 – Systemic control of blood sugars[22,23] and hypertension[24] reduces the risk of diabetic retinopathy progression. Elevated serum lipids[25] and serum triglyceride levels[26] are associated with a greater risk of developing more severe diabetic retinopathy. The ETDRS began enrollment of patients in 1980. Almost three decades ago 42% of patients in the ETDRS had a hemoglobin A1c ≥ 10%. Thirty-six percent of patients had a serum cholesterol ≥ 240 mg/100 ml. Twenty-six percent of patients had a low density lipoprotein cholesterol ≥ 160 mg/100 ml.[27] The DCCT demonstrated that the initial level of hemoglobin A1c was the greatest predictor of the risk of diabetic retinopathy progression. A 10% lower initial hemoglobin A1c was associated with a 45% decreased risk of diabetic retinopathy progression.[28] There was a 19% increased risk of retinopathy progressing ≥ 3 steps on the ETDRS scale for every 1% increase in baseline hemoglobin A1c.[29] We may be in a current medical environment where systemic medical factors are under better control. The DRCR.net reported results of its first clinical trial in 2007 in which the mean hemoglobin A1c was 8.2.[30] To date it has not been demonstrated that poor vs.

good control of systemic medical factors should change one's recommendation for treatment of clinically significant macular edema or proliferative diabetic retinopathy with high-risk characteristics.

However, some clinicians will logically defer therapy of diabetic macular edema if blood sugars or blood pressure is acutely out of control. Randomized clinical trials will usually collect information on systemic medical factors (Hgb A1c, blood pressure, lipid levels) to ascertain that such medical factors are evenly distributed among treatment groups. This implies that subclassifying diabetic retinopathy with regard to systemic medical factors may modify the response to therapy. One example of such subclassification arises from analysis of the ETDRS data for early scatter photocoagulation for patients with severe NPDR. For patients with severe NPDR, early scatter photocoagulation was beneficial only in patients with Type 2 diabetes mellitus but not in patients with Type 1 diabetes mellitus.[31]

Should systemic medical factors be utilized by clinicians to subclassify diabetic retinopathy?

Exercise 3 – Severe NPDR as characterized by the 4:2:1 rule requires four quadrants of > 20 hemorrhages or two quadrants of venous beading or one quadrant of IRMA. With extensive capillary closure, these fundus lesions may disappear producing what has been described as "featureless" retina. These patients have been described as being at significant risk for developing high-risk PDR. The following patient has been described by the Wisconsin Reading Center as "featureless" retina (Figs. 5.15–5.21).

How would this patient be characterized by the ETDRS? By the Global Diabetic Retinopathy Project?

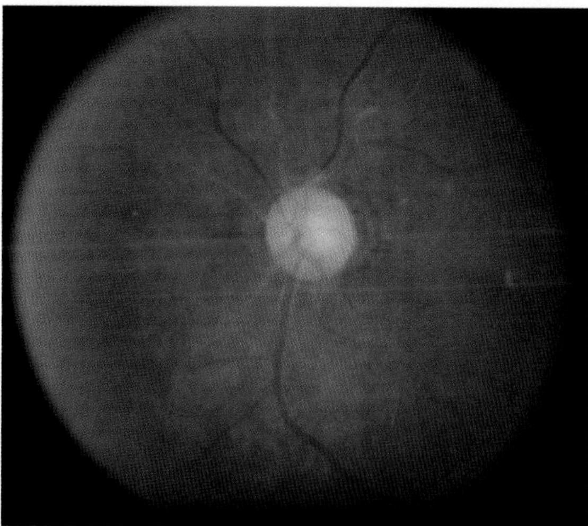

Fig. 5.15 Exercise 3: Field 1

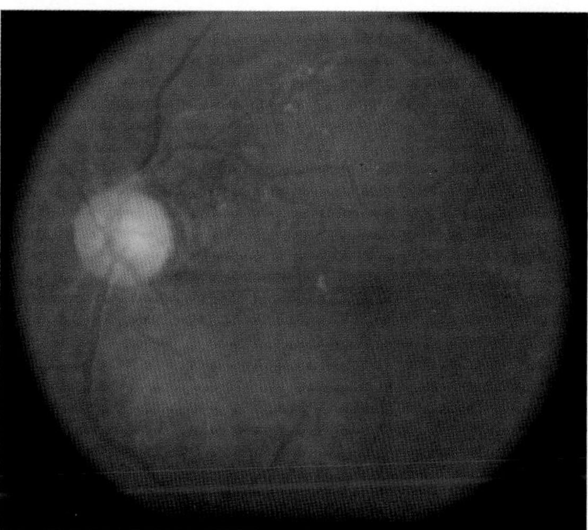

Fig. 5.16 Exercise 3: Field 2

Exercise 4

How many high-risk characteristics does this photograph demonstrate? (Fig. 5.22)

Would a fluorescein angiogram affect the classification?

Answer Key

Exercise 1 Answer:

Severe NPDR:

ETDRS definition 1: Soft exudates (SE), venous beading (VB), and intraretinal microvascular abnormalities (IRMA) all definitely present in at least two of fields 4 through 7 (Table 5.14).

ETDRS definition 2: Two of the preceding three lesions present in at least two of fields 4 through 7 and hemorrhages and microaneurysms present in these four fields, equaling or exceeding standard photograph 2A in at least one of them (Table 5.15).

ETDRS definition 3: Intraretinal microvascular abnormalities present in each of fields 4 through 7 and equaling or exceeding standard photograph 8A in at least two of them (Table 5.16).

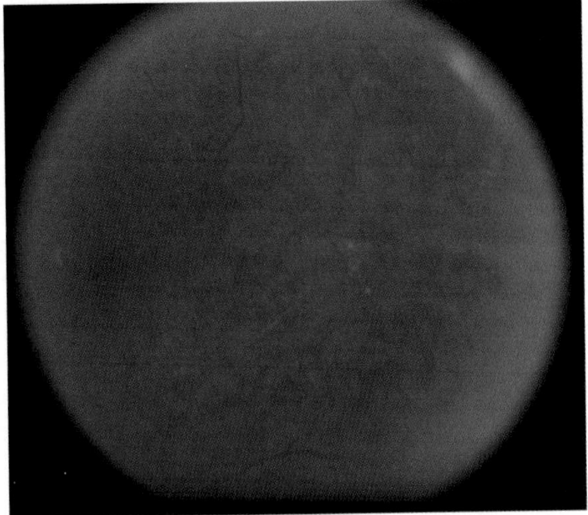

Fig. 5.17 Exercise 3: Field 3

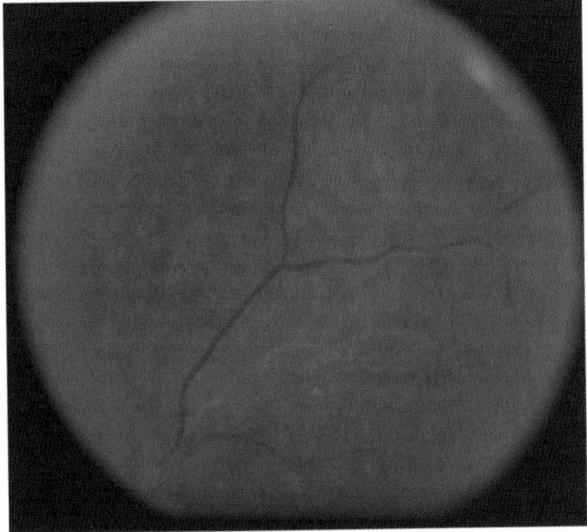

Fig. 5.18 Exercise 3: Field 4

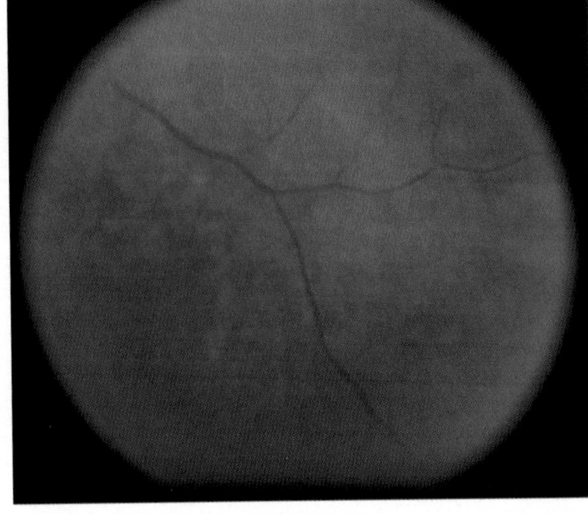

Fig. 5.19 Exercise 3: Field 5

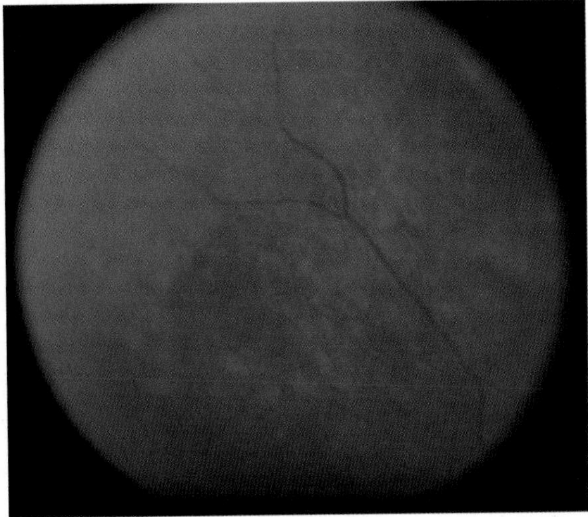

Fig. 5.20 Exercise 3: Field 6

DRS definition 1: Any three of the following: Soft exudates definitely present in ≥ 2 of photographic fields 4–7; IRMA definitely present in ≥ 2 of photographic fields 4–7; venous beading $\geq$ definitely present in ≥ 2 of photographic fields 4–7; hemorrhages/microaneurysms $\geq$ standard photo 2A in ≥ 1 of photographic fields 4–7 (Table 5.17).

4:2:1 rule: four quadrants of > 20 hemorrhages or two quadrants of venous beading or one quadrant of IRMA (Table 5.18).

Exercise 2 Answer:

Subclassification of diabetic retinopathy as to whether systemic medical factors are well controlled or poorly controlled has not undergone evaluation to determine whether such subclassification would change the response to therapy (it has been shown to affect the natural history). Such information would be helpful for clinicians to know.

Exercise 3 Answer:

ETDRS classification: Moderate NPDR

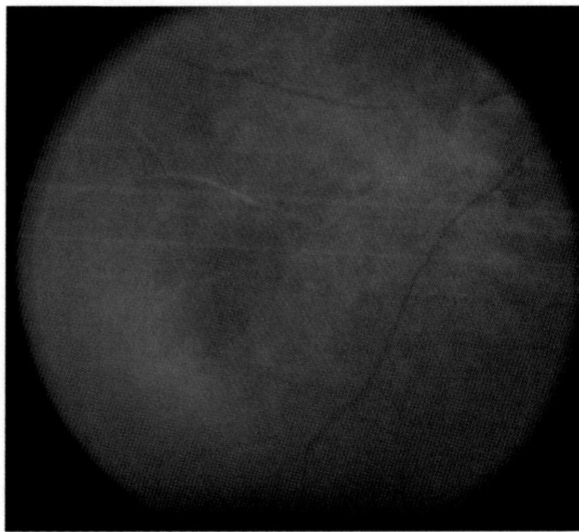

Fig. 5.21 Exercise 3: Field 7

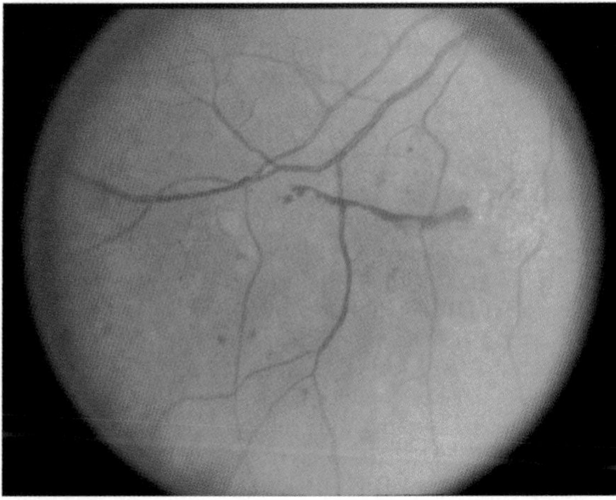

Fig. 5.22 Exercise 4

Table 5.14 Table with answers for grading fundus photographs using ETDRS definition 1 in exercise 1

Field	1	2	3	4	5	6	7
SE				No	**Yes**	No	No
VB				No	**Yes**	No	No
IRMA				**Yes**	No	No	No
Heme > 20				**Yes**	No	No	No

Table 5.15 Table with answers for grading fundus photographs using ETDRS definition 2 in exercise 1

Field	1	2	3	4	5	6	7
SE				No	**Yes**	No	No
VB				No	**Yes**	No	No
IRMA				**Yes**	No	No	No
Heme > 20				**Yes**	No	No	No

Table 5.16 Table with answers for grading fundus photographs using ETDRS definition 3 in exercise 1

Field	1	2	3	4	5	6	7
SE				No	**Yes**	No	No
VB				No	**Yes**	No	No
IRMA				**Yes**	No	No	No
Heme > 20				**Yes**	No	No	No

Table 5.17 Table with answers for grading fundus photographs using DRS definition 1 in exercise 1

Field	1	2	3	4	5	6	7
SE				No	**Yes**	No	No
VB				No	**Yes**	No	No
IRMA				**Yes**	No	No	No
Heme > 20				**Yes**	No	No	No

Table 5.18 Table with answers for grading fundus photographs using 4-2-1 rule in exercise 1

Field	1	2	3	4	5	6	7
SE				No	**Yes**	No	No
VB				No	**Yes**	No	No
IRMA				**Yes**	No	No	No
Heme > 20				**Yes**	No	No	No

Global Diabetic Retinopathy Project classification: Mild diabetic macular edema and moderate NPDR.

Exercise 4 Answer:

The preretinal hemorrhage present is the first high-risk characteristic. The presence of neovascularization is the second high-risk characteristic. The size of the neovascularization elsewhere being greater than 1/2 disc area is the third high-risk characteristic. A fluorescein angiogram may show disc neovascularization which would represent the fourth high-risk characteristic. The knowledge of whether or not the patient had the fourth high-risk characteristic would not change the recommendation that this patient stands to benefit from scatter laser photocoagulation. It may change the risk–benefit analysis in that the patient's natural history would be worse with four high-risk characteristics. A fluorescein angiogram may therefore be helpful if one is in doubt about the presence or absence of disk neovascularization.

References

1. Davis MD, Norton EWD, Meyers FL. The Airlie classification of diabetic retinopathy. In: Goldberg MF, Fine SL, eds. *Symposium on the Treatment of Diabetic*

Retinopathy. Washington, DC: US Government Printing Office; 1969:7–22. USPHS Publication #1890.
2. The Diabetic Retinopathy Study Research Group. A modification of the Airlie House classification of diabetic retinopathy: DRS Report 7. *Invest Ophthalmol Vis Sci*. 1981; 21:210–226.
3. Early Treatment Diabetic Retinopathy Study Group. Grading diabetic retinopathy from stereoscopic color fundus photographs: An extension of the modified Airlie house classification: ETDRS Report Number 10. *Ophthalmology*. 1991; 98: 786–806.
4. Early Treatment Diabetic Retinopathy Study Group. Fundus photographic risk factors for progression of diabetic retinopathy. ETDRS Report Number 12. *Ophthalmology*. 1991; 98: 823–833.
5. Early Treatment Diabetic Retinopathy Study Research Group. Early treatment Diabetic Retinopathy Study Design and baseline patient characteristics: ETDRS Report Number 7. *Ophthalmology*. 1991;98:741–756.
6. Wilkinson CP, Ferris FL III, Klein RE, et al. Proposed international clinical diabetic retinopathy and diabetic macular edema disease severity scales. *Ophthalmology*. 2003;110:1677–1682.
7. Early Treatment Diabetic Retinopathy Study Research Group. Early photocoagulation for diabetic retinopathy: ETDRS Report Number 9. *Ophthalmology*. 1991;98:766–785.
8. Patz A, Smith RE. The ETDRS and diabetes 2000. *Ophthalmology*. 1991;98:730–740.
9. Early Treatment Diabetic Retinopathy Study Group. Effects of aspirin treatment on diabetic retinopathy: ETDRS Report Number 8. *Ophthalmology*. 1991;98:758.
10. Gonzales ME, Gonzales C, Stern MP, et al. Concordance in diagnosis of diabetic retinopathy by fundus photography between retina specialists and a standardized reading center. *Arch Med Res*. 1995;26:127–131.
11. Early Treatment Diabetic Retinopathy Study Research Group. Photocoagulation for diabetic macular edema. ETDRS Report Number 4. *Int Ophthalmol Clin*. 1987;27:265–272.
12. Browning DJ, McOwen MD, Bowen RM Jr, et al. Comparison of the clinical diagnosis of diabetic macular edema with diagnosis by optical coherence tomography. *Ophthalmology*. 2004;111:712–715.
13. Browning DJ, Altaweel MM, Bressler NM, et al. Diabetic macular edema: what is focal and what is diffuse? *Am J Ophthalmol*. 2008;146:649–655.
14. Gangnon RE, Davis MD, Hubbard LD, et al. A severity scale for diabetic macular edema (DME) developed from ETDRS data. *IOVS*. 2008;49:5041–8.
15. Early Treatment Diabetic Retinopathy Study Research Group. Classification of diabetic retinopathy from fluorescein angiograms: ETDRS Report Number 11. *Ophthalmology*. 1991;98:807–822.
16. Early Treatment Diabetic Retinopathy Study Research Group. Fluorescein angiographic risk factors for progression of diabetic retinopathy: ETDRS Report Number 13. *Ophthalmology*. 1991;98:834–840.
17. Kylstra JA, Brown JC, Jaffe GJ, et al. The importance of fluorescein angiography in planning laser treatment of diabetic macular edema. *Ophthalmology*. 1999;106:2068–2073.
18. Early Treatment Diabetic Retinopathy Study Research Group. Treatment techniques and clinical guidelines for photocoagulation of diabetic macular edema: ETDRS Report Number 2. *Ophthalmology*. 1987;94:761–774.
19. Abu El, Asrar AM, Morse PH. Laser photocoagulation control of diabetic macular edema without fluorescein angiography. *Br J Ophthalmol*. 1991;75:97–99.
20. Diabetic Retinopathy Clinical Research Network. A phase II randomized clinical trial of intravitreal bevacizumab for diabetic macular edema. *Ophthalmology* 2007;114:1860–1867.
21. Friberg TR, Gupta A, Yu J, et al. Ultrawide angle fluorescein angiographic imaging: a comparison to conventional digital acquisition systems. *Ophthalmic Surg Lasers Imag*ing. 2008;39:304–311.
22. The Diabetes Control and Complications Trial/Epidemiology of Diabetes Intervention and Complications Study Research Group. Effects of intensive therapy on the microvascular complications of type I diabetes mellitus. *JAMA* 2002;287:2563–2569.
23. UK Prospective Diabetes Study Group. Effect of intensive blood-glucose control with metformin on complications in overweight patients with type 2 diabetes (UKPDS 34). *Lancet* 1988;352:854–865.
24. UK Prospective Diabetes Study Group. Tight blood pressure control and risk of macrovascular and microvascular complications in type 2 diabetes (UKPDS 38). *Br Med J*. 1998;317:703–713.
25. Lyons TJ, Jenkins AJ, Zhen D, et al. Diabetic retinopathy and serum lipoprotein subclasses in the DCCT/EDIC cohort. *Invest Ophthalmol Vis Sci*. 2004;45:910–918.
26. Kostraba JN, Klein R, Dorman JS, et al. The epidemiology of diabetes complications study. IV. Correlates of diabetic background and proliferative retinopathy. *Am J Epidemiol*. 1991;133:381–391.
27. Early Treatment Diabetic Retinopathy Study Research Group. Early Treatment Diabetic Retinopathy Study design and baseline patient characteristics: ETDRS Report Number 7. *Ophthalmology*. 1991;98:741–756.
28. Diabetes Control and Complications Research Group. The relationship of glycemic exposure (HbA1c) to the risk of development and progression of diabetic retinopathy in the diabetes control and complications trial. *Diabetes*. 1995;44:968–983.
29. Diabetes Control and Complications Trial/Epidemiology of Diabetes Interventions Complications Research Group. Prolonged effect of intensive therapy on the risk of retinopathy complications in patients with type 1 diabetes mellitus: 10 years after the diabetes control and complications trial. *Arch Ophthalmol*. 2008;126:1707–1715.
30. Diabetic Retinopathy Clinical Research Network. Comparison of modified-ETDRS and mild macular grid laser photocoagulation strategies for diabetic macular edema. *Arch Ophthalmol*. 2007;125:469–480.
31. Ferris F. Early photocoagulation in patients with type I or type II diabetes. *Trans Am Ophthalmol Soc*. 1996;94:505–537.

Chapter 6
Diagnostic Techniques in Clinical Practice – OCT, FA, Ultrasound

Keye Wong

If one follows the assumption that management of patients with diabetic retinopathy begins with an appropriate history and clinical examination then the purpose of ancillary diagnostic testing should be to add value to evaluation of the patient. Examples of such value may be to provide patient education to gain compliance with treatment recommendations (blood sugar control); to decide when additional intervention is beneficial either at baseline (detection of diabetic macular edema) or follow-up (response of diabetic macular edema to therapy); and to help establish prognosis such that appropriate follow-up schedules can be mutually agreed upon. In a research setting, there are additional purposes for ancillary testing but the emphasis in this chapter is on clinical care of patients with diabetic retinopathy.

6.1 Optical Coherence Tomography (OCT)

OCT measurements of macular structure provide both quantifiable measurements and morphologic information which are helpful in diagnosing and managing patients with diabetic macular edema.[1] Time domain OCT (Stratus OCT: Carl Zeiss Meditec, Inc., Dublin, CA) was proprietary and first to market. This technique has the ability to acquire images at a rate of 400 axial scans per second with an axial resolution up to 10 μm and transverse resolution up to 6 μm. By identifying the boundaries of the internal limiting membrane and the retinal pigment epithelium Stratus OCT software algorithms allow the calculation of the thickness of the retina at up to 512 points along a linear scan thereby generating a one-dimensional thickness map (see Fig. 6.1). By acquiring thickness measurements in two dimensions a topographical thickness map can be generated with various colors being assigned to numerical measurements (see Fig. 6.2).

Multiple linear scans in two dimensions are required to generate this two-dimensional map. The most commonly utilized software strategies to acquire these multiple linear scans are the "fast macular thickness" acquisition protocol and the "macular thickness" protocol. Both protocols obtain six radial line scans separated by two clock hours and centered on the foveola (see Fig. 6.1 – "Fundus Image").

The fast macular thickness protocol automatically obtains these six radial line scans. Each radial line scan obtains data from 128 axial measurements. At a scan rate of 400 scans per second the fast macular thickness protocol takes 1.92 s. In contrast, in the macular thickness acquisition protocol the operator obtains each of the six radial line scans individually as separate scans. Each line scan is obtained with 512 axial measurements so the lateral resolution of each component line scan is 4× higher than with the fast macular thickness protocol. Each individual scan takes 1.28 s. The potential advantage of this higher lateral resolution is that it gives more data points with which to interpolate thickness measurements. However, the disadvantage of the macular thickness protocol is that the quality of the scan is more reliant on patient fixation. If the center point of each individual line scan is not centered precisely on

K. Wong (✉)
University of South Florida, Sarasota, FL 34242, USA
e-mail: iskeye@yahoo.com

D.J. Browning (ed.), *Diabetic Retinopathy*, DOI 10.1007/978-0-387-85900-2_6,

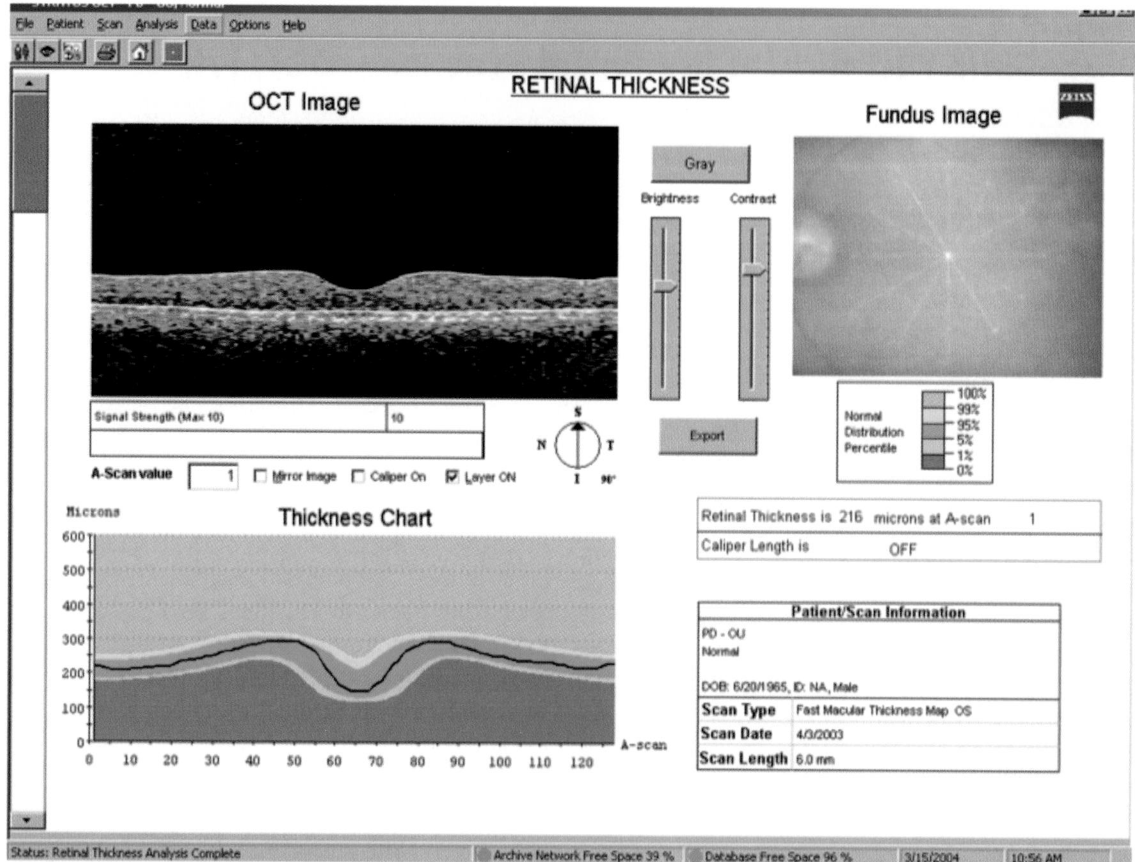

Fig. 6.1 By identifying the boundaries of the internal limiting membrane and the retinal pigment epithelium the Stratus OCT software generates a "Thickness Chart" (*bottom left*) by calculating the thickness of the retina (in μm) at each A-scan location (128 A-scans in the fast macular thickness protocol and up to 512 A-scans in the macular thickness protocol)

the foveal center (as in patients with poorer fixation) then the center point thickness measurement of each of the scans will vary and artifacts may be generated. This feature may lead to greater inter-operator variability and greater inter-visit variability.

Since OCT reliably[2] and reproducibly[3] measures the thickness of the macula it has found great clinical utility in diabetics in the management of macular edema.[4] Variable terminology has been used in reporting quantitative thickness measurements.[5] The quantitative measurements most commonly studied from both the fast macular thickness and the macular thickness acquisition protocols are the center point thickness and the central subfield mean thickness (CSMT) (see Fig. 6.2). The center point thickness represents the average thickness value of the center point of each of the six radial line scans. It therefore represents the average of six measurements. The central subfield mean thickness represents the average thickness value of all of the sampling points within the central 1 mm diameter circle surrounding fixation. With the protocol acquisition scans typically taking a 6.0 mm length scan the central subfield thickness averages the thickness measurements of 512 thickness measurements if using the macular thickness protocol and 128 thickness measurements if using the fast macular thickness protocol. Although there are more data points to average using the macular thickness protocol the central subfield mean thickness does not show significant variation from the fast macular thickness protocol for patients with macular edema.[6]

The initial normative data were obtained from 73 eyes of 41 volunteers.[7] The mean center point thickness was 152 ± 21 μm and the mean central retinal subfield thickness was 174 ± 18 μm. If one

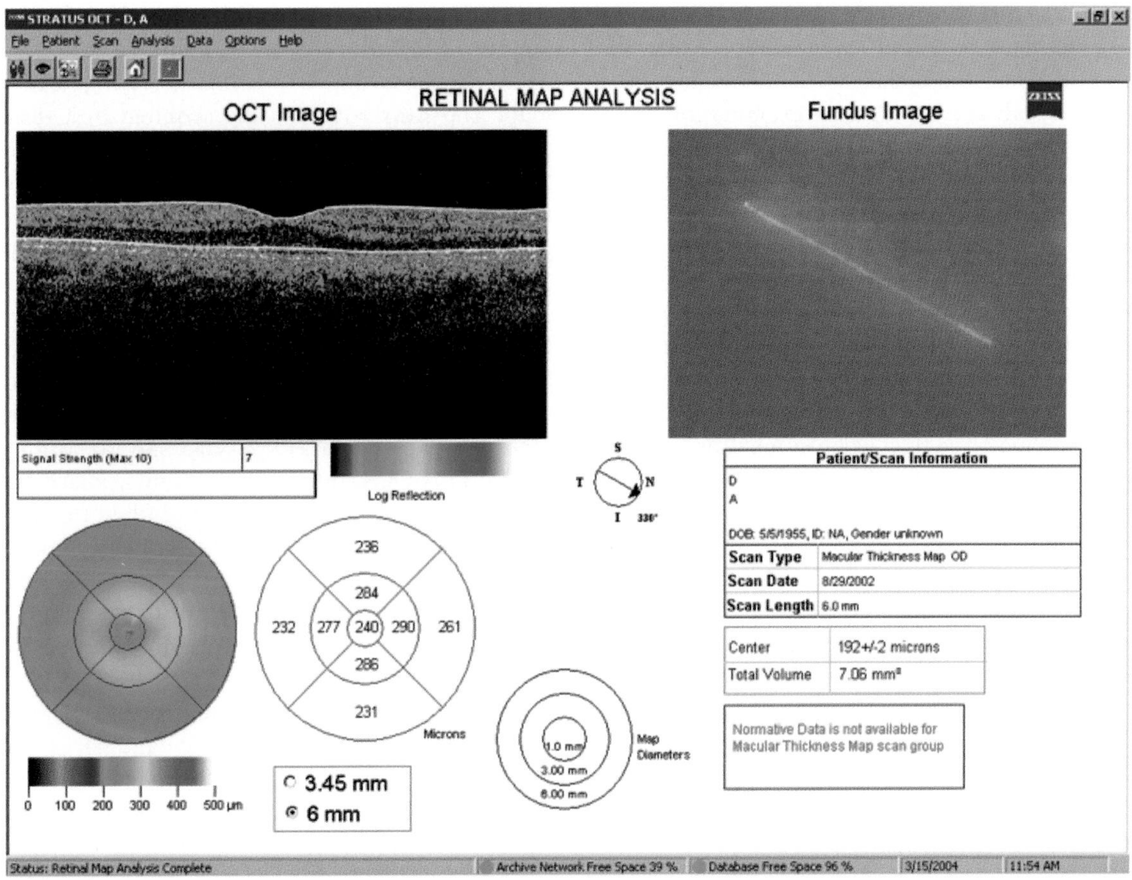

Fig. 6.2 The false color map (*lower left*) is generated by the Stratus OCT software applying an arbitrary color to each of the A-scan thickness measurements from each of the six individual line scans. By averaging the thickness measurements within the central 1.0 mm of each of the six line scans Stratus OCT software generates the "central subfield mean thickness" (240 µm in this example). By averaging the thickness at the very center of each of the six line scans a "center point thickness" measurement is generated (192 ± 2 µm in this example)

considers 95% of normals to be within two standard deviations above the mean then the upper limit for normals for CSMT would be 174 + 36 = 210 µm. Using the Stratus OCT in diabetics with minimal or no retinopathy[8] the CSMT was 201 ± 22 µm, considerably higher than that reported by Hee et al. with an older OCT version. The CSMT also varied with gender with the mean for men being 209 ± 18 µm and the mean for women being 194 ± 23 µm. Therefore 95% of normals for men would be less than 209 + 36 = 245 µm whereas 95% of normals for women would be less than 194 + 46 = 240 µm.

So how does *quantitative* OCT add value to and for the patient? Even with the advent of pharmacotherapy[9–11] the best evidence directing treatment of diabetic macular edema comes from the Early Treatment Diabetic Retinopathy Study.[12,13] Clinically significant macular edema is a subjective diagnosis made by slit lamp biomicroscopy but remains the only indication supported by level 1 evidence by which one should make the decision to treat with photocoagulation. In the ETDRS the presence or absence of "clinically significant macular edema" was determined by reading center grading of stereo fundus photographs. In the DRS and ETDRS the reading center agreed with experienced clinical investigators in the diagnosis of macular edema 55% of the time after correcting for the effects of chance agreement.[14]

The concordance between diabetic macular edema diagnosed by evaluation of stereo fundus photographs and by evaluation using OCT is moderate at best.[15] The concordance between clinically significant macular edema diagnosed by contact lens biomicroscopy and by evaluation using OCT is good when the edema is definitely present or definitely absent on clinical examination but is poor when the edema is clinically questionable. Brown et al.[16] examined the concordance between contact lens biomicroscopy and Stratus OCT in detecting patients with a clinical diagnosis of no edema, questionable edema, and definite edema involving the fovea. The concordance was high for patients without edema or with definite edema but significant disparity occurred in the patients with questionable edema. For patients with questionable foveal edema on contact lens examination over 50% of these patients had a central foveal thickness ≥300 μm. Browning et al.[17] found a similar lack of concordance if the diagnosis of CSME was performed using noncontact lens slit lamp biomicroscopy. For this subset of patients where clinical examination and OCT data are discordant, the data regarding natural history and response to therapy are not yet available.[18] Therefore, if one accepts that clinical examination with contact lens slit lamp biomicroscopy is the standard way to diagnose clinically significant macular edema then the lack of complete concordance between OCT and slit lamp biomicroscopy implies that the information obtained from OCT should remain as confirmatory.

On the contrary if one accepts that OCT measurements of diabetic macular edema are more accurate than clinical assessments then disparate information would be viewed as one's clinical examination representing false positives and false negatives and the OCT information as true positives and true negatives. Using OCT as a surrogate measure of contact lens-determined clinically significant macular edema would subsequently imply that a significant number of patients may be undertreated or overtreated in comparison to ETDRS guidelines. Currently there are no studies to compare the relative benefit of treatment for clinically significant macular edema diagnosed by contact lens biomicroscopy vs. OCT measurement of edema.

The recent advent of spectral (Fourier) domain OCT is a new technology which operates on a similar principle to the Stratus OCT but obtains axial scan rates of at least 20,000 scans per second with an axial resolution up to 5 μm. As compared to Stratus OCT the higher scan rate allows less fixation artifact. In addition this higher scan rate allows greater detail in generating a two-dimensional thickness map. The scans are typically acquired in a raster pattern with many more thickness measurements being acquired. Whereas the macular thickness protocol of the Stratus OCT obtains $6 \times 512 = 3{,}072$ thickness measurements within the macula, the default setting of Topcon spectral domain OCT acquires $128 \times 512 = 65{,}536$ thickness measurements with a central 6×6 mm square. Since the Stratus OCT samples thickness measurements only along the six radial scans at every two clock hours there are gaps of data between these radial lines. The Stratus OCT software allows interpolation of proximal thickness measurement to fill in the gaps. As compared to Stratus OCT the greater number of scans with spectral domain OCT allows for retinal thickness measurements to be calculated based on actual measurements in contrast to interpolation between actual measurements.

The algorithms for measuring retinal thickness may employ different anatomic landmarks and therefore the absolute quantitative measurement numbers may vary between Stratus OCT and spectral domain OCT systems. The Stratus time domain OCT system identifies retinal thickness as the distance between the internal limiting membrane and the junction of the photoreceptor outer segments and inner segments. In contrast the Cirrus spectral domain OCT identifies retinal thickness as the distance between the ILM and the retinal pigment epithelium. On average the quantitative measurements of retinal thickness within the various subfields of the Cirrus spectral domain OCT system are 30–55 μm greater as compared to the Stratus OCT consistent with histopathologic demonstration of the outer segments of photoreceptors measuring 50 μm in length.[19] Although the absolute numbers may vary between Stratus and Cirrus OCTs, the increased resolution from these spectral domain OCT systems should not theoretically change the principles of using OCT in management of DME.

Although spectral domain OCTs offer greater resolution the software algorithms for quantifying retinal thickness have not yet reached the acceptance level of Stratus OCT. In the absence of consistent quantitative data of spectral domain OCTs the clinician will have to rely upon comparing qualitative (morphologic) data on similarly registered scans.

To summarize the additional benefit of quantitative OCT over clinical examination, evaluation of stereo fundus photographs is the research standard by which macular thickening is classified as clinically significant or not clinically significant. Slit lamp biomicroscopy (either contact or noncontact) is an acceptable clinical surrogate for evaluation of stereo fundus photographs. The literature demonstrates a modest correlation between clinical determination of diabetic macular edema and OCT determination of diabetic macular edema with discordant results occurring primarily in cases of questionable clinical edema. Therefore in situations where subjective clinical examination and objective OCT findings are discordant one should make the decision to recommend initial treatment of diabetic macular edema based on clinical examination.

So if one's decision to treat is still based on clinical examination then when should an OCT be obtained? As compared to stereo photographs OCT is a more sensitive means of detecting change in retinal thickening.[20] Therefore in patients with clinically significant macular edema undergoing treatment the quantitative findings from the OCT may be of value to the patient in helping to make retreatment decisions. In all therapies in which a choice of treatments is available, clinicians attempt to categorize patients into "responders" and "non-responders" or "poor responders." In poor or non-responders decisions to repeat treatment or change treatment may logically improve patient outcome (although this premise has not been demonstrated by clinical trials). Obtaining an OCT at baseline and at time points where retreatment decisions are in question[21] may therefore be reasonable. One should realize, however, that the ultimate clinical goal is to provide the best visual outcome and that in patients with diabetic macular edema OCT correlates modestly with vision and changes in OCT in response to therapy correlates only modestly with changes in visual acuity.[22]

In patients with diabetic macular edema that is not yet clinically significant, obtaining an OCT was not helpful in predicting which patients would progress to clinically significant macular edema.[23] However, in those individuals with diabetic macular edema which is not yet clinically significant, obtaining an OCT may be helpful in confirming the progression to clinically significant macular edema.[24] This strategy provides added value to the patient if one believes that earlier diagnosis and treatment of clinically significant macular edema provides a better visual outcome, i.e., if chronic macular edema carries a poorer prognosis as compared to sub-acute macular edema.

Some clinicians believe that patients with proliferative diabetic retinopathy and high-risk characteristics may be at risk for worsening of macular edema in conjunction with scatter photocoagulation.[25] In the DRS 14% of patients treated with argon laser and 30% of patients treated with xenon laser suffered $\geq$ 1 line of vision loss at 2 years.[26] In the ETDRS, of the patients with baseline macular edema who underwent full-scatter photocoagulation, 4.5% suffered $\geq$ 3 lines of vision loss at 6 weeks and 9.7% suffered $\geq$ 3 lines of vision loss at 4 months.[27] The beneficial effect of scatter photocoagulation as outlined in the Diabetic Retinopathy Study is to help reduce the chance of deteriorating to vision <5/200 at two consecutive 4-month visits. However, in the current era patients may not consider their scatter photocoagulation treatment a "success" if their vision drops in conjunction with laser-induced macular edema. OCT documentation of this edema prior to scatter photocoagulation treatment may be helpful to serve as a baseline should visual decline occur and may incline the ophthalmologist to add adjunctive therapy such as intraocular or peribulbar triamcinolone or intraocular anti-VEGF therapy.[28,29] The documentation prior to therapy may be helpful in educating patients regarding their risk of suffering moderate visual loss. Should moderate visual loss occur then OCT quantification of macular edema may be helpful to follow the course of edema. Although the time course by which post-laser edema can be expected to improve is not known, if edema does not show improvement on sequential 3-month visits then additional therapy may be logical. Obtaining an OCT adds additional value to the patient by providing quantification of the improvement or lack of improvement of macular edema.

Besides *quantitative* information, OCT provides morphologic, *qualitative* information. Subclassifying diabetic macular edema by morphologic OCT patterns has been proposed:

(1) diffuse retinal thickening (see Fig. 6.3).
(2) cystoid macular edema (see Fig. 6.4)
(3) posterior hyaloidal traction (see Fig. 6.5)
(4) subretinal fluid (see Fig. 6.6)
(5) traction retinal detachment (see Fig. 6.7).[30–32]

There are intuitive reasons why the qualitative information of morphology may aid in altering prognosis or therapeutic approach over and above the quantitative information of retinal thickness measurements. Chronic fluid accumulation may result

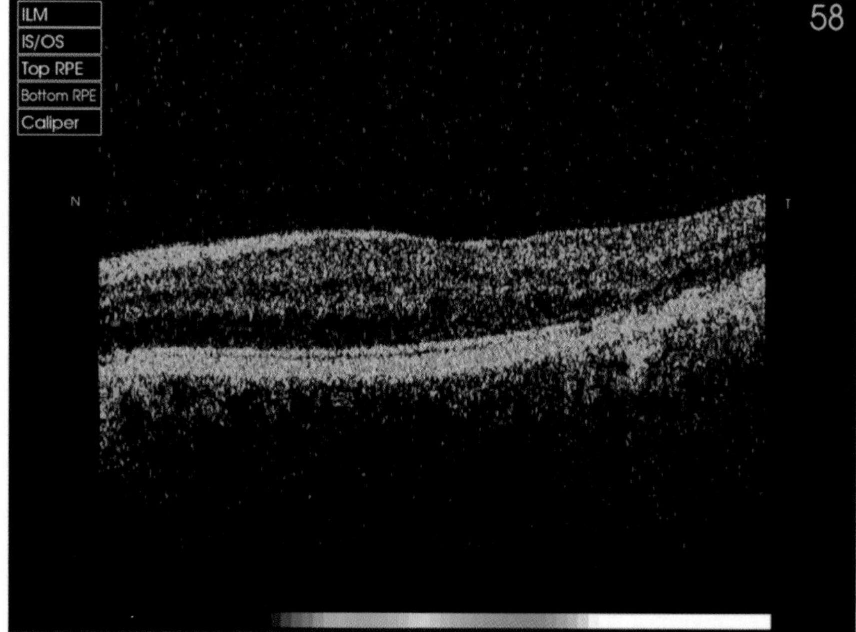

Fig. 6.3 Diffuse retinal thickening

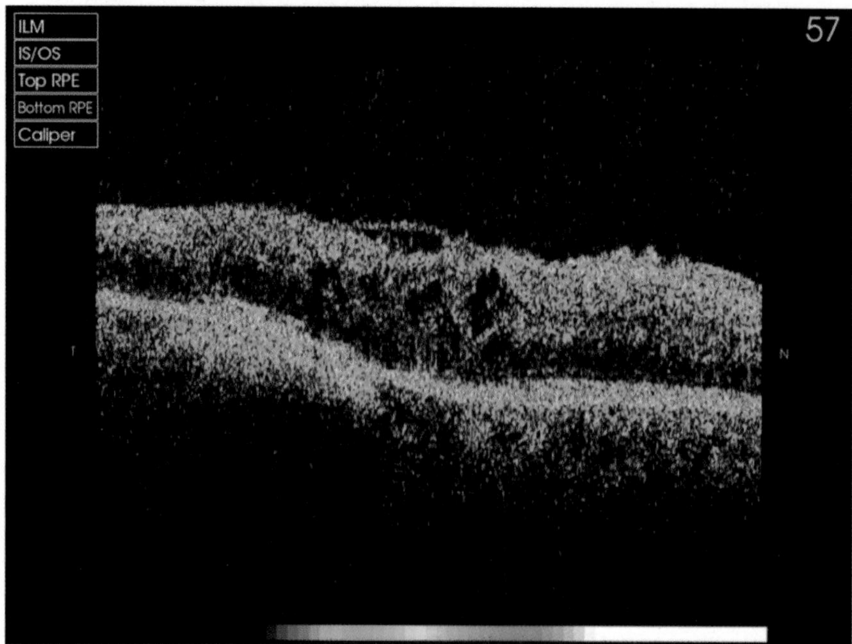

Fig. 6.4 Cystoid macular edema

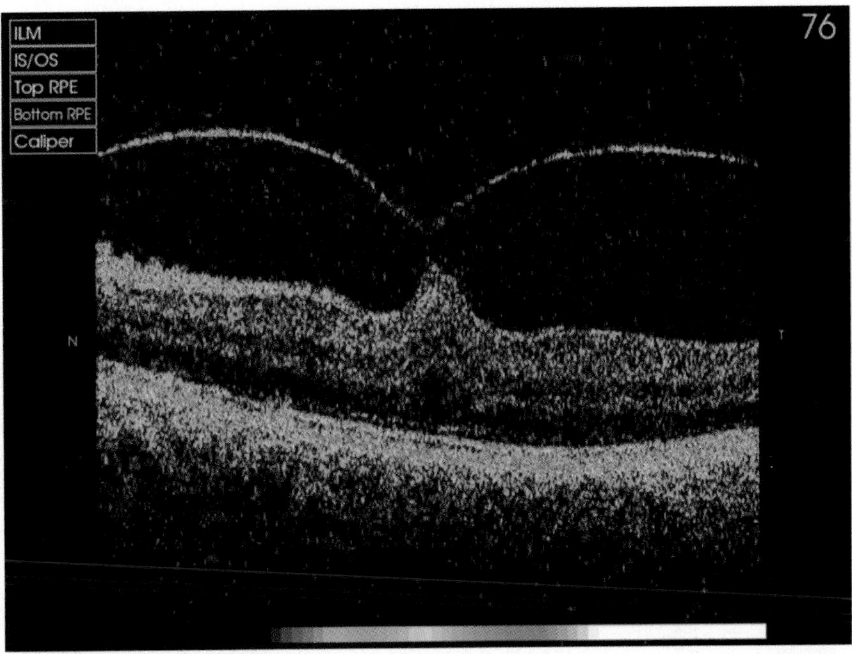

Fig. 6.5 Posterior hyaloidal traction

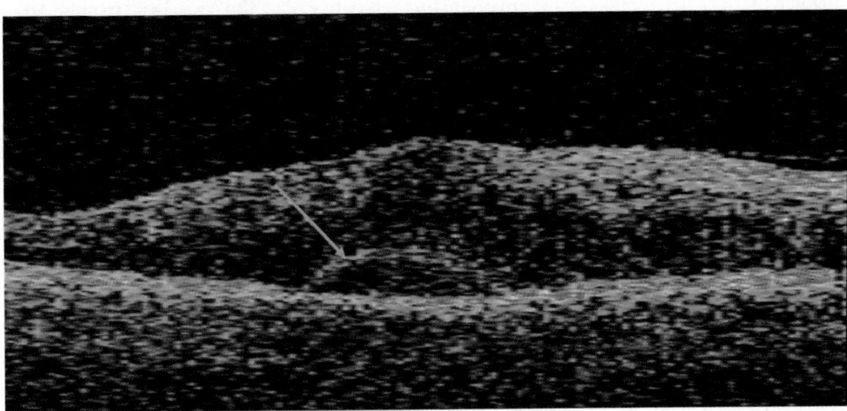

Fig. 6.6 Subretinal fluid indicated by an orange arrow

in Muller cell necrosis and accumulation of fluid in the extracellular space (presumably the "cystoid macular edema" OCT morphology pattern). The distinction of cystic vs. non-cystic retinal thickening may therefore imply Muller cell necrosis. On a functional basis this concept is supported by data indicating that an increased quantitative macular thickening shows a modest correlation with worse visual acuity.[33] Furthermore, with moderate thickening of the macula ($<\sim 400$ μm) the additional presence of cystoid changes correlates with a greater deficit in visual acuity.[34] However, although cystoid morphology may correlate with initially worse visual acuity it is unclear whether such morphology portends a poorer response to therapy. In the ETDRS the presence of cystoid changes did not eliminate the benefit of focal laser photocoagulation in reducing the risk of moderate visual loss.[35]

Likewise, the distinction of whether or not diabetic macular edema is caused by mechanical traction may intuitively alter the therapeutic approach. The demonstration of partially detached hyaloid which is exerting tangential traction on the macula in conjunction with subretinal fluid has been proposed as an indication to benefit from surgical

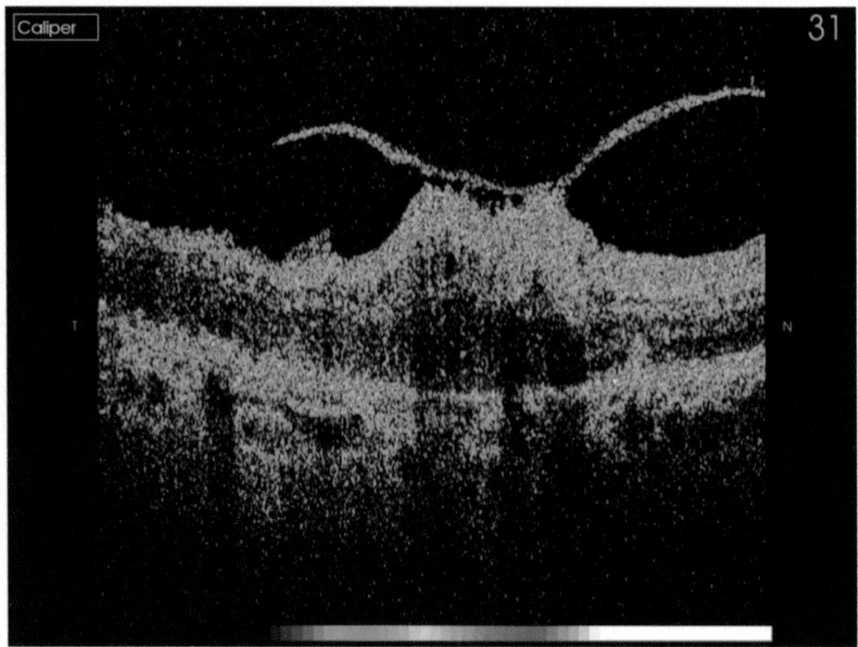

Fig. 6.7 Tractional retinal detachment

intervention.[36] Surgical intervention has also been proposed for a "taut" hyaloid membrane.[37] Diagnosis of a "taut" hyaloid membrane is clinically based on a "glistening" reflex from the surface of the macula in conjunction with fluorescein angiographic evidence of diffuse oozing from tissue deep in the retina. The OCT demonstration of an associated epiretinal membrane conceptually supports the potential benefit of surgical intervention for this "taut" hyaloid membrane. Although the morphologic information from OCT is very helpful in diagnosing both of these conditions, vitrectomy for diabetic macular edema is still not currently considered to be standard-of-care as evidenced by the current National Eye Institute-sponsored trial to evaluate vitrectomy for diabetic macular edema.[38]

6.2 Heidelberg Retinal Tomograph (HRT)

The Heidelberg Retinal Tomograph (HRT) (Heidelberg Engineering, Heidelberg, Germany) is a confocal laser scanning tomograph that sequentially acquires images in the x,y plane along the z-axis. The HRT II image contains 384 × 384 pixels in the central 4.5 × 4.5 mm square of the retina for a transverse resolution of approximately 12 μm. Given the sampling strategy of the HRT the transverse resolution is equivalent throughout the scanned area. As compared to the sampling strategy of OCT the HRT will provide more "edema" data points in the paracentral macula outside of the central 500 μm radius central subfield macular thickness (CSMT). However, it appears that global measures of diabetic macular edema consistently correlate with CSMT and provide no apparent differential information to modify treatment or prognosis.[39] Therefore the theoretical advantage of HRT sampling strategy may not be a clinically relevant advantage.

Unlike OCT in which retinal thickness is measured by computing the distance from the RPE reflection and the internal limiting membrane (ILM) reflection, the HRT measures a change in the distribution of the reflected light which is associated with retinal edema. An edema index can be generated for each scanned point of the macula. This edema index measures the optical effect of edema but does not quantify the distance between the RPE and ILM. When this edema index is compared to a clinically derived map drawn by retina specialists examining patients with diabetic macular edema (clinically significant macular edema), the HRT was 92% sensitive and 68% specific in detecting areas with edema[40] and as a consequence the HRT has not gained wide acceptance. In the absence of clinical trials it remains to be determined whether HRT adds value to the patient above clinical examination.

6.3 Retinal Thickness Analyzer (RTA)

The Retinal Thickness Analyzer (RTA; Talia Technology Ltd., Neve-Ilan, Israel) works on a principle of slit lamp biomicroscopy. Sixteen sequential vertical scans are rapidly generated across the central 3 × 3 mm of the macula to generate a topographical map of retinal thickness. The axial resolution is up to 50 μm and the transverse resolution is 187 μm. RTA software generates a foveal average thickness measurement. When this foveal average thickness measurement is compared to a clinically derived map drawn by retina specialists examining patients with diabetic macular edema (clinically significant macular edema) the RTA was 57% sensitive and 71% specific in detecting areas with edema.[40] This poor sensitivity and specificity translates into a reduced reliability in measuring macular edema as compared to stereo fundus photography[41] and OCT technology,[42] and as a consequence the RTA has not gained widespread use in clinical practice nor in clinical trials in managing diabetic macular edema. In the absence of clinical trials it remains to be determined whether RTA adds value to the patient above clinical examination.

6.4 Microperimetry

Retinal thickness measured by OCT correlates only modestly with visual acuity. Alternative explanations for visual loss (such as duration and severity of systemic diabetes and duration of edema) other than just the quantity of edema logically play a role. Fundus microperimetry is a scanning laser ophthalmoscope technology which maps fixation characteristics and sensitivity within the macula. Whereas visual acuity measures foveolar function, microperimetry can measure parafoveal visual function. In diabetic patients eccentric fixation and unstable fixation correlate with poorer visual acuity, mean OCT thickness, and a cystic OCT morphology.[43,44] The additional information provided by microperimetry over and above visual acuity data may logically allow diabetic macular edema to be subclassified into categories demonstrating differential response to therapeutic interventions. Such an investigation, however, has not yet been performed and it remains to be determined whether microperimetry adds value to the patient above clinical examination.

6.5 Color Fundus Photography

The large data set of the ETDRS demonstrates that stereoscopic color fundus photographs provide one with great predictive power to determine the risk of progression to proliferative diabetic retinopathy[45] (see Chapter 5). Dependent on the level of experience, ophthalmoscopy is often not as sensitive as slide film in detecting diabetic retinopathy.[46] Seven-field stereoscopic digital imaging is equally sensitive to slide film in detecting neovascularization of the disc, neovascularization elsewhere, and clinically significant macular edema.[47] Evaluation of stereoscopic digital images of fields 1 and 2 only with JPEG compression demonstrates a high correlation with seven-field stereoscopic slide film in detecting diabetic retinopathy.[48] Non-stereoscopic digital imaging has poor sensitivity in detecting clinically significant macular edema.[49] In summary, the acquisition of stereo color fundus photographs (either with slide film or digitally acquired) may add value to the evaluation of the diabetic patient dependent upon the experience of the examiner. These results may allow teleophthalmology strategies to effectively screen diabetic patients for appropriate referrals.

6.6 Fluorescein Angiography

Historically the development of fluorescein angiography (and fluorescein angiography conferences) defined the onset of medical retina as a distinct

Table 6.1 Cumulative 2-year rates of severe visual loss in eyes grouped by baseline severity of retinopathy and treatment assignment

Group	NVE	NVD	VH PRH	No. of NV-VH risk factors	Control SVL (%)	Control *N*	Treated SVL (%)	Treated *N*	*Z* value
A	0	0	0	0	3.6	195	3.0	182	0.4
B	0	0	+	1	4.2	11	0.0	16	1.0
C	< 1/2 DA	0	0	1	6.8	120	2.0	96	1.8
D	< 1/2DA	0	+	2	6.4	18	0.0	19	1.1
E	≥1/2 DA	0	0	2	6.9	125	4.3	141	1.0
F	≥1/2 DA	0	+	3	29.7	40	7.2	41	3.0
G	+ or 0	<10A	0	2	10.5	114	3.1	126	2.4
H	+ or 0	<10A	+	3	25.6	39	4.3	35	2.9
I	+ or 0	≥10A	0	3	26.2	150	8.5	174	4.7
J	+ or 0	≥10A	+	4	36.9	76	20.1	107	3.2
All eyes					15.9	897	6.4	946	7.2

NVD = new vessels on or within 1 disc diameter of the optic disc; NVE = new vessels elsewhere (i.e., outside of the area defined as NVD); VHPRH = vitreous and/or preretinal hemorrhage; SVL = severe visual loss (visual acuity < 5/200 at two or more consecutively completed follow-up visits scheduled at 4-month intervals); DA = disc area (NVE < 1/2 DA indicates that NVE does not equal or exceed one-half the area of the disc in any of the standard photographic fields, NVE ≥ 1/2 DA indicates that NVE equals or exceeds this area in at least one of these fields); 10A = Standard Photograph 10A of the Modified Airlie House Classification.
Reprinted with permission from DRS Research Group[58].

discipline.[50,51] Since its original descriptions in 1960s[52–54] fluorescein angiography remained the dominant imaging technique for managing retinal and choroidal vascular diseases until OCT became widely available at the start of the 21st century. By illustrating the competency of the retinal vascular and choroidal circulation the pathophysiology of diabetic retinopathy became much better understood. The landmark clinical trials of the Diabetic Retinopathy Study[55] and Early Treatment Diabetic Retinopathy Study used fluorescein angiography in classifying disease severity,[56] guiding laser therapy,[57] and evaluating the response to therapy.[35] With this historical background one may ask the question that in the 21st century does fluorescein angiography still add clinical value to the patient?

Regarding proliferative diabetic retinopathy the Diabetic Retinopathy Study (DRS) defined indications for benefiting from scatter photocoagulation.[58] Findings which placed the patient at high risk for losing vision were defined. These high-risk factors are (1) new vessels present, (2) new vessels located on or within 1 disc diameter of the disc, (3) new vessels moderate to severe (NVD ≥ standard photograph 10A or, for eyes without NVD, NVE ≥ 1/2 disc area), and (4) vitreous or preretinal hemorrhage present.[59] Determination and diagnosis of these features are based on clinical examination and not fluorescein angiography. In the DRS the cumulative 2-year rates of severe visual loss was as high as 36.9% in controls (see Table 6.1).

Groups F, H, I, and J have three or four high-risk factors and in those groups scatter photocoagulation significantly reduces the 2-year risk of severe visual loss. In groups with less than three high-risk factors, the difference between treatment and control groups was not significant and therefore prompt scatter photocoagulation was not advised. One can see that in a diabetic patient with vitreous hemorrhage but without clinically visible neovacularization (Groups B and D) the identification of neovascular tissue within the standard seven fields would change one's recommendation for *prompt* scatter photocoagulation. Therefore, in diabetic patients with vitreous hemorrhage but without identifiable neovascular tissue fluorescein angiography to attempt to identify leakage associated with occult NVE or NVD would change one's therapeutic recommendation.

In patients with nonproliferative diabetic retinopathy the indication to benefit from focal photocoagulation is clinically significant macular edema. As reviewed in Chapter 5 (Defining Diabetic Retinopathy Severity) this definition is a clinical diagnosis based on slit lamp biomicroscopy and does not rely on fluorescein angiography. Therefore the information obtained from fluorescein angiography should not change one's recommendation as to whether or not the patient should undergo laser therapy. However, the Early Treatment Diabetic Retinopathy Study utilized a combination of two laser strategies to treat diabetic macular edema. A focal treatment was applied directly to all leaking microaneurysms between 500 and 3,000 μm from the center of the fovea. (This pattern of leakage arising from microaneurysms was termed "focal" leakage in the ETDRS.) A grid treatment was subsequently applied to all areas of diffuse leakage and for areas of capillary nonperfusion. (This pattern of leakage was termed "diffuse" leakage in the ETDRS). Identification of microaneurysms, diffuse leakage, and areas of capillary nonperfusion are all features identified by fluorescein angiography. Fluorescein angiography is therefore indicated based on ETDRS data to help guide initial laser therapy.

The terms focal and diffuse fluorescein leakage are often used imprecisely.[60] Focal fluorescein leakage presumably arising from microaneurysms was differentiated in the ETDRS from diffuse fluorescein leakage presumably arising from leaking capillaries. The value of distinguishing between diffuse and focal diabetic macular edema is uncertain (see Sidebar in Chapter 7 Diabetic Macular Edema).[35]

Although ETDRS protocol utilized fluorescein angiography to guide therapy it is not clear whether such guidance is necessary to obtain beneficial results. Since the results of the ETDRS were released, interpretation of "ETDRS laser technique" in clinical practice varies. The Diabetic Retinopathy Clinical Research Network (DRCR.net) is a collaborative network involving 150 sites (both community and university based) with over 500 investigators.[61] Based on a survey of its investigators the initial protocol compared two prevalent laser treatment techniques for management of diabetic macular edema.[62] Microaneurysms were specifically treated in one laser treatment protocol (so-called modified ETDRS focal/gird [mETDRS]). The visual acuity results at 12 months were not statistically different from the protocol in which microaneurysms were specifically not treated (so-called modified macular grid treatment [MMG]). In a subsequent DRCR.net study comparing this "modified ETDRS" laser technique to intravitreal triamcinolone, fluorescein angiography was not required and performed only at investigator discretion.[63] This "modified ETDRS" laser treatment has not been compared to protocol ETDRS laser treatment in a clinical trial. However, there is support in the literature[64] and it appears that current clinical practice based on DRCR.net protocols demonstrates a positive treatment response when laser is not guided by fluorescein angiography. The ETDRS also found no fluorescein angiographic variable of prognostic importance for outcome.[35]

Retinal vascular diseases characterized by ischemia are associated with an upregulation of vascular endothelial growth factor[65] with a subsequent increased risk of retinal and iris neovascularization. Multiple clinical research protocols are currently investigating the benefit of anti-VEGF intravitreal injections in the management of proliferative diabetic retinopathy and diabetic macular edema.[66–68] As a means to document retinal circulation, fluorescein angiography is the best ancillary study to investigate ischemia. In contrast to ischemia of the macula, ischemia of the peripheral retina has a greater association with an increased production of VEGF and other vasoproliferative factors. If one could categorize peripheral retinal ischemia in diabetic retinopathy would this add value for the patient?

The technology currently exists to give us this information. Conventional fluorescein angiography images the retinal circulation within the posterior pole. Ultra wide-field fluorescein angiography is a technique which can visualize the peripheral retina far beyond the seven standard photographic fields of the Modified Airlie House Classification (see Fig. 6.8).

The results of the ETDRS are typically viewed with regard to its conclusions regarding the management of macular edema. One of the principal questions asked by the Early Treatment Diabetic Retinopathy Study (and perhaps why it was named "early treatment") was "when in the course of diabetic retinopathy is it most effective to initiate photocoagulation therapy?" Patients were eligible if they had mild, moderate, or severe nonproliferative retinopathy or early proliferative retinopathy. These patients were then randomized to early photocoagulation or deferral of photocoagulation until high-risk characteristics developed. In patients who received

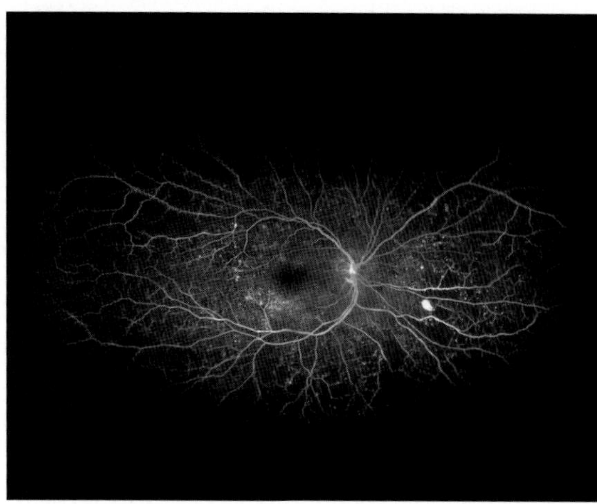

Fig. 6.8 Example of ultra wide field fluorescein in angiography taken with a scanning laser ophthalmoscope

early photocoagulation the pattern of scatter laser photocoagulation was randomized to either "mild" scatter or "full" scatter. About 1843 patients received a full-scatter treatment composed of 1,200–1,600 burns and 1,868 patients received a mild-scatter treatment composed of 400–650 burns.[27] At 5 years the rate of developing high-risk proliferative retinopathy was 18.4% in the full-scatter group and 28.7% in the mild-scatter group. Therefore, mild-scatter photocoagulation is not as effective as full-scatter photocoagulation in preventing progression to high-risk proliferative retinopathy. However, mild-scatter photocoagulation was better than observation in that 40.7% of patients in the observation group developed high-risk proliferative retinopathy at 5 years. The ETDRS therefore provides evidence that mild-scatter photocoagulation provides a reduction in the rate of progression to high-risk characteristics but not as great a rate as full scatter.

It is intuitive that if one were to have angiographic information from the retinal periphery which would subclassify diabetic retinopathy with regard to the extent of peripheral ischemia then this subclassification might allow the mild-scatter treatment protocol to achieve the degree of benefit demonstrated by full scatter without as great a risk of suffering moderate visual loss (9.7% at 4 months in full scatter vs. 6.4% at 4 months in mild scatter).[27] At this time a study using a subclassification of peripheral retinal ischemia to direct the extent of laser treatment has not been performed.

Table 6.2 Occurrence of moderate visual loss at 5 years

	Moderate vision loss		
	Early full scatter (%)	Early mild scatter (%)	Deferral (%)
Macular edema & less severe retinopathy	29.8	21.8	30.2
Macular edema & more severe retinopathy	24.1	25.7	32.1

Adapted with permission from ETDRS Research Group[27].

If one believes that a greater extent of peripheral retinal ischemia results in a greater upregulation of VEGF and a greater chance of diabetic macular edema then one might expect panretinal photocoagulation to provide some benefit for patients with diabetic macular edema. ETDRS data, however, do not support this hypothesis. The rate of moderate vision loss at 5 years in patients with macular edema who received scatter photocoagulation as a sole therapy was not much different from controls (see Table 6.2).

This data would therefore argue against the logic that wide-field fluorescein angiography would alter one's therapy. Therefore, although it makes intuitive sense, the information gained from wide-field fluorescein angiography currently has not been demonstrated to add value beyond classifying retinopathy based on fundus examination alone.

In retinal vascular diseases ischemia of the macula and an enlarged foveal avascular zone may be a mechanism associated with visual loss exclusive of macular edema.[69] The ETDRS categorized macular ischemia by grading the size of the foveal avascular zone, the features of the outline of the foveal avascular zone, and the areas of capillary loss <1,000 μm from the foveal center. There was only moderate agreement among the ETDRS professional graders in classifying capillary loss and abnormalities of the foveal avascular zone.[70] Schemes to classify severity of macular ischemia are inconsistent.[71,72] These inconsistencies between graders and between study centers make it difficult to know whether the additional information gained from fluorescein angiography of the macula adds therapeutic or prognostic value to patients. Since the classification schemes of the ETDRS and Global Diabetic Retinopathy Project (see Chapter 5) do not include the information from fluorescein angiography one can infer that the information regarding macular ischemia is not critical in providing prognostic information for patients.[73]

Upregulation of vascular endothelial growth factor resulting from retinal ischemia[74] correlates with development of iris neovascularization.[75] The detection of iris neovascularization in darkly pigmented irides can be challenging and iris fluorescein angiography[76] is therefore more sensitive than clinical examination in detecting abnormal iris vessels.[77] However, iris angiography is not widely utilized in clinical practice perhaps because of the lack of information as to the added value of this test above ophthalmoscopy, color fundus photography, and retinal fluorescein angiography.

6.7 Ultrasonography

In diabetic eyes ophthalmic ultrasound is a diagnostic tool with current utility primarily in eyes with opaque ocular media and vitreous hemorrhage.[78] Probe placement on the globe provides better resolution and is therefore preferable to placement on the lids. In diabetic eyes with vitreous hemorrhage precluding fundus examination ultrasonography is important in determining the presence or absence of retinal detachment, the location of the hemorrhage (vitreous, loculated between the vitreous and the retina, or subretinal), and the nature of associated traction. Traction retinal detachments are more commonly found along the vascular arcades and peripapillary retina. Knowledge of the extent of traction retinal detachment in addition to whether or not the macula is attached is helpful in planning surgical intervention and advising patients about the prognosis with surgery. Blood on the posterior cortical vitreous face can resemble a retinal detachment on ultrasound examination. The higher reflectivity exhibited with retinal tissue on A-scan ultrasonography in conjunction with the lack of attachment of the posterior cortical vitreous to the optic nerve seen with dynamic B-scan ultrasonography can be helpful in differentiating these two entities.

Anterior hyaloidal fibrovascular proliferation (AHFVP) is a severe complication following diabetic vitrectomy[79] which manifests with florid neovascularization from the peripheral retina growing along the anterior hyaloid to the posterior lens surface. Hypotony occurs from traction detachment of the ciliary body. The prognosis is poor if untreated and guarded if treated. In the setting of associated vitreous hemorrhage diagnosis of AHFVP depends on a high clinical suspicion. Ultrasonography to establish the extent and location of associated fibrovascular membranes is helpful.[80] High-frequency ultrasound biomicroscopy (UBM) provides greater resolution at the level of the pars plana[81] and may therefore be preferable to B-scan ultrasonography in demonstrating earlier fibrovascular proliferations at the sclerotomy sites.[82]

6.8 Multifocal ERG

Multifocal ERG allows simultaneous electrophysiologic testing of multiple small areas of the retina. Abnormal second-order wave forms can be detected prior to the development of clinical diabetic retinopathy implying a deficit in the inner retina. In comparison, patients with clinical diabetic retinopathy have abnormalities of both first-order and second-order wave forms implying a deficit in both the inner and outer retina. [83] A delay in multifocal ERG implicit times may correlate with the chance of diabetic retinopathy onset.[84] The clinical benefit of being able to predict which areas of the retina may develop changes of nonproliferative diabetic retinopathy (in the absence of finding clinically significant macular edema) has not been demonstrated.

6.9 Miscellaneous Modalities

Fluorescein does not leak from normal retinal vasculature. A breakdown of the blood retinal barrier can be measured by vitreous fluorophotometry and quantified by an instrument called the Retinal Leakage Analyzer.[85] Fine matrix mapping is a modified Humphrey field analyzer which assesses photopic and scotopic retinal function. These techniques may be useful as research tools but have not gained acceptance by clinicians in management of diabetic retinopathy.

6.10 Summary of Key Points

- Clinical examination (and not OCT) should determine the presence of clinically significant macular edema.
- OCT is helpful in determining the response of clinically significant macular edema to therapy.
- OCT morphology may alter prognosis (cystic changes indicative of chronicity and poorer response to therapy) or alter therapy (vitreomacular traction needing surgery).
- Stereoscopic color fundus photography is more sensitive than clinical examination in diagnosing diabetic retinopathy.
- Fluorescein angiography is indicated to help direct laser therapy of clinically significant macular edema but current clinical practice suggests benefit from laser therapy applied without fluorescein angiogram guidance.
- Determination of ischemia by fluorescein angiography is poorly reproducible.

6.11 Future Directions

- Determining whether the increased resolution and sampling strategy of spectral domain OCT provide additional benefit over Stratus OCT.
- Determination of the public health role of teleophthalmology in managing diabetic patients.

6.12 Practice Exercises

Exercise 1 – Hemorrhages vs. microaneurysms

The ETDRS laser protocol directed focal treatment to all microaneurysms between 500 and 3,000 μm from the foveola.

# Microaneurysms on fundus photo	# Microaneurysms on FA

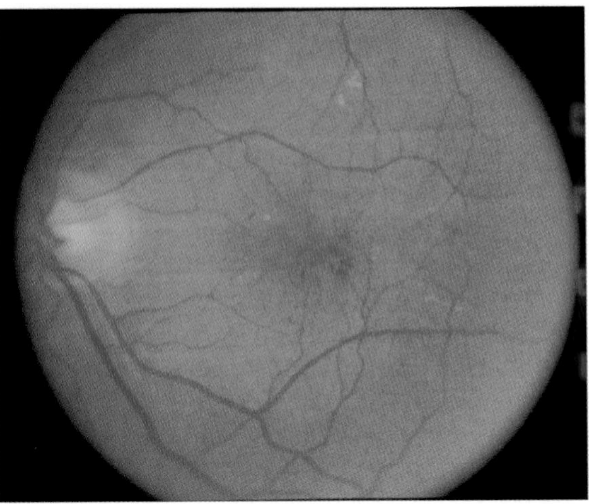

Fig. 6.9

This 54-year-old male has a 24-year history of type 1 diabetes mellitus. He complains of micropsia OS. His visual acuity OS is 20/25. Slit lamp biomicroscopy reveals clinically significant macular edema. Please identify and count on the color fundus photograph microaneurysms where focal laser would be applied (Fig. 6.9).

Microaneurysms are typically identified/confirmed in the transit phase of the fluorescein angiogram. Please identify and count on the fluorescein angiogram the microaneurysms where focal laser would be applied (Fig. 6.10).

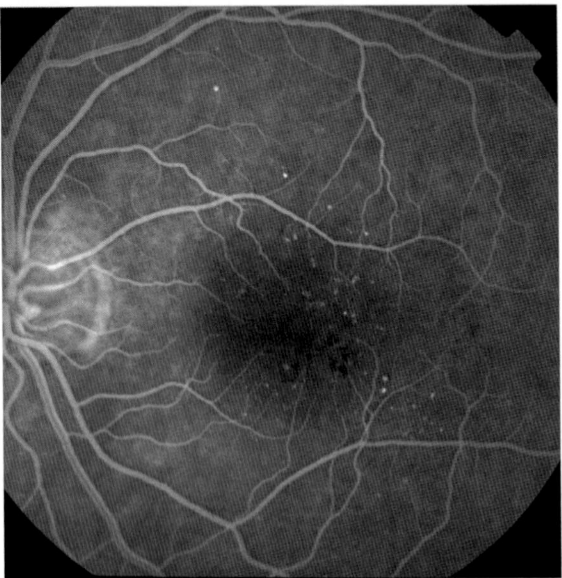

Fig. 6.10

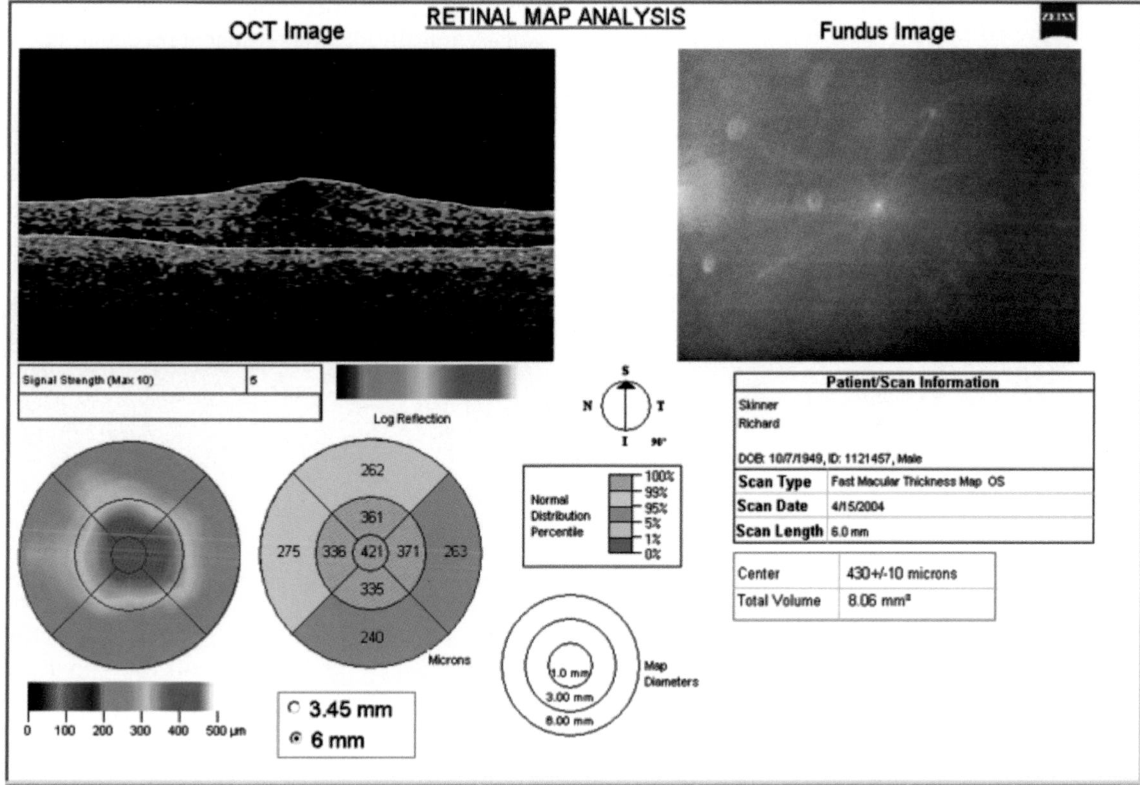

Fig. 6.11

Does the fluorescein angiogram change therapy?

Does the OCT change the pattern of laser? (Fig. 6.11)

Exercise 2 – Identify "focal" leakage

The ETDRS defined "focal" leakage as leakage arising from microaneurysms.

Does this angiogram (Figs. 6.10 and 6.12) reveal any leakage that is not "focal?" i.e., is there any region where grid laser would be applied?

Exercise 3 – The ETDRS defined areas of leakage which were not attributable to microaneurysms as "diffuse." The ETDRS laser protocol directed grid laser to these areas of "diffuse leakage" in addition to areas of capillary nonperfusion. This patient with type 1 diabetes mellitus has clinically significant macular edema (Figs. 6.13, 6.14, and 6.15).

Please identify the areas of capillary nonperfusion where grid laser treatment would be applied. Please identify the areas of leakage not attributable to microaneurysms ("diffuse" leakage) where grid laser treatment would be applied.

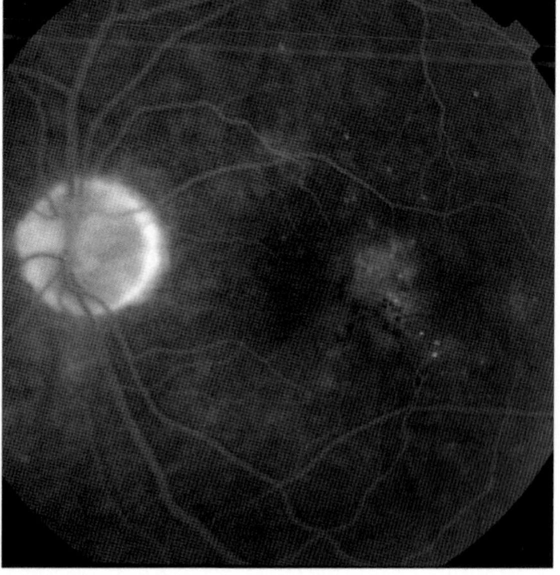

Fig. 6.12

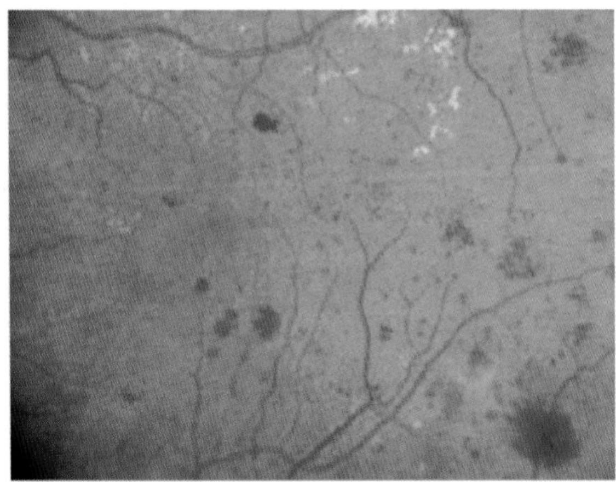

Fig. 6.13

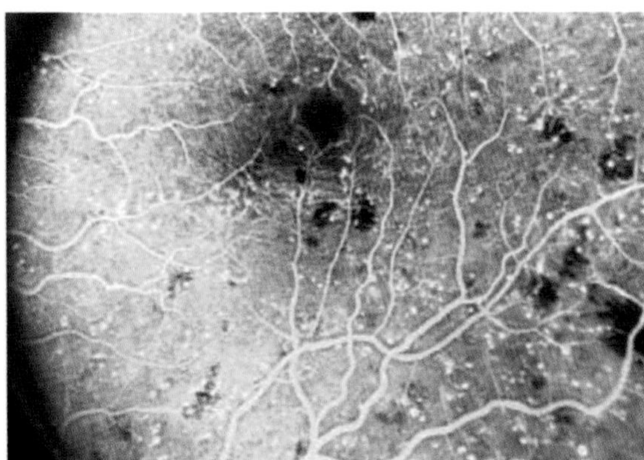

Fig. 6.14

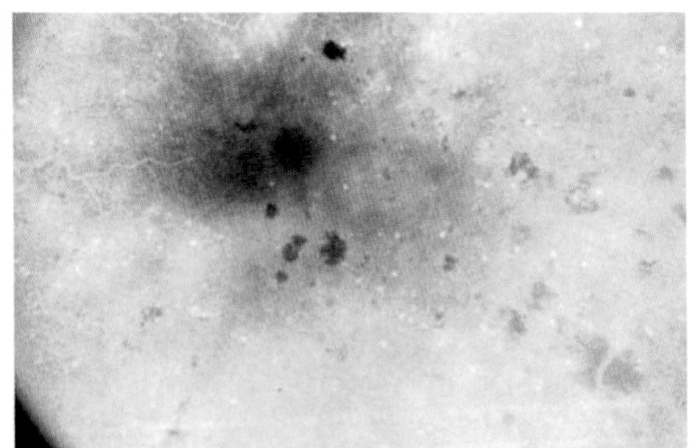

Fig. 6.15

Exercise 4 – This patient with type 1 diabetes mellitus has clinically significant macular edema. Please identify the areas of capillary nonperfusion where grid laser treatment would be applied. Please identify the areas of leakage not attributable to microaneurysms ("diffuse" leakage) where grid laser treatment would be applied (Figs. 6.16 and 6.17).

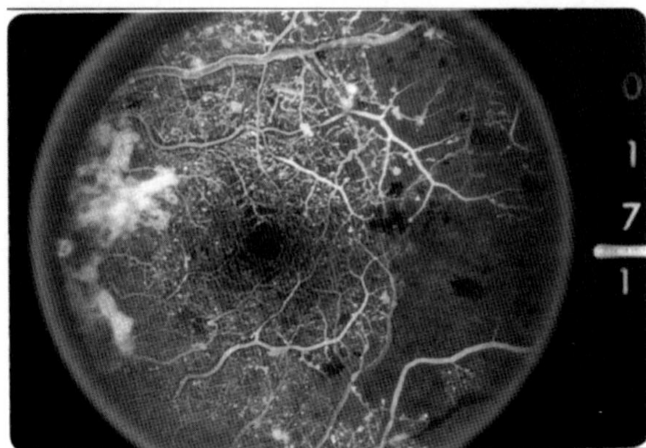

Fig. 6.16

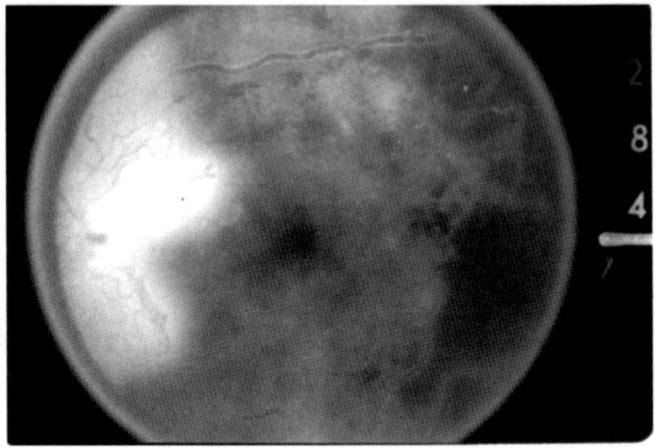

Fig. 6.17

References

1. Hee MR, Puliafito CA, Wong C, et al. Quantitative assessment of macular edema with optical coherence tomography. *Arch Ophthalmol*. 1995;113:1019–1029.
2. Tangelder GJ, Van der Heidje RG, Polak BC, et al. Precision and reliability of retinal thickness measurements in foveal and extrafoveal areas of healthy and diabetic eyes. *IOVS*. 208;49:2627–2634.

3. Diabetic Retinopathy Clinical Research Network. Reproducibility of macular thickness and volume using Zeiss optical coherence tomography in patients with diabetic macular edema. *Ophthalmology*. 2007;114:1520–1525.
4. Virgilia G, Menchini F, Dimastrogiovanni AF, et al. Optical coherence tomography versus stereo fundus photography or biomicroscopy for diagnosing diabetic macular edema: a systematic review. *IOVS*. 2007;48:4963–4973.
5. Browning DJ, Glassman AR, Aiello LP, et al. Optical coherence tomography measurements and analysis methods in optical coherence tomography studies of diabetic macular edema. *Ophthalmology*. 2008;115:1366–1371.
6. Degenring RF, Aschmoneit I, Kamppeter B, et al. Optical coherence tomography and confocal scanning laser tomography for assessment of macular edema. *Am J Ophthalmol*. 2004;138:354–162.
7. Hee MR, Pulafito CA, Duker JS, et al. Topography of diabetic macular edema with optical coherence tomography. *Ophthalmology*. 1998;105:360–370.
8. Bressler NM, Edwards AR, Antoszyk AN, et al. Retinal thickness on Stratus optical coherence tomography in people with diabetes and minimal or no diabetic retinopathy. *Am J Ophthalmol*. 2008;145:894–901.
9. Cunningham ET Jr., Adamis AP, Altaweel M, et al. A phase II randomized double-masked trial of pegaptanib, an anti-vascular endothelial growth factor aptamer, for diabetic macular edema. *Ophthalmology*. 2005;112: 1747–1757.
10. Chun DW, Heier JS, Topping TM, et al. A pilot study of multiple intravitreal injections of ranibizumab in patients with center-involving clinically significant diabetic macular edema. *Ophthalmology*. 2006;113: 1706–1712.
11. Shimura M, Nakazawa T, Yasuda K, et al. Comparative therapy evaluation of intravitreal bevacizumab and triamcinolone acetonide on persistent diffuse diabetic macular edema. *Am J Ophthalmol*. 2008;145:854–861.
12. Early Treatment Diabetic Retinopathy Study Research Group. Photocoagulation for diabetic macular edema: ETDRS Report Number 1. *Arch Ophthalmol*. 1985;103: 1796–1806.
13. Diabetic Retinopathy Clinical Research Network. A randomized trial comparing intravitreal triamcinolone acetonide and focal/grid photocoagulation for diabetic macular edema. *Ophthalmology*. 2008;115:1447–1459.
14. Bressler NM, Edwards AR, Antoszyk AN, et al. Retinal thickness on Stratus optical coherence tomography in people with diabetes and minimal or no diabetic retinopathy. *Am J Ophthalmol*. 2008;145:894–901.
15. Davis MD, Bressler SB, Aiello LP Jr, et al. Comparison of time-domain OCT and fundus photographic assessments of retinal thickening in eyes with diabetic macular edema. *IOVS*. 2008;49:1745–1752.
16. Brown JC, Solomon SD, Bressler SB, et al. Detection of diabetic foveal edema: Contact lens biomicroscopy compared with optical coherence tomography. *Arch Ophthalmol*. 2004;122:330–335.
17. Browning DJ, McOwen MD, Bowen RM Jr, et al. Comparison of the clinical diagnosis of diabetic macular edema with diagnosis by optical coherence tomography. *Ophthalmology*. 2004;111:712–715.
18. Diabetic Retinopathy Clinical Research Network. Subclinical Diabetic Macular Edema Study. http://public.drcr.net/DRCRnetstudies/studies/ProtocolG_subclinical/ProtGInfo.html. Accessed January 17, 2009.
19. Forooghian F, Cukras C, Meyerle CB, et al. Evaluation of time domain and spectral domain optical coherence tomography in the measurement of diabetic macular edema. *IOVS*. 2008;49:4290–4296.
20. Davis MD, Bressler SB, Aiello LP Jr, et al. Comparison of time-domain OCT and fundus photographic assessments of retinal thickening in eyes with diabetic macular edema. *IOVS*. 2008;49:1745–1752.
21. Diabetic Retinopathy Clinical Research Network. The course of response to focal photocoagulation for diabetic macular edema. http:www.drcr.net. Accessed January 17, 2009.
22. Diabetic Retinopathy Clinical Research Network. Relationship between optical coherence tomography-measured central retinal thickness and visual acuity in diabetic macular edema. *Ophthalmology*. 2007;114:525–536.
23. Browning DJ & Fraser CM. The predictive value of patient and eye characteristics on the course of subclinical diabetic macular edema. *Am J Ophthalmol*. 2008;145:149–154.
24. Browning DJ, Fraser CM, Propst BW. The variation in optical coherence tomography-measured macular thickness in diabetic eyes without clinical macular edema. *Am J Ophthalmol*. 2008;145:889–893.
25. Diabetic Retinopathy Clinical Research Network. An observational study of the development of diabetic macular edema following scatter laser photocoagulation. http://public.drcr.net/DRCRnetstudies/studies/ProtocolF_prp/ProtFInfo.html. Accessed January 17, 2009.
26. Diabetic Retinopathy Study Research Group. Photocoagulation treatment of proliferative diabetic retinopathy: clinical application of diabetic retinopathy study (DRS) findings. DRS Report #8. *Ophthalmology*. 1981;88:583–600.
27. Early Treatment Diabetic Retinopathy Study Research Group. Early photocoagulation for diabetic retinopathy. ETDRS report no. 9. *Ophthalmology*. 1991;98:766–785.
28. Zacks DN, Johnson MW. Combined intravitreal injection of triamcinolone acetonide and panretinal photocoagulation for concomitant diabetic macular edema and proliferative diabetic retinopathy. *Retina*. 2005;25:35–140.
29. Bandello F, Polito A, Pognuz DR, et al. Triamcinolone as adjunctive treatment to laser photocoagulation to laser panretinal photocoagulation for proliferative diabetic retinopathy. *Arch Ophthalmol*. 2006;124:643–650.
30. Otani T, Kishi S, Maruyama Y. Patterns of diabetic macular edema with optical coherence tomography. *Am J Ophthalmol*. 1999;127:688–693.
31. Kim BY, Smith SD, Kaiser PK. Optical coherence tomographic patterns of diabetic macular edema. *Am J Ophthalmol*. 2006;142:405–412.
32. Kang SW, Park CY, Ham DI. The correlation between fluorescein angiographic and optical coherence tomographic features in clinically significant diabetic macular edema. *Am J Ophthalmol*. 2004;137:313–322.

33. Diabetic Retinopathy Clinical Research Network. Relationship between optical coherence tomography-measured central retinal thickness and visual acuity in diabetic macular edema. *Ophthalmology*. 2007;114:525–536.
34. Kim BY, Smith SD, Kaiser PK. Optical coherence tomographic patterns of diabetic macular edema. *Am J Ophthalmol*. 2006;142:405–412.
35. Early Treatment Diabetic Retinopathy Study Research Group. Focal photocoagulation treatment of diabetic macular edema. Relationship of treatment effect to fluorescein angiographic and other retinal characteristics at baseline. ETDRS report no. 19. *Arch Ophthalmol*. 1995;113:1144–1155.
36. Lewis H. Abrams GW, Blumenkranz MS, et al. Vitrectomy for diabetic macular traction and edema associated with posterior hyaloidal traction. *Ophthalmology*. 1992;99:753–759.
37. Lewis H, Abrams GW, Blumenkranz MS, et al. Vitrectomy for diabetic macular traction and edema associated with posterior hyaloidal traction. *Ophthalmology*. 1992;99:753–759.
38. Diabetic Retinopathy Clinical Research Network. Evaluation of Vitrectomy for Diabetic Macular Edema. http://public.drcr.net/DRCRnetstudies/studies/ProtocolD_vitrectomy/ProtDInfo.html. Accessed January 17, 2009.
39. Browning DJ, Glassman AR, Aiello LP, et al. Optical coherence tomography measurements and analysis methods in optical coherence tomography studies of diabetic macular edema. *Ophthalmology*. 2008;115:1366–1371.
40. Guan K, Hudson C, Flanagan JG. Comparison of Heidelberg retinal tomography II and retinal thickness analyzer in assessment of diabetic macular edema. *IOVS*. 2004;45:610–616.
41. Strom C, Sander B. Comparison of objective retinal thickness analysis and subjective stereo fundus photography in diabetic macular edema. *IOVS*. 2004;45:1450–1455.
42. Neubauer AS, Priglinger S, Ullrich S, et al. Comparison of foveal thickness measured with the retinal thickness analyzer and optical coherence tomography. *Retina*. 2001;21:596–601.
43. Vujosevic S, Midena E, Pilotto E, et al. Diabetic macular edema: Correlation between microperimetry and optical coherence tomography findings. *IOVS*. 2006;47: 3044–1051.
44. Carpineto P, Ciancaglini M, Di Antonio L, et al. Fundus microperimetry patterns of fixation in type 2 diabetic patients with diffuse macular edema. *Retina*. 2007; 27:21–29.
45. ETDRS Research Group. Fundus photographic risk factors for progression of diabetic retinopathy. ETDRS Report # 12. *Ophthalmology*. 1991;98:823–833.
46. Whited JD. Accuracy and reliability of teleophthalmology for diagnosing diabetic retinopathy and macular edema: A review of the literature. *Diabetes Technol Ther*. 2006;8:102–111.
47. Tennant MT, Greve MD, Rudnisky CJ, et al. Identification of diabetic retinopathy by stereoscopic digital imaging via teleophthalmology: a comparison to slide film. *Can J Ophthalmol*. 2001;36:187–196.
48. Rudnisky CJ, Tennant MT, Weis E, et al. Web-based grading of compressed stereoscopic digital photography versus standard slide-film photography for the diagnosis of diabetic retinopathy. *Ophthalmology*. 2007;114:1748–1754.
49. Lim JI, LaBree L, Nichols T, et al. A comparison of digital nonmydriatic fundus imaging with standard 35-millimeter slides for diabetic retinopathy. *Ophthalmology*. 2000;107:866–870.
50. Gass JD. *Stereoscopic Atlas of Macular Diseases: Diagnosis and Treatment*. 4th ed. St. Louis: Mosby-Year Book; 1997.
51. Ryan SJ ed. *Retina: Volume Two Medical Retina*. 4th ed. St. Louis: Mosby; 2006.
52. Flocks M. Miller J, Chao P. Retinal circulation time with the aid of fundus cinephotography. *Am J Ophthalmol*. 1959;48:3–10.
53. MacLean Al, Maumenee AE. Hemangioma of he choroid. *Am J Ophthalmol*. 1960;50:3–11.
54. Novotny HR, Alvis DL. A method of photographing fluorescence in circulating blood in the human retina. *Circulation*. 1961;24:82–86.
55. Aiello L, Berrocal J. David M, et al. The diabetic retinopathy study. *Arch Ophthalmol*. 1973;90:347–348.
56. Early Treatment Diabetic Retinopathy Study Research Group. Classification of diabetic retinopathy from fluorescein angiograms: ETDRS report no. 11. *Ophthalmology*. 1991;98:807–822.
57. Early Treatment Diabetic Retinopathy Study Research Group. Treatment techniques and clinical guidelines for photocoagulation of diabetic macular edema. ETDRS report no. 2. *Ophthalmology*. 1987;94:761–774.
58. Diabetic Retinopathy Study Research Group. Indications for photocoagulation treatment of diabetic retinopathy. DRS report no. 14. *Int Ophthalmol Clin*. 1987;27:239–253.
59. Diabetic Retinopathy Study Research Group. Four risk factors for severe visual loss in diabetic retinopathy: the third report from the diabetic retinopathy study. *Arch Ophthalmol*. 1979;97:654–655.
60. Browning DJ, Altaweel MM, Bressler NM, et al. Diabetic macular edema: what is focal and what is diffuse? *Am J Ophthalmol*. 2008;146:649–655.
61. http://public.drcr.net/general/drcrnet_rationale.html
62. Diabetic Retinopathy Clinical Research Network Writing Group. Comparison of the modified early treatment diabetic retinopathy study and mild macular grid laser photocoagulation strategies for diabetic macular edema. *Arch Ophthalmol*. 2007;125:469–480.
63. Diabetic Retinopathy Clinical Research Network. A randomized trial comparing intravitreal triamcinolone acetonide and focal/grid photocoagulation for diabetic macular edema. *Ophthalmology*. 2008;115:1447–1459.
64. Abu El Asrar AM, Morse PH. Laser photocoagulation control of diabetic macular edema without fluorescein angiography. *Br J Ophthalmol*. 1991;75;97–99.
65. Aiello LP, Avery RL, Arrigg PG, et al. Vascular endothelial growth factor in ocular fluid of patients with diabetic retinopathy and other retinal disorders. *N Engl J Med*. 1994;331:1480–1487.

66. Efficacy Study of Lucentis in the Treatment of Diabetic Macular Edema. http://clinicaltrials.gov/ct2/show/NCT00387582. Accessed January 18, 2009.
67. Diabetic Retinopathy Clinical Research Network. Intravitreal Ranibuzumab or Triamcinolone Acetonide in Combination with Laser Photocoagulation for Diabetic Macular Edema. http://public.drcr.net/DRCRnetstudies/studies/ProtocolI_lrtdme/ProtIInfo.html. Accessed January 18, 2009.
68. Diabetic Retinopathy Clinical Research Network. Intravitreal Ranibuzumab or Triamcinolone Acetonide in as Adjunctive Treatment to Panretinal Photocoagulation for Proliferative Diabetic Retinopathy. http://public.drcr.net/DRCRnetstudies/studies/ProtocolJ_lrtpdr/ProtJInfo.html. Accessed January 18, 2009.
69. Branch Vein Occlusion Study Group. Argon laser photocoagulation for macular edema in branch vein occlusion. *Am J Ophthalmol.* 1984;98:271–282.
70. Early Treatment Diabetic Retinopathy Study Research Group. Classification of diabetic retinopathy from fluorescein angiograms. ETDRS report no. 11. *Ophthalmology.* 1991;98:807–822.
71. Pendergast SD, Hassan TS, Williams GA, et al. Vitrectomy for diffuse diabetic macular edema associated with a taut premacular posterior hyaloid. *Am J Ophthalmol.* 2000;130:178–186.
72. Chung EJ, Roh MI, Kwon OW, et al. Effects of macular ischemia on the outcome of bevacizumab therapy on diabetic macular edema. *Retina.* 2008;28:957–963.
73. Early Treatment Diabetic Retinopathy Study Research Group. Fluorescein angiographic risk factors for progression of diabetic retinopathy. ETDRS report no. 13. *Ophthalmology.* 1991;98:834–840.
74. Aiello LP, Avery RL, Arrigg PG, et al. Vascular endothelial growth factor in ocular fluid of patients with diabetic retinopathy and other retinal disorders. *N Engl J Med.* 1994;331:1480–1487.
75. Hamanaka T, Akabane N, Yajima T, et al. Retinal ischemia and angle neovascularization in proliferative diabetic retinopathy. *Am J Ophthalmol.* 2001;132:648–658.
76. Brancato R, Bandello F, Latanzio R eds. *Atlas of Iris Fluorescein Angiography.* Milano, Amsterdam, New York: Kugler, Ghendini; 1995.
77. Bandello F, Brancato R, Lattanzio R, et al. Biomicroscopy versus fluorescein angiography in the detection of diabetic iridopathy. *Graefes Arch Clin Exp Ophthalmol.* 1993;231:444–448.
78. Green RL & Byrne SF. Diagnostic ophthalmic ultrasound. In: Ryan SJ, ed. *Retina.* 4th ed. Philadelphia: Elsevier Mosby; 2006.
79. Lewis H, Abrams GW, Williams GA. Anterior hyaloidal fibrovascular proliferation after diabetic vitrectomy. *Am J Ophthalmol.* 1987;104:607–613.
80. Han DP, Lewandowski M, Mieler WF. Echographic diagnosis of anterior hyaloidal fibrovascular proliferation. *Arch Ophthalmol.* 1991;109:842–846.
81. Garcia JP & Rosen RB. Anterior segment imaging: optical coherence tomography versus ultrasound biomicroscopy. *Ophthalmic Surg Laser Imag.* 2008;39:476–484.
82. Bhende M, Agraharam SG, Gopal L, et al. Ultrasound biomicroscopy of sclerotomy sites after pars plana vitrectomy for diabetic vitreous hemorrhage. *Ophthalmology.* 2000;107:1720–1736.
83. Palmowski AM, Sutter EE, Bearse MA, et al. Mapping of retinal function in diabetic retinopathy using the multifocal electroretinogram. *IOVS.* 1997;38:2586–2596.
84. NG JS, Bearse MA, Schneck ME, et al. Local diabetic retinopathy prediction by multifocal ERG delays over 3 years. *IOVS.* 2008;49:1622–1628.
85. Lobo CL, Bernardes RC, Figueira JP, et al. Three-year follow-up of blood-retinal barrier and retinal thickness alterations in patients with type 2 diabetes mellitus and mild nonproliferative diabetic retinopathy. *Arch Ophthalmol.* 2004;122:211–217.

Chapter 7
Diabetic Macular Edema

David J. Browning

7.1 Epidemiology and Risk Factors

Diabetic retinopathy is the leading cause of blindness in persons under age 60 in the United States, and diabetic macular edema (DME) is the most common cause of visual loss in those with diabetic retinopathy.[1–3] Natural history studies of eyes with DME show that 24% will lose at least three lines of vision over a period of 3 years.[4] DME is increasing in prevalence throughout the world. In cross-sectional studies, the prevalence of DME in patients with diabetes has been reported to be 1.0–5.7%.[5,6] The prevalence of DME in patients with diabetic retinopathy has been reported to be 2.7–11.0%.[5,7–9] Suggestive data have been reported that the prevalence of DME relative to proliferative diabetic retinopathy (PDR) may vary by race with rates of DME relatively low in Native Americans relative to the rate of PDR.[10] Besides its adverse effects on affected patients, DME is associated with large economic costs. In a Medicare claims study, diagnosis of DME was associated with a 34 and 33% increase in 1- and 3-year direct medical costs after adjustment for demographic variables and baseline comorbid conditions.[11]

The prevalence of DME depends on the type of diabetes and the duration of the disease. For diabetes occurring in insulin-taking patients under age 30 (generally type 1 diabetics), DME begins to appear after 5 years and the prevalence thereafter increases to 30–40% after 30 years of disease (Fig. 7.1). For diabetes with onset after age 30 (generally type 2 diabetes), 3–5% of patients manifest DME at the time of diagnosis, presumably because of having undiagnosed diabetes for several years before diagnosis. Thereafter, prevalence increases with a plateau at approximately 30% after 25–30 years. In general, in this older onset group, noninsulin-taking diabetics have lower prevalence rates than insulin-taking diabetics (Fig. 7.1). Because of different prevalences according to diabetes type, and evidence that serum cholesterol is associated with retinopathy severity and severity of hard exudates in older onset diabetics using insulin (mostly type 2) but not in younger onset diabetics using insulin (type 1), there is conjecture that the pathophysiology of retinopathy and DME may differ between these categories of diabetes.[12,13] In the absence of further explorations of this possibility, in what follows we will discuss DME in both groups as though they have similar bases, understanding that this perspective may need modification as new information becomes available.

In population-based studies, certain systemic factors were associated with diabetic macular edema. In patients under age 30, associated factors were longer duration of diabetes, proteinuria, male sex, negative history of cardiovascular disease, use of diuretics, and higher hemoglobin A1C.[9] In patients 30 years of age and older, associated factors were longer duration of diabetes, higher systolic blood pressure, and higher hemoglobin A1C. Proteinuria was an associated risk factor in the insulin-taking older onset group, but not for the noninsulin-taking group. In type 1 diabetics, high serum lipids have been associated with an increased risk

D.J. Browning (✉)
Charlotte Eye Ear Nose & Throat Associates, Charlotte, NC 28210, USA
e-mail: dbrowning@ceenta.com

D.J. Browning (ed.), *Diabetic Retinopathy*, DOI 10.1007/978-0-387-85900-2_7,

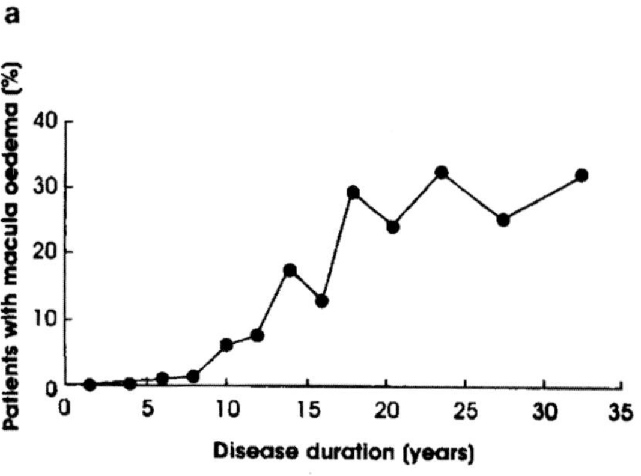

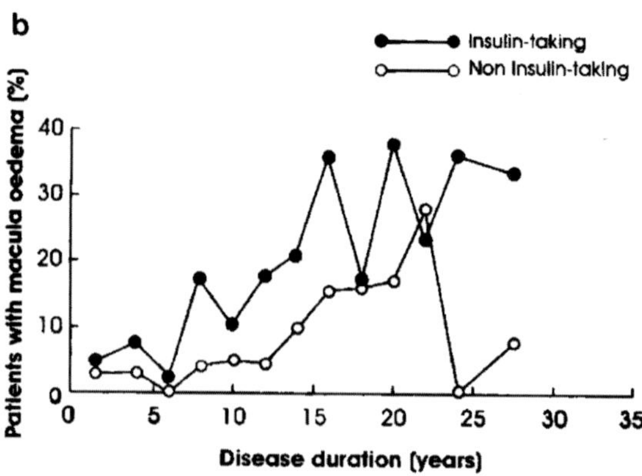

Fig. 7.1 The prevalence of diabetic macular edema by disease duration in (**a**) younger onset diabetics and (**b**) older onset diabetics. Reprinted with permission from Klein et al.[17]

of DME.[14] The onset of diabetes in patients with type 1 disease is usually easy to define, in contrast to patients with type 2 disease. As a result, one can measure in a meaningful way the duration of type 1 diabetes before which DME is not seen; a duration of 7 years has been reported.[15] Such is not possible in type 2 disease, in which it is common for patients to have the disease for years before diagnosis, and in which it is not rare to have patients present with blurred vision secondary to DME as the presenting sign that leads to the diagnosis of type 2 diabetes. The annual rate of incidence of DME has declined in recent years compared to earlier periods, perhaps as a result of tighter glycemic control. In the Wisconsin Epidemiologic Study of Diabetic Retinopathy, the annual rates of incidence of DME for the intervals 1980–1982 to 1984–1986 and 1994–1996 to 2005–2007 were 2.3 and 0.9%, respectively.[16] By comparison, the mean glycosylated hemoglobin values were 10.7 and 9.4%, respectively.[16]

The major ocular factor associated with DME and subclinical DME is diabetic retinopathy severity. Although DME can be seen at any level of diabetic retinopathy, increasing diabetic retinopathy severity is associated with increasing prevalence of both DME and subclinical DME.[3,16,18–20] The 14-year incidence of DME increases from 25 to 37% as baseline retinopathy severity increases from mild to moderate nonproliferative diabetic retinopathy (NPDR).[18] Point estimates of 4 and 15% for prevalence of subclinical DME in mild to moderate NPDR and severe NPDR to PDR, respectively, have been reported.[20]

7.2 Pathophysiology and Pathoanatomy

The reader should review Chapter 1 for a more detailed discussion of the pathophysiology of diabetic retinopathy. In this section, we emphasize only those aspects relevant to an understanding of diabetic macular edema.

7.2.1 Anatomy

The capillaries in the macula are distributed in two strata within the inner retina with the exception of the single-level arrangement bordering the foveal avascular zone (Fig. 7.2). This single level of capillaries

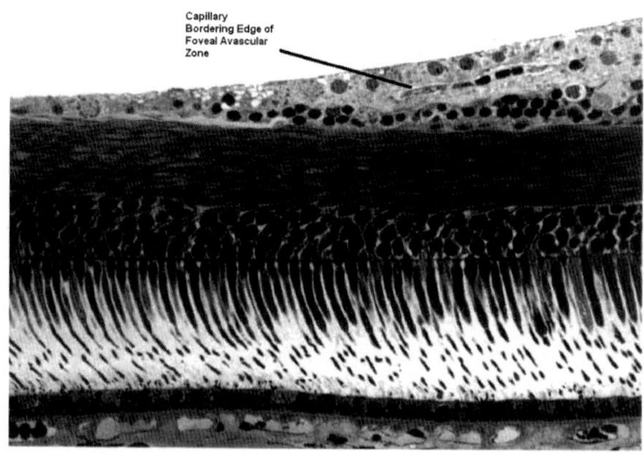

Fig. 7.2 Light micrograph of a section from the human macula. The *line* indicates a capillary comprising the foveal avascular zone border. The fovea lies to the *left* of the *line*. These capillaries are contained within the ganglion cell layer. Reprinted with permission from Iwasaki et al.[21]

is found within the ganglion cell layer.[21] Erythrocytes travel in the perifoveal capillaries in a pulsatile manner with speed in the range of 0.5–1.0 mm/s.[22] Farther from the fovea, the two levels of capillaries are found within the nerve fiber–ganglion cell layer and the inner nuclear cell layer. The more superficial capillary network is closer to the arteries, and the deeper network is closer to the venules. Arising from the disk and extending within the nerve fiber layer along the superotemporal and inferotemporal vascular arcades is the radial peripapillary capillary network, which seems to have sparse connections to the superficial capillary network of the ganglion cell layer (Fig. 7.3).[23] The outer retina throughout the macula is avascular and receives oxygenation by diffusion from the deeper choriocapillaris.[24] The maximum distance between capillaries in the inner retina is approximately 65–100 μm and the estimated maximal diffusion distance in the human macula consistent with normal function has been estimated to be approximately half this distance or approximately 45 μm.[21] Eighty percent of microaneurysms, which seem to be a microvascular response to vascular endothelial growth factor (VEGF) generated from hypoxic retinal tissue, originate in the inner nuclear layer and its border zones.[25] The larger microaneurysms tend to occur in this zone and smaller ones in the nerve fiber–ganglion cell layers. Microaneurysms range in size from 13 to 136 μm.[25] Microaneurysms are particularly frequent on the edges of nonperfused retina, consistent with the hypothesis that they are a secondary reaction to hypoxia and increased local vascular endothelial growth factor concentration, and not a primary change in diabetic retinopathy (Figs. 7.4 and 7.5). As defined by fluorescein angiography, microaneurysms in DME do not have a regional clustering. One study reported that, on average, 3% of the leaking microaneurysms discerned by fluorescein angiography were present in the central circular zone of 1-mm diameter, whereas the percentages in the inferior, nasal, superior, and temporal zones as defined by the Early Treatment Diabetic

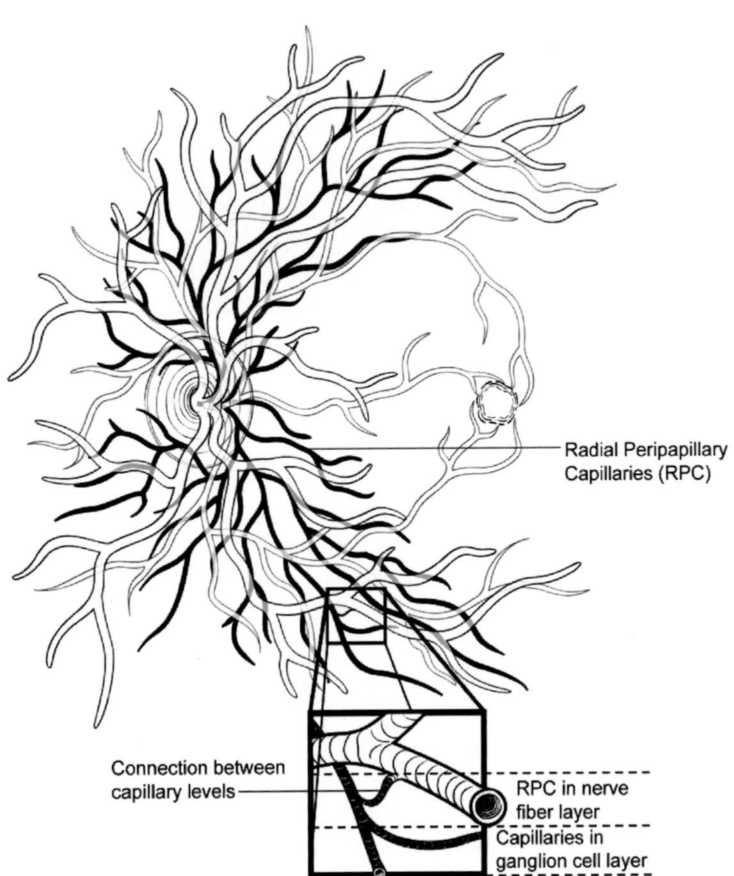

Fig. 7.3 Diagram indicating the distribution of the radial peripapillary capillary network, its location in the inner retina (primarily nerve fiber layer), and its sparse connections with deeper levels of capillaries

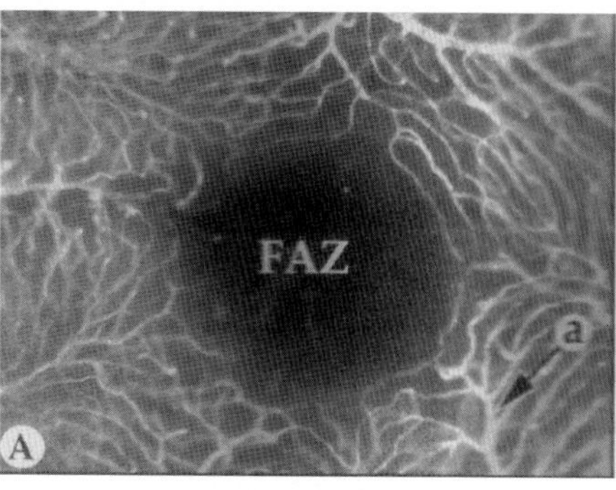

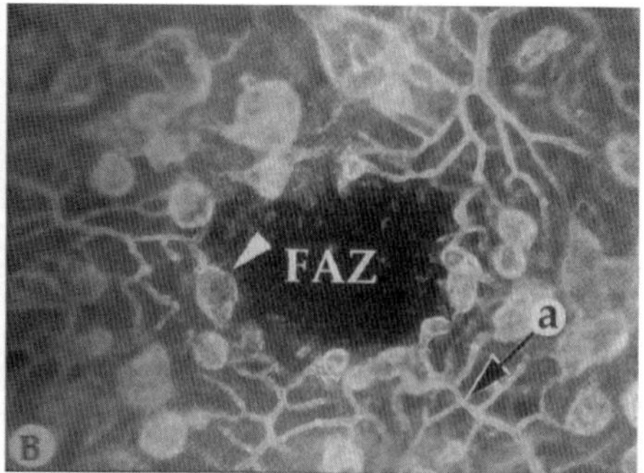

Fig. 7.4 The *left panel* (**a**) illustrates the foveal avascular zone (FAZ) of a normal macula from a cynomolgus monkey which has a similar anatomy to the human macula. The *right panel* (**b**) illustrates changes induced by intravitreal injection of VEGF. The microaneurysms resemble those seen in diabetic retinopathy. Reprinted with permission from Tolentino et al.[26]

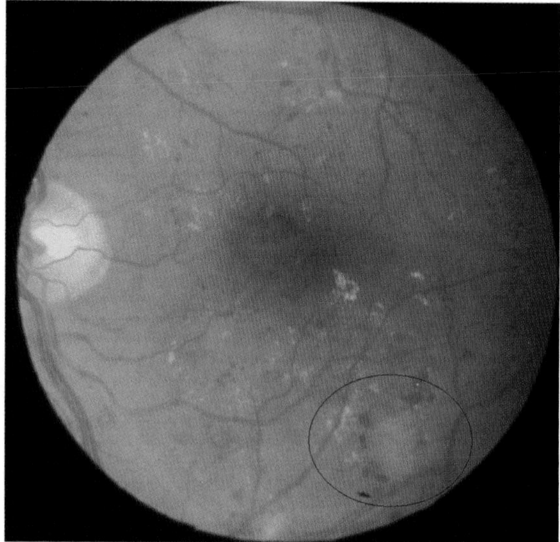

Fig. 7.5 The *circled zone* shows large microaneurysms and some dot hemorrhages that border an ischemic, *whitened zone* of retina

Retinopathy Study (ETDRS) grid were 26, 25, 23, and 24%, respectively.[27] The relationship of microaneurysms and DME is not straightforward. The retina is not necessarily thickened adjacent to microaneurysms and not all microaneurysms are leaky.[28,29] There is no increase in total microaneurysms or leaking aneurysms per unit area in progressively more thickened retina.[29] Nevertheless, ablation of leaky microaneurysms clearly improves DME.[4,30]

In center-involved macular edema, it is common for the central macula, including the foveal vascular zone, to be thickest, an inversion of the normal relationship. Although the underlying reason has not been established, one hypothesis is based on the avascularity at the center of the macula. In other regions of the macula, edema fluid can escape the extracellular space in two ways – outward to the choroid via the pumping mechanism of the retinal pigment epithelium, and back into the intravascular space through the walls of capillaries, the direction reverse to salt and water egress from intra to extravascular space in the more proximal microvasculature (Fig. 7.6). At the center of the macula, the only mechanism is that of the retinal pigment epithelial

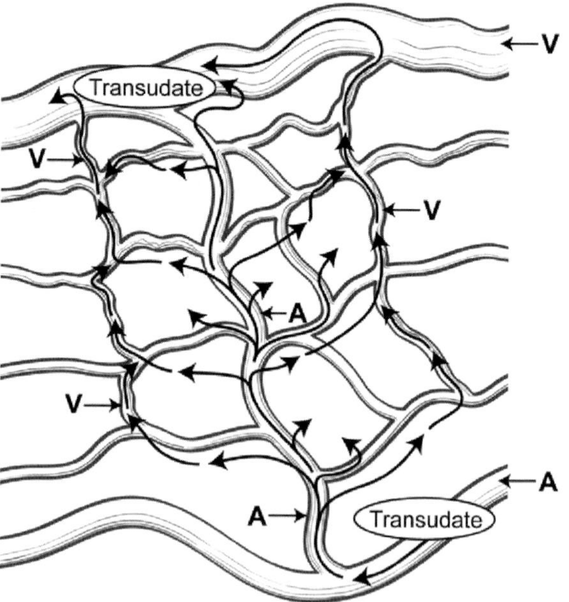

Fig. 7.6 Diagram indicating one pathway for salt and water within the retina. Under the influence of higher intravascular pressure in the arterioles, salt and water pass out of the vessels (transudate) and into the extracellular space of the retina, then returning to the intravascular space in part by entering the venular side of the circulation which has a lower intravascular pressure

(RPE) pump, which may explain the greater accumulation of edema fluid and increased retinal thickness at this location (Fig. 7.7). A fundus sign of the preferential accumulation of edema fluid in the center of the macula is the appearance of the macular lipid star commonly seen in cases of DME (Fig. 7.8). As the RPE pumps salt and water from the retinal extracellular space to the choroid, lipoproteins contained in the extracellular fluid are left behind as yellow exudates that must be cleared much more slowly by macrophages. In 15–30% of cases of DME, a serous retinal detachment is present which is usually localized under the fovea. Although the explanation for the subfoveal location of fluid is conjectural, one possibility posits an effect of impaired subfoveal choroidal circulation in DME.[31,32]

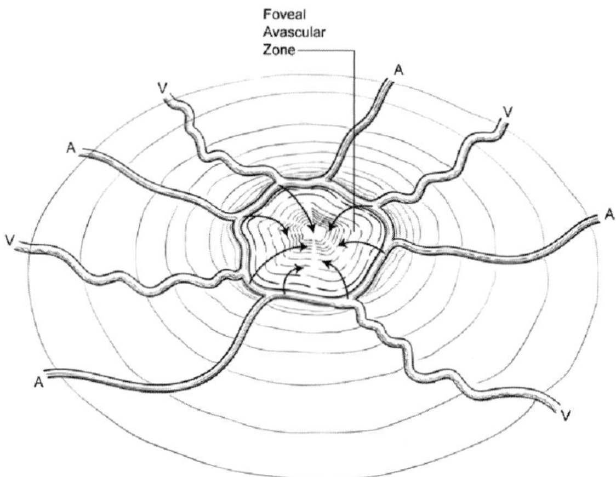

Fig. 7.7 Diagram indicating the different situation of the center of the macula. There is no venous side of the vasculature in this one location in the retina, thus salt and water can exit the vascular space from the capillaries, but can only leave the extracellular space via the action of the retinal pigment epithelial pump, and not via reentry into the venules which are missing in this location

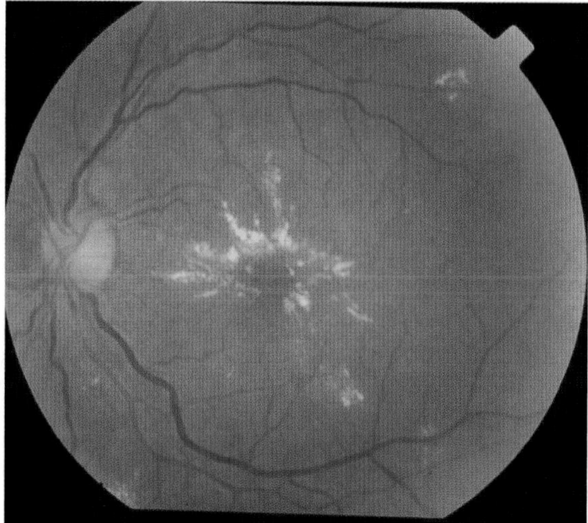

Fig. 7.8 A macular lipid star is a common fundus sign in diabetic macular edema and indicates that the center of the macula is a preferential site for accumulation of extracellular fluid

The Retinal Pigment Epithelial Pump

In most discussion of diabetic macular edema, the role of the retinal pigment epithelial pump is comparatively neglected, because it is difficult to study. Extracellular fluid travels from the retina outward toward the choroid primarily under the influence of the RPE pump action.[33] Figure 7.9 illustrates the current conception of ionic and fluid transport across the RPE into the choroid. An active sodium–potassium pump is present on the apical membrane of the RPE that exchanges three sodium ions toward the extracellular space for two potassium ions toward the RPE cytoplasm. An electrochemical gradient is generated by the asymmetry in the ionic exchange ratio, and this gradient powers other active transport mechanisms of which several have been described. Independent sodium–potassium-chloride and sodium-bicarbonate co-transport sites exist on the apical RPE membrane. An apical sodium-proton exchanger exists. These actively concentrate chloride and bicarbonate intracellularly. On the basal RPE membrane, separate sites exist for chloride and potassium ion egress as well as for a chloride–bicarbonate co-transporter.[33,34] Physiologic and pharmacologic modulation of fluid transport across the RPE is possible. Hypoxia decreases active transport across the RPE. Epinephrine applied to the apical RPE surface increases RPE transport. Acetazolamide increases transport, whereas furosemide decreases it. In extremely high concentrations not achieved clinically, digoxin reduces RPE transport. The possible influence of drugs commonly taken by patients with diabetes in altering the response to DME therapy has been completely unexplored to date.

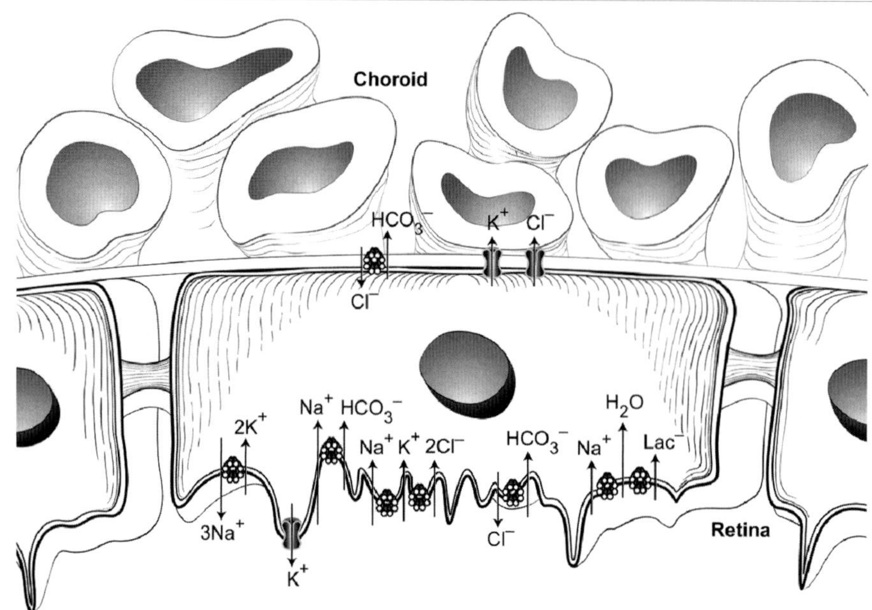

Fig. 7.9 Model of the retinal pigment epithelial pumping mechanism. The RPE cells are connected by zonula occludens which restrict the extracellular flow of ions and water back from the choroid toward the retina via the intercellular space between RPE cells. The primary energy dependent pump is the apical (retina side) sodium–potassium, electrogenic pump (*left side* of the cell). Other active transport systems derive the energy they require to run from the electrochemical gradients built up by this primary pump. In the apical membrane, independent sodium-bicarbonate, sodium–potassium-chloride, chloride–bicarbonate, and sodium-lactate–water transport sites have been described. In the basal membrane, a chloride–bicarbonate co-transporter exists. Passive conductance channels for potassium and chloride also exist as shown. Adapted with permission from La Cour[34] and Quintyn[33]

Tight junctions occur between capillary endothelial cells of the retina, the basis of the inner blood–retina barrier, and between the lateral walls of RPE cells, the outer blood–retina barrier. Diabetes causes a redistribution of occludin within the tight junctions of retinal vascular endothelium which may be the histologic correlate of the altered blood–retina barrier.[35] In a rat model of diabetes, the early breakdown of the blood–retinal barrier is selective for small venules and capillaries of the inner retina with sparing of the arterioles.[36] The inner blood–retina barrier rather than outer blood–retina barrier (RPE layer) breakdown is considered to be more important in the mechanism of DME even though RPE lesions can be seen shortly after induction of diabetes in the streptozotocin-treated rat model of the disease.[37,38] The amount of heparin sulfate proteoglycan is increased in the vascular endothelium of diabetic eyes compared to nondiabetic eyes. Muller cells are important in transporting water from the extracellular space into the retinal capillaries of the inner retina.[39] Their density in the macaque monkey is five times greater in the parafovea than the retinal periphery.[40] The colocalization of Muller cells with the retinal regions most affected by edema suggests that Muller cell dysfunction contributes to DME. Moreover, Muller cells proliferate in epiretinal membranes, which can exert traction on microvessels and possibly increase their permeability, exacerbating macular edema. Astrocytes, which wrap their end feet around microvessels, decrease their production of glial fibrillary acidic protein in diabetes, which may be important in the altered blood–retina barrier.[35] Within the retina, the synaptic portion of the outer plexiform layer and the entire inner plexiform layer comprise the two highest resistance barriers to the diffusion of interstitial fluid from the inner retina outward toward the choroid.[41] At these layers, the density of junctional complexes between cells and the tortuousness of cellular processes combine to impede most stringently the extracellular flow of water and solutes.[41] Diabetes also alters the structure of the vitreous which may play a role in increased traction on the macula with an increase in vascular permeability (Fig. 7.10).[42–44]

The vitreous and the vitreoretinal interface have significance in DME. Eyes containing vitreous have lowered oxygen tensions compared to eyes having had vitreous replaced with aqueous-like solutions, and presumably intraretinal oxygen tensions are secondarily affected.[45,46] In some cases of vitreous separation, the macula and the disk may adhere to the posterior hyaloid more firmly, and traction may contribute to blood–retinal barrier breakdown.[47] In eyes with DME, the internal limiting membrane (ILM) has more adherent cellular elements on its vitreous side, is thicker, and has more heparin sulfate proteoglycan compared to the ILM peeled from nondiabetic cases of macular holes. Amounts of fibronectin, laminin, and type I, III, IV, and V collagen are increased in the ILM of diabetic eyes.

7.3 Physiology

In DME the macula is thickened with increased extracellular fluid derived primarily from hyperpermeable retinal capillaries, but in perhaps 1% of cases from an abnormally permeable RPE as well.[49,50] Prolonged hyperglycemia produces secondary effects associated with increased leakage of salts, water, and macromolecules from the macular microcirculation into the extracellular space. Among these consequences of hyperglycemia are reduced inner retinal oxygen tension, venous dilation, increased VEGF concentration within the retina, leukocyte stasis, and dysregulated growth factor levels, which together are associated with increased exudation of serum out of the retinal vasculature and into the retinal extracellular space.[51,52] The RPE pump is overwhelmed by the exudation of serum and macular swelling results.[53] Because salt and water are pumped out from the retinal compartment out toward the choroid, but associated serum lipoproteins are not, hard exudates derived from the lipoproteins accumulate in the retina. They often appear in rings centered on leaking clusters of microaneurysms and dilated capillaries. In DME the permeability of the retinal capillaries increases approximately 12-fold, but the activity of the pigment epithelial pump increases only twofold, a mismatch resulting in extracellular fluid accumulation.[53,54]

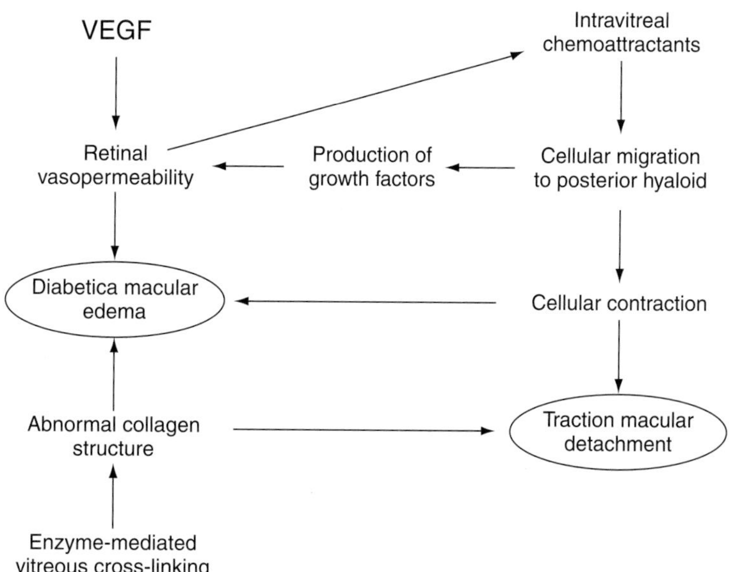

Fig. 7.10 Schematic of the multiple factors that may contribute to diabetic macular edema. Reprinted with permission from Lewis[48]

Poiseuille's Law

Poiseuille's law states that the change in the pressure drop over a length of a vessel will decrease markedly if the vessel dilates. Mathematically,

$$\Delta P = Q 8 \eta 1 / r^4$$

where

ΔP = change in intravascular pressure over the length of a vessel, Q = blood flow in volume per second, η = blood viscosity, l = vessel length, and r = vessel radius.

Thus, when a retinal arteriole dilates, there is less of a pressure drop over the length of the arteriole, leading to an increase in intravascular pressure experienced by the downstream capillaries. The significance of Poiseuille's law arises in the context of loss of autoregulation of the retinal vasculature in diabetes.[55,56] Loss of autoregulation results in widened arteriolar diameters such that the intravascular pressure transmitted to the retinal capillaries is greatly increased. Because of the fourth power dependence of the intravascular pressure gradient on vessel diameter, even minute changes in arteriolar diameter are associated with large increases in retinal capillary pressure.[54]

A useful framework for understanding the pathophysiology of diabetic macular edema is the oxygen theory.[24] According to this theory, hyperglycemia over prolonged periods leads to reduction in perfusion of the inner retina and decrease in inner retinal oxygen tension. The autoregulatory response of the retinal arterioles is dilation which leads to increased hydrostatic pressure in the intraretinal capillaries and venules as specified by Poiseuille's law (Box).[54] The elevated intravascular pressure experienced by the capillaries may itself damage them.[24,54] Concomitantly, the decrease in retinal oxygen tension leads to an increase in synthesis of VEGF and probably other permeability factors, which cause the microvasculature to become leakier. Besides increasing microvascular permeability, VEGF can also directly induce retinal venous dilation, a synergistic effect exacerbating extracellular edema.[57] By Starling's Law (Box), increased intravascular pressure and increased vascular permeability imply net flow of water, ions, and macromolecules from the intravascular space into the extravascular space. Extracellular fluid exits by reentering the retinal vessels further downstream or out into the choroid via the pumping action of the RPE. The relative contributions of these two pathways to the egress of macular extracellular fluid have not been quantitated. Clinical observations that retinal arteriolar dilation precedes DME fit well with this theory.[24,58]

Starling's Law

Starling's Law states that the equilibrium state of fluid transfer between intravascular and extravascular space is characterized by the equation

$$\Delta P – \Delta Q = 0$$

where ΔP = intravascular pressure within microvessels of retina minus the extravascular tissue pressure, and ΔQ = intravascular oncotic pressure minus the intraocular pressure. Arteriolar dilation causes ΔP to increase relative to its previous state of equilibrium, and thus fluid exits the vascular compartment and enters the extravascular, tissue compartment. The clinical significance of Starling's Law in DME has been recognized for decades in the form of observations that increased intraocular pressure is correlated with protection from exudates and hypotony with exacerbation of them.[59] An example of the clinical relevance of Starling's Law in DME is shown in the following case report.

Case Report

A 78-year-old woman with diabetes of 32 years duration and hypertension of 20 years duration had been treated with focal photocoagulation for DME with resolution 5 years before presenting with new blurred vision right eye in October 2008. The right eye had open angle glaucoma for which a mitomycin-assisted trabeculectomy had been performed in 2004. Between August 2008 and October 2008, the visual acuity dropped from 20/40 to 20/125 with recurrent DME. An intravitreal injection of triamcinolone and supplemental photocoagulation had little effect on the recurrent thickening (Fig. 7.11). At the December 2008 visit, the intraocular pressure was 8 mmHg and the fluorescein angiogram showed choroidal folds suggesting hypotony maculopathy. A decrease in intraocular pressure favors serous transudation across the macular capillaries according to Starling's Law. In this case, intravitreal triamcinolone and supplemental focal laser photocoagulation may not have addressed the responsible exacerbating factor for the recurrent macular edema. That is, recurrent DME may not have reflected an increase in retinal vascular permeability, but rather the low intraocular pressure.

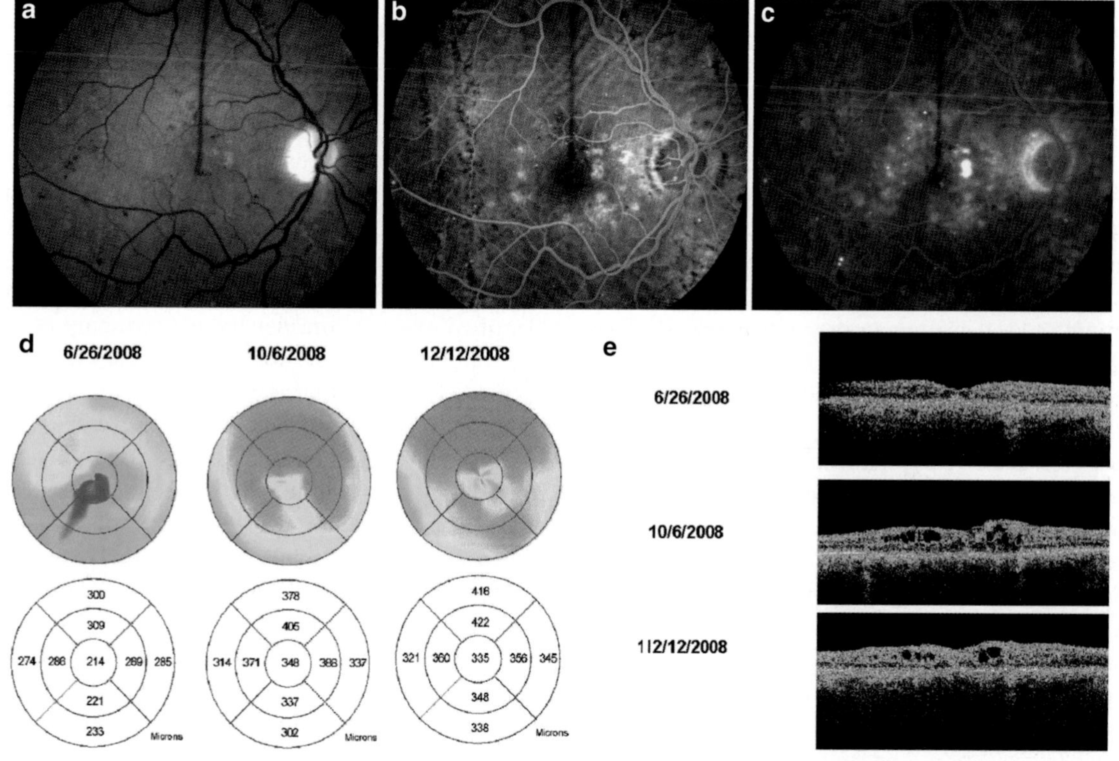

Fig. 7.11 (**a**) Development of hypotony with associated maculopathy (choroidal folds) in the presence of nonproliferative diabetic retinopathy inducing recurrent DME. (**b**) Mid-phase frame from the fluorescein angiogram showing leaky microaneurysms, old focal laser scars, and pigmented linear RPE scars from previous choroidal detachment subsequent to a mitomycin C trabeculectomy. (**c**) Late frame from the fluorescein angiogram showing late diffuse hyperfluorescence in the macula. (**d**) Recurrence of macular thickening as depicted in the macular false color map associated with onset of hypotony. (**e**) Radial line scans showing intraretinal cysts in the presence of the recurrent DME

Many variables have suspected importance in the breakdown of the blood–retina barrier. The duration of diabetes and the integrated elevation of blood glucose reflected in the HbA1C have proven pathophysiologic importance. Retinal neurons and glial cells increase their production of VEGF in diabetes, even before ophthalmoscopic evidence of capillary loss, and this is associated with increased occludin phosphorylation and reduced occludin content in capillary endothelial tight junctions.[35,60,61] Vitreous levels of VEGF are higher in eyes with DME than in diabetic eyes without retinopathy.[62] The diabetic retina shows leukostasis, accumulation of macrophages, intercellular adhesion molecule-1 activation, and prostacyclin upregulation which indicates a state of inflammation and is associated with capillary nonperfusion and breakdown of the blood–retina barrier.[52,63] Inflammatory cytokines such as tumor necrosis factor-beta and interleukin-1β may be important mediators of increased vascular permeability.[35,64,65] Pigment epithelium-derived growth factor, an antiangiogenic and possibly permeability decreasing cytokine, is lower in eyes with DME than diabetic eyes without retinopathy.[62] Many other small molecules and growth factors, including insulin-like growth factor, hepatocyte growth factor, and histamine, may be important in the mechanisms underlying DME, although the details of the pathways are incompletely understood.[64–68] High lipid levels may cause endothelial dysfunction and increased vascular permeability through a local inflammatory response, release of vascular permeability promoting cytokines, and higher levels of advanced glycation end products.[14,69]

Alterations in retinal and choroidal blood flow have been reported in diabetic retinopathy that may influence DME. Patients with diabetes have impaired retinal vascular reactivity to oxygen tension that worsens with retinopathy severity.[70,71] Retinal vascular autoregulation is impaired in diabetes with more severe dysfunction associated with more severe retinopathy.[55] The local factors primarily responsible for vascular autoregulation are nitric oxide and endothelin-1.[72] Vitreous nitric oxide concentration does not differ from vitreous concentrations in macular hole patients used as controls, but vitreous endothelin-1 concentration is significantly lower in DME than levels found in these controls.[72] It is possible that this loss of autoregulatory function may explain refractoriness of certain patients with DME to treatments that are effective in eyes retaining autoregulation. Reported decreases in foveal choroidal blood flow in type 2 diabetic patients with retinopathy may be relevant in the pathophysiology of DME as well, although the techniques for assessing choroidal blood flow have greater uncertainty. Eyes with DME have been reported to have a greater decrease in choroidal blood flow than eyes without DME, leading to suggestions of relative hypoxia of the RPE and outer retina and possible increased permeability of the outer blood retinal barrier on this basis.[31]

The vitreous has a role in the pathogenesis of DME. The diabetic vitreous differs from normal, and the increased cross-linking and glycation of the diabetic vitreous may explain the tendency to develop tangential macular traction, which may in turn induce or exacerbate DME.[42,44] Besides the direct effect of traction causing leakage from blood vessels or macular elevation with subretinal fluid, vitreous adherent to the macula may loculate chemical mediators of increased vessel permeability in proximity to macular capillaries and may impede oxygenation of the retina causing venous dilation and increased edema via Starling's Law or by upregulation of vascular endothelial growth factor.[45,58,73–75] Mean blood flow velocity in perifoveal capillaries increases after vitrectomy in eyes of diabetics with vitreous adhesion, which might be associated with improved macular oxygenation and lessened leakage.[76]

With all of the components that influence DME identified, we can consider the net economy of salt and water transport in subclinical and clinical DME. Figure 7.12 shows that the passive flux of salt and water out of retinal vessels and into the retinal interstitium increases monotonically as one traverses from the state of health to diabetic retinopathy without edema to subclinical DME and finally to clinically significant macular edema (CSME). Passive permeability increases 12-fold in going from health to CSME.[54] Correspondingly, the active transport of salt and water outward through the RPE increases, although less steeply, through the first three stages, but then falters going into CSME, such that active transport increases only twofold as one traverses from health to CSME.[54] The primary problem in DME, therefore, is the increase in passive permeability and not the RPE pumping mechanism.[54]

This account of the pathophysiology of DME informs our current understanding of how treatments for DME work and how nondiabetic factors can modulate severity of DME (Fig. 7.13). Pharmacologic blood pressure reduction reduces passive permeability of the inner blood–retinal barrier.[54] The beneficial effects of grid laser are thought to arise from the increase in oxygenation of the inner retina

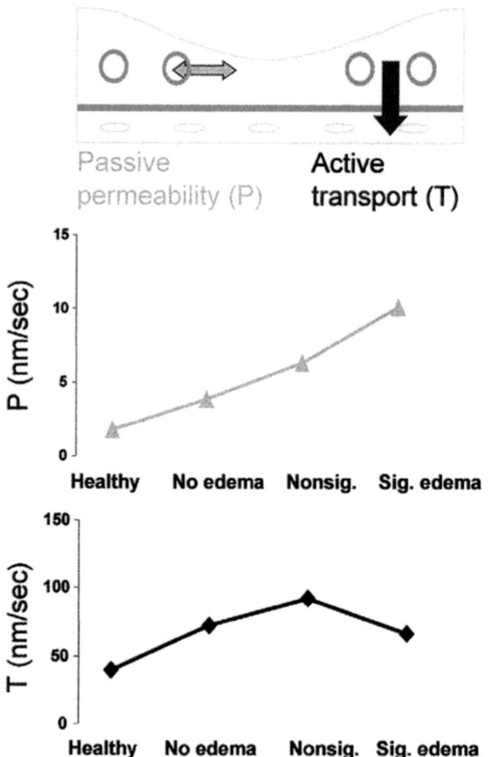

Fig. 7.12 Passive permeability primarily of the inner blood–retina barrier increases 12-fold in going from the state of health through the state of clinically significant macular edema. In contrast, active transport of salt and water outward via the RPE pump increases only doubles. P = passive permeability. T = active transport. Reproduced with permission from Lund-Andersen[54]

both by reduction in oxygen-consuming photoreceptors and by a shorter diffusion pathway to the inner retina for oxygen originating in the choroid.[24,77,78] Focal photocoagulation presumably works by directly destroying leakage sources such as microaneurysms. Focal/grid laser may also improve RPE pumping of salt and water outward toward the choroid.[24,79] In a rabbit model, focal/grid laser photocoagulation caused reduced expression of protein kinase C alpha, a regulatory protein for phototransduction and signal transmission in rod bipolar cells and increased labeling for glial fibrillary acidic protein in Muller cells throughout the retina, not just locally in the areas photocoagulated, implying more than a local effect of focal/grid laser treatment.[80] The macular thinning effect of focal/grid photocoagulation precedes significant documented closure of microaneurysms on fluorescein angiography suggesting that the grid effect begins immediately and the focal effect somewhat later. Eighty-nine percent of leaking microaneurysms have been reported to be closed by 12 weeks after a session of focal/grid laser, but less than 1% by 2 weeks post laser.[27] Anti-VEGF drugs work by blocking the permeability inducing effects of VEGF.[36] Although somewhat controversial, there is some evidence that corticosteroids reduce expression of the VEGF gene, thus reducing VEGF levels, and differentially regulate expression of the various VEGF receptors.[81,82] Corticosteroids may have other, non-VEGF-mediated effects resulting in reduction in permeability of retinal microvessels such as decreasing leukocyte recruitment and production of intercellular adhesion molecule-1.[83–85] Oral protein kinase C-β inhibitors such as ruboxistaurin block the biochemical pathway upregulated by VEGF binding to its receptor on retinal vascular endothelial cells.[86] Statins reduce serum lipid levels, possibly decreasing microvasculature leukostasis and secondary inflammation.[69,87] Vitrectomy may work by increasing intravitreal and secondarily inner retinal oxygen levels, leading to downregulation of VEGF synthesis and resulting in a decrease in permeability of microvessels.[24,78,88] In addition, vitrectomy may open up compartments of loculated cytokines and relieve traction exerted on the macula by an altered vitreous.[48,88,89] Peribulbar and intravitreal corticosteroids may exert beneficial effects on DME by blocking VEGF-mediated increases in retinal vascular permeability and through influences on non-VEGF-mediated pathways.[90] Endophthalmitis and other forms of uveitis that may coincidentally occur with diabetic retinopathy may exacerbate DME because inflammatory mediators increase microvasculature permeability.[91]

Our discussion of DME to this point has concerned extracellular edema, also called vasogenic edema. In addition to extracellular edema, a concept of intracellular edema exists which may be relevant for DME, although it has been less studied.[39,92] Water transport out of the retina occurs via retinal pigment epithelial active transport of potassium and chloride and passive co-transport of water across aquaporin1 channels. Less recognized, however, is transport of water into retinal microvessels via Muller cells. Muller cells possess a unidirectional potassium channel called Kir2.1 that allows extracellular potassium derived from neuronal firing to pass into

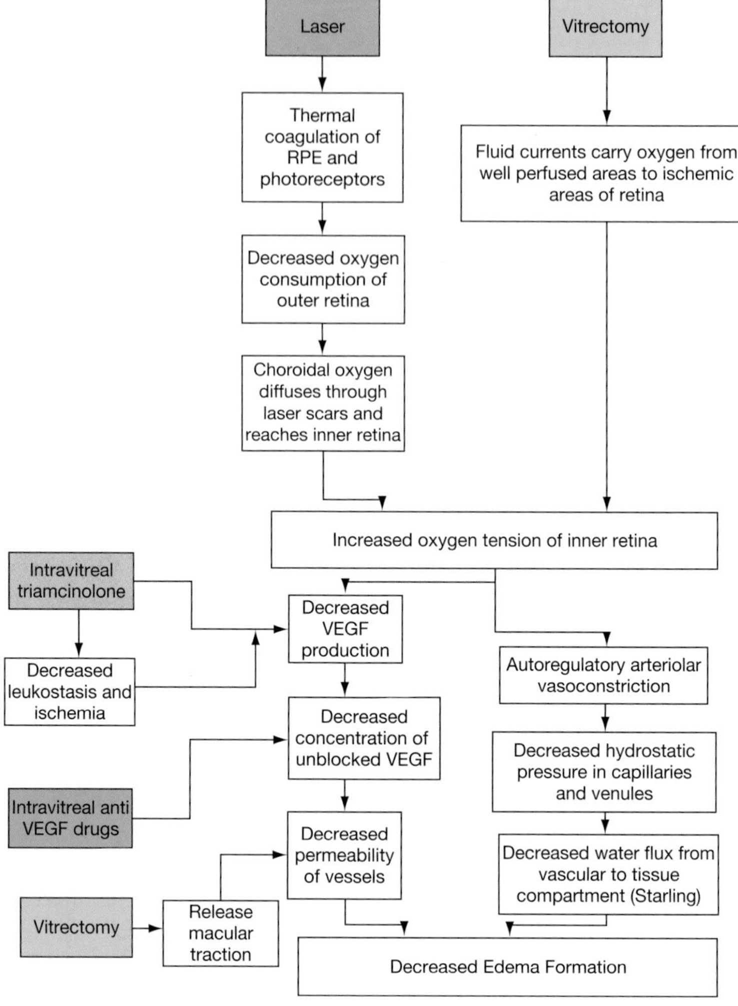

Fig. 7.13 Schematic summarizing the mechanisms of action of the various treatments for diabetic macular edema. The color-filled blocks represent different treatment modalities for DME. Adapted and expanded from Stefansson[24]

the Muller cell but not out of it. In addition, Muller cells have a bidirectional potassium channel called Kir4.1 that allows Muller cell intracellular potassium to flow into vessels around which Muller cell processes are wrapped (Fig. 7.14). In animal models of diabetes, there is downregulation of Kir4.1. Diabetic Muller cells in these models continue to take up potassium from the extracellular space but cannot discharge the potassium into the retinal microvessels. Because water osmotically follows solute, the Muller cells swell, a situation termed intracellular edema. In addition, a dysregulated polyol pathway activated by chronic hyperglycemia in diabetes is thought to be associated with accumulation of intracellular osmotically active solutes that draw in water and cause cellular swelling.[54,93] Whereas the evidence for intracellular edema appears to be substantial in diseases of the brain, models for intracellular edema in the retina have been less well investigated.[92,94]

7.4 Clinical Definitions

There are several definitions important for understanding the literature on diabetic macular edema.

Diabetic Macular Edema – retinal thickening within 1 disk diameter of the center of the macula or definite hard exudates in this region.[4] This definition used in the Early Treatment Diabetic Retinopathy Study (ETDRS) differs from some other definitions in which the radius may be 2 disk diameters

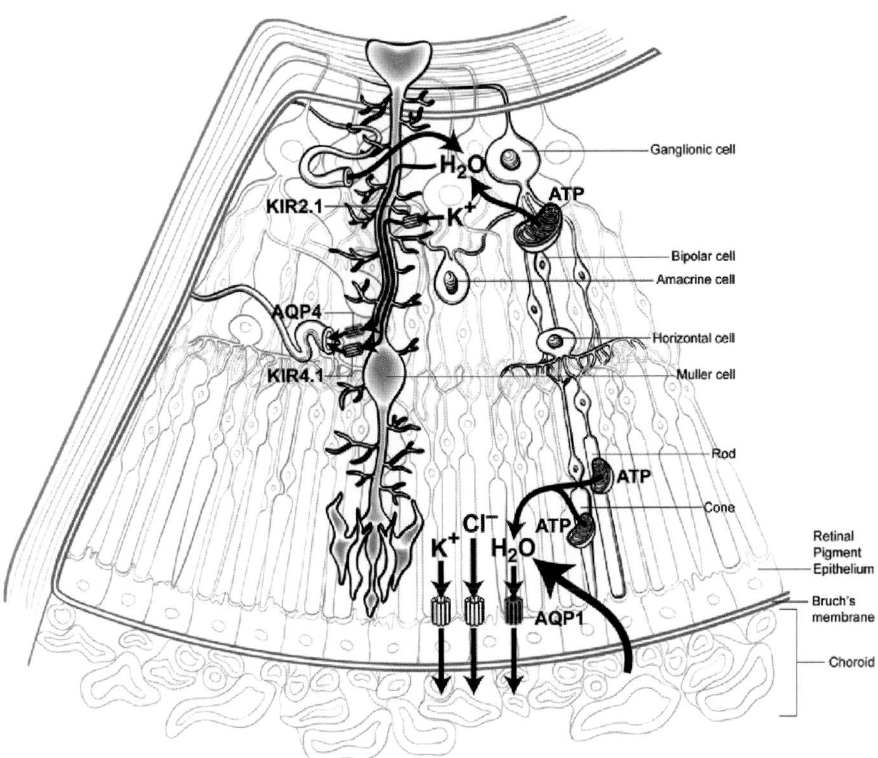

Fig. 7.14 Schematic depicting pathways for water transport in the retina. Water is generated in the retina by oxidative synthesis of adenosine 5′-triphosphate (ATP) that generates carbon dioxide and water (H_2O).The Muller cell has processes that wrap around retinal microvessels. Bidirectional potassium channels called Kir4.1 are present in the Muller cell membranes abutting these microvessels. Muller cells also possess unidirectional potassium channels called Kir2.1 abutting the extracellular space that allows passage of potassium from the neuroretinal cells into the Muller cell. Aquaporin 4 (AQ4) water channels allow the osmotic co-transport of water to follow potassium movement. The retinal pigment epithelium also actively transports potassium and chloride from the retina to the choroid with water co-transport occurring via aquaporin1 (AQ1) channels. In diabetes, the Kir4.1 channels are decreased, but not the KIR2.1 unidirectional potassium channels or the RPE potassium transport channels. The net effect is Muller cell swelling – intracellular edema. Reproduced with permission from Reichenbach and colleagues[92]

and in which the hard exudates criterion may be omitted. For epidemiologic purposes, some studies also classify an eye as having DME if there are macular photocoagulation scars to indicate previous treatment even if no macular thickening is present.[95]

Clinically Significant Macular Edema (CSME) – the situation in which at least one of the following criteria is fulfilled:

a. Retinal thickening within 500 μm of the center of the macula
b. Hard exudates within 500 μm of the center of the macula with adjacent retinal thickening
c. One disk area of retinal thickening any part of which is within 1 disk diameter of the center of the macula[4]

Clinically Significant Macular Edema – Terminologic Vagary

The definition of CSME was created in the ETDRS and was based on analysis of stereoscopic fundus photographs of the macula by trained nonphysician graders. The term, however, was used and continues to be used in a clinical sense as well. The eyes in the ETDRS were classified and randomized at baseline based on fundus photographic gradings, but at follow-up visits, retreatment decisions were made based on clinical examinations at the slit lamp. Thus, although there is one-term CSME, there are two methods of determining it.

The definition of CSME has been termed "complex" and "difficult to apply precisely in clinical practice" even by its originators.[96] Most published reproducibility statistics apply to the term as construed from color fundus photography.[97] There are no statistics published for the reproducibility of CSME as determined at the slit lamp by different clinicians, and yet the definition is widely used in clinical ophthalmology as the threshold for treatment of DME. To confidently extrapolate the results of the ETDRS trial to routine clinical practice, it would seem of interest to know how photographically graded CSME and clinically graded CSME compare. In one study on this topic, clinical diagnosis had a sensitivity of 24% relative to stereo photography.[96] In other studies, the chance corrected agreement between clinical diagnosis and stereo fundus photography has ranged from 0.31 to 0.55.[96,98] Among the disagreements between ophthalmoscopy and analysis of fundus photographs, undercalls by ophthalmoscopy were more common than overcalls (88 and 12%, respectively).[96] In the ETDRS itself, a much more tightly controlled study environment in which the retina specialists who were involved were the same ones who defined the term CSME, the kappa statistic for clinical examination with a fundus contact lens compared to analysis of stereo fundus photographs was 0.61.[99] In general, clinical detection of CSME is less sensitive than detection by analyzing stereo fundus photographs. The evidence suggests that treating DME based on clinical estimation of the presence of CSME probably leads to a degree of undertreatment compared to treatment decisions based on analysis of stereoscopic fundus photographs.

7.5 Focal and Diffuse Diabetic Macular Edema

The terms focal and diffuse are used frequently to differentiate two types of DME, although these terms have not been defined consistently in the literature.[100–121] Focal edema is said to arise from microaneurysms (Fig. 7.15), whereas diffuse edema is said to arise from generally dilated and hyperpermeable capillaries throughout the macula (Fig. 7.16).[122,123] The difficulty comes in translating this simple concept into an operationally reproducible methodology in clinical practice. Focal DME defined in a variety of ways has been reported to be more common than diffuse DME, but many cases of DME subjected to these definitions have mixed features making a clear distinction difficult (Fig. 7.17).[79,116,124–127] Additional confusion may arise because the term focal is used to describe a technique of applying laser directly to microaneurysms when treating DME with focal/grid photocoagulation.[4]

In general, paucity of lipid exudates has been associated with diffuse edema in ophthalmoscopic definitions, whereas presence of lipid and lipid rings has been associated with focal edema.[79,102,112,128–132] Definitions involving color fundus photographs often involve area criteria, and the criteria vary among studies.

In the ETDRS, DME was defined clinically from stereoscopic biomicroscopy without reference to focal or diffuse descriptions of that clinical examination. However, fluorescein angiograms were analyzed by a reading center and the source of fluorescein leakage was graded categorically by proportion of leakage originating from microaneurysms for classification of edema as focal or diffuse. Eyes with $\geq$ 67% of leakage associated with microaneurysms were classified as focal, those with 33–66% of leakage associated with microaneurysms as intermediate, and those with <33% of leakage associated with microaneurysms as diffuse.[133,134] The reproducibility of grading fluorescein angiograms for leakage source has been classified as only fair by the ETDRS authors.[133] Others are less circumspect. Blair and colleagues state "it is notoriously difficult to quantify leakage on fluorescein angiograms."[29]

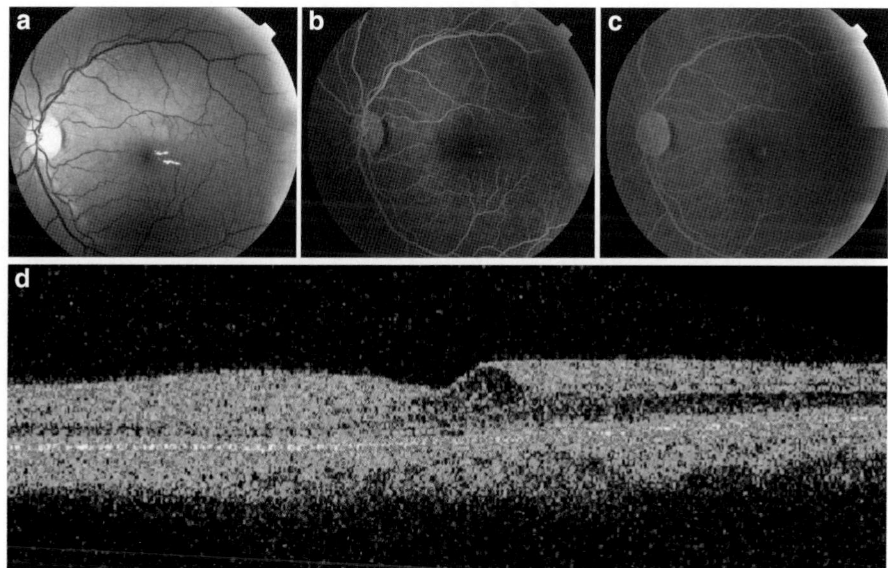

Fig. 7.15 (**a**) Focal diabetic macular edema is often described as arising from microaneurysms and having an association with lipid exudates, often in *circinate rings*. In this red-free photograph, lipid exudates surround a large microaneurysm temporal to the *center* of the macula. (**b**) The *mid*-phase fluorescein angiogram shows the microaneurysm responsible for the exudates. The exudates are not apparent on fluorescein angiography. (**c**) The *late*-phase fluorescein angiogram shows fluorescein leakage from the microaneurysm. (**d**) The *horizontal radial line* scan OCT image shows parafoveal cystoid thickening of the macula

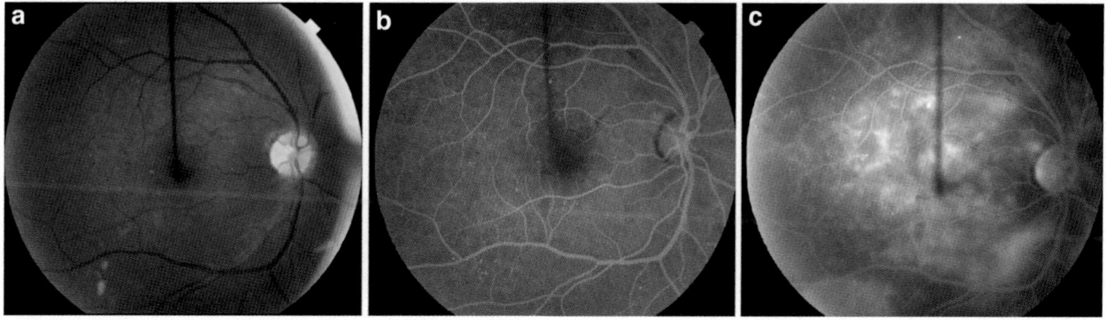

Fig. 7.16 (**a**) Diffuse diabetic macular edema is often described as arising from dilated capillaries throughout the posterior pole, but not from microaneurysms, involving large areas of the macula, involving the center of the macula, and associated with few lipid exudates.The usage of the term diffuse, however, is inconsistent in the published literature. This color fundus photograph shows few lipid exudates. (**b**) Relatively few microaneurysms are seen relative to the amount of fluorescein leakage shown in the late frame (see **c**). (**c**) Profuse late leakage of fluorescein is present

Optical coherence tomography (OCT) can also be used to define edema as focal or diffuse. In the false color map, isolated islands of hot colors surrounded by larger areas of cool colors give a sense of focality, but this is subjective. Some have suggested that diffuse DME be understood to imply an increasing number of elevated subfields on the map display.[135] This OCT-based characterization has not proven to explain additional variability in visual acuity over that explained by central subfield mean thickness, age, or fluorescein leakage in the inner subfields nor has it been predictive of visual acuity outcomes at 1 year after focal photocoagulation.[136]

When clinicians are asked to classify DME as focal or diffuse, evidence suggests that their assessments differ from classifications used by photographic

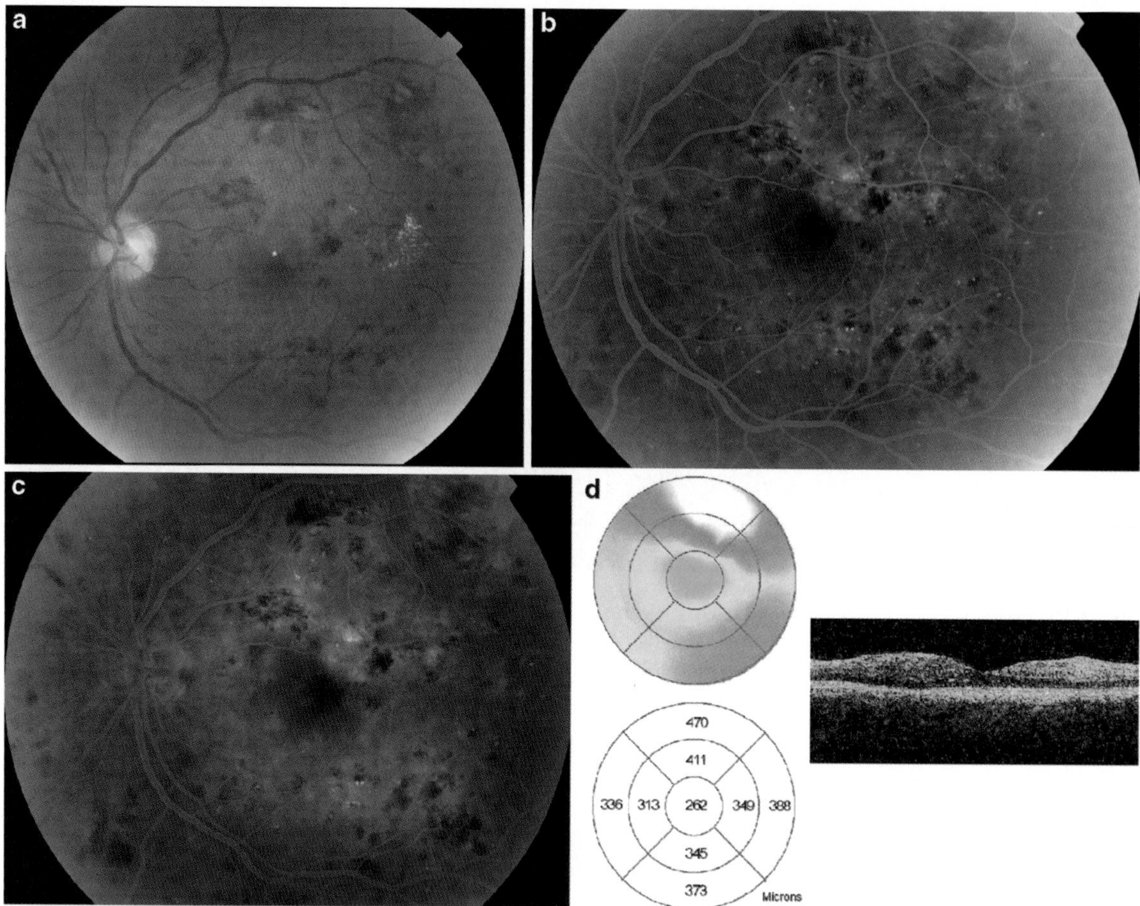

Fig. 7.17 Many eyes with diabetic macular edema have mixed characteristics with leakage from microaneurysms and dilated capillary segments, lipid exudates in some thickened areas and not others, and large areas of thickening, but not necessarily involving the center of the macula. An example is shown. (**a**) A *lipid ring* is present superotemporally but other regions of thickened macula are free of lipid. (**b**) A *mid-phase* frame of the fluorescein angiogram does not show more microaneurysms in the area of the lipid ring than in other areas without lipid. (**c**) A frame from the *late phase* of the fluorescein angiogram shows an area of leaky microaneurysms inferotemporal to the *center* of the macula without associated lipid of note. (**d**) The OCT shows that the fovea is only mildly thickened, a characteristic often associated with focal edema, yet with a large area of thickened macula, a characteristic often associated with diffuse edema

reading centers. In comparing a British prospective survey of laser treatment for DME in which clinicians graded DME and a Diabetic Retinopathy Clinical Research (DRCR) network clinical trial involving two methods of laser treatment for DME in which a reading center graded DME, there was a 27% discrepancy between fractions categorized as focal by the two studies.[137] Although this might reflect different samples, it could also suggest that the clinical and photographic methods capture different information about these eyes, and suggests that caution is required in implicitly comparing statements about focal DME defined in different ways.

Many authors have claimed that diffuse DME is refractory to macular photocoagulation and that diffuse DME is a prognostic factor for poorer visual acuity at follow-up, but the evidence for these claims has not come from prospective clinical trials and is weak.[115,138] In some cases, the literature has been misquoted, most frequently by claiming that the ETDRS showed that diffuse DME showed a poorer response to focal/grid laser than focal DME.[121,139] In fact, the ETDRS looked at the source of fluorescein leakage as a possible factor that might modify the beneficial effect of photocoagulation for DME on the development of moderate visual loss and found no difference when comparing eyes with leakage classified as predominantly focal with those classified as intermediate to diffuse. There were too few eyes with predominantly diffuse leakage for analysis.[134] Others have suggested that diffuse DME responds better to intravitreal triamcinolone injections, intravitreal bevacizumab injections, or vitrectomy and focal DME to focal laser photocoagulation.[121,123,140–142] The evidence to support the claims comes from qualitative comparisons across studies of different designs and is weak.[140,141]

It is possible that a concept of focal and diffuse edema, possibly expressed with a new vocabulary, will prove to be important in explaining baseline variance in visual acuity or in predicting treatment outcomes as has been claimed, but the usefulness of the concept has not yet been established despite its ubiquitous use.[137]

7.6 Subclinical Diabetic Macular Edema

Diabetic macular edema may be clinically recognized, yet not reach a severity satisfying the definition of CSME (Fig. 7.18). Clinical assessment of macular edema and OCT assessment of macular edema frequently disagree in this group of patients.[143,144] In addition, some eyes do not have clinically recognized DME, but macular thickening is detectable by OCT.[144] The term subclinical DME (SCDME) has been used to define both of these classes of DME that are less severe than clinically significant DME.[144,145]

7.7 Refractory Diabetic Macular Edema

Diabetic macular edema that has been treated with focal/grid photocoagulation and yet persists is defined as refractory.[146–148] Different authors use different criteria for the number of focal/grid treatments that are used before applying the term, but all require at least one. Eyes may be refractory to treatments other than focal/grid photocoagulation, and some eyes have edema refractory to all known treatments for DME. Refractory DME has been reported to produce more rapid visual acuity loss in older patients, and is associated with greater short-term variability in macular thickness than is seen in eyes without refractory DME.[149,150] It is also associated with higher levels of HbA1c than DME that resolves with focal/grid laser photocoagulation.[148]

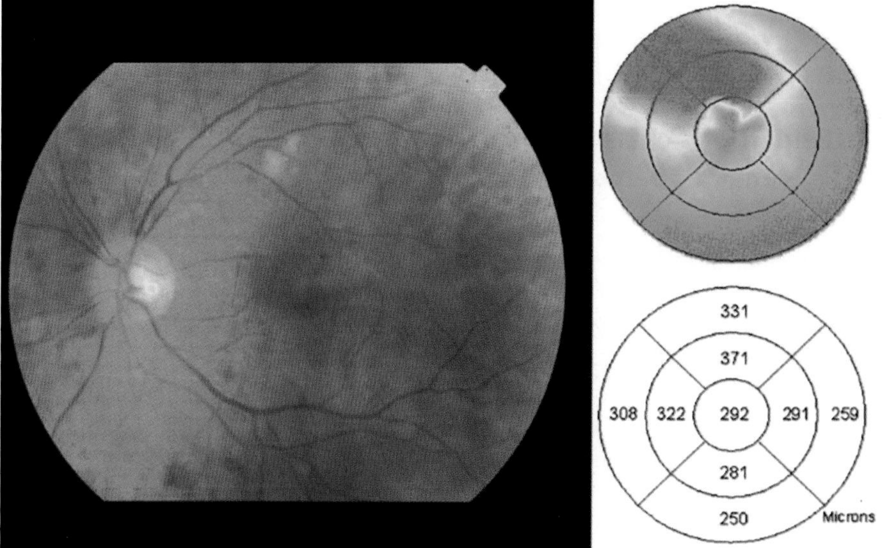

Fig. 7.18 Example of subclinical diabetic macular edema. No thickening of the macula was recognized on biomicroscopy, yet on OCT there is clearly abnormal thickening superonasal to the *center* of the macula

What Is the Rate of Visual Decline from Diabetic Macular Edema?

The rate of visual decline in the control group eyes with baseline visual acuity ≥ 20/40 in the ETDRS was 1 ETDRS letter per 48 days.[151] These eyes received no laser photocoagulation. In the PKC-DRS2 study, the treatment naïve eyes in the control group with severe DME and baseline visual acuity ≥ 20/40 also lost visual acuity at a rate of 1 ETDRS letter per 48 days.[152] Unpublished data of the author suggest an estimate of 1 ETDRS letter lost per 72 days of follow-up in eyes with refractory DME. It appears that the rate of visual acuity declines from DME may decrease over time but not to zero. Further studies are needed to properly address this suggestion.

7.8 Regressed Diabetic Macular Edema

Regressed diabetic macular edema is defined as the macular state in which DME was once present, was treated with focal/grid laser or other treatments, and is now absent. It is important to state the method for determining absence of the macular edema, as classifications may disagree using clinical methods and imaging methods such as OCT or fluorescein angiography.

7.9 Recurrent Diabetic Macular Edema

Regardless of the treatment used, cases exist in which DME vanishes after treatment, but subsequently recurs.[153] Although DME can resolve spontaneously without treatment, and then recur, the term recurrent DME is generally used with reference to treated eyes with recurrences.

7.10 Methods of Detection of Diabetic Macular Edema

Diabetic macular edema is most commonly assessed by stereoscopic slit-lamp examination using a fundus lens.[4] Examination with a contact lens is more sensitive, but takes more time and can degrade the view for subsequent photography.[154] Noncontact fundus lenses are more commonly used in daily practice, are faster and more compatible with subsequent fundus imaging, but have less sensitivity for detection of DME.[79] Direct ophthalmoscopy allows detection of lipid exudates, which may be a sign of DME, but suffers from lack of stereopsis. Although lipid presence suggests associated macular thickening, the two findings are not synonymous and, therefore, presence of lipid alone is an unreliable surrogate for DME.[155,156]

Stereoscopic fundus photographs can be used to assess presence of DME and grade its severity in clinical trials but not in clinical practice.[151,157] Compared to clinical examination with a contact fundus lens, stereo fundus photography with reading by trained nonphysicians is more sensitive for the detection of DME associated hard exudates, equally sensitive for detection of center-involved DME, and less sensitive for the detection of non-center-involved DME.[99] Because OCT is more reproducible and is more widely available, grading of DME by stereo fundus photography is a research tool used only in clinical trials, and even in this setting its use is declining.

Fluorescein angiography has been used to detect leakage of fluorescein from microaneurysms and other leakage sources in diabetic retinopathy. In some studies, fluorescein leakage has been used as a surrogate variable for macular thickening.[47] Because it does not assess the function of the retinal pigment epithelial pump, the correlation of fluorescein leakage with macular thickening is modest.[158,159] It was not used in the ETDRS for the detection of DME, but rather for guidance of focal/grid photocoagulation once DME had been diagnosed by slit-lamp stereo fundus biomicroscopy.[99]

As a practical matter, there appears to be a trend toward decreasing use of fluorescein angiography in management of DME. Immediately after the publication of the first ETDRS report, fluorescein angiography was considered as a necessary tool to guide focal/grid laser treatment.[160] Although no randomized trials have been done comparing focal/grid with and without use of fluorescein angiography for guidance, subsequent uncontrolled case series have reported similar results of focal/grid laser photocoagulation for DME whether fluorescein angiography is or is not used to guide the treatment.[112,161] The report that similar planned focal/grid treatment patterns result regardless of whether experienced retinologists use fluorescein angiography may have boosted a trend away from fluorescein angiography use.[162] For example, in a 1998 audit of DME management, only 19.5% of British ophthalmologists treating DME with focal laser photocoagulation obtained a fluorescein angiogram before treatment.[110] In a 2007 study from the DRCR Network, 50% of eyes were managed without fluorescein angiography.[163] In the year of diagnosis of DME, Medicare claims data indicate that a 60% of patients received a fluorescein angiogram over the 2000–2004 period. Despite investigation, there has been no evidence published to support assertions of necessity of fluorescein angiography for planning treatment or usefulnesss in predicting outcomes.[112,134,162] Oral fluorescein angiography has promise for detecting DME in the setting of a screening program, possibly reducing the numbers of patients requiring referral to ophthalmologists, but has not been adopted outside of a demonstration project. Compared to stereoscopic slit-lamp biomicroscopy, sensitivity of 92% and specificity of 81% have been reported for detection of DME with this technique.[164]

The importance of OCT in the diagnosis and management of DME can scarcely be overemphasized.[165] The clinical diagnosis of DME as practiced in the ETDRS era before OCT was beset by variability among clinicians actually carrying out the principles established in the clinical trial.[79] After accounting for the effects of chance, agreement between the clinical diagnosis of CSME by an investigator and the gold standard diagnosis based on stereoscopic viewing of color fundus photographs has been reported to be 31% in a setting representative of community care.[96] The importance of inaccuracy in disease detection and staging has been stressed as a factor explaining discrepancies in outcomes within clinical trials as compared to community settings.[166] Because detection and assessment of DME by OCT are more objective and reproducible than by clinical examination, more uniformity in intervention and outcomes of treatment may be possible than in the pre-OCT era.[143,144] Increasingly in both clinical trials and community care, an OCT component to a definition of DME is included based on normal databases of OCT values that have been published.[135,167] In the DRCR Network, central subfield mean thickness by Stratus OCT must be ≥ 250 μm to qualify for inclusion in DME trials and to be eligible for retreatment at specified reevaluation intervals. From Medicare claims analyses, 2.5% of patients with DME had an OCT ordered in the year after a diagnosis of DME in 2000, increasing to 40% in 2004.[11] The penetration of OCT machines into ophthalmic practice has continued to increase since 2004 and that percentage would undoubtedly be higher today.

There is no reproducibility data on clinical detection of DME, but there is a wealth of reproducibility data on OCT.[168–172] Variability in OCT measurements occur in several forms. Measurement variability is that variability noted between repeat measurements made within minutes of each other. Measurement variability has been found to be dependent on the macular thickness. In general, any change of macular thickness greater than 11% of a previous measurement exceeds OCT measurement variability and can be assumed to be a real change in macular thickness.[170] In addition to measurement variability, there is short-term fluctuation in macular thickness in DME. By this one refers to the variability noted over the course of days to even weeks when there is no trend in the changes.[173] Short-term fluctuation in DME is also dependent on macular thickness and is larger than measurement variability.[150] It is of particular importance in eyes with refractory DME and of little clinical importance in eyes with diabetic retinopathy but no previous history or present evidence of macular edema (Table 7.1).[173] Unpublished data of the author suggest that it is of intermediate magnitude and concern in eyes with regressed DME. Two clinical examples will help make concrete the clinical significance of short-term variation in macular thickness.

Table 7.1 Short-term variation in central subfield mean thickness in subgroups of eyes with diabetic retinopathy

Diabetic retinopathy group	Study	N	Baseline CSMT, median, IQR (µm)	Short-term variation in CSMT, median, (IQR), [range], (µm)
Diabetic retinopathy without DME	Browning[173]	56	219 (195–235)	18 (11–31) [2–172]
Treatment naïve DME	Toda[174]	8	374 (274–761)	137 (54–237) [27–299]
Refractory DME	Massin[150]	12	463 (407–541)	153 (80–296) [40–368]

IQR = interquartile range, µm = microns, CSMT = central subfield mean thickness

7.11 Case Report 1

A 67-year-old female with type 2 diabetes for 28 years had a history of DME in both eyes. She had had argon laser focal/grid photocoagulation of the right eye three times previously as well as vitrectomy and internal limiting membrane peeling when the DME did not resolve after laser treatment. Panretinal photocoagulation of the right eye had been administered for proliferative diabetic retinopathy with regression of the neovascularization. Despite multiple treatments, refractory DME of the right eye persisted (Fig. 7.19), yet her visual acuity was sufficient that she was able to read a newspaper and pass a drivers test. Treatment had been suspended as futile over the past 2 years, but she was monitored at 3–6-month intervals. The corrected visual acuity in March 2008 was right eye 20/50 and left eye 20/200. The central subfield mean thickness (CSMT) of the right eye was 273 µm. The left eye had chronic, more severe, refractory DME. She returned 6 months later and reported worse blurring of vision. At this time visual acuity was right eye 20/80 and left eye 20/200. The OCT-measured DME of the right eye had worsened with CSMT of 371 µm (Fig. 7.20). The fundus appearance and the fluorescein angiography for the right eye are shown in Figs. 7.21, 7.22, and 7.23. Loss of the ability to drive was feared, and reconsideration was therefore given to further intervention for the refractory DME. In attempting to decide the wisest

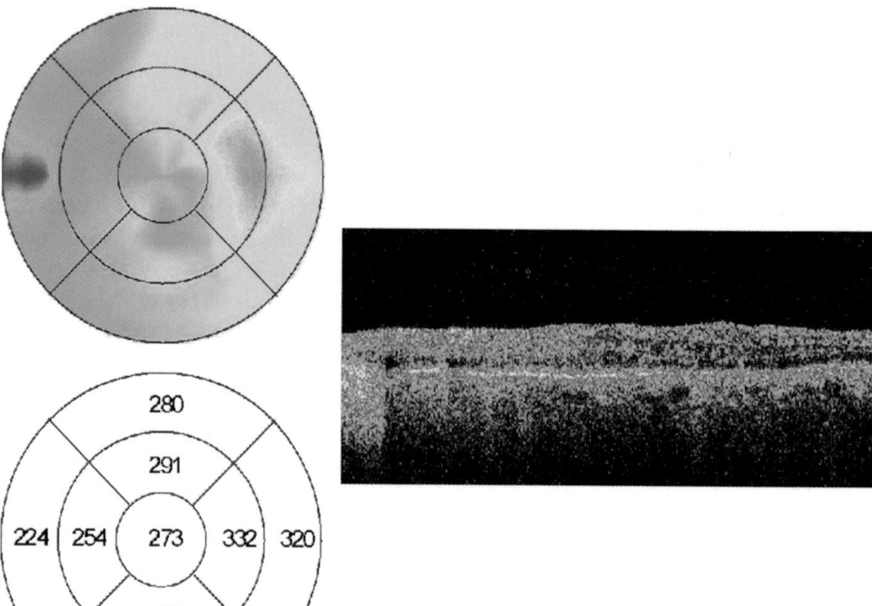

Fig. 7.19 Initial OCT images of the *right eye* of case report 1 in March 2008 when the patient could see sufficiently to pass a drivers license examination. The radial line scan is oriented vertically

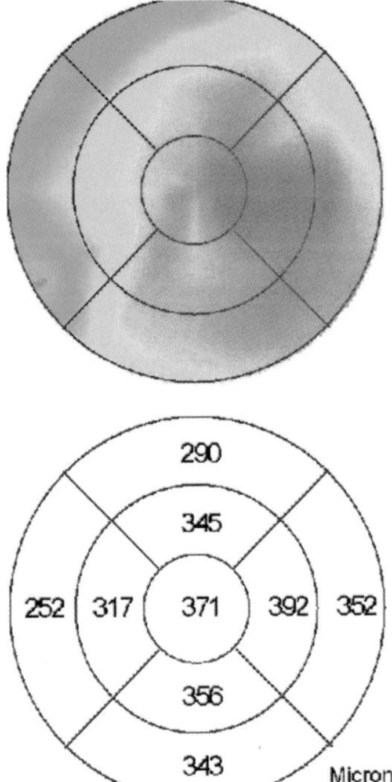

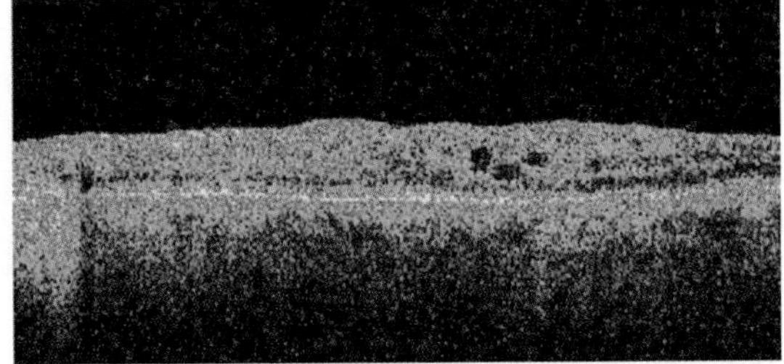

Fig. 7.20 OCT images of the *right eye* of case 1 in September 2008 when the patient had experienced deterioration of visual acuity, more difficulty driving, and was found to have increased diabetic macular edema. The radial line scan is oriented vertically

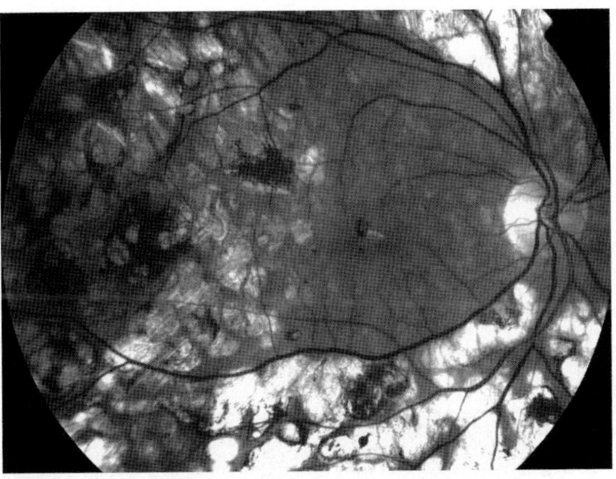

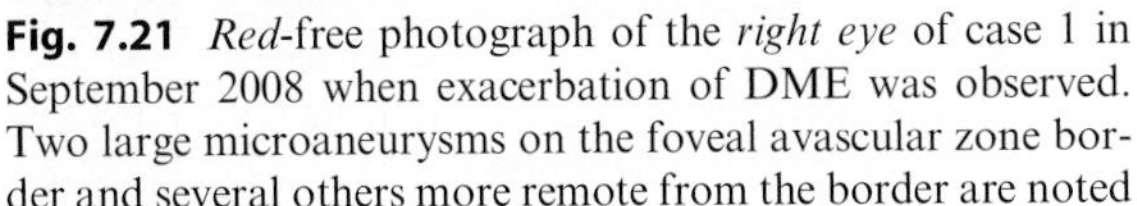

Fig. 7.21 *Red*-free photograph of the *right eye* of case 1 in September 2008 when exacerbation of DME was observed. Two large microaneurysms on the foveal avascular zone border and several others more remote from the border are noted

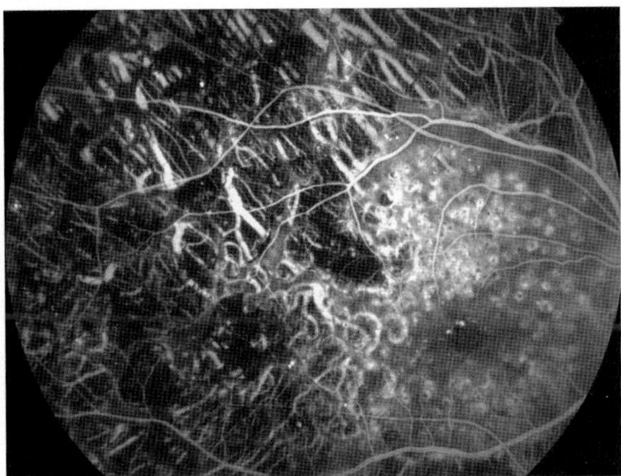

Fig. 7.22 *Mid-phase* fluorescein angiogram of the *right eye* of case 1 in September 2008. The location of two large microaneurysms on the border of the foveal avascular zone is documented

recommendation for this patient, the question arose whether the 98 μm thickening of the CSMT witnessed between the last two visits was within the expected range of short-term OCT variability for eyes with refractory DME. In other words, was she truly worsening – showing increasing macular thickening – or was this compatible with short-term variability of macular thickening in an eye with refractory DME?

The patient returned 1 month later, and the CSMT and visual acuity of the right eye had improved spontaneously to 178 μm and 20/60, respectively (Fig. 7.24). That is, as this case exemplifies, short-term fluctuation in CSMT in

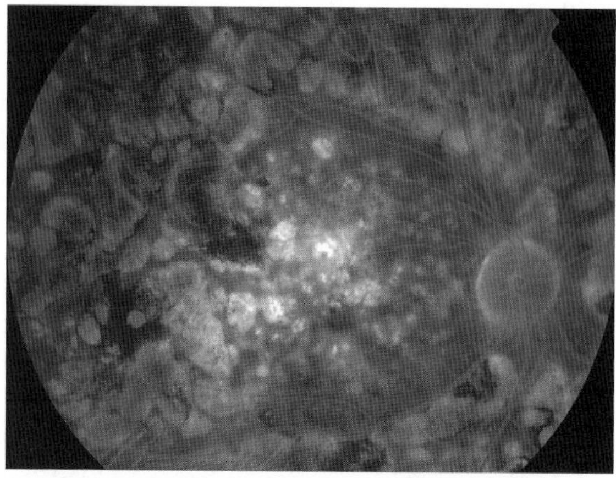

Fig. 7.23 *Late-phase* fluorescein angiogram of the *right eye* of case 1 in September 2008. There is petalloid hyperfluorescence most prominent superior and temporal to the fovea although the epicenter of the thickening on the OCT false color map is inferonasal to the fovea

refractory DME can be larger than OCT measurement variability, which for an eye with macular thickness of 273 μm would be approximately 30 μm. The clinician may need to include this factor of short-term variability of macular thickness in refractory DME in clinical decision making to avoid restarting previously futile styles of treatment and possibly inducing further side effects such as laser-induced paracentral scotomata or steroid-induced pressure elevation without benefiting visual acuity.[142,175]

7.12 Case Report 2

A 77-year-old man with diabetes of 10 years duration and hypertension of 1-year duration was examined in 2000 and found to have DME reducing visual acuity in the left eye to 20/50. No OCT was available in our clinic in 2000, but clinically significant macular edema was found on stereoscopic slit-lamp biomicroscopy with a noncontact fundus lens and two sessions ofargon laser focal/grid photocoagulation were given on 16 March 2000 and 28 January 2002. The DME resolved both on clinical examination and by OCT measurements once that instrument became available to the practice. During follow-up, four consecutive normal CSMTs were recorded between 25 January 2005 and 21 August 2007 in consonance with the clinical examination that showed no macular thickening on stereoscopic slit-lamp biomicroscopy. The appearance of the fundus at this time is shown in

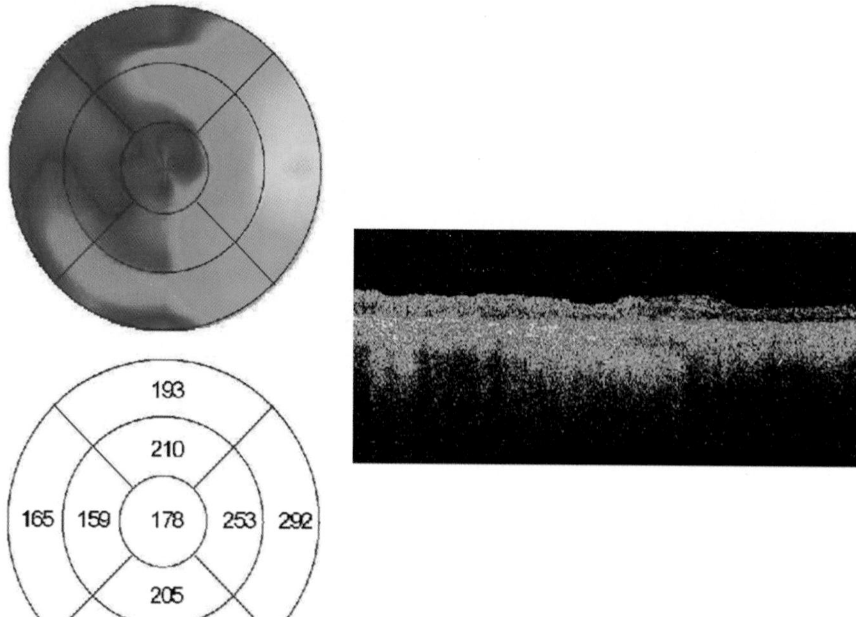

Fig. 7.24 OCT images of the *right eye* of case 1 in October 2008 when the patient had spontaneous regression of the exacerbated macular thickening. The radial line scan is oriented vertically

Fig. 7.25. At follow-up on 9 April 2008, the CSMT increased to 283 μm compared to the value of 205 μm on 21 August 2007 (Figs. 7.26 and 7.27). Clinically, the center of the macula was judged to be not thickened. The question arose whether the 78 μm increase in macular thickness represented a change in the macula in excess of the short-term fluctuation in macular thickness in an eye with regressed DME. In other words, was this recurrent DME and did it need to be treated?

The patient was observed without treatment and at follow-up on 11 November 2008 was noted to have spontaneous resolution of the macular thickening present at the previous examination. That is, as this case exemplifies, short-term fluctuation in CSMT in regressed DME is potentially larger than OCT measurement variability. For an eye with macular thickness of 205 μm, measurement

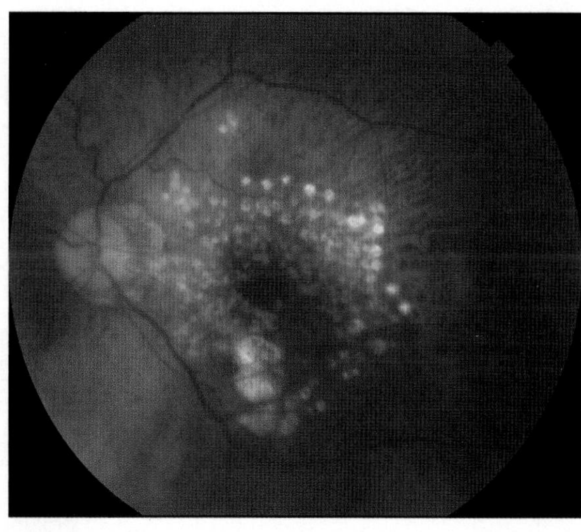

Fig. 7.25 Color fundus photograph documenting the appearance of the *left eye* of case 2 with regressed DME and a pattern of focal/grid laser scars

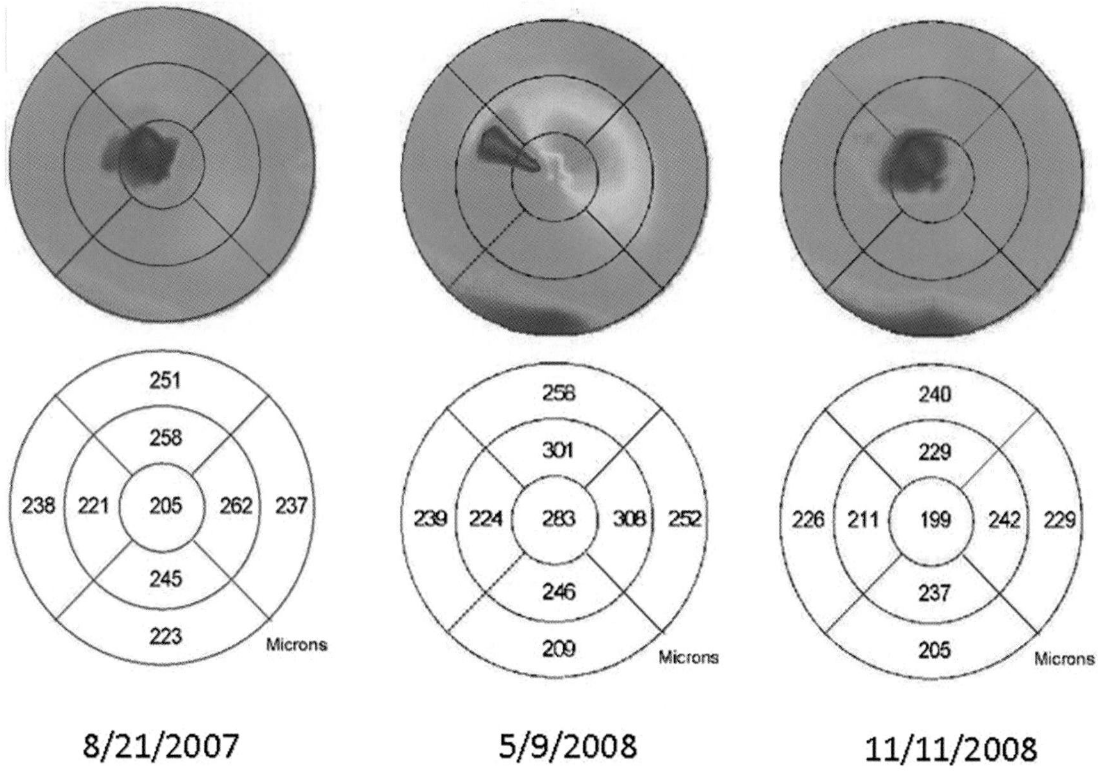

Fig. 7.26 Three OCT false color maps of the *left eye* of case report 2 documenting the regional pattern of macular thickness in a patient with regressed DME after two sessions of focal/grid photocoagulation given 7 years earlier. On 8 May 2008, there is OCT thickening that was not present at the 21 August 2007 visit. Without any therapy, there is spontaneous regression of this thickening as shown in the map from 11 November 2008

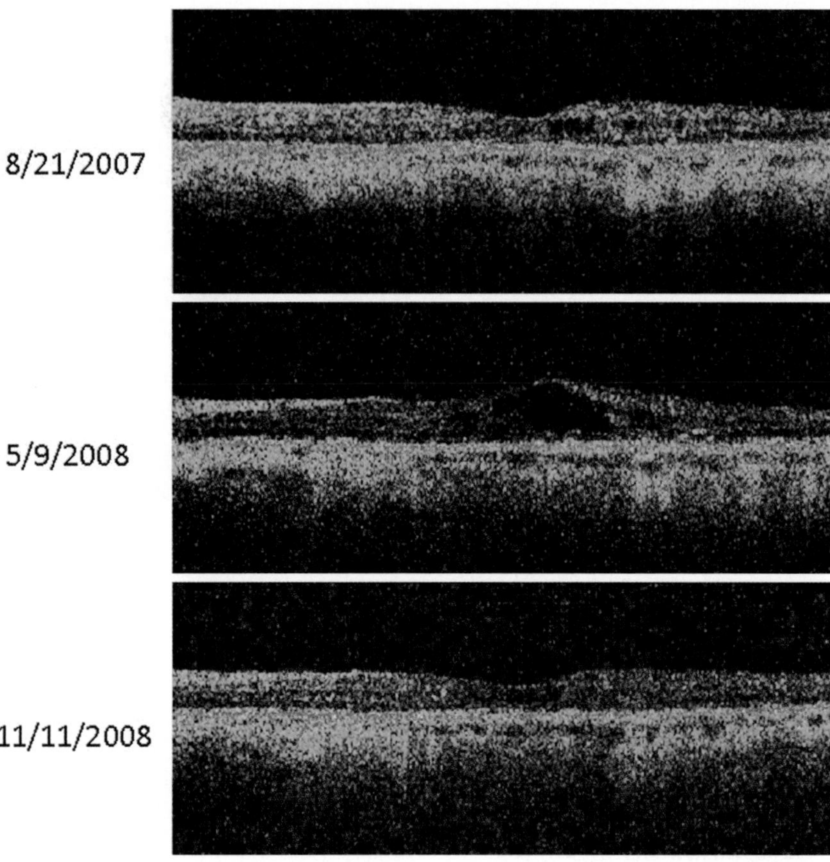

Fig. 7.27 Three OCT horizontal radial line scans documenting the macular morphology of the *left eye* of case report 2 on the same three dates shown in Fig. 7.25. On 9 May 2008, there is intraretinal cystoid change and thickening that was not present on 21 August 2007. The thickening has spontaneously resolved by the scan of 11 November 2008, although there is still some lesser degree of intraretinal cystoid change

variability would be approximately 21 μm. The clinician may be advised to include the larger short-term fluctuation factor for eyes with regressed DME in clinical decision-making.

Of the many OCT indices that can be followed in the course of DME, the central subfield mean thickness (CSMT) is the best single measure.[176,177] It is more reproducible than center point thickness, yet is highly correlated ($r = 0.99$) with the latter.[176,177] Total macular volume (TMV) correlates somewhat less well with CSMT($r = 0.76$), but there have been no conclusions drawn from analyzing TMV that would not have been drawn by studying CSMT instead.[146,157] Other variables such as maximal thickening of the inner zone and maximal thickening of the grid have not added value to analyses using CSMT.[157] OCT has also revealed the fact that serous retinal detachment is associated with DME in 9.7–26.0% of cases, a fact unappreciated in the ETDRS era.[68,132,178–180] Serous retinal detachment can be associated with mild or severe degrees of neural retinal thickening, with retinopathy featuring clustered microaneurysms or with few microaneurysms, and has little correlation with visual acuity impairment. It responds to treatments for DME, just as does the thickening of the neural retina, is not correlated with degree of capillary nonperfusion, and has little prognostic importance for outcome.[116] Serous retinal detachment is not seen in the absence of some degree of neural retinal edema.[180]

Methods of Analysis of OCT Data

OCT-measured changes in macular thickness can be analyzed in three ways – as absolute changes in thickness, relative changes in thickness, and relative changes in thickening, where thickening means excess retinal thickness compared to published normal values. Chan and Duker have stated that all studies of macular edema should employ the relative change in thickening method of analysis, but their recommendations were based on examples from the literature that were much thicker than the majority of eyes treated for DME.[177] The DRCR Network has shown that the relative change in thickening method of analysis is unstable for eyes with mild degrees of macular edema—for example, with thicknesses <300 μm (Fig. 7.28). For such eyes, the preferred method of analysis is absolute change in thickness.[176]

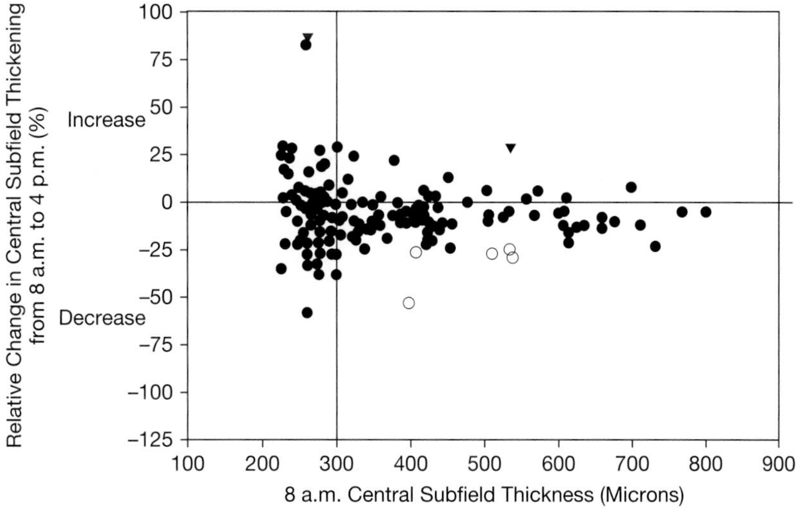

Fig. 7.28 Reproduced with permission from Browning.[176] Relative change in central subfield thickening from 8 a.m. to 4 p.m. by the 8 a.m. central subfield thickness in a study of diurnal variation of macular thickness in eyes with diabetic macular edema.[181] When the baseline thickening is small, the scatter in the relative change in thickening becomes large

Optical coherence tomography was originally developed using time domain acquisition of images (TD-OCT).[182] More recently, machines using spectral domain acquisition of images have been introduced (SD-OCT), and time domain machines, while prevalent in practice, are no longer being made. Spectral domain technology allows faster acquisition of images and denser sampling of the macula.[183–185] The normal values for SD-OCT and TD-OCT differ because the segmentation algorithms define the retina layers differently.[184,185] TD-OCT defines retinal thickness as the distance between the internal limiting membrane and the photoreceptor inner segment/outer segment boundary. SD-OCT defines retinal thickness as the distance between the internal limiting membrane and the retinal pigment epithelial layer. For this reason, retinal thickness values with SD-OCT are on average 50–60 μm thicker than values with TD-OCT and are tightly correlated ($r > 0.9$).[193–195] The axial resolution of SD-OCT is 2–7 μm compared to 10–15 μm with TD-OCT.[184,186,187] This leads to a more sensitive detection of cystoid changes in the macula with SD-OCT, such that prevalences of such morphologic findings must be qualified by describing the method of imaging in order to prevent potential confusion.[141,188] Reproducibility is better with SD-OCT because of the greater number of scans obtained per unit of area of retina. For the central subfield, the mean coefficients of variation of TD-OCT and SD-OCT have been reported to be 1.33 and 0.53–0.66%, respectively.[184,187]

OCT is an excellent tool for objectively measuring macular thickening, but macular thickening is only modestly correlated with visual acuity (r = 0.52–0.53), which is the more important clinical variable.[180,189] One potential explanation for the imperfect correlation is the effect of variable duration of edema, an elusive clinical variable to define.[119] Diabetes also causes apoptosis of retinal neurons before edema develops, and causes dysfunction of the glial cells of the retina, reflected in abnormalities in the electroretinogram (ERG) and thinning of the diabetic retina before edema develops.[35] Other confounders that impair correlation of macular thickening and visual acuity include variations in macular capillary perfusion, RPE dysfunction and scarring, and media opacities. The importance of these effects in degrading visual acuity varies from case to case and for some effects varies in ways that are currently impossible to measure.[35,68]

Besides its usefulness in the detection of macular edema, OCT has value as a method of longitudinally following DME, a chronic disease that follows a course of years to decades, and is subject to multiple interventions over time.[190] The important element in obtaining this function is the use of spreadsheet tabulation of the OCT with graphical capability (Fig. 7.29). A noncommercial program has been described using widely available spreadsheet software, and proprietary variations of this approach are appearing in electronic medical records products and the software that comes with OCT machines.[190]

OCT provides near histologic levels of detail in localizing edema within the retina and categorizing morphologic variations in edema. Specific cases can be seen in which cysts and edematous regions are present in any given layer of the retina, but in general DME is characterized by thickening of the outer rather than the inner retina.[68,132,178,191] Subretinal fluid has been seen in 9.7–26.0% of eyes with DME and is not seen in the absence of neuroretinal edema.[68,132,178–180] Various classifications of DME based on OCT morphology have been proposed. The most widely quoted classification proposes to grade DME into three OCT groups: sponge-like swelling, cystoid macular edema, and subfoveal fluid; others combine these categories into hybrid subgroups.[178,180] Because detection of CME is machine dependent, the reproducibility of interclinician grading using this scale is unknown, and no consensus or standardization of OCT classifications of DME has been achieved, the proposed scales are considered to be provisional.

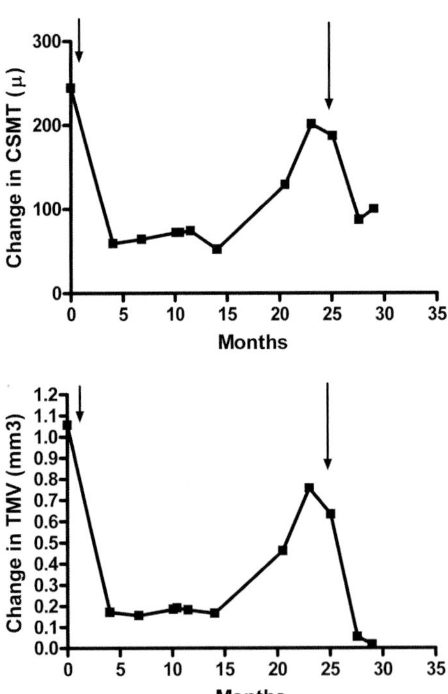

Fig. 7.29 Longitudinal plot of change in central subfield macular thickness (CSMT) in micrometers (top panel) and total macular volume (TMV) in mm^3 (bottom panel) of a patient with diabetic macular edema followed over 29 months. The short arrow indicates argon laser focal/grid laser treatment. The long arrow indicates vitrectomy, internal limiting membrane peeling. The longitudinal display allows easier recognition of signal (true changes in macular thickness) from noise (measurement variability, diurnal variation in macular thickness, and short-term variation in macular thickness). In addition, this format provides visualization of changes in OCT indices with interventions over time, a perspective difficult to achieve by flipping through sequential snapshot OCT images

Vitreous fluorometry has been used in research centers to assess permeability of the blood–retina barrier and has great appeal because it assesses a pathophysiologic variable directly responsible for DME.[192,193] Using this technique, it has been determined that the blood–retina barrier permeability increases 9–26% per 6 months in patients with nonproliferative diabetic retinopathy and no DME and that daily variation in permeability is approximately 20%.[50,193] The technique has been used to show that angiotensin converting enzyme inhibitor therapy (captopril) for 6 months in hypertensive diabetics and 18 months in normotensive diabetics with nonproliferative retinopathy can blunt this rise in permeability.[50,194] Limited evidence suggests that it has prognostic significance for visual loss in DME, but because it is not a clinically relevant ancillary study, and because interpretation of results is confounded by vitreous liquefaction, a common finding in patients with diabetic retinopathy, it currently has little impact in clinical care.[158] Fluorescein angiography does not provide equivalent information, because it is graded subjectively rather than objectively.

7.13 Other Ancillary Studies in Diabetic Macular Edema

Studies of multifocal electroretinography (mfERG) show that response density is decreased in eyes with DME, especially in the subclass of eyes with cystoid macular edema.[119] Full field cone b-wave amplitudes are also decreased in eyes with DME compared to normal controls. Microperimetry shows that DME can lead to unstable central fixation, that fixation may remain predominantly central, but can also become eccentric.[195,196] One study suggested that eyes with DME and eccentric fixation run the risk of treating the new area of fixation with supplemental focal/grid photocoagulation.[196] None of these ancillary studies is regularly used in clinical care of patients.[119]

7.14 Natural History

The ETDRS provided natural history data on a large number of eyes with DME. Over 3 years of follow-up, the rate of moderate visual loss (15 letters on the ETDRS chart) was 8% per year, such that by 3 years 24% of untreated eyes had suffered moderate visual loss.[4] Rates of visual loss increased according to the baseline visual acuity with worse-seeing eyes losing vision at a higher rate.[4] Rates of visual loss also increased according to baseline retinopathy severity with eyes having more severe retinopathy losing vision at higher rates than eyes with less severe retinopathy.[4] The median rate of visual loss in eyes with severe DME and baseline visual acuity of ≥20/40 was 0.63 ETDRS letters per month.[151] Rates of visual acuity gain of at least six ETDRS letters (at least one line on the ETDRS chart) in untreated eyes with DME and visual acuity of ≤20/40 (and thus capable of visual acuity improvement) over 3 years of follow-up were stable at 20–25%.[4] In the ETDRS, of eyes with DME less severe than CSME (one subset of what has been termed subclinical DME) and observed without treatment, 22 and 25% progress to DME with the center of the macula involved at 1 and 3 years of follow-up, respectively.[4] In the OCT era, in a retrospective case series, 31% of eyes with SCDME and serially observed progressed to CSME over a median follow-up of 14 months.[145]

Chronic, untreated DME and refractory DME can be associated with subretinal fibrosis, particularly if hard exudates are present, and by more subtle retinal pigment epithelial pigmentary changes (Fig. 7.30).[87,197]

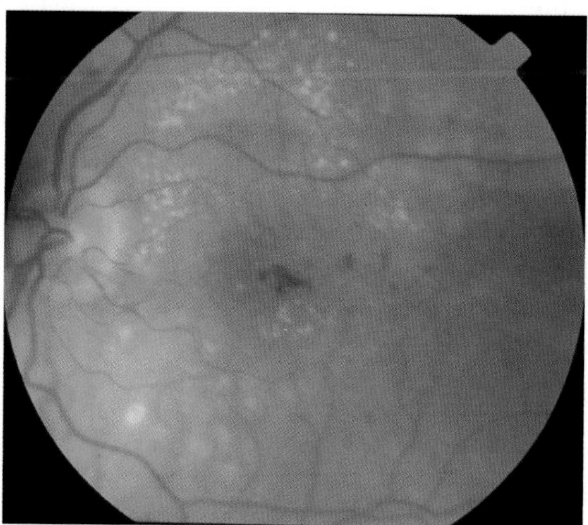

Fig. 7.30 Chronic extracellular fluid and subretinal fluid accumulation in the macula can trigger reactive retinal pigment epithelial hyperplasia manifested clinically as the stellate lesion in the center of the macula

7.15 Treatments

7.15.1 Metabolic Control and Effects of Drugs

Recognition of the risk factors for diabetic macular edema led to randomized clinical trials of better blood glucose and blood pressure control in attempts to reduce the prevalence of the condition. The Diabetes Control and Complications Trial (DCCT) showed that tight blood glucose control in patients with type 1 diabetes reduced the cumulative incidence of macular edema at 9 years follow-up by 29% and reduced the application of focal laser treatment for diabetic macular edema by half.[198,199] The effects of years of improved glycemic control persist even if control later deteriorates. In the Epidemiology of Diabetes Interventions and Complications (EDIC) study, an extension study of the DCCT in which the level of glycemic control of the former intensive and conventional control groups converged, the former intensive control group continued to fare better than the former conventional control group. Four years after the end of the DCCT, the former intensive control group had a 2% incidence of CSME compared to 8% for the former conventional control group ($P < 0.001$).[200] The UK Prospective Diabetes Study was an analogous randomized clinical trial of patients with type 2 diabetes. It showed that tighter blood glucose control reduced the requirement for laser treatment at 10 years follow-up by 29%, compared to looser control; 78% of the laser treatments were for DME.[201] It also showed that a mean systolic blood pressure reduction of 10 mmHg and a diastolic blood pressure reduction of 5 mmHg over a median follow-up of 8.4 years led to a 35% reduction in retinal laser treatments, of which 78% were for DME.[202] These clinical trial results make physiologic sense, as it has been shown that in eyes with retinopathy and a damaged blood–retina barrier, reduction of blood pressure not only reduces the driving force for egress of fluid to the extracellular space, but also decreases microvessel permeability, an effect documented before the appearance of microaneurysms and other morphologic stigmata of diabetic retinopathy.[50,196] In studies of blood–retina barrier permeability in patients with NPDR and hypertension, captopril with or without a diuretic has been shown to reduce permeability when used for 6 months. The effect was not immediate suggesting that a structural change in the blood–retinal barrier occurs that takes time to develop.[50,203] Over longer periods in normotensive patients with NPDR, captopril delayed the increase in BRB permeability seen in untreated patients.[194] There is suggestive evidence that level of glycemic control also influences responsiveness to therapy; higher glycosylated hemoglobin levels have been reported in patients with DME refractory to focal/grid laser photocoagulation.[148]

Multiple studies suggest a causal link between a patient's lipid profile and the presence of DME.[204] Increased serum cholesterol levels are associated with increased severity of retinal hard exudates at baseline, increased risk of developing DME during follow-up, and increased risk of losing visual acuity even after adjusting for presence or absence of macular edema (Fig. 7.31).[12,205] Patients with abnormally elevated triglycerides and HDL cholesterol had worse visual acuity outcomes after focal/grid photocoagulation than did patients with normal levels in one small prospective study.[206] Small studies have shown that 3-hydroxy-3-methylglutaryl coenzyme A inhibitors can reduce serum cholesterol levels and retinal hard exudates by themselves, and may reduce subfoveal lipid migration and improve regression rates of DME as adjunctive therapy to focal/grid laser.[87,207] Small clinical trials of clofibrate showed that macular exudates could be

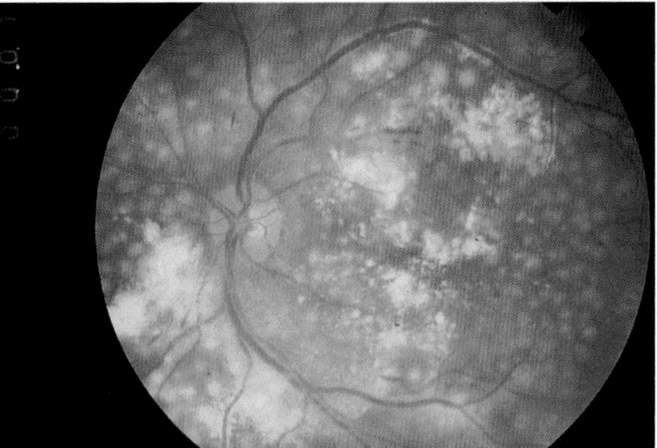

Fig. 7.31 Diabetic macular edema in a patient with marked elevation of serum cholesterol and triglycerides can be associated with more pronounced lipid exudates as illustrated in this case

reduced through their use, although visual acuity was not improved, possibly because of advanced disease and irreversible damage of the maculas at baseline.[204,208,209]

Pharmacologically induced diuresis, peritoneal dialysis, hemodialysis, and renal transplantation can all beneficially influence DME in patients with renal failure.[210–212] In a case report, plasmapheresis has been used in severe cases to lower serum lipids with improvement in macular edema and visual acuity.[69]

Certain drugs have been associated with induction of new DME or exacerbation of existing DME. Others have been associated with amelioration of DME. Thiazolidinediones are oral agents used to treat type 2 diabetes, often as adjuncts to other drugs. They are peroxisome proliferator-activated receptor γ agonists that work by enhancing insulin sensitivity. Pioglitazone and rosiglitazone are members of this class of drugs in common use. They have been associated with peripheral edema, pulmonary edema, and/or congestive heart failure, especially when used in combination with insulin. Plasma VEGF levels are higher in patients on thiazolidinediones than in patients not on these drugs.[213] Case reports and series suggest that they can be associated with new or worsened diabetic macular edema as well.[214–216] Although the reported association is controversial, it is worthwhile for ophthalmologists to monitor their patients using these drugs and to raise the possibility of a regimen change with the supervising internist if ocular intervention is being considered.

Ruboxistaurin is a protein kinase C-β antagonist that ameliorates diabetes-induced retinal circulatory abnormalities and suppresses VEGF-induced retinal vascular hyperpermeability in animal models.[217] In a clinical trial, treatment with ruboxistaurin for 36–46 months reduced the risk of moderate visual loss by 63% primarily affecting eyes with DME at baseline. In eyes with moderately severe to severe nonproliferative diabetic retinopathy, ruboxistaurin 32 mg/day reduced the risk of progression of DME to within 100 μm of the center of the macula in patients with CSME at baseline. In addition, compared to placebo, ruboxistaurin reduced the need for focal/grid photocoagulation for DME by 26%.[218] In a separate randomized, placebo-controlled clinical trial of varying doses of ruboxistaurin orally for 30 months in patients with DME >300 μm from the center of the macula, progression to sight-threatening DME or focal laser treatment was no different among groups.[219] Suggestive evidence for a beneficial neuroprotective effect of the 32-mg dose on secondary outcomes such as rate of visual decline in the presence of severe DME has led to further planned studies of this drug for DME.[152,219]

Improved metabolic control of diabetes, hypertension, and serum lipids is frequently underemphasized by the ophthalmologist because changes in management are made by the internist, yet there is an intimate connection between these changes and retinal effects. A multifactorial intervention aimed at reducing glycosylated hemoglobin, elevated blood pressure, and elevated serum lipids can produce measurable effects in OCT-measured macular thickness in as little as 6 weeks, and allows lower power laser treatment to be used when focal/grid photocoagulation is applied. Further collaborative studies taking this approach are needed as the published results involve small numbers of patients.[220]

There is a small subset of diabetic patients who undergo pancreas transplantation, sometimes in combination with kidney transplantation. Approximately 70% of such surgeries are successful in rendering patients euglycemic.[221] Approximately 20% of such patients have had focal laser photocoagulation for DME by the time they undergo transplantation. At an average follow-up of 14 months after surgery, 11.4% of eyes show progression of DME, a fraction similar to that in patients undergoing kidney transplantation alone and who remain insulin dependent.[221] In addition, other markers of retinopathy severity do not manifest improvements compared to similar patients who undergo isolated kidney transplantation and remain insulin dependent.[221] Thus in these patients who typically have advanced diabetic retinopathy and a significant prevalence of DME, normalization of glycemia via pancreas transplantation does not affect the retinopathy.

7.16 Focal/Grid Laser Photocoagulation

7.16.1 ETDRS Treatment of CSME

In the ETDRS model of treatment, a fluorescein angiogram was obtained to guide focal/grid argon laser treatment using either the argon blue-green or green wavelengths.[4] Initial focal treatment of microaneurysms, intraretinal microvascular abnormalities (IRMA), and other discrete leakage sites could extend from 500 μm of the center of the macula out as far as 2 disk diameters from the center of the macula. Fifty to hundred micrometers burns were used for this type of treatment. Fifty to two hundred micrometers burns could be used in a grid pattern to areas of diffuse fluorescein leakage and capillary nonperfusion. Burns were specified to be light to moderate in intensity, and photographs were published as examples of what this level of intensity meant (Fig. 7.32). In cases with CSME persisting at 4 months follow-up despite initial treatment and if visual acuity was less than 20/40, repeat treatments could extend to within 300 μm of the center of the macula if perifoveal capillary nonperfusion was not present.[222] Treatments were repeated at 4-month intervals if CSME persisted and treatable lesions or untreated, thickened, and nonperfused retina remained. It is important to conceive of ETDRS treatment as a regimen of repeated treatments, as the average patient in that study received between three and four focal/grid laser treatments.

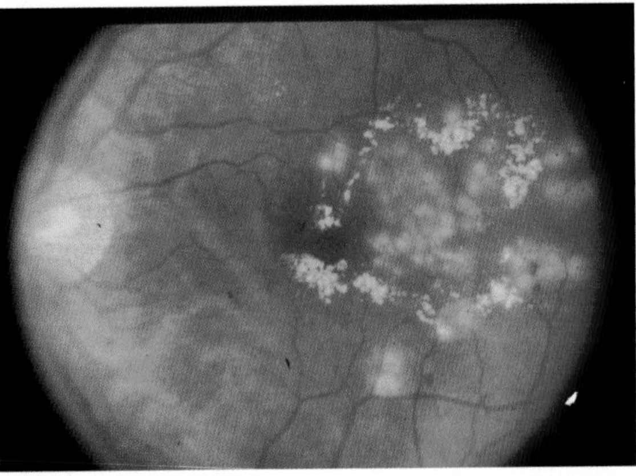

Fig. 7.32 This photograph of exemplary focal laser treatment from the ETDRS era would be considered too intense by contemporary standards

Potential Pitfalls in Applying ETDRS Focal/Grid Laser Criteria in Real Life

The ETDRS focal/grid laser protocol allows laser applications to microaneurysms within 300 μm of the center of the macula in cases of persistent CSME. Some have worried that such treatment could enlarge the diameter of the foveal avascular zone and induce loss of visual acuity. Others have worried that a microsaccade by the patient during laser treatment risks could cause a laser burn to the fovea.[121,222] There is evidence that direct laser to microaneurysms does not close the microaneurysms, despite the intent to do so; if true, the goal of such treatment is futile and the risk substantial.[223] There has been no subgroup study of such eyes from the ETDRS to see how they fared. Thus, although the ETDRS provides a rationale to manage such cases with direct focal laser to such parafoveal avascular zone (FAZ) microaneurysms, it is unknown if the benefit outweighs the risk. Figure 7.33 shows an eye in which these concerns were manifested, and illustrates the practical difficulty in defining the FAZ border under the best of circumstances.

The ETDRS showed that at 3 years follow-up, untreated eyes did worse than treated eyes by several different measures. For example, 24% of eyes in the untreated group had a doubling of the visual angle, compared to 12% in the treated group, and 12% of untreated eyes were legally blind compared to 7% of the treated group.[4] Obversely, more treated eyes had improved outcomes, again by several measures. For example, in patients with a presenting acuity of 20/40 or worse, visual acuity improved in 40% of treated eyes compared to 20% of untreated eyes at 3 years follow-up, and 36% of treated patients reported subjective improvement, compared to 14% of untreated patients at 1 year follow-up.[4] In general, these conclusions hold for different lengths of follow-up and across all baseline visual acuity levels, but the relative magnitude of the benefit conferred by focal laser treatment is smaller for better baseline visual acuities.[4] There is evidence from retrospective studies that increasing age has a negative influence on visual acuity outcomes after focal/grid laser for DME, but the prospective data

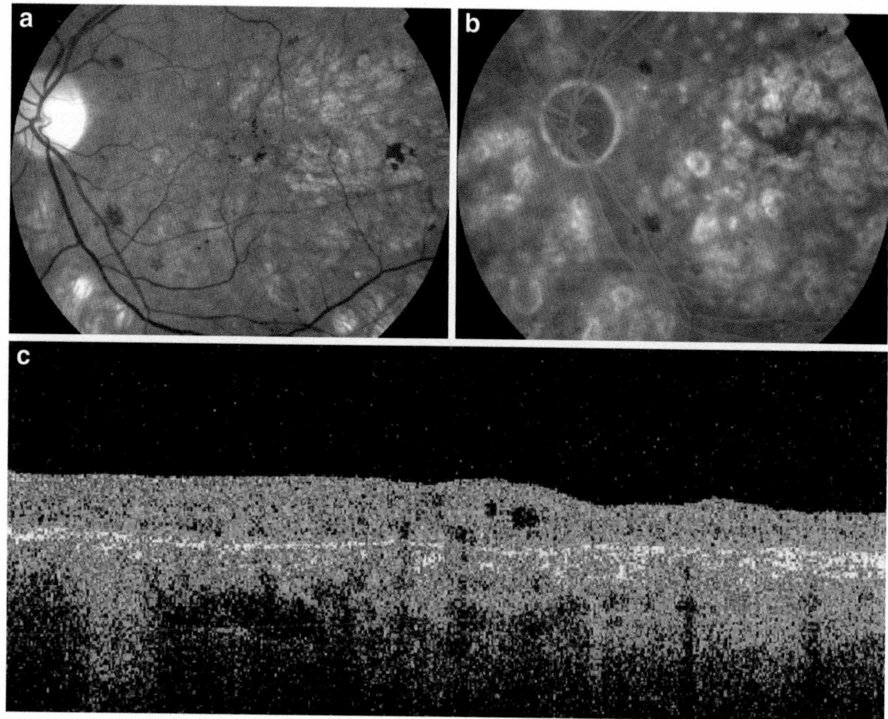

Fig. 7.33 (**a**) Example of an eye with persistent CSME despite previous focal/grid laser treatment. Microaneurysms within 300 μm of the *center* of the macula are present. (**b**) The *mid-phase* fluorescein angiogram shows many more laser spots than were visible on the red-free photograph which makes it difficult to assess the border of the foveal avascular zone. Some of the microaneurysms are perfused and some are nonperfused. (**c**) A *horizontal radial line* scan through the fovea shows loss of the foveal pit and presence of cystoid macular edema

contained in the ETDRS has not been explored in this regard to determine if this relationship is true.[224,225]

It has been commonly taught that focal/grid photocoagulation for DME rarely improves visual acuity.[54,222,226] To quote one of many sources, "Although clearly effective in saving many patients from blindness and severe visual impairment, photocoagulation cannot improve vision."[54] In fact, this was neither true in the ETDRS among eyes with subnormal baseline visual acuities nor has it been true in cohorts with DME treated with modified ETDRS focal/grid photocoagulation.[227] In the DRCR Network trial of intravitreal triamcinolone vs. focal/grid laser photocoagulation for DME, 31% of eyes in the focal/grid group gained 10 or more ETDRS letters at 2 years follow-up, and similar results were true of eyes with vision ≤20/40 in the ETDRS 20 years earlier.[227] A false impression of no visual acuity benefit conferred by focal laser treatment arose because most of the eyes in the ETDRS started with good vision, making any improvement difficult to achieve.

The Early Treatment Diabetic Retinopathy Study (ETDRS)

The ETDRS addressed important issues regarding DME, but also issues regarding when in the course of diabetic retinopathy it is appropriate to intervene with panretinal photocoagulation and whether aspirin use influences retinopathy progression, development of vitreous hemorrhage, or cataract development. Because of its singular importance in understanding management of DME, we include a summary table of its design and findings here, but some of the findings apply to issues addressed in the chapters on proliferative diabetic retinopathy and systemic considerations in diabetic retinopathy.

Table 7.2 Early treatment diabetic retinopathy study, 1979–1990

Major eligibility criteria
Visual acuity ≥20/40 (≥20/400 if reduction caused by macular edema)
Mild to severe nonproliferative diabetic retinopathy (NPDR) and/or non-high-risk proliferative diabetic retinopathy (PDR), with or without macular edema (ME)
Both eyes suitable for photocoagulation
Major design features
One eye of each patient assigned randomly to early photocoagulation and the other to deferral (careful follow-up and photocoagulation if high-risk PDR develops)
Patients assigned randomly to aspirin or placebo
Major conclusions
Focal photocoagulation (direct laser for focal leaks and grid laser for diffuse areas of leakage and nonperfusion) reduced risk of moderate visual loss (doubling of the visual angle) by ≥50% and increased the chance of a small improvement in visual acuity
Both early scatter with or without focal photocoagulation and deferral followed by low rates of severe visual loss (5-year rates in deferral subgroups 2–10%; in early photocoagulation groups, 2–6%)
Focal photocoagulation should be considered for eyes with clinically significant ME
Scatter photocoagulation not indicated for mild to moderate NPDR but should be considered as retinopathy approaches high-risk PDR and usually should not be delayed when this high-risk stage is present
Benefit of early scatter photocoagulation is more pronounced for patients with type 2 diabetes or with type 1 diabetes of long duration
Aspirin had no effect on progression of retinopathy, frequency of vitreous hemorrhage, or cataract development

Reproduced and adapted from Aiello.[228]

Focal/grid photocoagulation for DME has potential side effects. Macular visual fields show elevated thresholds after focal/grid laser treatment and cone thresholds increase using fine matrix mapping.[175,229] Laser scars can enlarge over time and paracentral scotomata from enlarging scars have been reported (Fig. 7.34).[230,231] Multifocal ERGs show prolonged implicit times and decreased amplitudes after focal/grid laser photocoagulation.[130] Some eyes develop subretinal fibrosis, but the relationship to the laser treatment as opposed to the edema is controversial (Fig. 7.35).[197,232,233] Some eyes develop secondary choroidal neovascularization, which has been associated with more intense, smaller burns (Fig. 7.36).[234]

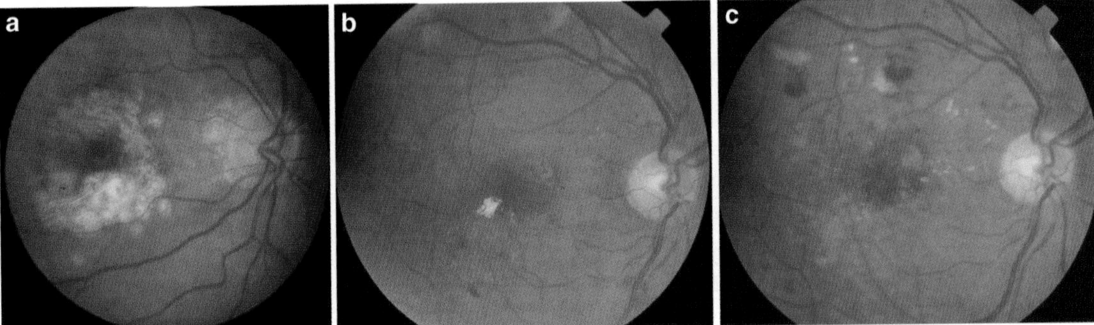

Fig. 7.34 (**a**) This eye was treated with a nonconfluent grid of laser spots that over 10 years expanded to produce a confluent zone of geographic retinal pigment epithelial atrophy. Smaller, lighter intensity laser burns are used now compared to the burns described as optimal at the time of the publication of ETDRS results, but evidence is lacking that these changes have resulted in avoidance of laser scar expansion. (**b**) Example of a laser scar on the superonasal border of the foveal avascular zone that expanded over 2 years of observation. (**c**) Note the larger diameter of the superonasal macular laser scar. Less obvious expansion of laser scars is seen in the inferotemporal macula by comparing **b** and **c**

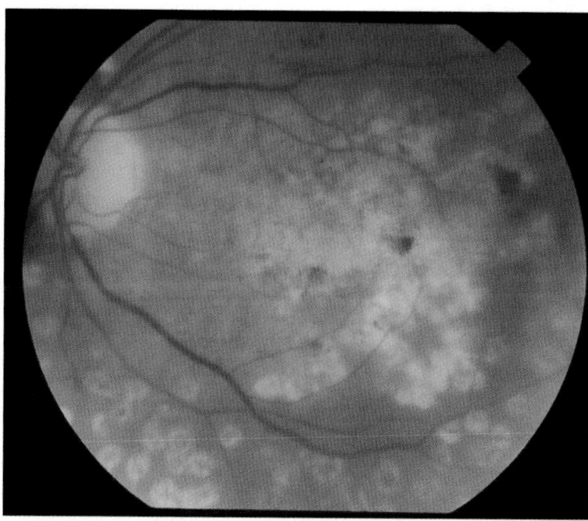

Fig. 7.35 This eye shows subfoveal retinal pigment epithelial metaplasia after focal photocoagulation for diabetic macular edema

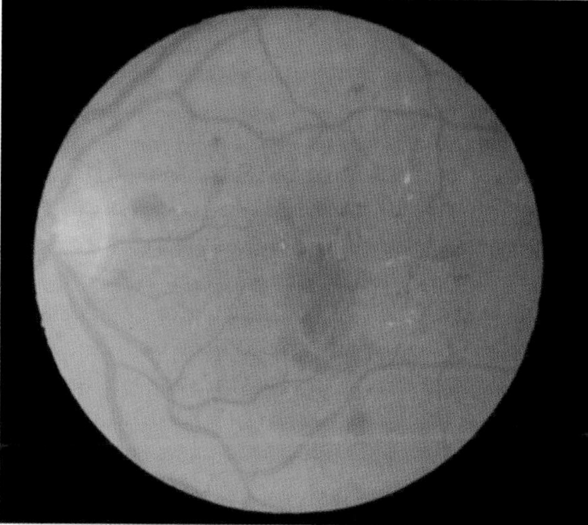

Fig. 7.36 A *gray* subretinal neovascular membrane with surrounding subretinal hemorrhage is shown arising from the site of a focal laser burn in the inferior perifoveal zone

7.17 Evolution in Focal/Grid Laser Treatment Since the ETDRS

The style of focal/grid argon laser treatment applied in the ETDRS has been modified over time. The most significant changes are embodied in the Diabetic Retinopathy Clinical Research Network (DRCR Network) protocols that employ focal/grid photocoagulation. Table 7.3 lists the major changes. Rather than burns that can vary from 50 to 200 μm, contemporary burns are 50 μm. The burns are lighter – light gray – rather than heavier intensity burns illustrated in ETDRS publications (Fig. 7.31).[222] The yellow wavelength (561–589 nm) laser is acceptable in addition to green (514–532 nm); blue-green (488 nm) is not used now because of the theoretical concern of absorption by macular luteal pigment, although it was allowed in the ETDRS. It is not necessary to darken microaneurysms as long as the subjacent retinal pigment epithelium is lightly blanched. The use of a fluorescein angiogram is now optional rather than required. Approximately 50% of eyes in DRCR Network studies, and up to 80% of eyes in other Western hemisphere countries, are treated without fluorescein angiography, and probably even higher percentages of eyes are treated without guiding fluorescein angiograms in less developed countries.[79,110,163] In eyes treated without fluorescein angiography, grid laser is applied to areas of thickening without focal lesions within 2 disk diameters of the center of the macula, and there is no provision for treating zones of capillary nonperfusion. The goal of these changes is to reduce the incidence of laser scar expansion and paracentral scotomata that have been reported to occur after ETDRS style focal/grid photocoagulation.[229] Figure 7.37 shows the type of post laser scarring intensity that could be seen with more intense laser technique 20 years after application compared with contemporary technique.

A continual problem with focal/grid laser photocoagulation for DME has been the decision regarding what constitutes maximal treatment. The decision is intrinsically subjective and makes it difficult to standardize.[235] For example, one study defines maximal focal laser treatment as "a point at which the investigator felt that additional laser treatment would be of no benefit based on clinical judgment and flurescein angiogram."[236] Other studies have graded focal/grid photocoagulation based on number of burns.[237,238] Heavy laser is defined as >300 burns, moderate as 126–300 burns, and light as <126 burns.[237,238] Unfortunately, these numerical definitions fail to capture the reality that spot sizes used in focal/grid laser vary from 50 to 200 μm, such that a specified number of burns may produce large differences in the area of photocoagulated macula.

Table 7.3 Changes in focal/grid laser from the ETDRS to the present

Avoid blue-green wavelength; addition of yellow wavelength as acceptable
Exclusive use of 50 μm burns
Fluorescein angiogram (FA) use to guide treatment now discretionary
Lighter burns – light gray and barely visible
If no FA use, grid is applied to diffuse areas of thickening without treatable lesions
Not necessary to darken microaneurysms. If not possible, lightly blanch the subjacent retinal pigment epithelium.

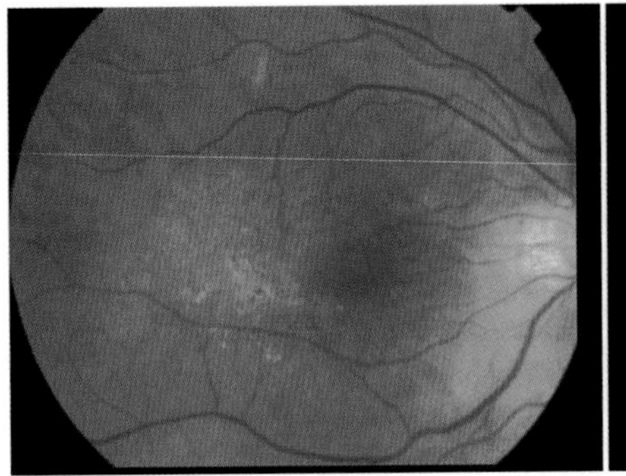
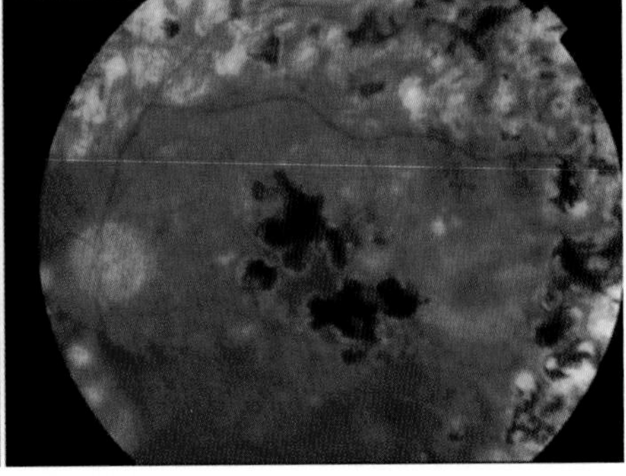

Fig. 7.37 The *left panel* shows the pigmentary pattern seen after contemporary focal/grid laser photocoagulation. The *right panel* shows the effects of more intense laser burns from an earlier era with laser scar expansion, retinal pigment epithelial hyperplastic scar formation, and paracentral scotoma induction

The interval for retreatment specified in the ETDRS has also been reevaluated. There is evidence that the macular thinning response to focal/grid laser takes longer than 4 months to reach an asymptote, which implies that a retreatment interval of 4 months for persistent edema could result in unnecessary overtreatment with the attendant side effects. A DRCR Network study showed that further reductions in macular thickness beyond 4 months occur in 42% of eyes with improved but persistent DME after a single session of focal/grid laser for DME (DRCR protocol K manuscript submitted for publication). This group amounted to 10% of all eyes (11 of 115) with DME receiving focal/grid laser in the study and evaluable at 32 weeks after laser. It is not known whether visual acuity outcomes would be improved by observation until OCT improvement stops or by retreatment for persistent DME 4 months after initial treatment as is the current convention in DRCR Network studies involving a laser arm for DME. A randomized trial would be necessary to answer this question.

A semiautomated patterned scanning laser has been developed that uses the argon green wavelength, shortens the pulse duration from the historically conventional 100–200 to 10–20 ms, and applies automatic patterns of laser with physician control of focusing.[239] Histologically, burns with this technology are indistinguishable from conventional argon green laser burns.[239] The advantage in the treatment of DME is faster treatment. A potential disadvantage of using patterned laser is that burn characteristics may change depending on the variable retinal thickness seen in DME such that a pattern of uniform powered spots applied to regionally varying retinal thickness may give varying thermal uptake over these regions. For scatter photocoagulation, an additional advantage is decreased pain associated with shorter pulse duration, but this advantage does not apply to focal/grid laser, which is painless using conventional laser machines.[239]

7.18 Macular Thickness Outcomes After Focal/Grid Photocoagulation

At the time the ETDRS was performed, there was no way to objectively measure macular thickness, but with OCT, this outcome has become important in following treatment. There is little information published on comparability of outcomes among different ophthalmologists performing ostensibly similar treatment, but what is available suggests rough comparability.[240] The biggest determinant of macular thinning effect after focal/grid laser treatment is the baseline macular thickness.[241] Table 7.4 shows a sample of the range of reported thinning effects as a function of baseline macular thickness. It is apparent that the greater the macular thickening before laser treatment, the greater the thinning response after focal/grid laser.

In general, the threshold for performing focal/grid laser photocoagulation occurs when the central subfield mean thickness attains 250 μm, and on average, for this threshold level of edema, one can expect approximately 25 μm of macular thinning after focal/grid laser at the usual first follow-up interval of 3–4 months. For every 100 μm of additional baseline macular thickening above this 250 μm threshold, one can expect that focal/grid laser will yield approximately 10 μm of additional macular thinning at the 3–4-month follow-up visit (Fig. 7.38). Visual acuity at this follow-up time is, on average, unchanged from baseline.[163,227,241,242]

7.19 Resolution of Lipid Exudates After Focal/Grid Laser Photocoagulation

The natural history of lipid exudates associated with DME is to spontaneously resolve over 2 years or longer.[243] Macrophages clear the exudates by phagocytosis.[69] Both serum lipid control and focal/grid photocoagulation can independently accelerate the clearance of lipid exudates in DME (Fig. 7.39).[87] A potential clinical problem is the subfoveal migration of hard lipid after focal/grid laser treatment,

Table 7.4 Macular thinning from a single session of focal/grid laser for diabetic macular edema at 3–4 months follow-up

References	*N*	Baseline macular thickness (mean±SD) or (median, IQR) in μm	Change in thickness at 12–17 weeks follow-up in μm
DRCR protocol H study[163]	19	441 (354, 512)	–40
DRCR protocol B study[227]	304	398 (329, 505)	–33
DRCR protocol K study	118	327 (279, 402)	–27
DRCR protocol E study[242]	38	324±70	–30
Browning[241]	122	271 (225, 362)	–26

N = number of eyes. SD = standard deviation. IQR = interquartile range.

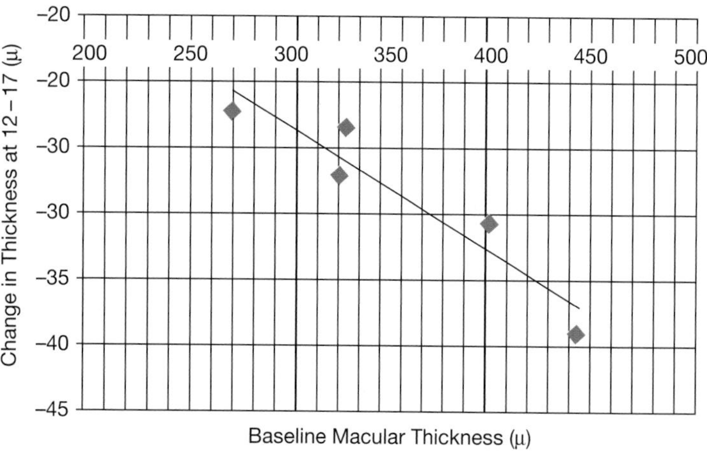

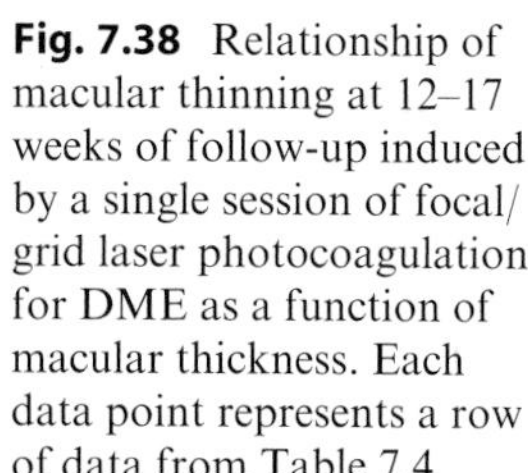
Fig. 7.38 Relationship of macular thinning at 12–17 weeks of follow-up induced by a single session of focal/grid laser photocoagulation for DME as a function of macular thickness. Each data point represents a row of data from Table 7.4

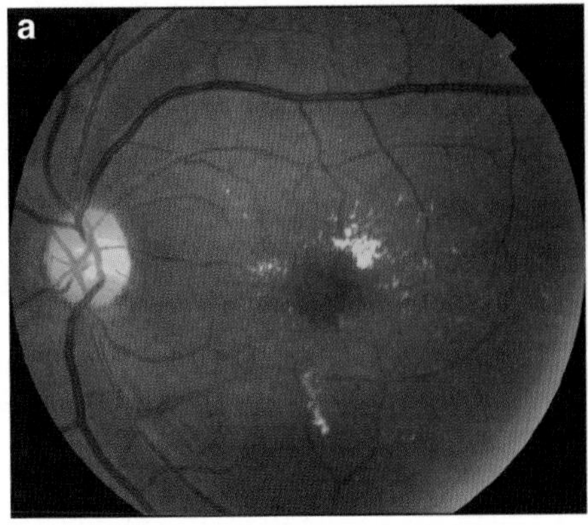

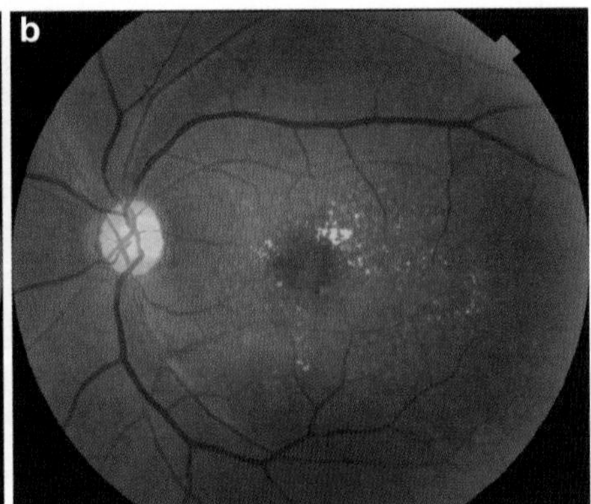

Fig. 7.39 Although spontaneous resolution of intraretinal lipid in DME can take ≥2 years, interventions can speed the process. (**a**) Lipid exudates present in the macula of an eye with DME before any treatment. (**b**) Five months after focal/grid laser treatment, a large fraction of the lipid has resolved, much faster than the natural history of lipid resolution. *Faint gray* focal laser scars are seen

particularly in patients with heavy lipid exudates before treatment. Adjunctive oral statin therapy in such patients has been reported to eliminate this problem in a small clinical trial.[87]

7.20 Inconsistency in Defining Refractory Diabetic Macular Edema

Focal/grid laser photocoagulation is the standard treatment for DME after optimization of metabolic control fails to eliminate DME. It is the only form of treatment that has been proven through a large, multicentered, randomized controlled trial. Moreover, it has been proven to be superior to serial intravitreal triamcinolone injections in a large, multicentered, randomized controlled clinical trial.[227] Thus, it becomes important to decide when an eye meets criteria for refractoriness to focal laser. This decision is linked to the clinician's sense of what constitutes maximal focal/grid laser photocoagulation, a conundrum already discussed. The mean number of focal/grid laser treatments in the ETDRS was 3.8. Yet, in some studies, investigators have labeled eyes as refractory to focal/grid laser after one or two sessions of laser, and used this term to justify moving on to alternative forms of therapy.[139,146,147,236] Some have termed eyes with persistent edema after three focal/grid treatments to be refractory and have used them in an observational control arm in testing other forms of therapy.[149] A recently initiated randomized clinical trial for refractory DME does not define how many laser treatments are required to qualify as refractory, and the same is true of another published randomized trial of intravitreal triamcinolone injection vs. placebo.[244,245] It is the norm for multiple focal/grid laser treatments to be necessary in the treatment of DME, and yet despite multiple treatments it is common for DME to persist. Of eyes with CSME at baseline and randomized to immediate focal photocoagulation, 35 and 24% of eyes continued to have DME with the center of the macula involved at 1 and 3 years, respectively.[246] In WESDR, 35 of 109 older onset diabetics with baseline DME returned for reexamination 10 years later. Of these 35, 5 (14.3%) had persistent DME and of these 5, 2 had refractory DME having received focal/grid laser photocoagulation after the baseline examination.[1]

7.21 Alternative Forms of Laser Treatment for Diabetic Macular Edema

Krypton red laser (647–670 nm) has been used in some clinical series and appears to have efficacy in DME; however, it is not the preferred wavelength, because it is poorly absorbed by red microaneurysms and other focal leaking sites, is absorbed more by the choroid than the RPE, and is associated with more pain for the patient.[247–249] Frequency doubled neodymium YAG and diode micropulse (532 and 810 nm, respectively) laser have been used as well in case series, again with some evidence of efficacy.[250,251] The advantage is an elimination of photoreceptor damage, reduction in retinal pigment epithelial scarring, and elimination of paracentral visual field scotomata.[252,253] The disadvantage is that there is no visible endpoint for treatment, making it difficult to determine where treatment has been given; treatment methods and settings have varied from study to study.[253] In addition, the treatment response is slower than with conventional laser treatment, and more treatments may be necessary to achieve elimination of edema.[252] Neither of these modalities has been widely used.

What Is Selective Micropulse Laser Treatment?

Micropulse laser treatment employs repetitive trains (50–500) of laser pulses of short duration (0.8–5.0 μs). Powers used have varied between 5 and 50 mW and energy per pulse between 70 and 175 μJ.[254] Wavelengths of 514, 524, 527, 532, and 810 nm have been used.[223,255–257] Individual microaneurysms are not targeted, in contrast to conventional focal/grid laser treatment. The intent of treatment is to lightly affect the retinal pigment epithelium alone, restricting the lateral spread of heat and thus sparing damage to the overlying photoreceptors and mid-retinal interneurons. The off period between pulses allows time for heat dissipation to achieve this goal. Although attractive as a concept, the practical problem remains that the clinician cannot tell where treatment has been applied, because the lesions are ophthalmoscopically invisible and can only be detected by fluorescein angiography (hyperfluorescence) or autofluorescence photography (hypoautofluorescence), both cumbersome ways of monitoring the distribution of lesions.[223,258] Methods of choosing power to use are ad hoc and variable and based on choosing a power that is some fraction of that producing a visible burn in an area remote from the macula. Moreover, the power setting is not changed, regardless of the presence of subretinal fluid or variable macular thickening, a concept that is counterintuitive to the stated goal of producing uniform lesions at the level of the RPE.[223] There are no microscotomata detectable by microperimetry over micropulse laser lesions by 3 months after treatment.[259]

7.22 Peribulbar Triamcinolone Injection

Peribulbar triamcinolone or methylprednisolone injections have been used to treat DME either as monotherapy or as adjunctive therapy to focal/grid laser, and short-term efficacy in thinning the macula and improving visual acuity has been demonstrated.[102,104,242,260] Evidence exists that peribulbar triamcinolone is less effective than intravitreal triamcinolone in improving visual acuity in DME over a 3-month period.[261,262] In a pilot prospective, randomized, multicentered clinical trial, neither peribulbar monotherapy nor combination therapy showed clinically important superiority over modified ETDRS focal/grid photocoagulation, and, therefore, a large-scale clinical trial was not done.[242] The complications of peribulbar triamcinolone injection include intraocular pressure elevation and ptosis in approximately 10 and 20% of cases, respectively.[242]

7.23 Intravitreal Triamcinolone Injection

Jonas and Sofker were the first to use intravitreal triamcinolone injection in the treatment of DME in 2001.[263] In a randomized clinical trial comparing intravitreal triamcinolone injection to observation, the efficacy of triamcinolone injections was established through 2 years of follow-up.[264] Many case series and a separate shorter term placebo controlled randomized trial have supported this conclusion.[142,150,245,265,266] The benefits of this form of therapy must be balanced by consideration of the side effects including surgical cataract formation in

51% of phakic eyes at 2 years follow-up and intraocular pressure elevation in 25–40% of eyes.[142,267,268] In a randomized clinical trial comparing serial intravitreal triamcinolone injection therapy using 1 or 4 mg to focal/grid photocoagulation, focal/grid photocoagulation showed superior efficacy and fewer side effects; thus, intravitreal triamcinolone therapy is a second line therapy for consideration when focal photocoagulation has failed.[227] In this study, the mean visual acuity was four–six ETDRS letters better in the laser group than in the 1 and 4 mg intravitreal triamcinolone groups after 2 years, and the improved visual outcomes persisted after discounting the effects of cataract progression in the triamcinolone groups.[227] The mean central subfield mean thickness decreased 53–62 μm more in the focal/grid group compared to the 1- and 4-mg triamcinolone groups at 2 years, respectively.[227] The 4-mg triamcinolone group was superior to the focal/grid laser group at the 4-month follow-up visit, but that short-term advantage of triamcinolone had vanished by 1 year follow-up, and at 2 years follow-up the focal/grid group had clearly superior outcomes.[227]

Many doses of intravitreal triamcinolone have been used, including 1, 2, 4, 5, 8, 13, and 20–25 mg. In general, there is inconclusive but suggestive evidence that duration of action is longer with higher doses and that frequency of intraocular pressure rise increases with higher doses.[140,238,269,270] There is no consistent evidence that higher doses are more effective for thinning the macula or improving visual acuity than lower doses, and some evidence exists that lower doses have greater efficacy for macular thinning than higher doses.[139]

In a small pilot randomized trial, intravitreal triamcinolone injection was associated with a higher rate of partial vitreous separation with foveal attachment or traction compared to eyes treated with focal/grid photocoagulation. Eyes with this change had worse visual outcomes.[271]

7.24 Intravitreal Dexamethasone Delivery System

A sustained release drug delivery system for dexamethasone inserted transclerally into the vitreous produced statistically significant visual acuity improvement for 90 days after insertion and was well tolerated for 180 days.[272] For the 700 μg device, the probability of a ≥10 letter improvement in visual acuity at 90 days was 2.8 times greater in the device group compared to the observation group. Mean central retinal thickness decreased by more than 160 μm at 90 days, but this figure included pooled results from other causes of macular edema besides DME. Eleven percent of treated patients had an intraocular pressure rise of 10 mmHg or higher. This device is presently undergoing further clinical trials.[272,273]

7.25 Intravitreal Injections of Anti-VEGF Drugs

Intravitreal injections of anti-VEGF drugs also produce reductions in macular thickening, but on average the magnitudes of the reductions and the durations of responses are less than with intravitreal triamcinolone injections, suggesting that biochemical pathways not involving VEGF are important in the pathogenesis of DME.[121,163,274–276] Intravitreal pegaptanib, bevacizumab, ranibizumab, and VEGF-trap all fall into this category.[109,121,274,277–279] Counterbalancing their lesser efficacy compared to steroids, the anti-VEGF drugs have a more favorable side effect profile, in particular without the tendency to cause cataract and raise intraocular pressure.[276] Instances have been reported in which intravitreal pegaptanib injected in one eye has been associated with regression in neovascularization in the fellow eye.[280] Similar concerns have been expressed for bevacizumab, but, despite study, no evidence of a fellow eye effect on DME has been found, suggesting that systemic absorption is negligible.[120] Limited data suggest that fears that intravitreal anti-VEGF drugs could worsen macular ischemia are unfounded.[121] No clinically important differences in effects on DME of 1.25 vs. 2.5 mg of bevacizumab have been reported in studies comparing the two.[163,109,281] Some evidence suggests that these drugs are more effective in treatment of naïve eyes than in eyes previously treated with focal/grid laser.[281] Further research will be necessary to better determine the role of these intravitreal injections in the therapy of DME, but they may find a role in phakic patients and patients with glaucoma.[275]

7.26 Combined Intravitreal Anti-VEGF Drugs and Triamcinolone

Combined intravitreal bevacizumab and triamcinolone as an initial injection followed by two intravitreal bevacizumab injections given at 6-week intervals was no more effective in decreasing DME than three consecutive intravitreal injections of bevacizumab given at 6-week intervals.[282,283] As the addition of triamcinolone would be expected to increase cataract development and intraocular pressure rise, there is little impetus to continue exploring the combination of steroids and anti-VEGF drugs for DME.

7.27 Combined Intravitreal and Peribulbar Triamcinolone and Focal Laser Therapy

Visual acuity outcomes are superior with focal laser photocoagulation than with observation alone in managing DME.[4] Serial injections of intravitreal triamcinolone therapy are also superior to observation at least over a period of 2 years follow-up.[264] A combination of intravitreal triamcinolone injection followed by focal laser photocoagulation is a form of therapy that has a theoretical rationale for being possibly superior to focal laser alone or serial intravitreal triamcinolone injections alone. Preceding the focal/grid photocoagulation by steroid treatment might reduce inflammation associated with the photocoagulation, reduce the macular thickness allowing less powerful laser applications, and thereby reduce unnecessary collateral retinal damage and laser-induced scarring.[284,285] The photocoagulation part of the combined regimen theoretically provides sustainability to the treatment effect that an injection alone lacks.[174] The preponderance of the evidence suggests that combination therapy may reduce macular thickening somewhat better than serial intravitreal triamcinolone injections in the short term and have a faster onset of action than focal laser alone.[266,285,286] Similar improved results of combined peribulbar triamcinolone plus focal photocoagulation have been reported.[102,122] Not enough patients have been studied prospectively for a sufficiently long time to make conclusions on this point, but the DRCR Network is engaged in a clinical trial that should answer whether combination therapy is superior to focal/grid laser alone.

7.28 Vitrectomy

The idea that vitreomacular adhesion might promote DME arose from the observation that eyes with DME have a lower prevalence of posterior vitreous detachment than eyes without DME.[47] The subsequent observation that resolution of DME could occur after posterior vitreous detachment strengthened the plausibility that surgical induction of a vitreomacular separation might improve DME.[287,288] Vitrectomy for DME was first reported by Lewis and colleagues in 1992.[289] Since then, many small retrospective and prospective case series, several small clinical trials, one large retrospective case series, but no large, multicentered, randomized, controlled trials of the approach have been published.[48,74,76,146,147,149,153,229,238,290–301] Vitrectomy was introduced for eyes with a taut posterior hyaloid adherent to the macula, often associated with shallow traction macular detachment, which had futile previous focal/grid laser.[73,75,153,289,290,302] Later, it was explored as a therapy for eyes with an attached but nonthickened, nontaut posterior hyaloid or for eyes with persistent DME despite previous focal laser or intravitreal triamcinolone injection regardless of the status of the posterior hyaloid.[147,153,291–293,300,301] Most recently, the treatment has been studied as a potential primary therapy in eyes with more severe edema, greater visual acuity loss at presentation, and characteristics considered to mitigate against effectiveness of focal/grid.[74,294,296,299] The relative frequencies of the various candidate groups have been reported as follows: refractory DME in eyes with attached but nontaut posterior hyaloid 68%, refractory DME in eyes with posterior vitreous detachment 22%, refractory DME in eyes with a taut posterior hyaloid 5%, and refractory DME in eyes with an epiretinal membrane 5%.[237] Other categories for which primary vitrectomy has been applied include eyes with microaneurysms too close to the fovea to receive focal laser, eyes with enlarged foveal avascular zones, and eyes with cystoid edema.[121]

Although the concept of a taut hyaloid has been widely discussed, the term is not consistently defined in the literature. On biomicroscopy, a taut hyaloid has been defined as a thickened, glistening, posterior hyaloid without stria.[237] In addition to a biomicroscopic appearance, others define the term based on an OCT-visualized attachment of the hyaloid layer to the macula with adjacent partial vitreomacular detachment and accompanying submacular fluid. Finally, some define the term based on intraoperative findings even when preoperative biomicroscopic and OCT examinations are negative.[289,303,304] Because submacular fluid has been seen in cases of DME with no macular traction by clinical examination or OCT, submacular fluid cannot be considered specific for the taut hyaloid syndrome.[116,305,306]

Some groups distinguish a taut hyaloid with its hypothesized tangential traction in DME from the vitreomacular traction syndrome with its hypothesized anterior–posterior traction, but others do not.[146,289,290,292] Diffuse, deep intraretinal fluorescein leakage has been commonly associated with a taut hyaloid, but is also not specific for this condition, as it can be seen in eyes after vitrectomy.[289,293] Some authors have required more than simple OCT identification of a vitreomacular point of contact, requiring, for example, that the slope of the elevated macula be steep and that the OCT-defined posterior hyaloid be thicker than normal and hyperreflective, although a cutpoint for "thicker" and a definition of hyperreflective have not been given.[75] Others report an associated large central macular cyst in tractional cases.[146] When eyes have been classified by biomicroscopic signs, OCT evidence of partial vitreomacular separation, and OCT evidence of submacular fluid, different groupings of eyes result. Some eyes have all three signs, some any two of the three, and some only one of the three.[304] Several groups have reported inability to predict OCT or intraoperative signs of vitreomacular traction and adhesion based on clinical biomicroscopy.[146,290] Eyes with DME in association with a taut hyaloid are uncommon, with estimates that they comprise 3.1–18.0% of cases of DME.[304,306] Lewis has suggested that the presence of a shallow macular traction detachment on OCT is a conservative way to determine if a suspected taut hyaloid is truly contributory in a specific case of DME and perhaps indicative that vitrectomy surgery might be helpful, but Massin and colleagues report numerous cases of DME with taut hyaloid yet no traction macular detachment on OCT.[48,307] Among reports in which vitrectomy was effective in thinning the macula, the magnitude of the treatment effect has been greater in eyes with OCT signs of macular traction.[146]

Taut Hyaloid Syndrome – Is It More Than Vitreomacular Traction Syndrome?

The novice to the literature on the taut hyaloid syndrome may be excused if he deduces that tangential traction, said to be characteristic of the taut hyaloid, and anterior–posterior traction, said to be characteristic of vitreomacular traction syndrome, can be distinguished with slit-lamp biomicroscopy.[289,290] In fact, if one puts the illustrative OCTs of these two conditions side by side, it is difficult to distinguish them. Below are published OCTs from the two conditions (Fig. 7.40). Which OCT goes with which condition? (For the answer, see Fig. 7.40)

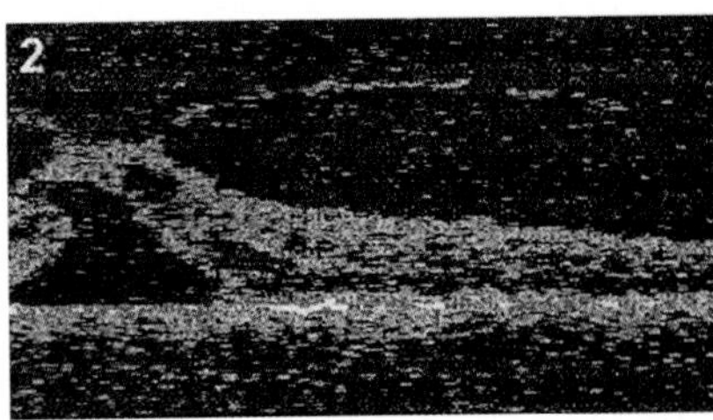

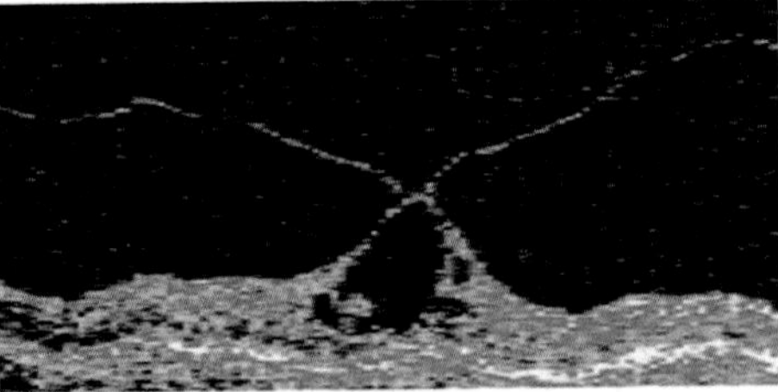

Fig. 7.40 It is difficult to distinguish OCTs published to exemplify the taut hyaloid syndrome in diabetic macular edema and the vitreomacular traction syndrome. The *left panel* shows DME with a taut hyaloid and the *right* from a case of nondiabetic vitreomacular traction syndrome. The *left panel* is reproduced with permission from Kaiser et al.[73] and *right panel* is reproduced with permission from Johnson et al.[308]

It is likely that many cases exist in which vitreous traction on the macula contributes to microvessel hyperpermeability but is not the sole problem. The clinical issue is frequently whether to attempt focal laser treatment or intravitreal injectional therapy alone or in combination first to address the non-tractional component of the problem or whether to proceed directly to a treatment involving vitrectomy with peeling of frequently associated epiretinal membranes and the adherent posterior hyaloidal face.[309] Although eyes with a taut hyaloid are frequently refractory to focal/grid photocoagulation, it is typical for clinicians to attempt these less invasive treatments first in hopes of substantial improvement without needing to proceed to vitrectomy.[289]

A controversy exists regarding the effects of vitrectomy for DME. Several groups of investigators have reported that vitrectomy reduces macular thickening but does not improve visual acuity.[297,310,311] Others report improved visual acuities simultaneous with decreases in macular thickening or lagging behind macular thinning by a few months.[146,271,294,301,303] Still others report improved visual acuity in cases with macular traction, but no visual improvement in cases without traction.[75,305] Ancillary tests of macular function, such as cone thresholds by fine matrix mapping, have been reported to improve in parallel with macular thinning after vitrectomy surgery.[146] Even when investigators report that both morphology and visual acuity improve, the morphologic improvement has consistently been more pronounced than visual acuity improvement, presumably because of permanent damage to the macula due to ischemia, subfoveal exudates and pigment epithelial metaplasia, damage from previous extensive focal/grid laser, or long duration of edema.[89,238]

Because the types of eyes chosen for application of vitrectomy could influence the outcomes, it is difficult to compare the results of different series. Table 7.5 lists the characteristics of included eyes in various studies of vitrectomy for DME to assist in the comparison. Some studies report that a history of previous focal/grid laser or presence of submacular fluid at baseline is a negative influence on visual acuity outcome.[240,312] Longer duration of edema has been reported to negatively influence visual outcomes.[111] Duration of DME is difficult to quantitate, however, because of ambiguity regarding date of onset before clinical diagnosis.[75,189]

Vitrectomy surgery for DME potentially involves multiple steps that could affect DME. Creating a posterior vitreous separation with or without enzymatic adjuncts, internal limiting membrane peeling with or without staining, supplemental or de novo panretinal laser photocoagulation, supplemental or de novo focal laser photocoagulation, concomitant cataract extraction, and concomitant injection of intravitreal triamcinolone or anti-VEGF drugs could all be important variables affecting the response to the intervention.[299] Different groups have employed different procedures (Table 7.5).[302,310] Internal limiting membrane (ILM) peeling with the use of indocyanine green (ICG) staining has been considered potentially toxic to the macula and optic nerve with loss of visual field after its use in cases of DME.[313] Two groups reported no advantage in outcomes in eyes receiving internal limiting membrane peeling.[310,311] The largest study reported an improved visual outcome in the group with ILM peeling at 6 months and 1 year but not at 5 years.[301] Others report improved OCT outcomes but not visual acuity outcomes with ILM peeling.[297] Terasaki and colleagues reported that ILM removal was associated with delayed recovery of the focal macular electroretinogram b-wave after surgery.[294] In the absence of a randomized clinical trial, it is difficult to determine which steps are important in reducing macular edema.

A consensus on the kinetics of macular thinning after vitrectomy for DME is lacking. In support of slow change, Terasaki and colleagues found that thinning progressively occurred over 12 months of follow-up. For 19 eyes for which posterior hyaloid separation was induced, the reduction in thickening observed was 61, 69, and 82% of the baseline macular thickening at 3, 6, and 12 months, respectively.[294] Tachi and Ogino likewise found that progressive macular thinning occurred from 6 to 12 months after vitrectomy.[293] Yanyali and colleagues found progressive reduction in thickening over follow-up time through 6 months. Reduction in thickening observed was 61 and 85% at 1 and 6 months, respectively.[296] Yamamoto and colleagues found that macular thinning continues at least through 4 months after vitrectomy.[298] In support of faster equilibration, Recchia

Table 7.5 Selected studies of vitrectomy surgery for diabetic macular edema

A

Study	Year	Prospective?	Controlled?	Number of eyes	Previous focal	Taut hyaloid	Previous IVTA
Terasaki	2003	N	N	19	Not stated	Some	N
Yanyali	2005	Y	Y	12	N	N	N
Stolba	2005	Y	Y	25	Y	Y	N
Recchia	2005	Y	N	11	Y	N	N
Tachi	1996	N	N	58	Some	N	N
Otani	2002	Y	Y	7	Some	Some	N
Rosenblatt	2004	N	N	26	Y	N	N
Yamamoto	2007	N	N	69	Some	Some	N
Asami	2004	N	N	10	N	N	N
Kadonoso	2000	Y	N	9	N	N	N
Patel	2006	Y	N	12	Y	Some	N
Shimonagano	2007	N	N	46	Some	N	Not stated
Figueroa	2008	Y	N	42	Some	N	N
Hartley	2008	N	N	9	Some	Some	Some
Bardak no ILM peel group	2006	Y	N	11	Y	Some	Not stated
Bardak ILM peel group	2006	Y	N	13	Y	Some	Not stated
Higuchi	2006	N	N	3	Y	Y	Y
Mochizuki VTX only	2006	N	N	13	N	Some	N
Mochizuki VTX +IVTA	2006	N	N	22	N	Some	N
Mochizuki VTX +ILM peel	2006	N	N	22	N	Some	N
Patel	2006	Y	Y	6	Y	Some	N
la Heij	2001	N	N	21	Some	N	N
Patel, no ILM peel group	2006	Y	N	8	Y	N	N
Patel, ILM peel group	2006	Y	N	10	Y	N	N
Thomas	2006	Y	Y	15	Y	N	N
DRCR network	2009	Y	N	87	Some	Y	Some

B

Study	Previous PRP	Active NV	Peel hyaloid	Peel ILM	IVTA	PRP	Focal
Terasaki	Some	Not stated	Y	N	N	Y	N
Yanyali	Some	Not stated	Y	Y	N	N	N
Stolba	Not stated	N	Y	Y	N	N	N
Recchia	Some	Not stated	Y	Y	N	N	N
Tachi	Y		Y	N	N	N	N
Otani	Y	N	Y	N	N	N	N
Rosenblatt	Not stated	Not stated	Y	Y	N	Y	N
Yamamoto	Some	Some	Y	N	N	N	N
Asami	Some	Some	Y	Y	N	Y	N
Kadonoso	Y	Not stated	Y	N	N	N	N
Patel	Some	Not stated	Y	N	N	N	N
Shimonagano	Some	Not stated	Y	N	N	All	None
Figueroa	Not stated	Not stated	Y	Some	Some	None	None
Hartley	Some	Not stated	Y	Y	N	N	N
Bardak no ILM peel group	Not stated	Not stated	Y	Y	N	Y	N

Table 7.5 (continued)

B

Study	Previous PRP	Active NV	Peel hyaloid	Peel ILM	IVTA	PRP	Focal
Bardak ILM peel group	Not stated	Not stated	Y	N	Y	Y	N
Higuchi	N	Not stated	Y	N	N	N	N
Mochizuki VTX only	Y	Not stated	Y	N	N	N	N
Mochizuki VTX + IVTA	Y	Not stated	Y	N	Y	N	N
Mochizuki VTX + ILM peel	Y	Not stated	Y	Y	N	N	N
Patel	Some	N	Y	N	N	N	N
la Heij	Some	N	Y	N	N	N	N
Patel, no ILM peel gp	N	N	Y	N	N	N	N
Patel, ILM peel gp	Some	N	Y	Y	N	N	N
Thomas	Some	Not stated	Y	Y	N	N	N
DRCR network	Some	Some	Y	Some	Some	Some	Some

C

Study	Baseline CSMT	6 mo CSMT	12 mo CSMT	Baseline logMAR VA	6 mo chge ETDRS letters	12 mo chge ETDRS letters
Terasaki	548	282	232	0.63		8
Yanyali	439	220		0.75	11	
Stolba	543	484		0.28	2	
Recchia	445	252		1.25	28	
Tachi				1.029		14
Otani	622	269		0.7	10	
Rosenblatt	599	325		0.982	0.75	
Yamamoto	464	275	224	0.78	7	9
Asami	456	260		0.78	8	
Kadonoso	283	216		0.951	30	
Patel	334		280	0.7		13
Shimonagano	516	331	271	0.78	6.5	10
Figueroa	409	312	280	0.7	10	–3
Hartley	406	297	283	0.66	1	
Bardak no ILM peel group				1.3	20	
Bardak ILM peel group				1.4	20	
Higuchi	533		230	0.699		14
Mochizuki VTX only				0.99	3	
Mochizuki VTX + IVTA				0.9	7	
Mochizuki VTX + ILM peel				0.74	2	
Patel	364	277	337	0.25	2	2
la Heij				1.1		15
Patel, no ILM peel group	233		213	0.7		13
Patel, ILM peel group	400		275	0.4		2
Thomas	272		199	0.72		–3
DRCR network	491			0.7	3	

Y = yes, N = no, IVTA = intravitreal triamcinolone, PRP = panretinal photocoagulation, ETDRS = early treatment diabetic retinopathy, VTX = vitrectomy, ILM = internal limiting membrane, DRCR = diabetic retinopathy clinical research, mo = month, chge = change, VA = visual acuity, CSMT = central subfield mean thickness, NV = neovascularization, logMAR = logarithm of the minimal angle of resolution.

and colleagues and the DRCR Network studies reported completion of the macular thinning response by 3 months after surgery[153] (DRCR Vitrectomy study submitted for publication).

The reported amplitude of the macular thinning to vitrectomy surgery has been variable, but more thinning occurs with vitrectomy than single session macular grid laser.[237,241] The average macular thinning effect of single session focal laser at 6 months is –69 μm for an eye with CSMT of 410 μm.[241] In contrast, the average thinning produced by vitrectomy surgery in eyes of this baseline thickness was –144 μm.[241] Vitrectomy surgery is rarely done for eyes with macular thickness less than 300 μm. For eyes of 300 μm, the average response to vitrectomy surgery is macular thinning of approximately 60 μm at 6 months (Table 7.5 and Fig. 7.40). For each additional 100 μm of baseline macular thickness, vitrectomy surgery on average yields an additional 70 μm of macular thinning at 6-month follow-up (Fig. 7.41).[241] The median change in visual acuity at 6-month follow-up after vitrectomy surgery for DME is eight ETDRS letters, IQR (2,11), based on analysis of the data in Table 7.5. There are no important relationships between the baseline macular thickening and the change in visual acuity at 6 months or between change in macular thickness at 6 months and change in visual acuity at 6 months (data not shown, but based on Table 7.5).

As has been reported for other treatments for DME, recurrence of edema after initial improvement, incomplete resolution of macular thickening, and failure to respond also occur with vitrectomy. Recchia and colleagues found recurrence of initially improved edema in 18% of eyes by 6-month follow-up and employed intravitreal triamcinolone injection to manage such cases.[153] Rosenblatt and colleagues found that macular thickening increased despite vitrectomy in 7% of eyes.[147] Massin and colleagues found that macular thickening resolved in all seven patients with vitreomacular traction treated with vitrectomy over a mean follow-up of 19 months, but persistent thickening was present in 75% of eyes without vitreomacular traction.[75] Kadonoso and colleagues found that 22% of eyes failed to show macular thinning after vitrectomy for DME.[76]

Although there is general acceptance that vitrectomy has a role in the management of at least some cases of DME, there is also consensus that it has no role in many cases, including cases of mild edema with minimal visual compromise and in cases with large submacular hard exudates, in which chronic retinal pigment epithelial atrophic changes limit the potential for improvement even after specifically removing these exudates through small retinotomies.[89,314] Prospective, multicentered, randomized clinical trials have been published regarding focal/grid photocoagulation and intravitreal triamcinolone injection for DME. A similar large study is needed to define the role of vitrectomy surgery in the management of DME. The many retrospective studies make a case that vitrectomy for DME has a

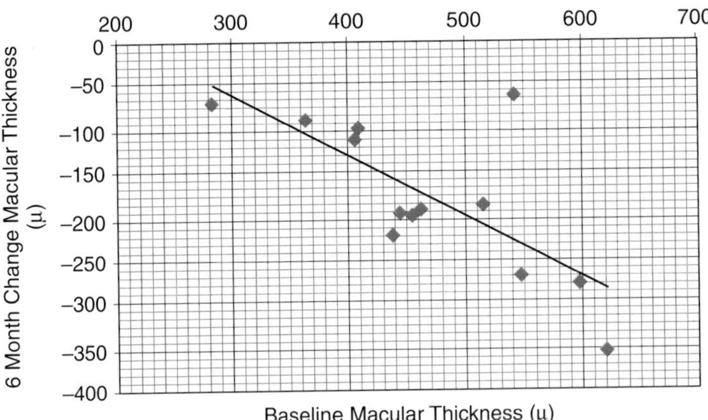

Fig. 7.41 Relationship of macular thinning induced at 6 months by vitrectomy surgery for DME and the baseline macular thickness. The thinning effect increases with increasing baseline macular thickness. Each data point represents one study in Table 7.5 for which a baseline mean or median central subfield mean thickness and a 6-month change in central subfield mean thickness were reported

role, but a large-scale clinical trial is necessary to clarify what that role is. Such a trial has been frequently advocated in the past, although not unanimously.[237] A multicentered, randomized clinical trial (the TIME Study) comparing observation vs. vitrectomy with internal limiting membrane peeling vs. intravitreal injection(s) of triamcinolone 4 mg once is underway.[244]

7.29 Supplemental Oxygen and Hyperbaric Oxygenation

Hyperbaric oxygenation reduced breakdown of the blood–retinal barrier in a rat model of diabetic retinopathy.[315] In a small clinical series, 10–30 hyperbaric oxygen treatments resulted in no morphologic change in DME.[316] Three months of supplemental oxygen therapy by nasal cannula improved macular thickness in nine eyes of five patients with DME refractory to conventional focal/grid laser treatment.[317] Three eyes showed ≥ 2 lines improvement in visual acuity and five of nine eyes worsened after cessation of supplemental oxygen. More experience is needed with these therapies before any recommendations for use can be considered.

7.30 Resection of Subfoveal Hard Exudates

Lipid exudates in DME primarily occur in the outer plexiform layer, often in a perivascular distribution.[69] However, in advanced and chronic cases of DME, large plaques of hard exudates can accumulate in the subfoveal space and stimulate formation of fibrotic scars.[197,318] Several case series have examined whether surgical removal of these plaques is beneficial. The conclusions of the series are inconsistent with some series reporting improvements compared to nonrandomly selected comparison groups not undergoing surgery and others suggesting improvements over the natural course.[314,319] Because the effect size of the surgery based on these case series is modest, a randomized controlled trial of a large number of patients would be needed to decide whether this type of surgery is worthwhile, an unlikely prospect given the relative infrequency of such cases in practice.

7.31 Subclinical Diabetic Macular Edema

The ETDRS included several groups of patients that provided useful estimates of the rate of development of CSME in patients without DME at baseline. In eyes with severe NPDR or early PDR and no macular edema, an estimate of the rate of development of CSME was 4% per year over a follow-up period of 7 years.[320] For eyes with severe NPDR or early PDR and macular edema, but not CSME, an estimate for the rate of development of CSME was 12% per year over 5 years of follow-up.[320] A similar estimate for the eyes with mild to moderate nonproliferative diabetic retinopathy and macular edema, but not CSME, was 14% per year over 5 years of follow-up.[320]

With known effective treatments for DME, the clinical problem of following patients with macular edema insufficient to lead to a recommendation for focal/grid laser treatment is important.[4,79,135] The management of patients with less than clinically significant DME was investigated in the ETDRS in an era without the assistance of retinal thickness measurements by OCT.[4,320] Studies have shown that clinical assessment of macular edema and OCT assessment of macular edema frequently disagree in this group of patients.[143,144] The macular status of such patients as followed in the OCT era is not well understood.[143,144] Subclinical DME refers to eyes with macular edema recognized clinically, but of severity less than the threshold characterized by the term clinically significant, as well as edema not detected clinically but detected by OCT.[144,145] Clinically important questions concerning these patients include the following: Are there factors that predict rates of progression of patients with subclinical DME to reach CSME? And, how frequently should patients be followed with subclinical DME in order to promptly detect conversion to CSME and institute treatment?

In one study of a cohort of eyes with SCDME followed over a median duration of 14 months, 31.4% of the eyes reached clinically significant

DME and received treatment.[145] An analysis looking for any patient characteristics or eye characteristics that predicted the eventual need for treatment revealed none. In particular, no OCT indices were predictive of progression. The median time to treatment for the eyes eventually receiving treatment was 13 months, and only 11% needed treatment within 4 months of the baseline visit.[145] Thus, the generally observed slow change in OCT values and delayed time to treatment suggest that a 4–6 month follow-up interval would be unlikely to miss progression from SCDME to clinically significant DME. Figure 7.42 shows an example of an eye that progressed from SCDME to CSME over a period of 28 months of periodic observation.

Patients with subclinical DME merit periodic examination with stereoscopic slit-lamp biomicroscopy to determine when the threshold for intervention is reached. This threshold continues to be defined by the concept of CSME proposed by the ETDRS. Where OCT is available, it should be used in the care of these patients, because of evidence that stereoscopic slit-lamp biomicroscopy alone results in errors of both underdiagnosis and overdiagnosis of DME.[143,144] Subclinical DME does not inexorably progress, and when it progresses, tends to do so

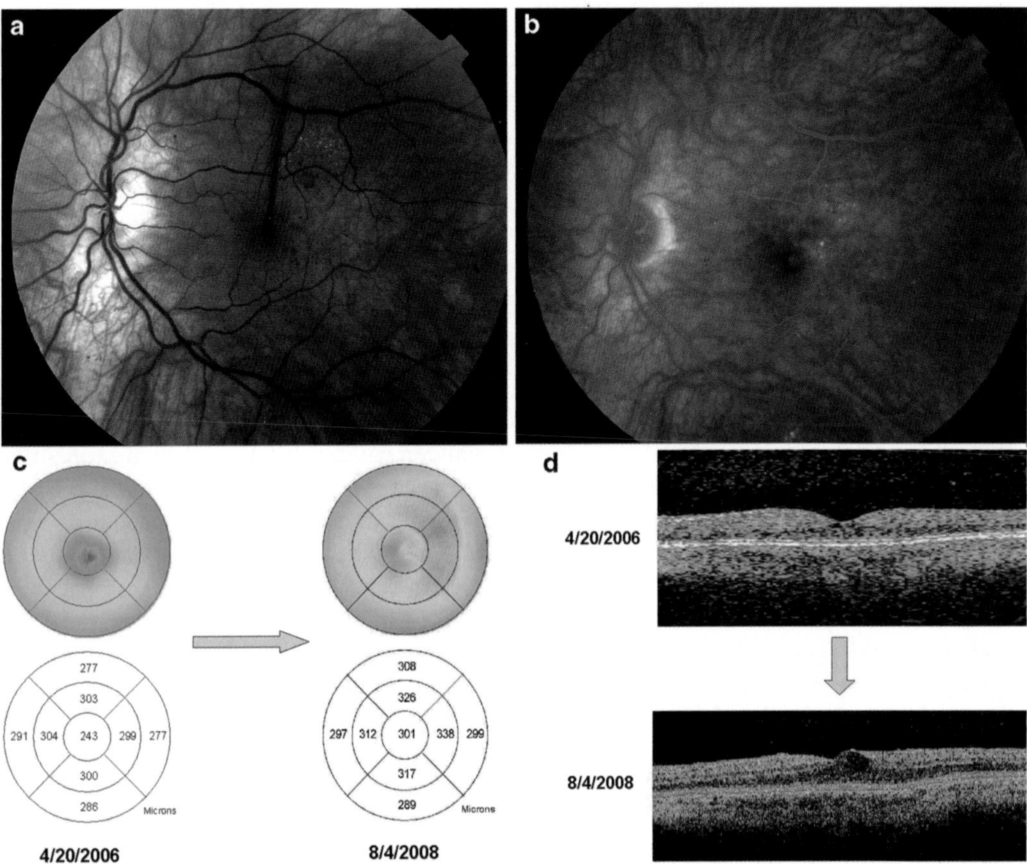

Fig. 7.42 (**a**) Red-free fundus photograph of the *left macula* manifesting CSME on 24 August 2008. Microaneurysms are present temporal to the macula with a lipid ring superotemporal to the center of the macula. (**b**) Late-phase fluorescein angiogram shows leakage of fluorescein from the microaneurysms temporal to the macula. (**c**) OCT map images of the *left eye* over time. In 2006, the central subfield mean thickness is at the upper limit of normal and the inner paracentral fields are more than two standard deviations above normal, but there was no clinically recognized edema (i.e., the eye manifests SCDME). Over the ensuing 28 months, all subfields increased in thickness and edema became clinically apparent. (**d**) Horizontally oriented OCT line scans of the *left eye* of a patient with SCDME. The morphology is initially normal, with a preserved foveal depression. Over the ensuing 28 months of follow-up cystoid thickening developed

slowly. A substantial fraction of eyes with subclinical DME show spontaneous improvement in macular edema over time.[145] There is no rationale to push intervention earlier than the present standard of clinically significant DME.[145]

7.32 Cases with Simultaneous Indications for Focal and Scatter Laser Photocoagulation

In some cases of diabetic retinopathy, both clinically significant diabetic macular edema and a level of retinopathy equal to or more severe than severe nonproliferative retinopathy are present (Fig. 7.43). In these eyes, there are indications to begin both focal and panretinal laser photocoagulation, giving rise to the question of how the two types of treatments should be administered. Should therapy be sequential, and if so, in what order? Should therapy be combined in some cases?

No large randomized clinical trials have been performed that give evidence favoring the best management approach in every clinical scenario, but evidence does exist that suggests reasonable approaches in many situations. The ETDRS compared five treatment approaches in eyes with macular edema and either severe nonproliferative or early proliferative retinopathy: deferral of photocoagulation, immediate focal/immediate mild scatter, immediate mild scatter/delayed focal, immediate focal/immediate full scatter, and immediate full scatter/delayed focal.[320] The approach with the lowest rates of $\geq$15 ETDRS letters visual acuity loss (moderate visual loss) was immediate focal/immediate mild scatter. Approximately, 5% of patients with this approach will have moderate visual loss shortly after treatment, a greater percentage than with deferral, but this short-term inferior outcome is effaced by 4 months compared to deferral, and thereafter the intervention is superior to deferral.[320] For eyes with high-risk PDR and macular edema, Maia and colleagues reported a small randomized trial of 22 patients with symmetric disease in which both eyes received focal/grid plus three sitting scatter laser treatments separated by 1 week. One eye of the two in each patient was randomized to receive a 4 mg intravitreal triamcinolone injection after the third sitting. Both macular thickness and visual acuity were better in the intravitreal triamcinolone group at 12 months.[321] Other case series and reasoning based on pathophysiology suggest that simultaneous focal/grid with panretinal photocoagulation supplemented in some cases by a preparatory intravitreal injection of an anti-VEGF drug is a reasonable treatment alternative.[224,322] A DRCR Network randomized trial comparing focal/grid plus panretinal laser, adjunctive intravitreal ranibizumab followed by focal/grid plus panretinal laser and repeat ranibizumab at 4 weeks, and adjunctive intravitreal triamcinolone followed by focal/grid plus panretinal laser is underway.

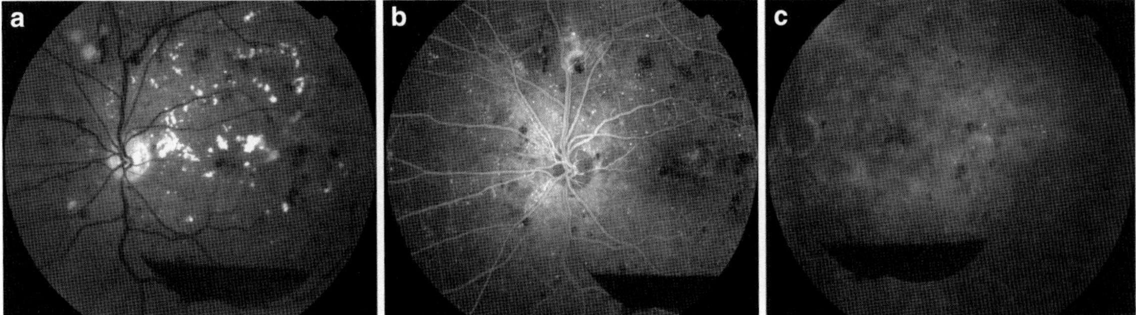

Fig. 7.43 (**a**) Red-free photograph of a pseudophakic eye with high-risk proliferative diabetic retinopathy (new vessels along the superior arcade plus preretinal hemorrhage inferiorly) and concomitant clinically significant diabetic macular edema. (**b**) Frame from the mid-phase fluorescein angiogram showing mid-peripheral capillary nonperfusion and rather many leaky microaneurysms and capillary segments. (**c**) Frame from the late-phase fluorescein angiogram showing widespread fluorescein leakage

7.33 Exacerbation of Diabetic Macular Edema by Scatter Photocoagulation

Scatter photocoagulation can induce DME in eyes without preexisting DME and can exacerbate DME in eyes with concomitant DME.[320,323,324] Hydrogen peroxide increases in the vitreous after scatter laser photocoagulation which is in turn associated with increased adhesion molecules in the vascular endothelium. Leukocytes therefore stagnate in the macular microcirculation and reduce blood flow leading to release of oxygen-free radicals, proteolytic enzymes, nitric oxide, and inflammatory cytokines.[325,326] The risk of scatter photocoagulation-induced DME increases for eyes with subclinical DME compared to eyes with normal macular thickness.[327,328] Because these are eyes for which clinical examination alone is frequently unreliable for detecting increased thickening, it is worthwhile to obtain a macular OCT study for any eye for which scatter photocoagulation is being considered.[328,329] If thickening is detected, consideration should be given to pretreating the eye with a peribulbar or intravitreal injection of triamcinolone or an intravitreal injection of an anti-VEGF drug.[328,330,331] If the indications for scatter photocoagulation are not so pressing, dividing the treatment into smaller sessions separated over time may decrease the treatment-associated inflammation and reduce the chance of induced DME.[327] Some evidence exists that panretinal laser that emphasizes more peripheral treatment and avoids treatment closer to the perimacular vascular arcades may reduce the chance of exacerbating concomitant DME.[332] There is no good evidence that dividing sessions of scatter laser in eyes without increased macular thickening is useful in preventing induction of new DME.[333]

7.34 Factors Influencing Treatment of Diabetic Macular Edema

Increasing duration of DME with cell death has been hypothesized as a negative influence on treatments for DME, but because of inability to determine duration, its effects have not been adequately assessed.[30,151] Increased macular ischemia has been reported to negatively influence results of vitrectomy and intravitreal bevacizumab therapy for DME and has been suspected as a negative influence in other therapies for DME.[121,238,334] These studies suggest that if vitrectomy and intravitreal bevacizumab therapy were applied to cases with less macular ischemia, the visual outcomes might be better. Macular ischemia is difficult to quantitate, gradable with only modest reproducibility, and associated with low rates of interpretable fluorescein angiograms in eyes with DME which often have concomitant cataract. Macular ischemia has been infrequent in most cases with DME making it difficult to assess the modifying effects of macular ischemia on treatments for DME. Presence of subretinal fluid and subretinal hard lipid exudates have both been reported as negative prognostic factors for cases treated with vitrectomy.[306,335]

7.35 Sequence of Therapy

Four different interventions for DME are in current use by ophthalmologists: focal laser photocoagulation, intravitreal injection of triamcinolone acetonide (IVTA), injection of anti-VEGF drugs, and vitrectomy surgery.[4,163,267,289] In general, focal laser is applied initially, followed by intravitreal triamcinolone or anti-VEGF drug injection if response is suboptimal or transitory, and vitrectomy surgery is reserved for the worst cases in which less invasive techniques have failed or for which intravitreal triamcinolone injections are contraindicated.[147] This paradigm has evolved by the historical development of treatments and their relative risks, and not by conscious design. As these treatments improve and risks change with modification of techniques, it is possible that the conventionally accepted sequence of interventions may change, with factors affecting the surgical decisions depending on particulars of anatomy, visual acuity, lens status, and other clinical variables. The targeted abnormalities for all of these treatments are the thickening of the macula anatomically and decreased visual acuity ultimately. Reconsidering the rationale underpinning the optimal sequence of intervention in diabetic macular edema has been suggested.[241] Groups of investigators have already begun to study alternative sequences of intervention, including intravitreal triamcinolone therapy and vitrectomy surgery as initial treatments.[75,227,310] When traction of the vitreous on the macula has been judged to be important, vitrectomy surgery is sometimes chosen as the initial treatment, although the criteria are often subjective and unstated for deciding that vitreous traction is of primary importance.[75,300] One articulated rationale has been that visual outcomes in cases undergoing vitrectomy without previous focal/grid photocoagulation have, in some series, been superior to those in eyes with previous focal/grid photocoagulation.[238,292]

The four interventions for DME are not currently applied to comparable groups of eyes. The best seeing eyes with the least macular thickening generally receive focal laser treatment. More severely affected eyes, with thicker maculas and often having failed focal laser, receive intravitreal triamcinolone injection. The most severely affected eyes, with the thickest maculas and often having failed the first two treatments, receive vitrectomy surgery or combined treatments.[336] For example, in the DRCR Network studies of focal/grid laser therapy, intravitreal triamcinolone injections, and vitrectomy surgery for DME, the median CSMTs were 327, 398, and 491 μm, respectively[227] (DRCR vitrectomy study submitted for publication, DRCR protocol K submitted for publication).

For the purpose of considering an optimal sequence of intervention, treatments for DME can be characterized by their effect sizes with respect to macular thickening and visual acuity at specific times after treatment, the slope of the effect with respect to time, and rates of paradoxical thickening. Table 7.6 shows such a comparison using 6 months as the reference interval after treatment.

Differences in effect size, stability, and duration of effect, and rates of paradoxical thickening associated with the three interventions have been reported.[241] Focal/grid laser has a modest, stable effect. IVTA has a more pronounced early effect, but it wears off, and the same is true of intravitreal anti-VEGF therapy. Vitrectomy surgery has an early effect midway between focal laser and IVTA, but the effect appears to increase to a stable ceiling over time.[241] Prospective studies are needed to put these provisional observations in truer context.

The observed differences in treatment effects have to do in part with the differences in baseline characteristics of the groups to which the interventions are applied. Thus, the effect size of IVTA and vitrectomy may in part reflect the opportunity in these groups for the macula to thin more after an intervention because these groups typically have thicker maculas. For example, the macular thinning effects of focal laser, IVTA, and vitrectomy all vary directly with the baseline CSMT (Fig. 7.41).[241] In addition, the treatments work by different mechanisms, which makes the concept of combined therapy more attractive for severe cases.

In mild cases of DME, focal/grid laser remains the gold standard treatment. In more severe cases, this approach is also worth an initial trial, understanding that persistent thickening of the center of the macula may be seen in approximately 35% of cases after 1 year of repetitive treatments at 4-month intervals.[4] Because persistent DME is associated with progressive loss of visual acuity, which is faster the more severe the edema, at some point an alternative combined treatment may be prudent.[151]

In view of the small effect size and 25.4% rate of paradoxical thickening induced by focal laser, and the consistent, but transient thinning induced by peribulbar or intravitreal triamcinolone, a combined approach with initial steroid adjunct followed by

Table 7.6 Summary of the magnitude of reduction in thickness and of change in visual acuity of three interventions for diabetic macular edema at 6 months follow-up

Intervention	Macular thinning at 6 months (μm)	Change in ETDRS letters read at 6 months	Slope of the effect at 6 months	Fraction with paradoxical thickening at 6 months (%)
Untreated	0	0	Flat	40.4
Focal	–28	0	Flat	25.4
IVTA	–83	+3	Decreasing	3.8
Vitrectomy	–92	–1	Increasing	19.0

IVTA = intravitreal triamcinolone acetonide. Note that the treatments on average are applied to groups with different baseline thickening in relative order focal laser< IVTA< Vitrectomy. Paradoxical thickening refers to the fact that thinning is expected with treatment, but in a proportion of cases, the macula actually thickens.
Reproduced with permission from Browning.[241]

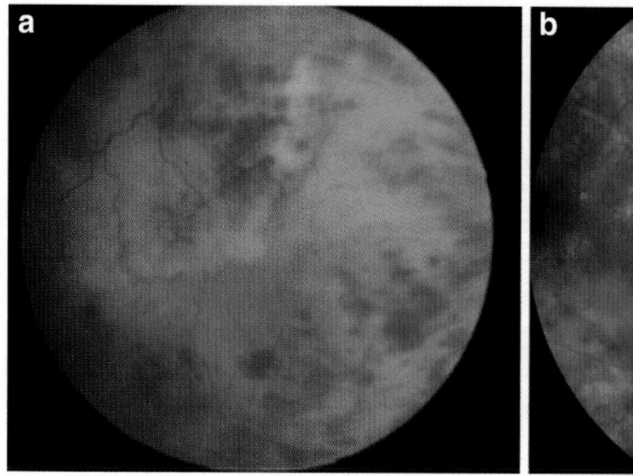

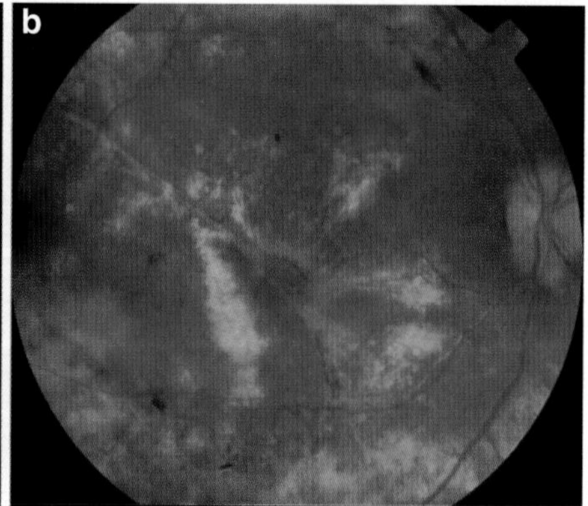

Fig. 7.44 Example of the effect of vitrectomy and panretinal photocoagulation alone without focal laser and without adjunctive intravitreal pharmacotherapy in causing regression of severe diabetic macular edema. (**a**) Preoperative severe diabetic macular edema. The macula is so thickened and ischemic that focal laser burns cannot be achieved without using unreasonably high power settings likely to rupture Bruch's membrane. The patient underwent vitrectomy, separation of the posterior hyaloid, and panretinal laser photocoagulation. The purpose of panretinal photocoagulation was to reduce the vitreous concentration of VEGF by ablating ischemic retina. (**b**) Postoperative resolution of the diabetic macular edema with residual subretinal scarring. No focal laser has been given, nor has there been any use of intraocular triamcinolone or any anti-VEGF drug

focal laser may be a rational step in improving attempts to treat more severe cases of DME.[122,285] For the most severely affected eyes, perhaps with visual acuity of 20/100 or worse, earlier use of vitrectomy surgery may be a rational step and worthwhile investigating (Fig. 7.44).[336] Better seeing eyes should probably not be exposed to the risks of vitrectomy surgery, which are higher than the risks of focal laser or intravitreal triamcinolone injection. Further clinical trials are needed to better define preferred practices.

7.36 Interaction of Cataract Surgery and Diabetic Macular Edema

Cataract surgery can induce diabetic macular edema in eyes with diabetic retinopathy and no preexisting edema and exacerbate DME when it predates cataract surgery. Pseudophakic cystoid macular edema, a post-surgical inflammatory condition distinct from DME, also occurs more frequently after cataract surgery in eyes of patients with diabetes, even if the eye is free from clinical retinopathy. From a public health perspective, this topic is so important that a separate chapter in this book is devoted to its review and analysis. The reader is directed to chapter 10 for further information.

7.37 Summary of Key Points

- The prevalence of diabetic macular edema is increasing worldwide, mainly because of increasing type 2 diabetes.
- Types 1 and 2 diabetes both lead to diabetic macular edema, but the clinical profiles and risk factors of the cases in these two types differ.
- Understanding retinal anatomy helps in analyzing clinical presentations of diabetic macular edema based on the effects of the avascularity of the central macula, the locations of the microvessels in the inner retinal layers, the importance of the pigment epithelial layer, and the role of the vitreoretinal interface.
- The oxygen theory of DME is the most comprehensive pathophysiologic schema, and VEGF is the single most important, although not the sole, mediator in that pathway. Impaired retinal vascular autoregulation, breakdown of the inner blood–retina barrier, dysregulation of retinal signaling pathways, and vitreoretinal traction are important factors in understanding DME.
- Optical coherence tomography is ascending in importance as a clinical ancillary study in managing diabetic macular edema. Fluorescein angiography is less often used.

- Macular thickening has an imperfect correlation with visual acuity, probably due to factors currently difficult to assess, such as duration of edema and degree of macular ischemia. Visual acuity outcome for now remains the primary clinical focus, and macular thickening outcomes cannot be viewed as surrogates.
- Metabolic control of blood glucose, blood pressure, and serum lipids is the foundation of therapy for diabetic macular edema, and specific ocular treatments are most effective when this foundation is optimized first.
- Focal/grid photocoagulation is the benchmark ocular treatment for diabetic macular edema of all degrees of severity, but evidence for the efficacy of intravitreal injections of triamcinolone and anti-VEGF drugs and of vitrectomy surgery is increasing. These other therapies are likely to have a role in managing many cases, and may prove to be useful in combination. The best sequence of application of these therapies is as yet undefined.

7.38 Future Directions

Although fraught with uncertainty, it is interesting to hazard some predictions about directions of future research into the causes and best management of DME. Genetic mutations rendering patients more or less susceptible to DME as a complication of diabetes are likely to be defined. The physiologic pathways contributing to DME and not mediated by VEGF are a likely focus of future research. Most patients with DME take many medications, and many of them, such as certain classes of antihypertensive drugs, newer oral agents for management of diabetes, and statins, have theoretical bearing on retinal physiology. The interactions of drugs with DME are presently unexplored and should be clarified in the next years. Using SD-OCT, it should be possible to define at almost histologic levels the retinal changes occurring in DME and determine which, if any, changes associate with visual outcomes. Newer methods of laser photocoagulation are likely to become increasingly tested against conventional photocoagulation. The semiautomated production of laser patterns that is currently found in certain commercial laser machines may overcome the problem with micropulse laser of not knowing where treatment has been applied. Refinements in the best methods of application of focal/grid photocoagulation and the role of alternative therapies such as pharmacologic adjuncts, combined therapies, and vitrectomy will likely flow from clinical trials. Trials using visual acuity as the primary endpoint are expensive and lengthy. The quest for surrogate clinical endpoints that correlate well with visual acuity and could allow randomized trials to be simplified and shortened continues. OCT-measured macular thickness has not been the hoped-for surrogate, but other endpoints, such as retinal vessel diameter, are being evaluated.[54,189]

References

1. Klein R, Klein B, Moss S, Cruickshanks K. The Wisconsin epidemiologic study of diabetic retinopathy: the long-term incidence of macular edema. *Ophthalmology*. 1995;102: 7–16.
2. Klein R, Klein BE, Moss SE, Linton KL. The Beaver Dam eye study. retinopathy in adults with newly discovered and previously diagnosed diabetes mellitus. *Ophthalmology*. 1992;99:58–62.
3. Mohamed Q, Gillies MC, Wong TY. Management of diabetic retinopathy. A systematic review. *JAMA*. 2007; 298:902–916.
4. Early Treatment Diabetic Retinopathy Study Research Group. Photocoagulation for diabetic macular edema. *Arch Ophthalmol*. 1985;103:1796–1806.
5. Xie XW, Xu L, Wang YX, Jonas JB. Prevalence and associated factors of diabetic retinopathy. The Beijing eye study 2006. *Graefe's Arch Clin Exp Ophthalmol*. 2008;246:1519–1526.
6. Wong TY, Cheung N, Tay WT, Wang JJ, Aung T, Saw SM, et al. Prevalence and risk factors for diabetic retinopathy. The Singapore Malay eye study. *Ophthalmology*. 2008;115:1869–75.
7. Rubino A, Rousculp MD, Davis K, Wang J, Girach A. Diagnosed diabetic retinopathy in France, Italy, Spain, and the United Kingdom. *Prim Care Diabetes*. 2007;1:75–80.
8. Wong TY, Klein R, Islam FMA, Cotch MF, Folsom AR, Klein BEK, et al. Diabetic retinopathy in a multi-ethnic cohort in the United States? *Am J Ophthalmol*. 2006;141:446–455.
9. Varma R, Torres M, Pena F, Klein R, Azen SP, Los Angeles Latino eye study group. Prevalence of diabetic retinopathy in adult latinos. *Am Acad Ophthalmol*. 2004;111:1298–1306.
10. Wolfe JA, Horton MB, McAteer MB, Szuter CF, Clayton T. Race, macular degeneration, and diabetic maculopathy. *Arch Ophthalmol*. 1993;111:1603–1604.

11. Shea AM, Curtis LH, Hammill BG, Kowalski JW, Ravelo A, Lee PP, et al. Resource use and costs associated with diabetic macular edema in elderly persons. *Arch Ophthalmol.* 2008;126:1748–1754.
12. Klein BEK, Moss SE, Klein R, Surawicz TS. The Wisconsin epidemiologic study of diabetic retinopathy XIII. Relationship of serum cholesterol to retinopathy and hard exudate. *Ophthalmology.* 1991;98: 1261–1265.
13. Sigelman J. Diabetic macular edema in juvenile and adult onset diabetes. *Am J Ophthalmol.* 1980;90:287–296.
14. Miljanovic B, Glynn RJ, Nathan DM, Manson JE, Schaumberg DA. A prospective study of serum lipids and risk of diabetic macular edema in type 1 diabetes. *Diabetes.* 2004;53:2883–2892.
15. Vitale S, Maguire MG, Murphy RP, Hiner CJ, Rourke L, Sackett C, et al. Clinically significant macular edema in type 1 diabetes incidence and risk factors. *Ophthalmology.* 1995;102:1170–1176.
16. Klein R, Knudtson MD, Lee KE, Gangnon R, Klein BEK. The Wisconsin epidemiologic study of diabetic retinopathy XXIII. The twenty-five year incidence of macular edema in persons with type 1 diabetes. *Ophthalmology.* 2009;116:497–503.
17. Klein R, Klein BE, Moss SE, David MD, DeMets DL. The Wisconsin epidemiologic study of diabetic retinopathy IV. Diabetic macular edema. *Ophthalmology.* 1984; 91:1464–1474.
18. Klein R, Klein BEK, Moss SE, Cruickshanks KJ. The 14-year incidence and progression of diabetic retinopathy and associated risk factors in type 1 diabetes. *Ophthalmology.* 1998;105:1801–1815.
19. Lattanzio R, Brancato R, Pierro L, Bandello F, Iaccheri B, Fiore T, et al. Macular thickness measured by optical coherence tomography (OCT) in diabetic patients. *Eur J Ophthalmol.* 2002;12:482–487.
20. Browning DJ, Fraser CM, Clark S. The relationship of macular thickness to clinically graded diabetic retinopathy severity in eyes without clinically detected diabetic macular edema. *Ophthalmology.* 2007;115: 533–539.
21. Iwasaki M, Inomata H. Relation between superficial capillaries and foveal structures in the human retina. *Invest Ophthalmol Vis Sci.* 1986;27:1698–1705.
22. Riva C, Petrig B. Blue field entoptic phenomenon and blood velocity in the retinal capillaries. *Opt Soc Am.* 1980;70:1234–1238.
23. Henkind P. Symposium on glaucoma: joint meeting with the national society for the prevention of blindness: new observations on the radial peripapillary capillaries. *Invest Ophthalmol Vis Sci.* 1967;6:103–108.
24. Stefansson E. Ocular oxygenation and the treatment of diabetic retinopathy. *Surv Ophthalmol.* 2006;51: 364–380.
25. Moore J, Bagley S, Ireland G, Mcleod D, Boulton ME. Three dimensional analysis of microaneurysms in the human diabetic retina. *J Anat.* 1999;194:89–100.
26. Tolentino MJ, McLeod DS, Taomoto M, Otsuji T, Adamis AP, Lutty GA. Pathologic features of vascular endothelial growth factor-induced retinopathy in the nonhuman primate. *Am J Ophthalmol.* 2002;133:373–385.
27. Sachdev N, Gupta V, Abhiramurthy V, Singh R, Gupta A. Correlation between microaneurysm closure rate and reduction in macular thickness following laser photocoagulation of diabetic macular edema. *Eye.* 2008; 22: 975–977.
28. Nishikawa H, Shahidi M, Vitale S, Alexander J, Asrani S, Mori M, et al. Relation between retinal thickening and clinically visible fundus pathologies in mild nonproliferative diabetic retinopathy. *Ophthalmic Surg Lasers.* 2002; 33:127–134.
29. Blair NP, Shahidi M, Lai WW, Zelkha R. Correlation between microaneurysms and retinal thickness in diabetic macular edema. *Retina.* 2008;28:1097–1103.
30. DiabeticRetinopathy Clinical Research Network. Comparison of the modified early treatment diabetic retinopathy study and mild macular grid laser photocoagulation strategies for diabetic macular edema. *Arch Ophthalmol.* 2007;125:469–480.
31. Nagaoka T, Kitaya N, Sugawara R, Yokota H, Mori F, Hikichi T, et al. Alteration of choroidal circulation in the foveal region in patients with type 2 diabetes. *Br J Ophthalmol.* 2004;88:1060–1063.
32. Fryczkowki AW, Hodes BL, Walker J. Diabetic choroidal and iris vasculature scanning electron microscopy findings. *Int Ophthalmol.* 1989;13:269–279.
33. Quintyn JC, Brasseur G. Subretinal fluid in primary rhegmatogenous retinal detachment: physiopathology and composition. *Surv Ophthalmol.* 2004;49:96–108.
34. LaCour M. The retinal pigment epithelium. In: Kaufman PL, ed. *Adle's Physiology of the Eye: Clinical Application.* St. Louis: Mosby; 2003:348–357.
35. Gardner TW, Antonetti DA, Barber AJ, LaNoue KF, Levison SW, Penn State Retina Research Group. Diabetic retinopathy: more than meets the eye. *Surv Ophthalmol.* 2002;47:S253–S262.
36. Qaum T, Xu Q, Joussen AM, Clemens MW, Qin W, Miyamoto K, et al. VEGF-initiated blood-retinal barrier breakdown in early diabetes. *Invest Ophthalmol Vis Sci.* 2001;42:2408–2413.
37. Vinores SA, McGehee R, Lee A, Gadegbeku C, Campochiaro P. Ultrastructural localization of blood-retinal barrier breakdown in diabetic and galactosemic rats. *J Histochem Cytochem.* 1990;38:1341–1352.
38. Tso M, Cunha-Vaz J, Shih C, Jones C. Clinicopathologic study of blood-retinal barrier in experimental diabetes mellitus. *Arch Ophthalmol.* 1980;98:2032–2040.
39. Bringmann A, Uckermann O, Pannicke T, Iandiev I, Reichenbach A, Wiedemann P. Neuronal versus glial cell swelling in the ischemic retina. *Acta Ophthalmol Scand.* 2005;83:528–538.
40. Distler C, Dreher Z. Glia cells in the monkey retina-II. Muller cells. *Vision Res.* 1996;36:2381–2394.
41. Antcliff R J, Hussain AA, Marshall J. Hydraulic conductivity of fixed retinal tissue after sequential excimer laser ablation-barriers limiting fluid distribution and implications for cystoid macular edema. *Arch Ophthalmol.* 2001;119:539–544.
42. Sebag J, Buckingham B, Charles A, Reiser K. Biochemical abnormalities in vitreous of humans with proliferative diabetic retinopathy. *Arch Ophthalmol.* 1992;110: 1472–1476.

43. Sebag J, Nie S, Reiser K, Charles MA, Yu NT. Raman spectroscopy of human vitreous in proliferative diabetic retinopathy? *Invest Ophthalmol Vis Sci.* 1994;35:2976–2980.
44. Sebag J, Balazs EA. Pathogenesis of cystoid macular edema: consideration of vitreoretinal adhesions. *Surv Ophthalmol.* 1984;28:S493–S498.
45. Holekamp NM, Shui YB, Beebe DC. Vitrectomy surgery increases oxygen exposure to the lens: a possible mechanism for nuclear cataract formation. *Am J Ophthalmol.* 2005;139:302–310.
46. LeGoff MM, Bishop PN. Adult vitreous structure and postnatal changes. *Eye.* 2008;22:1214–1222.
47. Nasrallah FP, Jalkh AE, Coppenolle FV, Kado M, Trempe CL, McMeel JW, et al. The role of the vitreous in diabetic macular edema. *Ophthalmology.* 1988;95: 1335–1339.
48. Lewis H. The role of vitrectomy in the treatment of diabetic macular edema. *Am J Ophthalmol.* 2001;131: 123–125.
49. Weinberger D, Fink-Cohen S, Gaton DD, Priel E, Yassur Y. Non-retinovascular leakage in diabetic maculopathy. *Br J Ophthalmol.* 1995;79:728–731.
50. Parving HH, Larsen M, Hommel E, Lund-Andersen H. Effect of antihypertensive treatment on blood-retinal barrier permeability to fluorescein in hypertensive Type 1 (insulin-dependent) diabetic patients with background retinopathy. *Diabetologia.* 1989;32:440–444.
51. Miyamoto K, Khosrof S, Bursell SE, Moromizato Y, Aiello LP, Ogura Y, et al. Vascular endothelial growth factor (VEGF)-induced retinal vascular permeability is mediated by intercellular adhesion molecule-1 (ICAM-1). *Am J Pathol.* 2000;156:1733–1739.
52. Miyamoto K, Khosrof S, Bursell SE, Rohan R, Murata T, Clermont AC, et al. Prevention of leukostasis and vascular leakage in streptozotocin-induced diabetic retinopathy via intercellular adhesion molecule-1 inhibition. *Proc Natl Acad Sci USA.* 1999;96:10836–10841.
53. Sander B, Larsen M, Lund-Andersen H. Diabetic macular edema: passive and active transport of fluorescein through the blood-retina barrier. *Invest Ophthalmol Vis Sci.* 2001;42:433–438.
54. Lund-Andersen H. Mechanisms for monitoring changes in retinal status following therapeutic intervention in diabetic retinopathy. *Surv Ophthalmol.* 2002;47:S270–S277.
55. SinclairSH, Grunwald JE, Riva CE, Braunstein SN, Nichols CW, Schwartz SS. Retinal vascular autoregulation in diabetes mellitus. *Ophthalmology.* 1982;89:748–750.
56. Harris A, Cuilla TA, Chung HK, Martin B. Regulation of retinal and optic nerve blood flow. *Arch Ophthalmol.* 1998;116:1491–1495.
57. Clermont AC, Aiello LP, Mori F, Aiello LM, Bursell SE. Vascular endothelial growth factor and severity of nonproliferative diabetic retinopathy mediate retinal hemodynamics in vivo: a potential role for vascular endothelial growth factor in the progression of nonproliferative diabetic retinopathy. *Am J Ophthalmol.* 1997;124:433–446.
58. Kristinsson JK, Gottfredsdottir MS, Stefansson E. Retinal vessel dilatation and elongation precedes diabetic macular oedema. *Br J Ophthalmol.* 1997;81:274–278.
59. Igersheimer J. Intraocular pressure and its relation to retinal extravasation. *Arch Ophthalmol.* 1944;32:50–55.
60. Amin RH, Frank RN, Kennedy A, Eliott D, Puklin JE, Abrams GW. Vascular endothelial growth factor is present in glial cells of the retina and optic nerve of humans with nonproliferative diabetic retinopathy. *Invest Ophthalmol Vis Sci.* 1997;38:36–47.
61. Harba jNS, Felinski EA, Wolpert EB, Sundstrom JM, Gardner TW, Antonetti DA. VEGF activation of protein kinase C stimulates occludin phosphorylation and contributes to endothelial permeability. *Invest Ophthalmol Vis Sci.* 2006;47:5106–5115.
62. Funatsu H, Yamashita H, Nakamura S, Mimura T, Eguchi S, Noma H, et al. Vitreous levels of pigment epithelium-derived factor and vascular endothelial growth factor are related to diabetic macular edema. *Ophthalmology.* 2006;113:294–301.
63. Joussen AM, Murata T, Tsujikawa A, Kirchhof B, Bursell SE, Adamis AP. Leukocyte-mediated endothelial cell injury and death in the diabetic retina. *Am J Pathol.* 2001;158:147–152.
64. Kent D, Vinores SA, Campochiaro PA. Macular edema: the role of soluble mediators. *Br J Ophthalmol.* 2000;84: 542–545.
65. Patel JI, Hykin PG, Cree IA. Diabetic cataract removal: postoperative progression of maculopathy-growth factor and clinical analysis. *Br J Ophthalmol.* 2006;90:697–701.
66. Gardner T, Eller A, Friberg T, D'Antonio J, Hollis T. Antihistamines reduce blood-retinal barrier permeability in type I (insulin-dependent) diabetic patients with nonproliferative retinopathy. *Retina.* 1995;15:134–140.
67. Kaiser PK. Antivascular endothelial growth factor agents and their development: therapeutic implications in ocular diseases? *Am J Ophthalmol.* 2006;142:660–668.
68. Johnson MW. Etiology and treatment of macular edema. *Am J Ophthalmol.* 2009;147:11–21.
69. Cusick M, Chew EY, Chan CC, Kruth HS, Murphy RP, Ferris FL III. Histopathology and regression of retinal hard exudates in diabetic retinopathy after reduction of elevated serum lipid levels. *Ophthalmology.* 2003;110: 2126–2133.
70. Hickam JB, Sieker HO. Retinal vascular reactivity in patients with diabetes mellitus with atherosclerosis. *Circulation.* 1960;22:243–246.
71. Hickam JB, Frayser R. Studies of the retinal circulation in man. Observations on vessel diameter, arterio-venous oxygen difference, and mean circulation time. *Circulation.* 1966;33:302–316.
72. Patel JI, Saleh GM, Hykin PG, Gregor ZJ, Cree IA. Concentration of hemodynamic and inflammatory related cytokines in diabetic retinopathy. *Eye.* 2008;22: 223–228.
73. Kaiser PK, Riemann CD, Sears JE, Lewis H. Macular traction detachment and diabetic macular edema associated with posterior hyaloidal traction. *Am J Ophthalmol.* 2001;131:44–49.
74. Otani T, Kishi S. A controlled study of vitrectomy for diabetic macular edema. *Am J Ophthalmol.* 2002;134: 214–219.
75. Massin P, Duguid G, Erginay A, Haouchine B, Gaudric A. Optical coherence tomography for evaluating diabetic macular edema before and after vitrectomy. *Am J Ophthalmol.* 2003;135:169–177.

76. Kadonosono K, Itoh N, Ohno S. Perifoveal microcirculation before and after vitrectomy for diabetic cystoid macular edema. *Am J Ophthalmol*. 2000;130:740–744.
77. YuD Y, Cringle SJ, Su E, Yu PK, Humayun MS, Dorin G. Laser-induced changes in intraretinal oxygen distribution in pigmented rabbits. *Invest Ophthalmol Vis Sci*. 2005;46:988–999.
78. Stefansson E, Landers M, Wolbarsht M. Increased retinal oxygen supply following pan-retinal photocoagulation and vitrectomy and lensectomy. *Trans Am Ophthalmol Soc*. 1981;129:308–321.
79. Browning DJ. Diabetic macular edema: a critical review of the early treatment diabetic retinopathy study (ETDRS) series and subsequent studies. *Comp Ophthalmol* Update 1. 2000;1:69–83.
80. Wallenten KG, Malmsjo M, Andreasson S, Wackenfors A, Johansson K, Ghosh F. Retinal function and PKC alpha expression after focal laser photocoagulation. *Graefe's Arch Clin Exp Ophthalmol*. 2007;245: 1815–1824.
81. Zhang X, Bao S, Lai D, Rapkins RW, Gillies MC. Intravitreal triamcinolone acetonide inhibits breakdown of the blood-retinal barrier through differential regulation of VEGF-A and its receptors in early diabetic rat retinas. *Diabetes*. 2008;57:1026–1033.
82. Gao H, Qiao X, Gao R, Mieler WF, McPherson AR, Holz ER. Intravitreal triamcinolone does not alter basal vascular endothelial growth factor mRNA expression in rat retina. *Vision Res*. 2004;44:349–356.
83. Nauck M, Karaliulakis G, Perruchoud AP, Papakonstantinou E, Roth M. Corticosteroids inhibit the expression of the vascular endothelial growth factor gene in human vascular smooth muscle cells. *Eur J Pharmacol*. 1998;341:309–315.
84. Tamura H, Miyamoto K, Kiryu J, Miyahara S, Katsuta H, Hirose F, et al. Intravitreal injection of corticosteroid attenuates leukostasis and vascular leakage in experimental diabetic retina. *Invest Ophthalmol Vis Sci*. 2005;46:1440–1444.
85. Cunningham MA, Edelman JL, Kaushal S. Intravitreal steroids for macular edema: the past, the present, and the future. *Surv Ophthalmol*. 2008;53:139–149.
86. Aiello LP, Clermont A, Arora V, Davis MD, Sheetz MJ, Bursell SE. Inhibition of PKC Beta by oral administration of ruboxistaurin is well tolerated and ameliorates diabetes-induced retinal hemodynamic abnormalities in patients. *Invest Ophthalmol Vis Sci*. 2006;47: 86–92.
87. Gupta A, Gupta V, Thapar S, Bhansali A. Lipid-lowering drug atorvastatin as an adjunct in the management of diabetic macular edema. *Am J Ophthalmol*. 2004;137:675–682.
88. Stefansson E, Landers MB. How does vitrectomy affect diabetic macular edema. *Am J Ophthalmol*. 2006;141: 984–985.
89. Laidlaw DAH. Vitrectomy for diabetic macular edema? *Eye*. 2008;22:1337–1341.
90. Edelman JL, Lutz D, Castro MR. Corticosteroids inhibit VEGF-induced vascular leakage in a rabbit model of blood-retinal and blood-aqueous barrier breakdown. *Exp Eye Res*. 2005;80:249–258.
91. Dev S, Pulido JS, Tessler HH, Mittra RA, Han DP, Mieler WF, et al. Progression of diabetic retinopathy after endophthalmitis. *Ophthalmology*. 1999;106:774–781.
92. Reichenbach A, Wurm A, Pannicke T, Iandiev I, Wiedemann P, Bringmann A. Muller cells as players in retinal degeneration and edema? *Graefe's Arch Clin Exp Ophthalmol*. 2007;245:627–636.
93. Lorenzi M. The polyol pathway as a mechanism for diabetic retinopathy: attractive, elusive, and resilient. *Exp Diabetes Res*. 2007.
94. Luan H, Roberts R, Sniegowski M, Goebel DJ, Berkowitz BA. Retinal thickness and subnormal retinal oxygenation response in experimental diabetic retinopathy. *Invest Ophthalmol Vis Sci*. 2006;47:320–328.
95. Moss SE, Klein R, Klein BEK. The 14-year incidence of visual loss in a diabetic population. *Ophthalmology*. 1998;105:998–1003.
96. Emanuele N, Klein R, Moritz T, Davis MD, Glander K, Anderson R, et al. Comparison of dilated fundus examinations with seven-field stereo fundus photographs in the Veterans Affairs Diabetes Trial. *J Diabetes Complicat*. 2009;23:323–9.
97. Early Treatment Diabetic Retinopathy Study Group. Grading diabetic retinopathy from stereoscopic color fundus photographs – an extension of the modified Airlie house classification, ETDRS Report No. 10. *Ophthalmology*. 1991;98:786–806.
98. Kiri A, Dyer DS, Bressler NM, Bressler SB, Schachat AP. Detection of diabetic macular edema: Nidek 3Dx stereophotography compared with fundus biomicroscopy. *Am J Ophthalmol*. 1996;122:654–662.
99. Kinyoun J, Barton FB, Fishner MR, Hubbard LD, Aiello LP, Ferris FL, et al. Detection of diabetic macular edema: ophthalmoscopy versus photography-early treatment diabetic retinopathy study report number 5. *Ophthalmology*. 1989;96:746–751.
100. Krepler K, Wagner J, Sacu S, Wedrich A. The effect of intravitreal triamcinolone on diabetic macular edema. *Graefe's Arch Clin Exp Ophthalmol*. 2004;243:478–481.
101. NegiA K, Vernon SA, Lim CS, Owen-Armstrong K. Intravitreal triamcinolone improves vision in eyes with chronic macular edema refractory to laser photocoagulation. *Eye*. 2005;19:747–751.
102. Tunc M, Onder HI, Kaya M. Posterior sub-tenon's capsule triamcinolone injection combined with focal laser photocoagulation for diabetic macular edema. *Ophthalmology*. 2005;112:1086–1091.
103. Ciardella AP, Klancik J, Schiff W, Barile G, Langton K, Chang S. Intravitreal triamcinolone for the treatment of refractory diabetic macular edema with hard exudates: an optical coherence tomography study. *Br J Ophthalmol*. 2004;88:1131–1136.
104. Knudsen LL. Retrobulbar injection of methylprednisolone in diffuse diabetic macular edema. *Retina*. 2004; 24:905–909.
105. Avci R, Kaderli B. Intravitreal triamcinolone injection for chronic diabetic macular edema with severe hard exudates. *Graefe's Arch Clin Exp Ophthalmol*. 2006;244:28–35.
106. Jonas JB, Kreissig I, Sofker A, Degenring RF. Intravitreal injection of triamcinolone for diffuse diabetic macular edema. *Arch Ophthalmol*. 2003;121:57–61.

107. McDonald HR, Schatz H. Grid photocoagulation for diffuse macular edema. *Retina*. 1985;5:65–72.
108. Haritoglou C, Kook D, Neubauer A, WOlf A, Priglinger S, Strauss R, et al. Intravitreal bevacizumab (Avastin) therapy for persistent diffuse diabetic macular edema? *Retina*. 2006;26:999–1005.
109. Arevalo JF, Fromow-Guerra J, Quiroz-Mercado H, Sanchez JG, Wu L, Maia M, et al. Primary intravitreal bevacizumab (Avastin) for diabetic macular edema. Results from the Pan-American Collaborative Retina Study Group at 6-month follow-up. *Ophthalmology*. 2007;114:743–750.
110. Bailey CC, Sparrow JM, Grey RHB, Cheng H. The national diabetic retinopathy laser treatment audit I. Maculopathy. *Eye*. 1998;12:69–76.
111. Kumar A, Sinha S, Azad R, Sharma YR, Vohra R. Comparative evaluation of vitrectomy and dye-enhanced ILM peel with grid laser in diffuse diabetic macular edema. *Graefe's Arch Clin Exp Ophthalmol*. 2006;245:360–368.
112. Abu El Asrar AM, Morse PH. Laser photocoagulation control of diabetic macular edema without fluorescein angiography. *Br J Ophthalmol*. 1991;75:97–99.
113. Aylward GW. Progressive changes in diabetics and their management. *Eye*. 2005;19:1115–1118.
114. Zein WM, Noureddin BN, Jurdi FA, Schakal A, Bashshur ZF. Panretinal photocoagulation and intravitreal triamcinolone acetonide for the management of proliferative diabetic retinopathy with macular edema. *Retina*. 2006;26:137–142.
115. Bresnick GH. Diabetic macular edema. A review? *Ophthalmology*. 1986;93:989–997.
116. Gaucher D, Sebah C, Erinay A, Haouchine B, Tadayoni R, Gaudric A, et al. Optical coherence tomography features during the evolution of serous retinal detachment in patients with diabetic macular edema. *Am J Ophthalmol*. 2008;145:289–296.
117. Bardak Y, Cekic O, Tig SU. Comparison of ICG-assisted ILM peeling and triamcinolone-assisted posterior vitreous removal in diffuse diabetic macular oedema. *Eye*. 2006;20:1357–1359.
118. Zander E, Herfurth S, Bohl B, Heinke P, Herrmann U, Kohnert KD, et al. Maculopathy in patients with diabetes mellitus type 1 and type 2: associations with risk factors. *Br J Ophthalmol*. 2000;84:871–876.
119. Yamamoto S, Yamamoto T, Hayashi M, Takeuchi S. Morphological and functional analyses of diabetic macular edema by optical coherence tomography and multifocal electroretinograms. *Graefe's Arch Clin Exp Ophthalmol*. 2001;239:96–101.
120. Velez-Montoya E, Fromow-Guerra J, Burgos O, Landers MB III, Morales-Caton V, Quiroz-Mercado H. The effect of unilateral intravitreal bevacizumab (Avastin) in the treatment of diffuse bilateral diabetic macular edema. A pilot study. *Retina*. 2009; 29:20–26.
121. Kook D, Wolf A, Kreutzer T, Neubauer A, Strauss R, Ulbig M, et al. Long-term effect of intravitreal bevacizumab (Avastin) in patients with chronic diffuse diabetic macular edema. *Retina*. 2009;28: 1053–1060.
122. Verma LK, Vivek MB, Kumar A, Tewari HK, Venkatesh P. A prospective controlled trial to evaluate the adjunctive role of posterior sub-tenon triamcinolone in the treatment of diffuse diabetic macular edema. *J Ocul Pharmacol Ther*. 2004;20:277–284.
123. Lee SJ, Choi MG. Association of manganese superoxide dismutase gene polymorphism (V16A) with diabetic macular edema in Korean type 2 diabetic patients. *Metabolism*. 2006;55:1681–1688.
124. Berman DH, Friedman EA. Partial absorption of hard exudates in patients with diabetic end-stage renal disease and severe anemia after treatment with erythropoietin. *Retina*. 1994;14:1–5.
125. Greenstein VC, Chen H, Hood DC, Holopigian K, Seiple W, Carr RE. Retinal function in diabetic macular edema after focal laser photocoagulation. *Invest Ophthalmol Vis Sci*. 2000;41:3655–3664.
126. Greenstein VC, Holopigian K, Hood DC, Seiple W, Carr RE. The nature and extent of retinal dysfunction associated with diabetic macular edema. *Invest Ophthalmol Vis Sci*. 2000;41:3643–3654.
127. Gaucher D, Tadayoni R, Erginay A, Haouchine B, Gaudric A, Massin P. Optical coherence tomography assessment of the vitreoretinal relationship in diabetic macular edema. *Am J Ophthalmol*. 2005;139:807–813.
128. Schatz H, Patz A. Cystoid maculopathy in diabetics? *Arch Ophthalmol*. 1976;94:761–768.
129. Jensen DB, Knudsen LL. Stereoscopic fluorescein angiography in diabetic maculopathy. *Retina*. 2006; 26:153–158.
130. Gibran SK, Cullinane A, Jungkim S, Cleary PE. Intravitreal triamcinolone for diffuse diabetic macular edema. *Eye*. 2006;20:720–724.
131. Jeppesen P, Bek T. Impaired retinal autoregulation in small retinal arterioles before and after focal laser treatment for diabetic maculopathy. *Br J Ophthalmol*. 2006; 90:198–201.
132. Catier A, Tadayoni R, Paques M, Erginay A, Haouchine B, Gaudric A, et al. Characterization of macular edema from various etiologies by optical coherence tomography. *Am J Ophthalmol*. 2005;140:200–206.
133. Early Treatment Diabetic Retinopathy Study Group. Classification of diabetic retinopathy from fluorescein angiograms. ETDRS Report Number 11. *Ophthalmology*. 1991;98:807–822.
134. Early Treatment Diabetic Retinopathy Study Research Group. Focal photocoagulation treatment of diabetic macular edema-relationship of treatment effect to fluorescein angiographic and other retinal characteristics at baseline: ETDRS report number 19. *Arch Ophthalmol*. 1995;113:1144–1155.
135. Browning DJ, Fraser C. Regional patterns of sight-threatening diabetic macular edema. *Am J Ophthalmol*. 2005;140:117–124.
136. Browning DJ, Apte RS, Bressler SB, Chalam KV, Danis RP, Davis MD, et al. Association of the extent of diabetic macular edema as assessed by optical coherence tomography with visual acuity and retinal outcome variables. *Retina*. 2009;29:300–305.
137. Browning DJ, Altaweel MM, Bressler NM, Bressler SB, Scott IU, Diabetic Retinopathy Clinical Research

Network. Diabetic macular edema: what is focal and what is diffuse. *Am J Ophthalmol.* 2008;146:649–655.

138. Lee CM, Olk RJ. Modified grid laser photocoagulation for diffuse diabetic macular edema long-term visual results. *Ophthalmology.* 1991;98:1594–1602.
139. Hauser D, Bukelman A, Pokroy R, Katz H, Len A, Thein R, et al. Intravitreal triamcinolone for diabetic macular edema. Comparison of 1, 2 and 4 mg.? *Retina.* 2008;28:825–830.
140. Spandau UHM, Derse M, Schmitz-Valckenberg P, Papoulis C, Jonas J. Dosage dependency of intravitreal triamcinolone acetonide as treatment for diabetic macular edema. *Br J Ophthalmol.* 2005;89:999–1003.
141. Chieh JJ, Roth DB, Liu M, Belmone J, Nelson M, Regillo C, et al. Intravitreal triamcinolone acetonide for diabetic macular edema. *Retina.* 2005;25:828–834.
142. Martidis A, Duker JS, Greenberg PB, Rogers AH, Puliafito CA, Reichel E, et al. Intravitreal triamcinolone for refractory diabetic macular edema. *Ophthalmology.* 2002;109:920–927.
143. Browning DJ, McOwen MD, Bowen RM Jr, O'Marah TL. Comparison of the clinical diagnosis of diabetic macular edema with diagnosis by optical coherence tomography. *Ophthalmology.* 2004;111:712–715.
144. Brown JC, Solomon SD, Bressler SB, Schachat AP, DiBernardo C, Bressler NM. Detection of diabetic foveal edema; contact lens biomicroscopy compared with optical coherence tomography. *Arch Ophthalmol.* 2004;122:330–335.
145. Browning DJ, Fraser CM. The predictive value of patient and eye characteristics on the course of subclinical diabetic macular edema? *Am J Ophthalmol.* 2008; 145:149–154.
146. Patel JI, Hykin PG, Schadt M, Luong V, Fitzke F, Gregor ZJ. Pars plana vitrectomy for diabetic macular oedema: OCT and functional correlations. *Eye.* 2006;20:674–680.
147. Rosenblatt BJ, Shah GK, Sharma S, Bakal J. Pars plana vitrectomy with internal limiting membranectomy for refractory diabetic macular edema without a taut posterior hyaloid. *Graefe's Arch Clin Exp Ophthalmol.* 2005;243:20–25.
148. Do DV, Shah SM, Sung JU, Haller JA, Nguyen QD. Persistent diabetic macular edema is associated with elevated hemoglobin A1c. *Am J Ophthalmol.* 2005; 139:620–623.
149. Stolba U, Binder S, Gruber D, Krebs I, Aggermann T, Neumaier B. Vitrectomy for persistent diffuse diabetic macular edema. *Am J Ophthalmol.* 2005; 140:295–301.
150. Massin P, Audren F, Haouchine B, Erginay A, Bergmann JF, Benosman R, et al. Intravitreal triamcinolone acetonide for diffuse diabetic macular edema; preliminary results of a prospective controlled trial. *Ophthalmology.* 2004;111:218–225.
151. Gangnon R, Hubbard LD, Aiello LM, Chew EY, Ferris FL, Fisher MR, et al. A severity scale for diabetic macular edema developed from ETDRS data. *Invest Ophthalmol Vis Sci.* 2008;49:5041–5047.
152. Davis MD, Sheetz MJ, Aiello LP, Milton RC, Danis RP, Zhi X, et al. Effect of ruboxistaurin on the visual acuity decline associated with longstanding diabetic macular edema. *Invest Ophthalmol Vis Sci.* 2009;50:1–4.
153. Recchia FM, Ruby AJ, Recchia CAC. Pars plana vitrectomy with removal of the internal limiting membrane in the treatment of persistent diabetic macular edema. *Am J Ophthalmol.* 2005;139:447–454.
154. Brun SC, Bressler SB, Maguire MG. A comparison of fundus biomicroscopy and 90 diopter lens examination in the detection of diabetic macular edema. *Invest Ophthalmol Vis Sci.* 1993;34:72.
155. Rudniskey CJ, Tennant MTS, de Leon AP, Hinz BJ, Greve MDJ. Benefits of stereopsis when identifying clinically significant macular edema via teleophthalmology. *Can J Ophthalmol.* 2006;41:727–732.
156. Bresnick GH, Mukamel DB, Dickinson JC, Cole DR. A screening approach to the surveillance of patients with diabetes for the presence of vision-threatening retinopathy. *Ophthalmology.* 2000;107:19–24.
157. Davis MD, Bressler SB, Aiello LP, Bressler NM, Browning DJ, Flaxel CJ, et al. Comparison of time-domain OCT and fundus photographic assessments of retinal thickening in eyes with diabetic macular edema. *Invest Ophthalmol Vis Sci.* 2008;49:1745–1752.
158. Sander B, Hamann P, Larsen M. A 5-year follow-up of photocoagulation in diabetic macular edema: the prognostic value of vascular leakage for visual loss. *Graefe's Arch Clin Exp Ophthalmol.* 2008;246:1535–1539.
159. Sander B, Thornit DN, Colmorn L, Strom C, Girach A, Hubbard LD, et al. Progression of diabetic macular edema: correlation with blood-retinal barrier permeability, retinal thickness, and retinal vessel diameter. *Invest Ophthalmol Vis Sci.* 2007;48:3983–3987.
160. Chew EY, Benson WR, Boldt HC, Chang TS, Lobes LA, Miller JW, et al. Diabetic retinopathy preferred practice guidelines. San Franciso: American Academy of Ophthalmology; 2003.
161. Browning DJ, Elmore C. Is the outcome of focal photocoagulation for diabetic macular edema influenced by using preoperative fluorescein angiography(FA). (Abstract). American Academy of Ophthalmology Annual Meeting. 1998.
162. Kylstra JA, Brown JC, Jaffe GJ, Cox TA, Gallenmore R, Greven CM, et al. The importance of fluorescein angiography in planning laser treatment of diabetic macular edema. *Ophthalmology.* 1999;106:2068–2073.
163. Diabetic Retinopathy Clinical Research Network, Scott IU, Edwards AR, Beck RW, Bressler NM, Chan CK, et al. A phase II randomized clinical trial of intravitreal bevacizumab for diabetic macular edema? *Ophthalmology.* 2007;114:1860–1867.
164. Razvi FM, Kritzinger EE, Tsaloumas MD, Ryder REJ. Use of fluorescein angiography in the diagnosis of diabetic macular edema within a diabetic retinopathy screening program. *Diabetes Med.* 2001;18:1003–1006.
165. Massin P, Girach A, Erginay A, Gaudric A. Optical coherence tomography: a key to the future management of patients with diabetic macular edema. *Acta Ophthalmol Scand.* 2006;84:466–474.
166. Lee P, Blumberg DM. Understanding the critical importance of diagnosis in the measurement of quality of care. *Arch Ophthalmol.* 2008;126:426–427.

167. Bressler NM, Edwards AR, Antoszyk AN, Beck RW, Browning DJ, Ciardella AP, et al. Retinal thickness on stratus optical coherence tomography in people with diabetes and minimal or no diabetic retinopathy. *Am J Ophthalmol*. 2008;145:894–901.
168. Browning DJ. Interobserver variability in optical coherence tomography for macular edema. *Am J Ophthalmol*. 2004;137:1116–1117.
169. Browning DJ, Fraser CM. Intraobserver variability in optical coherence tomography. *Am J Ophthalmol*. 2004; 138:477–479.
170. Diabetic Retinopathy Clinical Research Network. Reproducibility of macular thickness and volume using Zeiss optical coherence tomography in patients with diabetic macular edema. *Ophthalmology*. 2007; 114:1520–1525.
171. Massin P, Viaut E, Haouchine B, Erginay A, Paques M, Gaudric A. Reproducibility of retinal mapping using optical coherence tomography. *Arch Ophthalmol*. 2001; 119:1135–1142.
172. Koozekanani D, Roberts C, Katz SE, Herderick EE. Intersession repeatability of macular thickness measurements with the Humphrey 2000 OCT. *Invest Ophthalmol Vis Sci*. 2000;41:1486–1491.
173. Browning DJ, Fraser C, Propst BW. The variation in optical coherence tomography-measured macular thickness in diabetic eyes without clinical macular edema. *Am J Ophthalmol*. 2008;145:889–893.
174. Toda J, Fukushima H, Kato S. Injection of triamcinolone acetonide into the posterior sub-tenon capsule for treatment of diabetic macular edema.? *Retina*. 2007;27: 764–769.
175. Striph GG, Hart WM, Olk RJ. Modified grid laser photocoagulation for diabetic macular edema-the effect on the central visual field. *Ophthalmology*. 1988;95: 1673–1679.
176. Browning DJ, Glassman AR, Aiello LP, Bressler NM, Bressler S, Danis RP, et al. Optical coherence tomography measurements and analysis methods in optical coherence tomography studies of diabetic macular edema. *Ophthalmology*. 2008;115:1366–1371.
177. Chan A, Duker JS. A standardized method for reporting changes in macular thickening using optical coherence tomography. *Arch Ophthalmol*. 2005;123:939–943.
178. Otani T, Kishi S, Maruyama Y. Patterns of diabetic macular edema with optical coherence tomography. *Am J Ophthalmol*. 1999;127:68–693.
179. Kang SW, Park CY, Ham DI. The correlation between fluorescein angiographic and optical coherence tomographic features in clinically significant diabetic macular edema. *Am J Ophthalmol*. 2004;137:313–322.
180. Ozdek SC, Erdinc MA, Gurelik G, Aydin B, Bahceci U, Hasanreisoglu B. Optical coherence tomographic assessment of diabetic macular edema: comparison with fluorescein angiographic and clinical findings. *Ophthalmologica*. 2004;219:86–92.
181. Diabetic Retinopathy Clinical Research Network. Diurnal variation in retinal thickening measurement by optical coherence tomography in center-involved diabetic macular edema. *Arch Ophthalmol*. 2006;124: 1701–1707.
182. Hee MR, Puliafito CA, Wong C, Duker JS, Reichel E, Rutledge B, et al. Quantitative assessment of macular edema with optical coherence tomography. *Arch Ophthalmol*. 1995;113:1019–1029.
183. Forooghian F, Cukras C, Meyerle CB, Chew EY, Wong WT. Evaluation of time domain and spectral domain optical coherence tomography in the measurement of diabetic macular edema. *Invest Ophthalmol Vis Sci*. 2008;49:4290–4296.
184. Kakinoki M, Sawada O, Sawada T, Kawamura H, Ohji M. Comparison of macular thickness between Cirrus HD-OCT and Stratus OCT. *Ophthalmic Surg Lasers Imaging*. 2008;39:S37–S42.
185. Legaretta JE, Gregori G, Punjabi OS, Knighton RW, Lalwani GA, Puliafito CA. Macular thickness measurements in normal eyes using spectral domain optical coherence tomography? *Ophthalmic Surg Lasers Imaging*. 2008;39:S43-S49.
186. Drexler W. Cellular and functional optical coherence tomography of the human retina? *Invest Ophthalmol Vis Sci*. 2007;48:5340.
187. Menke MN, Dabov S, Knecht P, Sturm V. Reproducibility of retinal thickness measurements in healthy subjects using spectralis optical coherence tomography. *Am J Ophthalmol*. 2009;147:467–472.
188. Brasil OFM, Smith SD, Galor A, Lowder CY, Sears JE, Kaiser PK. Predictive factors for short-term visual outcome after intravitreal triamcinolone acetonide injection for diabetic macular edema: an optical coherence tomography study. *Br J Ophthalmol*. 2006;91:761–765.
189. Diabetic Retinopathy Clinical Research Network. Relationship between optical coherence tomography–measured central retinal thickness and visual acuity in diabetic macular edema. *Ophthalmology*. 2007;114:525–536.
190. Browning DJ, Fraser CM, Powers ME. A spreadsheet template for the analysis of optical coherence tomography in the longitudinal management of diabetic macular edema. *Ophthalmic Surg Lasers Imaging*. 2006;37: 399–405.
191. Otani T, Kishi S. Correlation between optical coherence tomography and fluorescein angiography findings in diabetic macular edema. *Ophthalmology*. 2007;114: 104–107.
192. Sander B, Larsen M, Engler C, Moldow B, Larsen N, Lund. Diabetic macular edema: a comparison of vitreous fluorometry, angiography, and retinopathy. *Br J Ophthalmol*. 2002;86:316–320.
193. Bungay PM, Roy MS, Bonner RF. Posterior vitreous fluorophotometry. I. Description of a new analysis procedure and results in normal subjects. *Arch Ophthalmol*. 1989;107:1321–1327.
194. Larsen M, Hommel E, Parving HH, Lund-Andersen H. Protective effect of captopril on the blood-retina barrier in normotensive insulin-dependent diabetic patients with nephropathy and background retinopathy. *Graefe's Arch Clin Exp Ophthalmol*. 1990;228:505–509.
195. Grenda P, Lupo S, Domanico D, Vingolo EM. Efficacy of intravitreal triamcinolone acetonide in long standing diabetic macular edema. A microperimetry and optical coherence tomography study. *Retina*. 2008;28: 1270–1275.

196. Vujosevic S, Midena E, Pilotto E, Radin PP, Chiesa L, Cavarzeran F. Diabetic macular edema: correlation between microperimetry and optical coherence tomography findings. *Invest Ophthalmol Vis Sci.* 2006;47: 3044–3051.
197. Fong D, Segal P, Myers F, Ferris F, Hubbard L, Davis M. Subretinal fibrosis in diabetic macular edema.? *Arch Ophthalmol.* 1997;115:873–877.
198. Diabetes Control and Complications Trial Research Group. Progression of retinopathy with intensive versus conventional treatment in the diabetes control and complications trial. *Ophthalmology.* 1995;102:647–661.
199. Diabetes Control and Complications Trial Research Group. Early worsening of diabetic retinopathy in the diabetes control and complications trial. *Arch Ophthalmol.* 1998;116:874–886.
200. The writing team for the diabetes control and complications trial/Epidemiology of diabetes interventions and complications research group. Effect of intensive therapy on the microvascular complications of type 1 diabetes mellitus. *JAMA.* 2002;287:2563–2569.
201. UK Prospective Diabetes Study (UKPDS) Group. Intensive blood-glucose control with sulphonylureas or insulin compared with conventional treatment and risk of complications in patients with type 2 diabetes (UKPDS 33). *Lancet.* 1998;352:837–853.
202. UK Prospective Diabetes Study Group. Tight blood pressure control and risk of macrovascular and microvascular complications in type 2 diabetes: UKPDS 38. *BMJ.* 1998;317:703–714.
203. Engler CB, Parving HH, Methiesen ER, Larsen M, Lund-Andersen H. Blood-retina barrier permeability in diabetes during acute ACE-inhibition. *Acta Ophthalmol.* 1991;69:581–585.
204. Chowdhury TA, Hopkins D, Dodson PM, Vafidis GC. The role of serum lipids in exudative diabetic maculopathy: is there a place for lipid lowering therapy. *Eye.* 2002;16:689–693.
205. Chew EY, Klein ML, Ferris FL, Remaley NA, Murphy RP, Chantry K, et al. Association of elevated serum lipid levels with retinal hard exudate in diabetic retinopathy-early treatment diabetic retinopathy study (ETDRS) report 22. *Arch Ophthalmol.* 1996;114: 1079–1084.
206. Kremser BG, Falk M, Kieselbach GF. Influence of serum lipid fractions on the course of diabetic macular edema after photocoagulation? *Ophthalmologica.* 1995;209:60–63.
207. Gordon B, Chang S, Kavanagh M, Berrocal M, Yannuzzi L, Robertson C, et al. The effects of lipid lowering on diabetic retinopathy? *Am J Ophthalmol.* 1991;112: 385–391.
208. Harrold BP, Marmion VJ, Gough KR. A double -blind controlled trial of clofibrate in the treatment of diabetic retinopathy. *Diabetes.* 1969;18:285–291.
209. Duncan LJP, Cullen JF, Ireland JF, Nolan J, Clarke BF, Oliver MF. A three-year trial of Atromid therapy in exudative diabetic retinopathy. *Diabetes.* 1968;17:467.
210. Perkovich BT, Meyers SM. Systemic factors affecting diabetic macular edema. *Am J Ophthalmol.* 1988;105: 211–212.
211. Ramsay RC, Knobloch WH, Barbosa JJ, Sutherland DE, Kjellstrand CM, Najarain JS, et al. The visual status of diabetic patients after renal transplantation. *Am J Ophthalmol.* 1979;87:305–310.
212. Ciardella AP. Partial resolution of diabetic macular edema after systemic treatment with furosemide. *Br J Ophthalmol.* 2004;88:1224–1225.
213. Emoto M, Sato AT, Tanabe K, Tanizawa Y, Matsutani A, Oka Y. Troglitazone treatment increases plasma vascular endothelial growth factor in diabetic patients and its mRNA in 3T3-L1 adipocytes. *Diabetes.* 2001; 50:1166–1170.
214. Liazos E, Broadbent DM, Beare N, Kumar N. Spontaneous resolution of diabetic macular oedema after discontinuation of thiazolidenediones. *Diabet Med.* 2008; 25:860–882.
215. Colucciello M. Vision loss due to macular edema induced by rosiglitazone treatment of diabetes mellitus. *Arch Ophthalmol.* 2005;123:1273–1275.
216. Ryan EH, Han DP, Ramsay RC, Cantrill HL, Bennett SR, Dev S, et al. Diabetic macular edema associated with glitazone use. *Retina.* 2006;26:562–570.
217. Aiello LP, Bursell SE, Clermont A, Duh E, Ishii H, Takagi C, et al. Vascular endothelial growth factor-induced retinal permeability is mediated by protein kinase C in vivo and suppressed by an orally effective B-isoform-selective inhibitor. *Diabetes.* 1997;46: 1473–1480.
218. PKC-DRS2 Group. Effect of Ruboxistaurin on visual loss in patients with diabetic retinopathy. *Ophthalmology.* 2006;113:2221–2230.
219. The PKC-DMES Study Group. Effect of ruboxistaurin in patients with diabetic macular edema. Thirty-month results of the randomized PKC-DMES clinical trial. *Arch Ophthalmol.* 2007;125:318–324.
220. Singh R, Abhiramamurthy V, Gupta V, Gupta A, Bhansali A. Effect of multifactorial intervention on diabetic macular edem. *Diabetes Care.* 2006;29:463–464.
221. Wang Q, Klein R, Moss SE, Klein BEK, Hoyer C, Burke K, et al. The influence of combined kidney-pancreas transplantation on the progression of diabetic retinopathy; a case series. *Ophthalmology.* 1994;101: 1071–1076.
222. Early Treatment Diabetic Retinopathy Study Research Group. Treatment techniques and clinical guidelines for photocoagulation of diabetic macular edema-Early treatment diabetic retinopathy study report number 2. *Ophthalmology.* 1987;94:761–774.
223. Roider J, Brinkmann R, Wirbelauer C, Laqua H, Birngruber R. Subthreshold (retinal pigment epithelium) photocoagulation in macular diseases: a pilot study. *Br J Ophthalmol.* 2000;84:40–47.
224. Browning DJ, Zhang Z, Benfield JM. The effect of patient characteristics on response to focal laser treatment for diabetic macular edema. *Ophthalmology.* 1997;104:466–472.
225. Gupta A, Gupta V, Dogra MR, Pandav SS. Risk factors influencing the treatment outcome in diabetic macular oedema. *Ind J Ophthalmol.* 1996;44:145–148.
226. Shimonagano Y, Makiuchi R, Miyazaki M, Doi N, Uemura A, Sakamoto T. Results of visual acuity and

foveal thickness in diabetic macular edema after vitrectomy. *Jpn J Ophthalmol.* 2007;51:204–209.
227. Diabetic Retinopathy Clinical Research Network. A randomized trial comparing intravitreal triamcinolone acetonide and focal/grid photocoagulation for diabetic macular edema. *Ophthalmology.* 2008; 1447–1459.
228. Aiello LM. Perspectives on diabetic retinopathy. *Am J Ophthalmol.* 2003;136:122–135.
229. Patel JI, Hykin PG, Schadt M, Luong V, Bunce C, Fitzke F, et al. Diabetic macular oedema: pilot randomised trial of parts plana vitrectom. *vs.* macular argon photocoagulation? *Eye.* 2006;20:873–881.
230. Schatz H, Madeira D, McDonald R, Johnson R. Progressive enlargement of laser scars following grid laser photocoagulation for diffuse diabetic macular edema. *Arch Ophthalmol.* 1991;109:1549–1551.
231. Framme C, Roider J. Immediate and long-term changes of fundus autofluorescence in continuous wave laser lesions of the retina. *Ophthalmic Surg Lasers Imaging.* 2004;35:131–138.
232. Guyer DR, D'Amico DJ, Smith CW. Subretinal fibrosis after laser photocoagulation for diabetic macular edema. *Am J Ophthalmol.* 1992;113:652–656.
233. Han DP, Mieler WF, Burton TC. Submacular fibrosis after photocoagulation for diabetic macular edema. *Am J Ophthalmol.* 1992;113:513–521.
234. Lewis H, Schachat AP, Haimann MH, Haller JA, Quinlan P, Von Fricken MA, et al. Choroidal neovascularization after laser photocoagulation for diabetic macular edema. *Ophthalmology.* 1990;97:503–511.
235. Ip MS, Edwards AR, Beck RW, Bressler NM. Author reply. *Ophthalmology.* 2009;116:596–507.
236. Kim JE, Pollack JS, Miller DG, Mittra RA, Spaide RF, ISIS Study Group. ISIS-DME. A prospective, randomized, dose-escalation intravitreal steroid injection study for refractory diabetic macular edema. *Retina.* 2008;28:735–740.
237. Thomas D, Bunce C, Moorman C, Laidlaw DAH. A randomized controlled feasibility trial of vitrectomy versus laser for diabetic macular edema? *Br J Ophthalmol.* 2005;89:81–86.
238. Pendergast SD, Hassan TS, Williams GA, Cox MS, Margherio RR, Ferrone PJ, et al. Vitrectomy for diffuse diabetic macular edema associated with a taut premacular posterior hyaloid. *Am J Ophthalmol.* 2000;130:178–186.
239. Blumenkranz MS, Yellachich D, Andersen DE, Wiltberger MW, Mordaunt D, Marcellino GR, et al. Semiautomated patterned scanning laser for retinal photocoagulation. *Retina.* 2006;26:370–376.
240. Browning DJ, Antoszyk AN. The effect of the surgeon and the laser wavelength on the response to focal photocoagulation for diabetic macular edema. *Ophthalmology.* 1999;106:243–248.
241. Browning DJ, Fraser CM, Powers ME. Comparison of the magnitude and time course of macular thinning induced by different interventions for diabetic macular edema: implications for sequence of application. *Ophthalmology.* 2006;113:1713–1719.
242. Diabetic Retinopathy Clinical Research Network. Randomized trial of peribulbar triamcinolone acetonide with and without focal photocoagulation for mild diabetic macular edema. A pilot study. *Ophthalmology.* 2007;114:1190–1196.
243. King RC, Dobree JH, Kok DA, Foulds WS, Dangerfield WG. Exudative diabetic retinopathy. Spontaneous changes and effects of a corn oil diet. *Br J Ophthalmol.* 1963;47:666–672.
244. Joussen AM, Weiss C, Bauer D, Hilgers RD, the TIME Study Group. Triamcinolone versus inner-limiting membrane peeling in persistent diabetic macular edema (TIME study): design issues and implications. *Graefe's Arch Clin Exp Ophthalmol.* 2007;245:1781–1787.
245. Dehghan MH, Ahmadieh H, Ramezani A, Entezari M, Anisian A. A randomized, placebo-controlled clinical trial of intravitreal triamcinolone for refractory diabetic macular edema? *Int Ophthalmol.* 2008;28:7–17.
246. Early Treatment Diabetic Retinopathy Study Research Group. Photocoagulation therapy for diabetic eye disease. *JAMA.* 1985;254:3086.
247. Khairallah M, Brahim R, Allagui M, Chachia N. Comparative effects of argon green and krypton red laser photocoagulation for patients with diabetic exudative maculopathy. *Br J Ophthalmol.* 1996;80:319–322.
248. Olk RJ, Wallow IH, Poulsen GL. Argon green (514 nm) versus krypton red (647 nm) modified grid laser photocoagulation for diffuse diabetic macular edema. *Ophthalmology.* 1990;1101–1112.
249. Smiddy WE, Fine SL, Quigley HA, Dunkelberger G, Hohman RM, Addicks EM. Cell proliferation after laser photocoagulation in primate retina. an autoradiographic study. *Arch Ophthalmol.* 1986;104:1065–1069.
250. Larsen ML, Moeller F, Sander B, Sjoelie AK. Subthreshold micropulse diode laser treatment in diabetic macular edema? *Br J Ophthalmol.* 2004;88:1173–1179.
251. Luttrull JK, Musch DC, Mainster A. Subthreshold diode micropulse photocoagulation for the treatment of clinically significant diabetic macular oedema. *Br J Ophthalmol.* 2005;89:74–80.
252. Akduman L, Olk RJ. Subthreshold (invisible) modified grid diode laser photocoagulation in diffuse diabetic macular edema (DDME). *Ophthalmic Surg Lasers Imaging.* 1999;30:706–714.
253. Figueira J, Khan J, Nunes S, Sivaprasad S, Rosa A, Faria de Abreu J, et al. Prospective randomized controlled trial comparing subthreshold micropulse diode laser photocoagulation and conventional green laser for clinically significant diabetic macular oedema. *Br J Ophthalmol.* 2009;93:1341–1344.
254. Framme C, Schule G, Roider J, Birngruber R, Brinkmann R. Influence of pulse duration and pulse number in selective RPE laser treatment. *Ophthalmic Surg Lasers Imaging.* 2004;34:206–215.
255. Roider J, Hillenkamp F, Flotte T, Birngruber R. Microphotocoagulation: selective effects of repetitive short laser pulses. *Proc Natl Acad Sci USA.* 1993;90:8643–8647.
256. Friberg TR, Karatza EC. The treatment of macular disease using a micropulsed and continuous wave 810-nm diode laser. *Ophthalmology.* 1997;104:2030–2038.
257. Roider J, Michaud NA, Flotte TJ, Birngruber R. Response of the retinal pigment epithelium to selective photocoagulation. *Arch Ophthalmol.* 1992;110:1786–1792.

258. Framme C, Brinkmann R, Birngruber R, Roider J. Autofluorescence imaging after selective RPE laser treatment in macular diseases and clinical outcome: a pilot study. *Br J Ophthalmol.* 2002;86:1099–1106.
259. Roider J, Brinkmann R, Wirbelauer C, Laqua H, Birngruber R. Retinal sparing by selective retinal pigment epithelial photocoagulation. *Arch Ophthalmol.* 1999; 117:1028–1034.
260. Shima C, Ogata N, Minamoto K, Yoshikawa T, Matsuyama K, Matsumura M. Posterior sub-tenon injection of triamcinolone acetonide as pretreatment for focal laser photocoagulation in diabetic macular edema patients. *Jpn J Ophthalmol.* 2008;52:265–268.
261. Bonini-Filho MA, Jorge R, Barbosa JC, Calucci D, Cardillo JA, Costa RA. Intravitreal injection versus sub-tenon's infusion of triamcinolone acetonide for refractory diabetic macular edema: a randomized clinical trial. *Invest Ophthalmol Vis Sci.* 2005;46:3845–3849.
262. Cardillo JA, Melo LAS, Costa RA, Skaf M, Belfort R Jr, Souza-Filho AA, et al. Comparison of intravitreal versus posterior sub-tenon's capsule injection of triamcinolone acetonide for diffuse diabetic macular edema. *Ophthalmology.* 2005;112:1557–1563.
263. Jonas JB, Sofker A. Intraocular injection of crystalline cortisone as adjunctive treatment for diabetic macular edema. *Am J Ophthalmol.* 2001;132:425–426.
264. Gillies MC, Sutter FK, Simpson JM, Larsson J, Ali H, Zhu M. Intravitreal triamcinolone for refractory diabetic macular edema: two-year results of a double-masked, placebo-controlled, randomized clinical trial. *Ophthalmology.* 2006;113:1533–1538.
265. Audren F, Lecleire-Collet A, Erginay A, Haouchine B, Benosman R, Bergmann JF, et al. Intravitreal triamcinolone acetonide for diffuse diabetic macular edema: phase 2 trial comparing 4 mg vs. 2 mg. *Am J Ophthalmol.* 2006;142:794–799.
266. Avitabile T, Longo A, Reibaldi A. Intravitreal triamcinolone compared with macular laser grid photocoagulation for the treatment of cystoid macular edema. *Am J Ophthalmol.* 2005;140:695–702.
267. DRCR Network. A Randomized Trial Comparing Intravitreal Triamcinolone Acetonide and Laser Photocoagulation for Diabetic Macular Edema. www.DRCR.net, 3-1. 2008.
268. Jonas JB. Intravitreal triamcinolone acetonide for diabetic retinopathy. *Dev Ophthalmol.* 2007;39:96–100.
269. Audren F, Lecleire-collet A, Erginay A, Haouchine B, Benosman R, Bergmann JF, et al. Intravitreal triamcinolone acetonide for diffuse diabetic macular edema: phase 2 trial comparing 4 mg vs. 2 mg. *Am J Ophthalmol.* 2006;142:794–799.
270. LamD SC, Chan CKM, Mohamed S, Lai TYY, Li KKW, Li PSH, et al. A prospective randomised trial of different doses of intravitreal triamcinolone for diabetic macular edema. *Br J Ophthalmol.* 2007;91:199–203.
271. Sivaprasad S, Ockrim Z, Massaoutis P, Ikeji F, Hykin PG, Gregor ZJ. Posterior hyaloid changes following intravitreal triamcinolone and macular laser for diffuse diabetic macular edema. *Retina.* 2008;28:1435–1442.
272. Kuppermann BD, Blumenkranz MS, Haller JA, Williams GA, Weinberg DV, Chou C, et al. Randomized controlled study of an intravitreous dexamethasone drug delivery system in patients with persistent macular edema. *Arch Ophthalmol.* 2007;125:309–317.
273. Haller JA, Dugel P, Weinberg DV, Chou C, Whitcup SM. Evaluation of the safety and performance of an applicator for a novel intravitreal dexamethasone drug delivery system for the treatment of macular edema. *Retina.* 2009;29:46–51.
274. Macugen Diabetic Retinopathy Study Group. A phase II randomized double-masked trial of pegaptanib, an anti-vascular endothelial growth factor aptamer, for diabetic macular edema. *Ophthalmology.* 2005;112: 1747–1757.
275. Shimura M, Nakazawa T, Shiono T, Iida T, Sakamoto T, Nishida K. Comparative therapy evaluation of intravitreal bevacizumab and triamcinolone acetonide on persistent diffuse diabetic macular edema. *Am J Ophthalmol.* 2008;145:854–861.
276. Roh MI, Byeon SH, Kwon OW. Repeated intravitreal injection of bevacizumab for clinically significant diabetic macular edema. *Retina.* 2008;28: 1314–1318.
277. Do DV, Nguyen QD, Shah SM, Browning DJ, Haller JA, Chu K, et al. An exploratory study of the safety, tolerability and bioactivity of a single intravitreal injection of vascular endothelial growth factor (VEGF) trap-eye in patients with diabetic macular edema. *Br J Ophthalmol.* 2009;93:144–149.
278. Chun DW, Heier JS, Topping TM, Duker JS, Bankert JM. A pilot study of multiple intravitreal injections of ranibizumab in patients with center-involving clinically significant diabetic macular edema. *Ophthalmology.* 2006;113:1706–1712.
279. Ozkiris A. Intravitreal bevacizumab (Avastin) for primary treatment of diabetic macular edema. *Eye.* 2009; 23:616–620.
280. Macugen Diabetic Retinopathy Study Group. Changes in retinal neovascularization after pegaptanib (Macugen) therapy in diabetic individuals. *Ophthalmology.* 2006;113:23–28.
281. Lam DSC, Lai TYY, Lee VYW, Chan CKM, Liu DTL, Mohamed S, et al. Efficacy of 1.25 mg versus 2.5 mg intravitreal bevacizumab for diabetic macular edema. Six month results of a randomized controlled trial. *Retina.* 2009;29:292–299.
282. Ahmadieh H, Ramezani A, Shoeibi N, Bijanzadeh B, Tabatabaei A, Azarmina M, et al. Intravitreal bevacizumab with or without triamcinolone for refractory diabetic macular edema; a placebo-controlled, randomized trial. *Graefe's Arch Clin Exp Ophthalmol.* 2008; 246:483–489.
283. Soheilian M, Ramezani A, Bijanzadeh B, Yaseri M, Ahmadieh H, Dehghan MH, et al. Intravitreal bevacizumab (Avastin) injection alone or combined with triamcinolone versus macular photocoagulation as primary treatment of diabetic macular edema. *Retina.* 2007;27:1187–1195.
284. Iida T. Combined triamcinolone acetonide injection and grid laser photocoagulation: a promising treatment for diffuse diabetic macular edema. *Br J Ophthalmol.* 2007;91:407–408.

285. Kang SW, Sa HS, Cho HY, Kim JI. Macular grid photocoagulation after intravitreal triamcinolone acetonide for diffuse diabetic macular edema. *Arch Ophthalmol.* 2006;124:653–658.
286. Lam DSC, Chan CKM, Mohamed S, Lai TYY, Lee VYW, Liu DTL, et al. Intravitreal triamcinolone plus sequential grid laser versus triamcinolone or laser alone for treating diabetic macular edema. Six-month outcomes. *Ophthalmology.* 2007;114: 2162–2167.
287. Hikichi T, Fujio N, Akiba J, Azuma Y, Takahashi M, Yoshida A. Association between the short-term natural history of diabetic macular edema and the vitreomacular relationship in type II diabetes mellitus. *Ophthalmology.* 1997;104:473–478.
288. Yamaguchi Y, Otani T, Kishi S. Resolution of diabetic cystoid macular edema associated with spontaneous vitreofoveal separation. *Am J Ophthalmol.* 2003;135: 116–118.
289. Lewis H, Abrams GW, Blumenkranz MS, Camp RV. Vitrectomy for diabetic macular traction and edema associated with posterior hyaloidal traction. *Ophthalmology.* 1992;99:753–759.
290. Harbour JW, Smiddy WE, Flynn HW, Rubsamen PE. Vitrectomy for diabetic macular edema associated with a thickened and taut posterior hyaloid membrane. *Am J Ophthalmol.* 1996;121:405–413.
291. Ikeda T, Sato K, Katano T, Hayashi Y. Improved visual acuity following pars plana vitrectomy for diabetic cystoid macular edema and detached posterior hyaloid. *Retina.* 2000;20:220–222.
292. La Heij, Hendrikse F, Kessels AGH, Derhaag PJM. Vitrectomy results in diabetic macular oedema without evident vitreomacular traction. *Graefe's Arch Clin Exp Ophthalmol.* 2001;239:264–270.
293. Tachi N, Ogino N. Vitrectomy for diffuse macular edema in cases of diabetic retinopathy. *Am J Ophthalmol.* 1996;122:258–260.
294. Terasaki H, Kojima T, Niwa H, Piao CH, Ueno S, Kondo M, et al. Changes in focal macular electroretinograms and foveal thickness after vitrectomy for diabetic macular edema? *Invest Ophthalmol Vis Sci.* 2003;44:4465–5572.
295. Yamamoto T, Akabane N, Takeuchi S. Vitrectomy for diabetic macular edema: the role of posterior vitreous detachment and epimacular membrane. *Am J Ophthalmol.* 2001;132:369–377.
296. Yanyali A, Nohutcu AF, Horozoglu F, Celik E. Modified grid laser photocoagulation versus pars plana vitrectomy with internal limiting membrane removal in diabetic macular edema. *Am J Ophthalmol.* 2005; 139:795–801.
297. Patel JI, Hykin PG, Schadt M, Luong VY, Fitzke F, Gregor ZJ. Pars plana vitrectomy with and without peeling of the inner limiting membrane for diabetic macular edema. *Retina.* 2006;26:5–13.
298. Tamamoto T, Hitani K, Tsukahara I, Yamamoto S, Kawasaki R, Yamashita H, et al. Early postoperative retinal thickness changes and complications after vitrectomy for diabetic macular edema. *Am J Ophthalmol.* 2003;135:14–19.
299. Asami T, Terasaki H, Kachi S, Nakamura M, Yamamura K, Nabeshima T, et al. Ultrastructure of internal limiting membrane removed during plasmin-assisted vitrectomy from eyes with diabetic macular edema. *Ophthalmology.* 2004;111:231–237.
300. Hartley KL, Smiddy WE, Flynn HW Jr, Murray TG. Pars plana vitrectomy with internal limiting membrane peeling for diabetic macular edema. *Retina.* 2008;28: 410–419.
301. Kumagai K, Furukawa M, Ogino N, Larson E, Iwaki M, Tachi N. Long-term follow-up of vitrectomy for diffuse nontractional diabetic macular edema. *Retina.* 2009;29:464–472.
302. Gandorfer A, Messmer EM, Ulbig MW, Kampik A. Resolution of diabetic macular edema after surgical removal of the posterior hyaloid and the inner limiting membrane. *Retina.* 2000;20:126–133.
303. Higuchi A, Ogata N, Jo N, Wada M, Matsumura M. Pars plana vitrectomy with removal of posterior hyaloid face in treatment of refractory diabetic macular edema resistant to triamcinolone acetonide. *Jpn J Ophthalmol.* 2006;50:529–531.
304. Thomas D, Bunce C, Moorman C, Laidlaw AH. Frequency and associations of a taut thickened posterior hyaloid, partial vitreomacular separation, and subretinal fluid in patients with diabetic macular edema. *Retina.* 2005;25:883–888.
305. Shah SP, Laidlaw DA. Vitrectomy for diabetic macular edema. *Am J Ophthalmol.* 2006;141:225.
306. Shah SP, Patel M, Thomas D, Aldington S, Laidlaw DAH. Factors predicting outcome of vitrectomy for diabetic macular edema: results of a prospective study. *Br J Ophthalmol.* 2006;90:33–36.
307. Massin P, Haouchine B, Gaudric A. Macular traction detachment and diabetic edema associated with posterior hyaloidal traction? *Am J Ophthalmol.* 2001; 132:599.
308. Johnson MW. Tractional cystoid macular edema: a subtle variant of the vitreomacular traction syndrome? *Am J Ophthalmol.* 2005;140:184–192.
309. Gaudric A. Macular cysts, holes, and cavitations. *Graefe's Arch Clin Exp Ophthalmol.* 2008;246: 1071–1079.
310. Figueroa MS, Contreras I, Noval S. Surgical and anatomical outcomes of pars plana vitrectomy for diffuse nontractional diabetic macular edema. *Retina.* 2008;28: 420–426.
311. Mochizuki Y, Hata Y, Enaida H, Yoshiyama K, Mitazaki M, Ueno A, et al. Evaluating adjunctive surgical procedures during vitrectomy for diabetic macular edema. *Retina.* 2006;26:143–148.
312. Heij ECL, Hendrikse F, Kessels AGH, Derhaag PJFM. Vitrectomy results in diabetic macular oedema without evident vitreomacular traction. *Graefe's Arch Clin Exp Ophthalmol.* 2001;239:264–270.
313. Ando F, Yasui O, Hirose H, Ohba N. Optic nerve atrophy after vitrectomy with indocyanine green-assisted internal limiting membrane peeling in diffuse diabetic macular edema. *Graefe's Arch Clin Exp Ophthalmol.* 2004;242:995–999.
314. Takaya K, Suzuki Y, Mizutani H, Sakuraba T, Nakazawa M. Long-term results of vitrectomy for removal of

submacular hard exudates in patients with diabetic maculopathy. *Retina*. 2004;24:23–29.
315. Chang YH, Chen PL, Tai MC, Chen CH, Lu DW, Chen JT. Hyperbaric oxygen therapy ameliorates the blood-retinal barrier breakdown in diabetic retinopathy. *Clin Exp Ophthalmol*. 2006;34:584–589.
316. Krott R, Heller R, Aisenbrey S, Bart-Schmidt KU. Adjunctive hyperbaric oxygenation in macular edema of vascular origin. *Undersea Hyperb Med*. 2000;27: 195–204.
317. Nguyen QD, Shah SM, Anden EV, Sung JU, Vitale S, Campochiaro PA. Supplemental oxygen improves diabetic macular edema: a pilot study. *Invest Ophthalmol Vis Sci*. 2004;45:617–624.
318. Sigurdsson R, Begg I. Organised macular plaques in exudative diabetic maculopathy. *Br J Ophthalmol*. 1980; 64:392–397.
319. Avci R, Inan UU, Kaderli B. Long-term results of excision of plaque-like foveal hard exudates in patients with chronic diabetic macular edema. *Eye*. 2008;22: 1099–1104.
320. Early Treatment Diabetic Retinopathy Study Research Group. Early photocoagulation for diabetic retinopathy-ETDRS report number 9. *Ophthalmology*. 1991;98: 766–785.
321. Maia OO Jr, Takahashi BS, Costa RA, Scott IU, Takahashi WY. Combined laser and intravitreal triamcinolone for proliferative diabetic retinopathy and macular edema: one-year results of a randomized clinical trial. *Am J Ophthalmol*. 2009;147:291–297.
322. Mason JO III, Nixon PA, White MF. Intravitreal injection of bevacizumab (Avastin) as adjunctive treatment of proliferative diabetic retinopathy. *Am J Ophthalmol*. 2006;142:685–688.
323. McDonald HR, Schatz H. Macular edema following panretinal photocoagulation. *Retina*. 1985;5:5–10.
324. McDonald H, Schatz H. Visual loss following panretinal photocoagulation for proliferative diabetic retinopathy. *Ophthalmology*. 1985;92:388–393.
325. Nonaka A, Kiryu J, Tsujikawa A, Yamashiro K, Nishijima K, Kamizuru H, et al. Inflammatory response after scatter laser photocoagulation in nonphotocoagulated retina. *Invest Ophthalmol Vis Sci*. 2002;43(4):1204–1209.
326. Er H, Doganay S, Turkoz Y, Cekmen M, Daglioglu MC, Gunduz A, et al. The levels of cytokines and nitric oxide in rabbit vitreous humor after retinal laser photocoagulation. *Ophthalmic Surg Lasers*. 2000;31(6):479–483.
327. Shimura M, Yasuda K, Nakazawa T, Kano T, Ohta S, Tamai M. Quantifying alterations of macular thickness before and after panretinal photocoagulation in patients with severe diabetic retinopathy and good vision. *Ophthalmology*. 2003;110:2386–2394.
328. Shimura M, Yasuda K, Nakazawa T, Tamai M. Visual dysfunction after panretinal photocoagulation in patients with severe diabetic retinopathy and good vision. *Am J Ophthalmol*. 2005;140:8–15.
329. Browning DJ. Visual dysfunction after panretinal photocoagulation in patients with severe diabetic retinopathy and good vision. *Am J Ophthalmol*. 2005;140: 127–128.
330. Shimura M, Yasuda K, Shiono T. Posterior sub-tenon's capsule injection of triamcinolone acetonide prevents panretinal photocoagulation-induced visual dysfunction in patients with severe diabetic retinopathy and good vision. *Ophthalmology*. 2006;113:381–387.
331. Mason JO III, Yunker JJ, Vail R, McGwin G Jr. Intravitreal bevacizumab (Avastin) prevention of panretinal photocoagulation-induced complications in patients with severe proliferative diabetic retinopathy. *Retina*. 2008;28:1319–1324.
332. Blankenship G. A clinical comparison of central and peripheral argon laser panretinal photocoagulation for proliferative diabetic retinopathy. *Ophthalmology*. 1988;95:170–177.
333. Diabetic Retinopathy Clinical Research Network. Observational study of the development of diabetic macular edema following panretinal (scatter) photocoagulation given in 1 or 4 sittings. *Arch Ophthalmol*. 2009;127:132–140.
334. Chung EJ, Roh MI, Kwon OW, Koh HJ. Effects of macular ischemia on the outcome of intravitreal bevacizumab therapy for diabetic macular edema. *Retina*. 2008;28:957–963.
335. Yang CM. Surgical treatment for severe diabetic macular edema with massive hard exudates? *Retina*. 2000; 20:121–125.
336. Kang SW, Park SC, Cho HY, Kang JH. Triple therapy of vitrectomy, intravitreal triamcinolone, and macular laser photocoagulation for intractable diabetic macular edema. *Am J Ophthalmol*. 2007;144:878–885.

Chapter 8
Diabetic Macular Ischemia

Scott E. Pautler

8.1 Introduction

Diabetic retinopathy encompasses many interrelated pathological changes that occur in the retina of diabetic patients. Retinal ischemia has received much attention as a primary risk factor for the development of proliferative diabetic retinopathy.[1] Ischemia affecting the macula has received less attention in the literature likely due to difficulty in detection and lack of treatment options.[2] Retinal capillary nonperfusion was first described by Ashton using India ink preparations of the diabetic retina (Fig. 8.1).[3] Subsequent histological studies revealed acellular capillaries in zones of nonperfusion (Fig. 8.2).[4–7] Clinically, diabetic macular ischemia is detected by fluorescein angiography as a lack of filling of the macular capillaries, which correlates well with reported histological changes.[1,7–9] Although capillary obstruction occurs in the early stages of diabetic retinopathy, precapillary arteriolar and larger arteriolar occlusions become increasingly evident in more advanced stages.[3] The cause and sequence of evolution are not well understood, but the risk factors for DMI are likely those of diabetic retinopathy in general. These include degree and duration of hyperglycemia and hypertension.[10–12] Small studies of DMI identify increased risk of macular ischemia with diabetic macular edema, increased stage of diabetic retinopathy, and other factors that likely relate to severity of diabetes, such as age of onset.[2,13,14] Prevalence data are not available as major population studies of diabetic retinopathy are not geared to identify macular ischemia.[15,16] Despite these gaps in understanding, diabetic macular ischemia is recognized as an important cause of visual disability and poor response to treatment of diabetic macular edema and proliferative diabetic retinopathy.[7,17,18]

8.2 Pathogenesis, Anatomy, and Physiology

Anatomic changes in diabetic macular ischemia include a variety of cellular and extracellular abnormalities resulting in a loss of neuroretinal tissue and occlusion of the microvasculature. These anatomic changes occur in the late stages of diabetic retinopathy along with other complications of diabetic retinopathy, such as macular edema and fibrovascular proliferation. Thus, it is difficult to study macular ischemia in isolation. Furthermore, there are myriad physiological and anatomical alterations with complicated and arcane interactions that have not been fully elucidated to date.

Factors involved in the occlusion of macular capillaries include changes in the vascular lumen itself, as well as interactions with the extraluminal neurosensory retina and intraluminal blood constituents. Diabetes affects both the cellular and extracellular components of the retinal capillary wall. Among the earliest pathological abnormalities are alterations in the retinal capillary basement membrane, which represents the shared basement membrane of the pericytes and endothelial cells.

S.E. Pautler (✉)
Department of Ophthalmology, University Community Hospital, University of South Florida, Tampa, FL 33607, USA
e-mail: pautlers@aol.com

D.J. Browning (ed.), *Diabetic Retinopathy*, DOI 10.1007/978-0-387-85900-2_8,

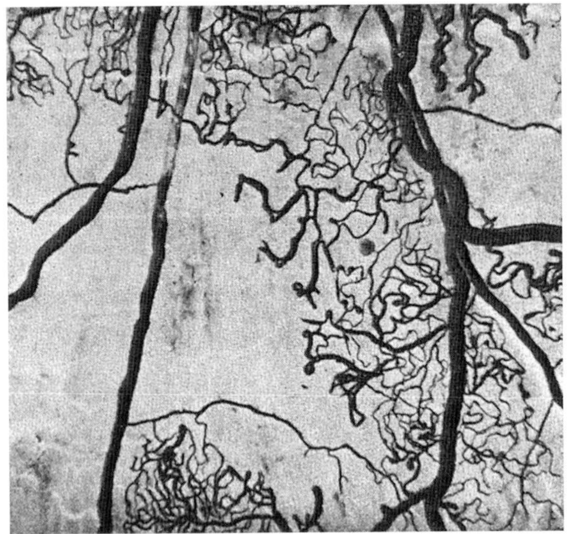

Fig. 8.1 India ink preparation demonstrating capillary loss in diabetic retinopathy. (Reprinted with permission from Ashton.[3] Copyright © 1953 British Journal of Ophthalmology. All rights reserved)

Normally, the basement membrane is primarily composed of a thin, smooth deposition of type IV collagen with macromolecules, which interact with the endothelium. The basement membrane may serve as a skeleton to support cellular components, as a molecular sieve, and metabolically as an inhibitor of proliferation. In diabetic retinopathy, there is thickening of the retinal capillary basement membrane with increased type IV collagen deposition, vacuolization, deposition of fibrillar type III collagen, and decreased heparin sulfate BM-1 proteoglycan.[19–21] The alteration of macromolecules within the basement membrane may result in direct deleterious effects on endothelial cells.[20] The cause of these basement membrane changes appears to be related to the aldose reductase metabolic pathway, advanced glycation end products (AGE) formation, and vascular endothelial growth factor (VEGF).[19,21–25] Retinal cellular dysfunction may result in the formation of abnormal basement membrane by the endothelium.[23,26] Conversely, it is conceivable that basement membrane pathology may be causally related to further subsequent cellular changes. For example, a thickened basement membrane may decrease access of nutrients and oxygen to pericytes and neurosensory retina in a manner analogous to thickening of Bruch's membrane in age-related macular degeneration.[27–29] Low oxygen tension induces the expression of VEGF and its receptors.[25]

Pericytes surround the abluminal capillary surface and play important roles in capillary function. As pericytes are derived from smooth muscle cell precursors, they may regulate vascular tone.[30–32] Pericytes produce structural elements of the extracellular matrix and basement membrane.[30] Pericytes regulate endothelial proliferation and differentiation.[30,33] They are well seen on enzymatic digest preparations with prominent round nuclei on the outer surface of the capillary wall, and loss of pericytes is revealed as empty balloon-like spaces (Fig. 8.3).[6] Pericyte apoptosis occurs early in diabetic retinopathy. Pericytes have a relatively lower rate of proliferation relative to endothelial cells, which are also lost through apoptosis. Consequently,

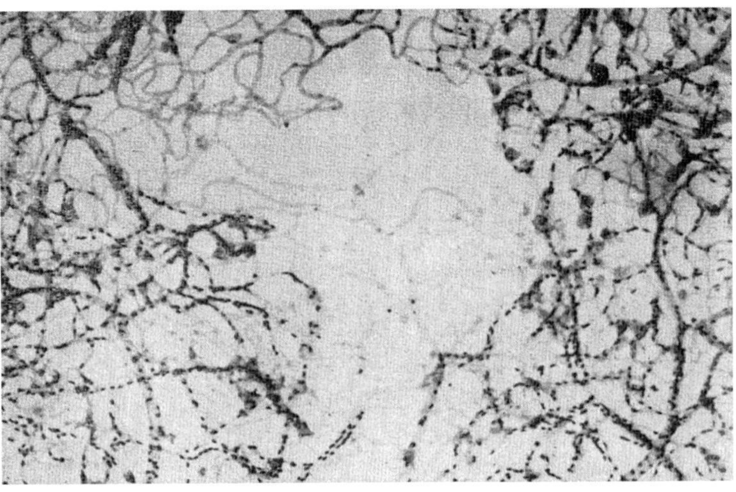

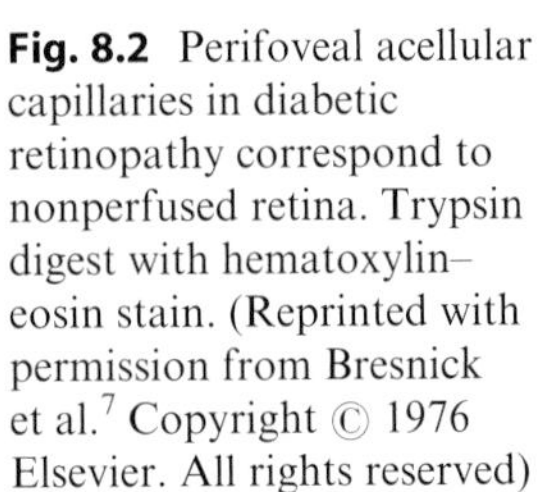

Fig. 8.2 Perifoveal acellular capillaries in diabetic retinopathy correspond to nonperfused retina. Trypsin digest with hematoxylin–eosin stain. (Reprinted with permission from Bresnick et al.[7] Copyright © 1976 Elsevier. All rights reserved)

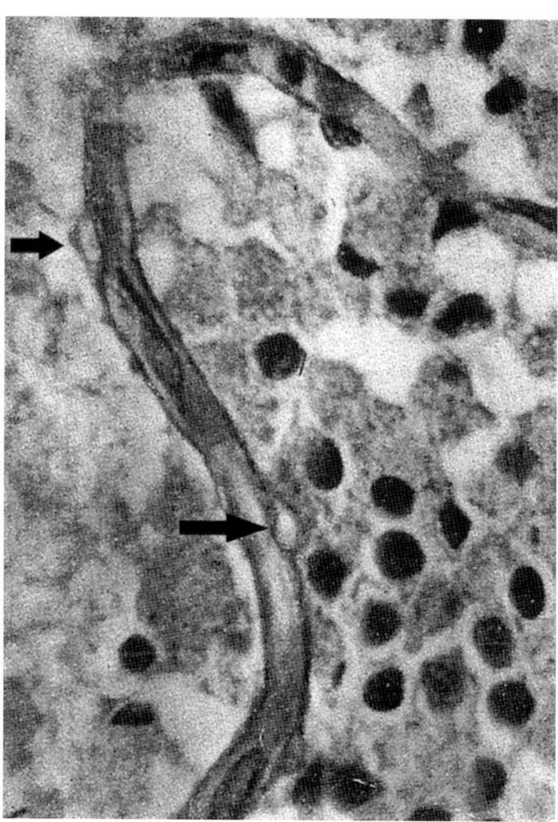

Fig. 8.3 Flat section reveals former pericytes as clear spaces on the outer surface of the capillary wall. (Reproduced with permission from Cogan et al.[5] Copyright © 1961 American Medical Association. All rights reserved)

pathological specimens often show a greater loss of pericytes relative to endothelial cells.[34] A newer concept explaining the loss of pericytes is angiopoietin-induced migration of pericytes from the capillary wall.[35] Because pericyte loss occurs to a much greater degree in the retina than in other tissues, local retinal factors are implicated in the pathogenesis.[4] Additional factors implicated in pericyte loss include impaired adhesion to abnormal basement membrane and adverse effects of hyperglycemia on cell replication.[36,37] The loss of pericytes may lead to closure of capillary lumen though the loss of cytokine interaction with the endothelium.[38] The presence of antipericyte antibodies may represent a risk factor for diabetic macular ischemia; it is unknown whether this is a cause of or a result of tissue damage.[39–41]

The endothelial cell plays a central role in diabetic retinopathy. The endothelium interacts with many humoral and cellular elements, and loss of endothelial cells is associated with capillary closure. The endothelium is a continuous monocellular lining of the luminal wall of retinal capillaries and with intercellular tight junctions creates a barrier to the diffusion of macromolecules (the blood–ocular barrier). Its function is affected by surrounding elements in the capillary wall, the neurosensory retina, and the blood components.[23,26,38] The molecular mechanisms involved in endothelial damage and macular ischemia are complex and include the sorbitol pathway, AGE formation, protein kinase C, renin–angiotensin system, inflammation, oxidation, and alterations in gene expression and in the release of numerous cytokines.[42–54] There may be a balance of angiogenic cytokines, which appear to protect against apoptosis of the endothelium, and anti-angiogenic cytokines, which may induce apoptosis.[55,56] In diabetes, factors in the blood stream that lead to endothelial damage include increased platelet aggregation and adherence, as well as leukostasis resulting from less deformability, increased activation, and increased adhesion.[57–61] Decreased red blood cell deformability and increased aggregation occur with hyperglycemia as well.[62] Normal platelet–endothelial interaction maintains the endothelial vascular integrity through the release of humoral factors that stabilize the tight junctions.[33] Platelets also mediate endothelial–leukocyte interaction and help suppress blood–ocular breakdown when the endothelium becomes damaged.[63,64] The degradation of extracellular matrix in diabetic retinopathy releases fibronectin and associated fragments that stimulate endothelial cell proliferation and adhesion, likely involved in microaneurysm formation and neovascularization.[65] Endothelial cell proliferation may play a role in the pathogenesis of microaneurysms, and hypertrophy may result in capillary occlusion.[66] Subsequent apoptosis of the endothelium may also result in obliteration of the capillary lumen and neurosensory nonperfusion.[7,9,34] Platelet–fibrin thrombi likely contribute to obliteration of the capillary lumen in association with endothelial cell loss.[67] Integrin-mediated leukocyte entrapment is increasingly recognized as a cause of arteriolar occlusion and downstream damage to the capillary bed.[68–71] Following acute occlusion, retinal glial cells invade and proliferate within the vascular lumen.[72]

The Role of VEGF in the Early and Late Stages of Diabetic Retinopathy

VEGF is one of many cytokines that plays a prominent role in diabetic retinopathy and is induced by ischemic neurosensory retina.[73,74] VEGF is a marker of oxidative stress and induces hyperpermeability of macular capillaries contributing to macular edema.[75–77] VEGF also induces endothelial proliferation and migration consistent with clinical findings of microaneurysm and neovascular membrane formation.[53] VEGF prevents apoptosis of capillary endothelial cells.[56] When neurosensory cell death occurs, VEGF production might be expected to decrease with the result of apoptotic endothelial cell loss, capillary occlusion, resolution of macular edema, and involution of neovascularization. Indeed, this clinical picture is seen late in the course of diabetic retinopathy.[78,79] In addition, VEGF offers protection against apoptotic neuroretinal cell death in ischemic retinal conditions.[80] This raises concern regarding the use of multiple injections of anti-VEGF agents in the treatment of eyes with ischemic diabetic retinopathy.[81] The possibility exists that anti-VEGF therapy may help preserve vision in the short term by reducing macular edema and proliferative complications at the long-term expense of eventual neuroretinal apoptosis and capillary dropout. Supporting this hypothesis is the finding that intravitreal bevacizumab (IVB) injections for diabetic macular edema (DME) may result in a decrease in visual acuity in eyes with macular ischemia despite a decrease in macular thickness/edema.[81] Also, a case report demonstrated the acute loss of vision and rapid enlargement of the FAZ following IVB injection in an eye with diabetic macular ischemia.[82] In another report, IVB for severe PDR with traction retinal detachment resulted in acute loss of vision to no light perception.[83] However, in a retrospective case series of DME treated with multiple IVB injections, no progressive change in FAZ diameter was reported.[84] Furthermore, in a small prospective clinical trial of bevacizumab for DME in eyes with severe macular ischemia, no change in perfusion was detected over a 1-year follow-up period.[85] Indeed, some researchers reported subtle evidence of limited improvement in perfusion of the retina following bevacizumab injection, though this apparent change may be due to a reversal of shunting of blood flow through neovascular channels in PDR.[83,86,87] Additional research is needed to better define the role of VEGF in diabetic retinopathy.

There is evidence to suggest that the neurosensory retina plays a role in the evolution of retinal microangiopathy.[88] Prior to the development of diabetic retinopathy, neurosensory retinal dysfunction is evident on testing with ERG, hue discrimination, and contrast sensitivity.[89–97] Early functional changes in neurotransmission are reversible and may be due to hyperglycemia or hypoxia.[92,98,99] Although there is an adaptive response by the retina to hyperglycemia, over time permanent neurosensory damage occurs and may lead to further microvascular changes of diabetic retinopathy.[90,100–102] For example, the hypoxic retina produces VEGF, among other cytokines, in response to hypoxia.[73,103,104] VEGF production may represent an adaptive response to metabolic stress in order to promote neuronal survival.[88] VEGF protects against apoptosis and induces endothelial proliferation, migration, and vasopermeability that may lead to microaneurysm formation, neovascularization, and edema.[53,56,105] Glutamate excitotoxic damage may ultimately lead to neurosensory apoptosis leading to a reduction in cytokine production and resultant retinal capillary cellular apoptosis and capillary closure.[89,106] In addition, lipid mediators are released from the neurosensory retina in response to oxidative stress. These prostanoids contribute to neurovascular injury and directly induce endothelial cell death with subsequent closure of the capillary bed.[67,107] Thus, a number of pathways have been identified to support the role of neurosensory damage in contributing to capillary dropout. In addition, there are examples of retinal vasculopathy secondary to neuronal cell loss in conditions without diabetes. Capillary microangiopathy secondary to neurosensory damage has rarely been described in a laboratory model of glaucoma and in retinitis pigmentosa.[102,108] These data suggest a contributory role of neuroretinal cell loss in causing retinal capillary microangiopathy.

In the final stages of diabetic macular ischemia, neurosensory cellular apoptosis is seen in association with retinal capillary occlusion. Glutamate excitotoxicity appears to play a role in ischemia-associated neuroretinal cell death.[109] Plasminogen activators and oxidative damage contribute to the accumulation of glutamate.[110,111] Clinically, this is manifested by thinning of the macula, which is readily demonstrated on optical coherence tomography (Fig. 8.4).

8.3 Natural History

The natural history of diabetic macular ischemia is not well described. One explanation for the lack of information is the relative rarity of clinically identifiable macular ischemia in large prospective clinical trials using standard fluorescein angiography.[112] Video-fluorescein angiography with the scanning laser ophthalmoscope reveals macular capillary dropout prior to the development of microaneurysms.[113] The Early Treatment Diabetic Study provided some degree of information on the short-term natural history of diabetic macular ischemia. DMI was graded in 1,243 eyes over a 5-year period. However, the study was limited by attrition (36%)

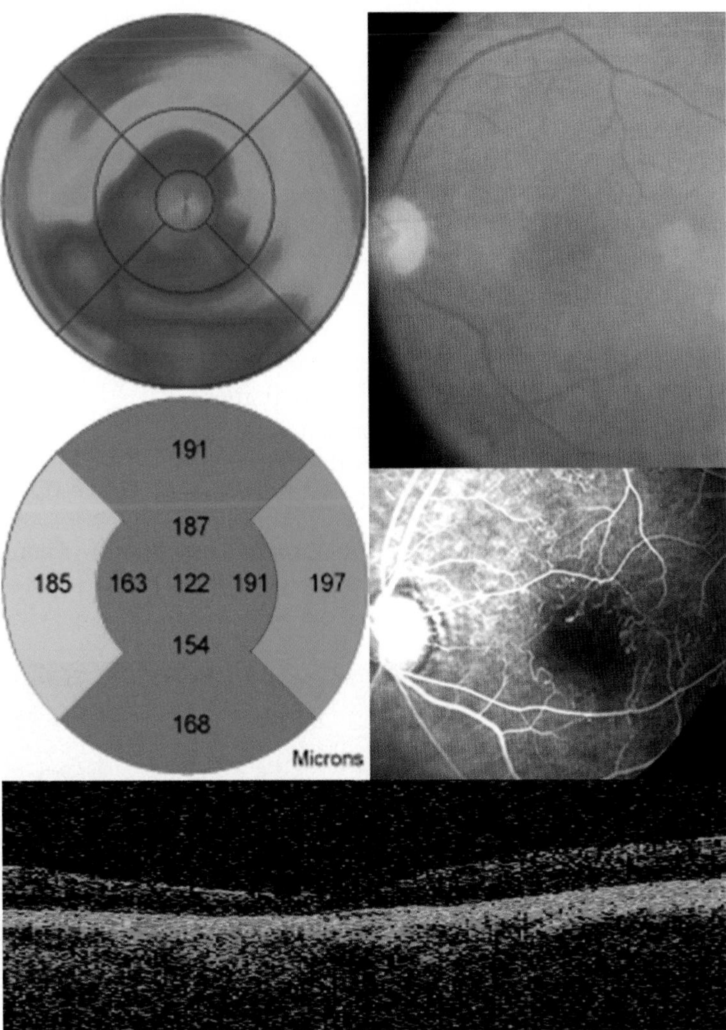

Fig. 8.4 Clinical example of severe diabetic macular ischemia. The time-domain optical coherence tomogram shows thinning of the macula (a dramatic increase in *blue* on the false color map and reduced subfield thickness measurements) and loss of architectural detail (as seen on the line scan at *bottom*). The photograph with fluorescein angiogram demonstrates capillary dropout with an enlarged foveal avascular zone (5.21 mm^2). The visual acuity was 20/125, J10

and by the inclusion of only a few cases of severe macular ischemia. Analysis of the data demonstrated no change in the distribution of severity of diabetic macular ischemia over the 5-year study period.[114] Over the long term, however, diabetic macular ischemia is known to progress. The perifoveal intercapillary area and size of foveal avascular zone increase with advancing stages of diabetic retinopathy.[13,113,115,116] Retinal vascular remodeling may result in limited revascularization at the border of ischemic retina and may result in visual improvement.[68,117] The presumed mechanism appears to be intraretinal neovascularization.[117,118] The potential for improvement in DMI is unknown, but is probably very low. There are no definitive data on the bilaterality or symmetry of DMI. Macular nonperfusion has been reported to occur sooner after the diagnosis of type 2 diabetes than type 1 diabetes.[119] The higher prevalence of coexisting systemic hypertension in patients with type 2 diabetes may offer an explanation of this finding.[10,120–122] However, the true date of onset in type 2 diabetes is more difficult to assess than in type 1 diabetes. The time between the true onset and the diagnosis of type 2 diabetes may be less in young patients than in older patients. In addition, the prevalence of diabetic retinopathy was reportedly higher in type 1 than in type 2 diabetes mellitus in a study of an adolescent cohort.[122] Thus, it appears likely that diabetic macular ischemia develops and progresses as an integral part of diabetic retinopathy related to severity and duration of hyperglycemia.

8.4 Clinical Evaluation

Various modes of clinical study provide information on the structural and functional effects of diabetic macular ischemia. Fundoscopy and fundus photography demonstrate "featureless" areas of ischemic retina in which no microaneurysms, blot hemorrhages, or exudates are present (Fig. 8.5). Surrounding the area of ischemia is the hypoxic penumbra where there are dilated ectatic capillaries and other typical findings of diabetic retinopathy.[68] Larger caliber vessels traversing ischemic areas are attenuated, sheathed, or appear as ghost vessels (Fig. 8.6).[7,123,124] As seen in other ischemic retinopathies, focal depressions in the macula are due to ischemic infarcts.[125]

Fluorescein angiography (FA) is the gold standard in the clinical diagnosis of diabetic macular ischemia. FA displays relative hypofluorescent areas of retina where there is absence of blood flow through the macular capillaries. At the edges of ischemic retina, associated angiographic findings include arteriolar changes and capillary dilatation. The hallmark findings include enlargement and irregularity of the foveal avascular zone (FAZ) and widened, non-uniform spaces between macular capillaries indicative of intervening capillary loss (Fig. 8.7).[7,8,13,115,126] In the late phase of the fluorescein angiogram, the relative hypofluorescent patches of ischemia are surrounded by hyperfluorescent leakage (Fig. 8.8).[8] The normal FAZ as determined by trypsin digestion studies is reported to have an average longest diameter of 0.65 mm with a considerable range from 0.12 to 1.2 mm

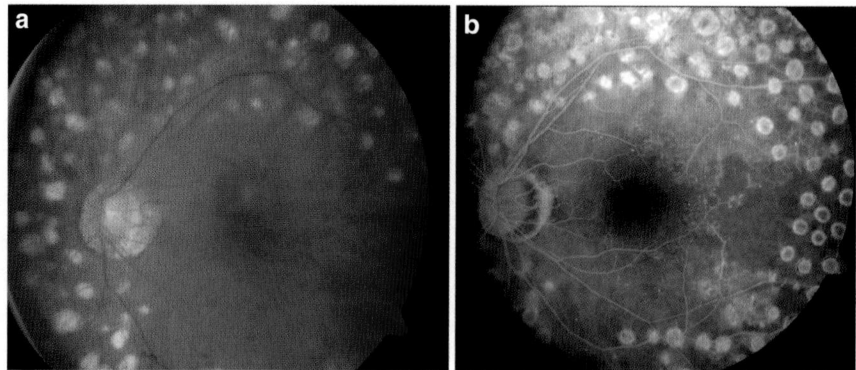

Fig. 8.5 (**a**) Fundus photograph showing featureless temporal macula without microaneurysms or blot hemorrhages in ischemic temporal macula (**b**) Fluorescein angiogram demonstrating capillary dropout in temporal macula

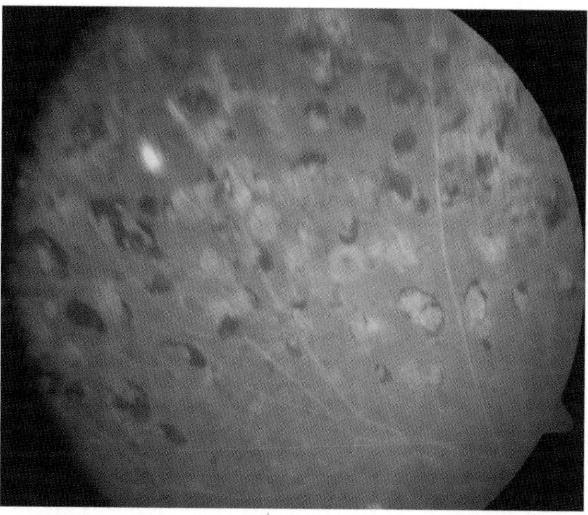

Fig. 8.6 Severely ischemic retina in which sclerotic major retinal vessels appear as white "ghost vessels"

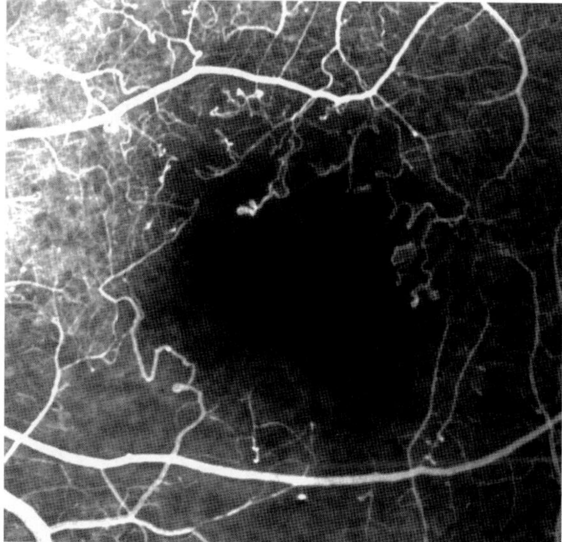

Fig. 8.7 Enlarged, irregular foveal avascular zone with widened spaces between macular capillaries resulting in increased perifoveal intercapillary area (PIA)

area of the FAZ.[127] When measured by fluorescein angiography, the mean diameter (the average of two perpendicular measurements) is 0.53–0.73 mm.[126,128] In diabetic retinopathy the average longest diameter of the FAZ was reported to be 0.94 mm with a range from 0.74 to 1.02 mm.[126] The mean diameter in diabetic eyes was 0.79 with a range of 0.66–0.91 mm.[126] Given the irregularity

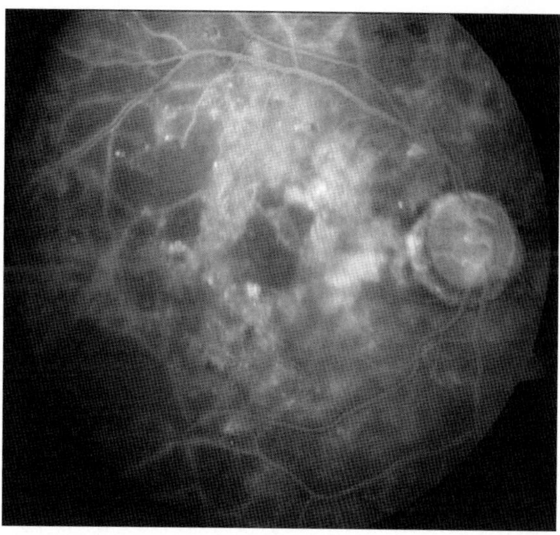

Fig. 8.8 Late-phase fluorescein angiogram demonstrating diabetic macular ischemia as areas of relative hypofluorescence surrounded by diffuse intraretinal fluorescein leakage

of the FAZ in diabetic retinopathy[126], the FAZ area may be a more reliable measurement of ischemia than FAZ diameter. The normal FAZ area is 0.205–0.405 mm^2, similar to that reported in mild-to-moderate NPDR.[2,13,113,115,116,126,129,130] However, the high end of the normal range of FAZ measurements exceeds 2 mm^2 in area.[115,126,131] In severe NPDR and PDR, the reported range of the FAZ is 0.42–0.96 mm^2.[2,13,115,126,129] Certainly, there are cases of severe macular ischemia that exceed these reported ranges (Fig. 8.4). For comparison, one disk areais equal to 1.77 mm^2, assuming one disk diameter equals 1,500 μm.

Grading the degree of diabetic macular ischemia by fluorescein angiography is useful for clinical studies, but is limited by media opacity and lacks uniformity among published reports. The proportion of ungradable angiograms in the ETDRS was low (2%), but selection bias might suggest that media opacity may prevent detailed evaluation in the clinical setting.[114] In a subsequent study in which the ETDRS scheme of grading DMI was used by Goebel et al., fluorescein angiograms were ungradable in 11% of eyes despite the exclusion of eyes with advanced cataract and corneal opacities.[132] Assessment of macular ischemia by evaluating the perifoveal capillaries is appropriate as they appear particularly susceptible to occlusion from diabetes and

FAZ dimensions are strongly positively correlated with the severity of capillary nonperfusion in the posterior retina.[7,126] Various measures of DMI include presence/absence of enlarged or irregular FAZ, nonperfusion within 1,500 μm from foveal center, gradations of areas of ischemia based on disk area, and computerized calculations of the area of ischemia.[13,81,133–135] The measured perimeter of the foveal avascular zone and the FAZ area may be a reasonable substitute for the ETDRS method of assessment, although it does not take into account the impact of ischemia outside the FAZ.[13] The ETDRS approached assessment of macular ischemia by the use of reference photographs that demonstrated the boundaries of the grading groups. For example, standard photograph 1A represented the lower boundary of medium grade capillary loss (Fig. 8.9).[114] Ischemic changes that were graded by the ETDRS included the degree of capillary loss, the size of the FAZ, capillary dilatation, and abnormalities of the arterioles. Capillary loss within 1,500 μm from the fovea was evaluated by dividing the area into five subfields. Each subfield was graded by severity: grade 0 (absence of capillary loss), grade 1 (questionable capillary loss), grade 2 (definite capillary loss, but less than standard photo 1A), grade 3 (moderate capillary loss, equal to or greater than standard photo 1A, but less than standard photo 2), and grade 4 (severe capillary loss, equal to or greater than standard photo 2).[8] The reader is directed to Fig. 8.10 for ETDRS standard photograph 2. The size of the foveal avascular zone was quantified by linear dimension: grade 0 (less than 300 μm), grade 1 (equal to 300 μm), grade 2 (300–500 μm), grade 3 (greater than 500 μm), and grade 8 (cannot grade, e.g., severely irregular FAZ). The outline of the FAZ was also graded by the degree of destruction of the normally smooth round to oval contour: grade 0 (normal), grade 1 (questionable), grade 2 (less than one-half is destroyed), grade 3 (more than one-half of FAZ destroyed, but some remnants remain), grade 4 (FAZ completely destroyed), and grade 8 (cannot grade). Capillary dilatation was graded by standard photographs with the same five-step grading scale as that used for capillary loss. Arteriolar abnormalities associated with ischemia were graded by severity and included focal narrowing, pruning, staining, broadening, and blurred contour. Focal arteriolar narrowing of perpendicular side branches is usually seen in smaller, terminal, or near-terminal branches (Fig. 8.11). Pruning is a short arteriolar stump

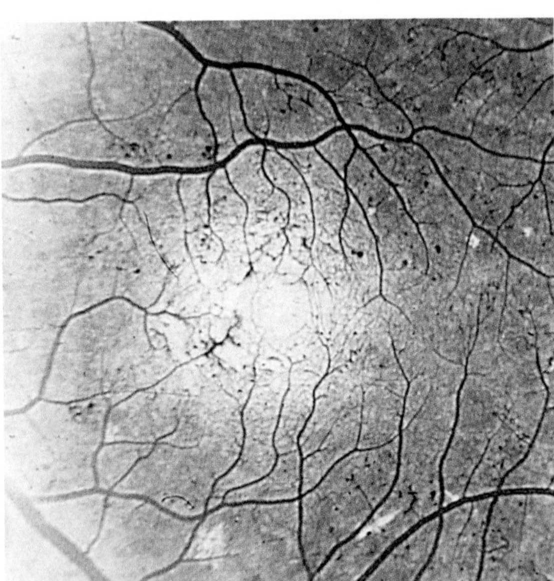

Fig. 8.9 ETDRS standard photograph 1A. Lower boundary of macular ischemia for medium grade capillary loss. (Reproduced with permission from the Early Treatment Diabetic Retinopathy Study Research Group)

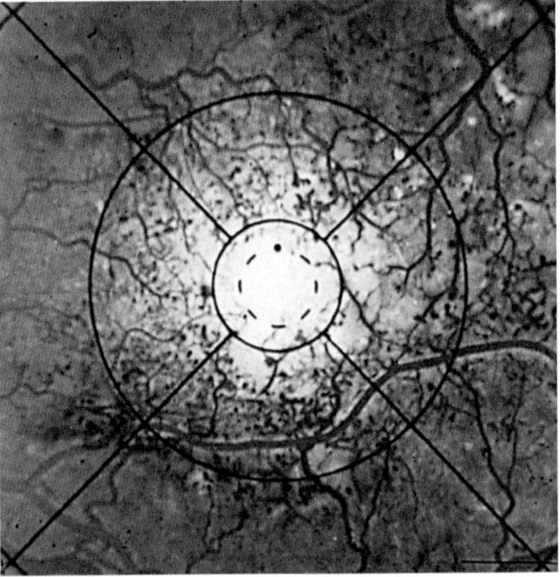

Fig. 8.10 ETDRS standard photograph 2. Lower boundary of macular ischemia for severe grade capillary loss. (Reproduced with permission from the Early Treatment Diabetic Retinopathy Study Research Group)

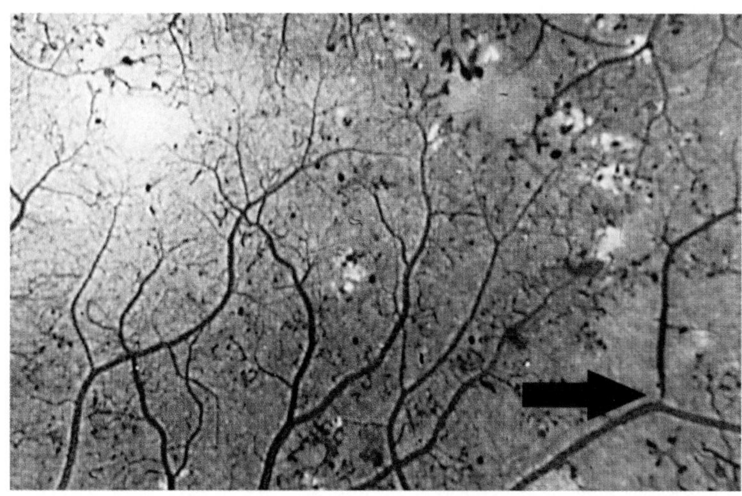

Fig. 8.11 Focal arteriolar narrowing (see *arrow*). (Standard photograph 5A, reproduced with permission from the Early Treatment Diabetic Retinopathy Study Research Group)

directed to an area of capillary loss (Fig. 8.12). Staining is described as narrow fluorescent lines visible on each side of the arteriolar blood column. Staining may also be seen as an arteriolar segment appearing more fluorescent than neighboring segments (Fig. 8.13). Broadening of an arteriolar segment is due to staining of the arteriolar wall and is frequently preceded by a side branch or by focal narrowing of the arteriole. Broadening of an arteriolar segment and blurring of arteriolar contour are due to abnormal fluorescein leakage due to increased permeability. Despite the use of standard photographs, clear definitions, highly trained angiographers, and expert clinicians, there was only moderate inter-observer agreement on grading the degree of DMI in the Early Treatment Diabetic Retinopathy Study (weighted kappa = 0.41–0.60).[8] In the clinical setting, the ETDRS method of grading diabetic macular ischemia may be impractical and of limited clinical use. A recently proposed International Classification of Diabetic Retinopathy did not include grading of macular ischemia.[136]

Optical coherence tomography can accurately and reliably quantify macular thickness in diabetic retinopathy.[137] In diabetes before clinical detection of retinopathy, pericentral retinal thickness may be

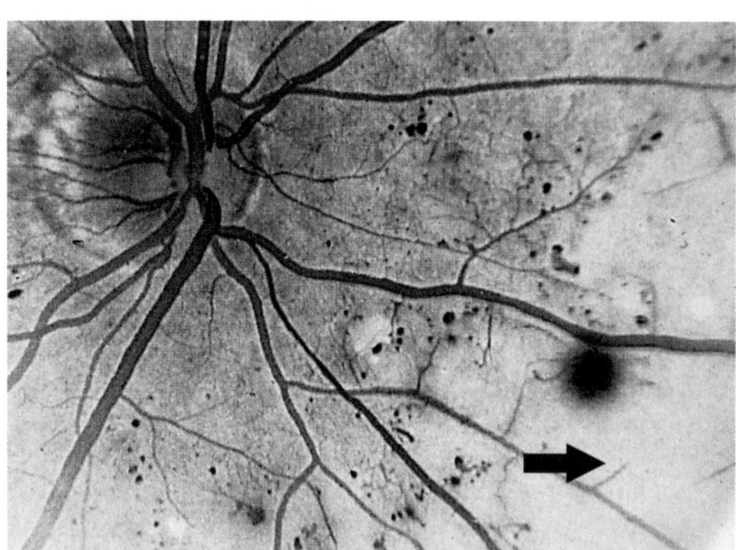

Fig. 8.12 Arteriolar pruning (see *arrow*). (Standard photograph 7, reproduced with permission from the Early Treatment Diabetic Retinopathy Study Research Group)

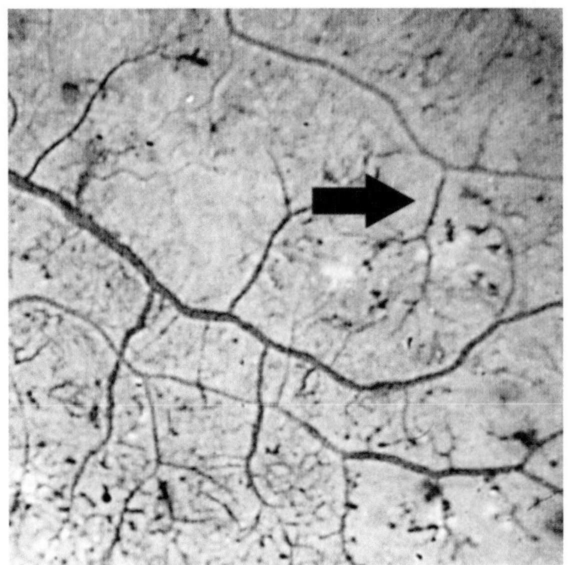

Fig. 8.13 Arteriolar staining/broadening (see *arrow*). (Standard photograph 4, reproduced with permission from the Early Treatment Diabetic Retinopathy Study Research Group)

reduced due to ischemic neurosensory tissue loss.[138,139] Retinal nerve fiber layer thickness is significantly reduced in preproliferative diabetic retinopathy.[140] In specific areas of retinal ischemia there is a disturbance of the inner retina and high-reflective deposit between the outer segments and the retinal pigment epithelium (Fig. 8.14).[141] In the absence of edema, the ischemic areas in the macula appear thin on OCT (Fig. 8.4). Coexisting macular pathology is common in diabetic retinopathy and may complicate the interpretation of OCT.[142] Idiopathic preretinal membranes may cause macular thickening and small retinal cysts.[143] Although the quality and quantity of cystic changes may be helpful in differentiating between diabetic macular edema from preretinal membrane, both cause retinal thickening that may offset neuroretinal thinning from DMI.[141,143–145] This may explain the finding that macular ischemia confounds the correlation of visual acuity with macular thickness in diabetic macular edema (Fig. 8.15).[132,146]

Perimetry provides useful information on functional loss of vision in diabetic retinopathy beyond that of visual acuity.[147] Various methods of perimetry show significant reduction of retinal sensitivity in diabetic eyes prior to the development of clinical findings of retinopathy and these findings are predictive of future development of diabetic retinopathy.[97,148–150] Short-wave automated perimetry (SWAP) isolates the blue–yellow neural pathway and appears more sensitive than standard white-on-white automated perimetry (SAP).[147,151,152] Areas of decreased retinal sensitivity on perimetry reliably correlate well with angiographic areas of capillary dropout.[153–155] With regard to central macular ischemia, mean thresholds of SWAP show abnormalities before loss of visual acuity and the findings correlate well with increasing size of foveal avascular zone and perifoveal intercapillary area.[147,155] Worsening of functional defects on SAT and SWAP correlates well with progression of diabetic retinopathy.[152] Furthermore, visual field defects detected by SWAP are more common in eyes with macular edema, but may reflect ischemic damage rather than macular edema itself.[156] If confirmed, SWAP may be helpful in stratifying patients with diabetic macular edema for potential visual return with treatment. Microperimetry offers the option to test retinal sensitivity while directly observing the fundus and demonstrates loss of retinal sensitivity in areas of ischemia and reduced sensitivity at the border of ischemia.[141,157] Although perimetry may provide helpful information on the functional effect of DMI, it is primarily employed in research at this time.

Considerations in the Management of Glaucoma in Patients with Diabetes

The functional visual field defects and thinning of the nerve fiber layer in diabetic retinopathy may confound the interpretation of diagnostic testing in eyes with coexisting glaucoma.[101,149,158] This complication may also be encountered in patients without any clinical sign of diabetic retinopathy.[101,149,159] In addition, young diabetic women may demonstrate a significant depression in visual field threshold sensitivity in the luteal phase of the menstrual cycle, further exacerbating the problem of fluctuating field loss in glaucomatous eyes.[160]

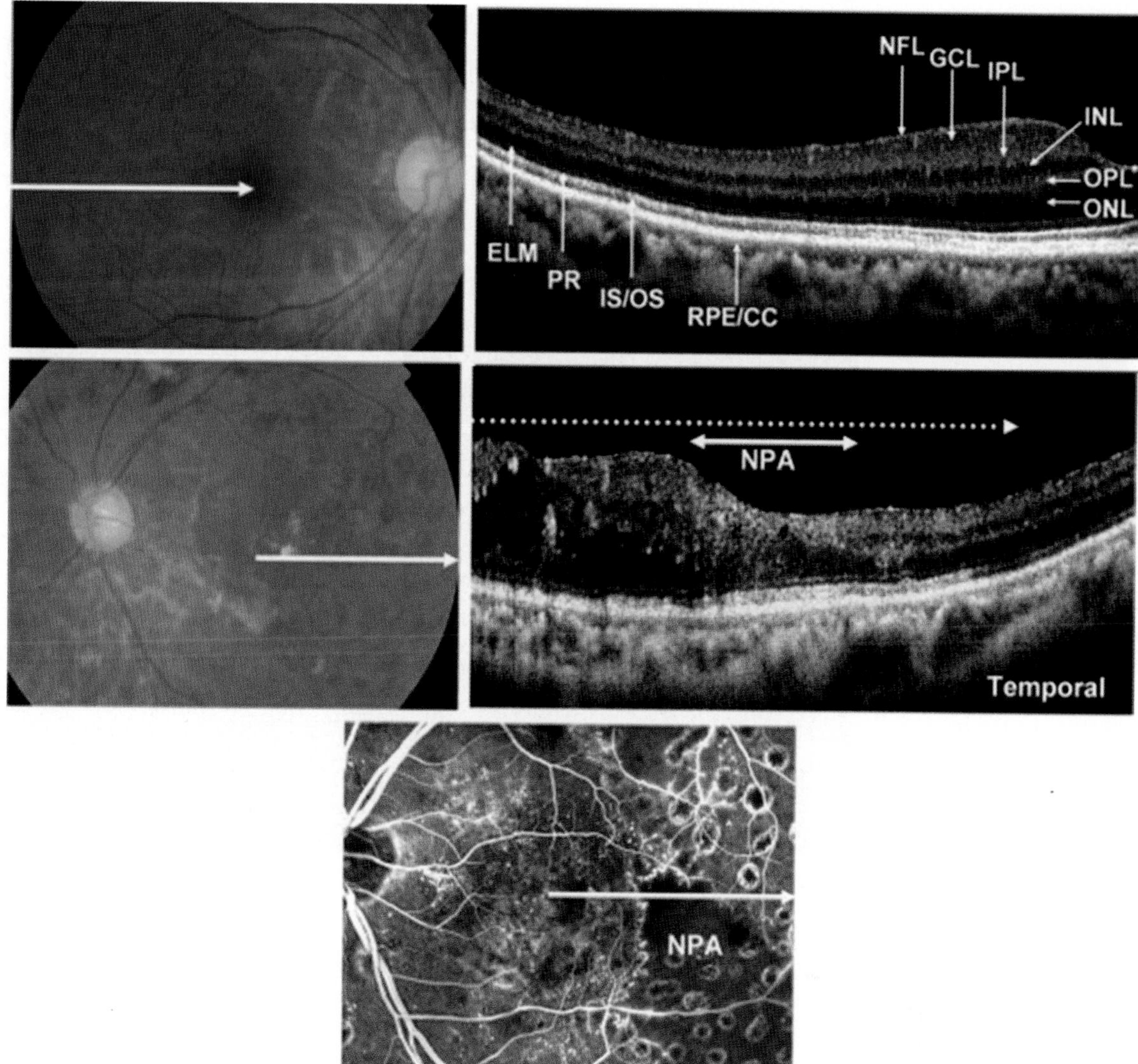

Fig. 8.14 Comparison of normal (*top*) fundus and spectral-domain optical coherence tomography (SD OCT) and severe nonproliferative diabetic retinopathy (*middle*). The *white arrow* in the fundus photos shows the direction of SD OCT scans. *Top right SD OCT scan* shows all ten layers of the normal retina: innermost hyperreflective retinal nerve fiber layer (RNFL), the hyporeflective ganglion cell layer (GCL), the hyperreflective inner plexiform layer (IPL), the hyporeflective inner nuclear layer (INL), the hyperreflective outer plexiform layer (OPL), the hyporeflective outer nuclear layer (ONL), the hyperreflective external limiting membrane (ELM), the hyporeflective photoreceptor cell layer (PR), the hyperreflective photoreceptor inner/outer segment junction (IS/OS), and the hyperreflective retinal pigment epithelium/choriocapillaris (RPE/CC). The *middle right* image demonstrates thinning of inner retinal layers and abnormal high OCT reflectivity between the IS/OS and the RPE/CC on the SD OCT scan in the nonperfused area (NPA, *double-sided arrow*) of the retina. The *bottom image* shows the NPA on the corresponding fluorescein angiogram. (Reprinted from Unoki et al.[141] Copyright © 2007, with permission from Elsevier)

The electroretinogram (ERG) provides an objective measurement of retinal function in diabetes. Prior to the development of clinical or angiographic findings of diabetic retinopathy, ERG most consistently shows an increase in the oscillatory potential implicit time (OP1, suggesting dysfunction among bipolar, amacrine, and ganglion cells possibly related to preclinical circulatory insufficiency), and other functional inner retinal abnormalities are variably described.[90] Progressive retinal dysfunction on ERG correlates with and may be predictive of progressive diabetic microangiopathy seen

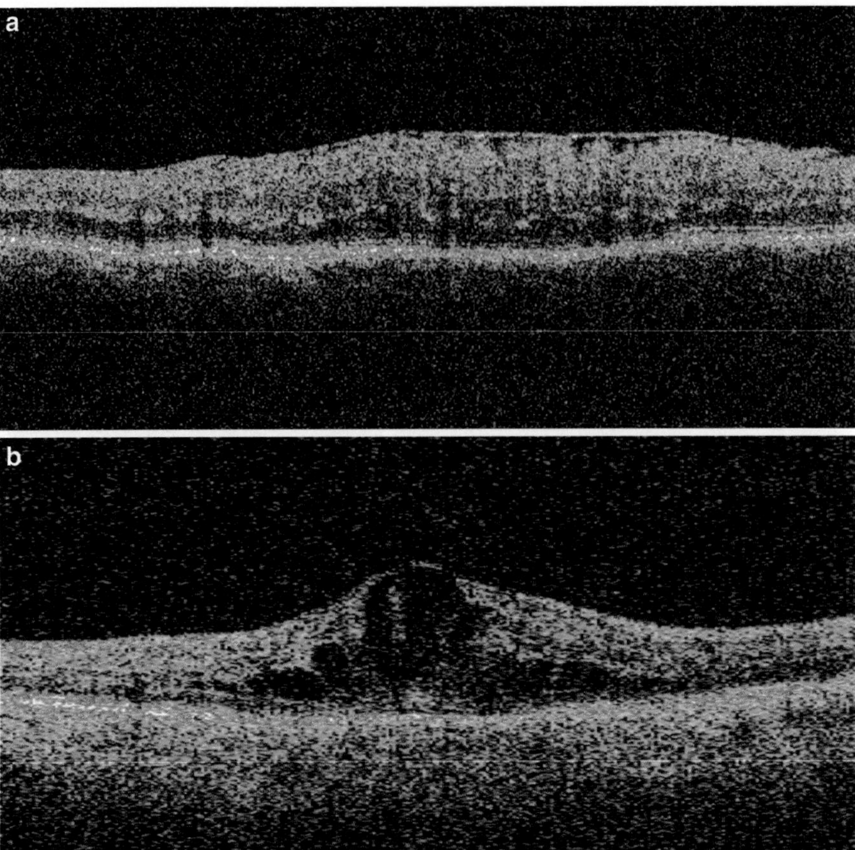

Fig. 8.15 Retinal thickening from premacular membrane (**a**) or diabetic macular edema (**b**) may obscure macular thinning induced by diabetic macular ischemia

clinically.[90] Macular dysfunction studied by multifocal ERG (mfERG) is inconsistently localized to specific areas of apparent pathologic fundus lesions, perhaps due to the presence of occult macular ischemia.[161,162] Foveal cone ERG parameters may be abnormal in diabetic retinopathy with or without edema, but severity of dysfunction on mfERG seems to correlate with degree of retinal thickness.[163,164] The wealth of information on ERG and diabetic retinopathy includes, but does not clearly separate, the effects of diabetic macular ischemia and edema.[90] Electroretinography is not used in the routine clinical management of PDR.

Color perception testing reveals a variety of defects in diabetic retinopathy beginning before significant visual loss.[96,165] Approximately 50% of patients enrolled in the ETDRS had abnormal color vision on the Farnsworth-Munsell 100 hue test.[166] Tritan color defects are the most common color deficiency in diabetic retinopathy and may relate to an S-cone (blue cone) pathway dysfunction or S-cone cell loss.[167–169] In the ETDRS, factors associated with impaired hue discrimination included age, diabetic macular edema, and neovascularization.[170] The severity of macular ischemia and altered retinal blood flow has also been shown to correlate with a tritan defect.[171,172] At this time, little useful clinical information is gleaned by color vision testing.

Contrast sensitivity testing reveals abnormal function before visual acuity testing and may be more sensitive and specific for degree of retinopathy than color vision testing.[94] Contrast sensitivity loss correlates well with fluorescein angiographic evidence of capillary dropout and macular edema.[173,174] Impaired contrast sensitivity may be reversed with improvement in metabolic control in non-ischemic nonproliferative diabetic retinopathy.[175] Oxygen supplementation partially reverses abnormalities in contrast sensitivity and hue discrimination, suggesting retinal hypoxia plays a role in these tests of early functional defects.[98,176] From a clinical standpoint, contrast sensitivity testing does not offer critical information for the clinical decision-making process.

The blue-field entopic phenomenon demonstrates reduced capillary blood flow in diabetic retinopathy.[177] The entopic phenomenon may be used to evaluate the macular capillary hemodynamics as well as measure the size and shape of the foveal avascular zone.[131,178,179] This subjective method of assessment is rarely applied clinically.

8.5 Clinical Significance of Diabetic Macular Ischemia

Although there is no established treatment of diabetic macular ischemia, management decisions are complicated by its presence. DMI is important as it relates to visual function. The ETDRS baseline visual acuity showed little tendency to decrease with worsening of ischemia, except in the group with severe ischemia. However, the number of eyes classified as moderate or severe DMI was small and there was no attempt to control for differences in edema among the groups.[114] Some investigators report that visual acuity correlates well with measures of DMI, including enlargement of the foveal avascular zone ($R^2 = 0.51$) and the parafoveal intercapillary area ($R^2 = 0.24$).[129] Visual acuity less than 20/50 was found to be consistent with an FAZ $\geq$ 0.55 mm^2 or perifoveal intercapillary area $\geq$ 14,000 μm^2 (Fig. 8.16).[129] DMI, as measured by degree of destruction of the FAZ, is better correlated with visual acuity ($R = 0.69$, $P = 0.0014$) than with retinal thickening, as judged by stereo fundus photography.[180] The ETDRS described retinal changes consistent with macular ischemia as the primary cause of decreased acuity in only 10 of 149 eyes with persistent severe visual loss.[181] Others also report profound DMI is a cause of severe visual loss and may limit visual return after treatment of diabetic retinal complications, such as macular edema and traction retinal detachment.[84,124,182] DMI may be underappreciated. Severe DMI is associated with advanced PDR which may be associated with complications of hemorrhage, macular edema, retinal detachment, and neovascular glaucoma, which may overshadow the associated presence of DMI.[181]

Not surprisingly, diabetic macular ischemia portends a poor prognosis in diabetic retinopathy. Capillary loss, in general, is associated with progression from nonproliferative to proliferative diabetic retinopathy.[1] Although capillary dropout is usually most severe outside the macula,[1,183] the presence of DMI has also been reported to be a risk factor for macular edema, PDR, poor visual outcome after vitrectomy, and presence of nephropathy.[114,126,133,183–187] The 1-year risk of developing PDR was 18.2% in NPDR without DMI compared with 41.3% risk in eyes with severe DMI.[1]

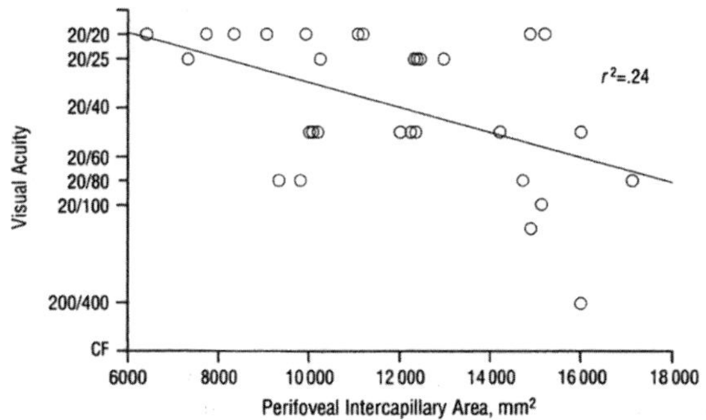

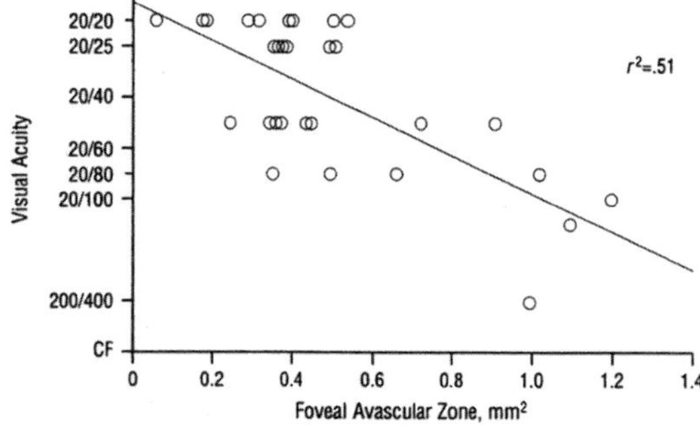

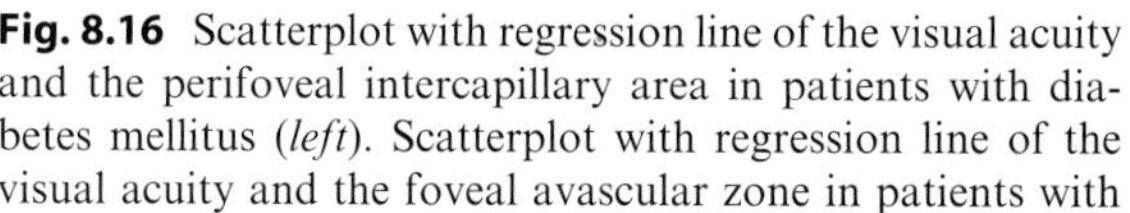

Fig. 8.16 Scatterplot with regression line of the visual acuity and the perifoveal intercapillary area in patients with diabetes mellitus (*left*). Scatterplot with regression line of the visual acuity and the foveal avascular zone in patients with diabetes mellitus (*right*). (Reprinted from the Arend et al.[129] Copyright © 1995 American Medical Association. All rights reserved)

Furthermore, the rate of progression of capillary dropout appears to be greater in eyes with predominant posterior capillary dropout compared with eyes with predominant peripheral or midperipheral involvement, although no statistical analysis is available for review.[126,186]

Macular ischemia may be present in eyes with potentially treatable macular pathology and may impart a poor response to treatment. The ETDRS protocol recommended focal treatment up to 300 μm from the foveal center for persistent CSME and visual acuity less than 20/40.[188] The study demonstrated a trend toward less treatment effect of focal/grid laser for diabetic macular edema in eyes with macular ischemia. This trend did not reach statistical significance possibly as a result of the small number of cases with moderate to severe macular ischemia. At baseline there were 1,243 eyes in the study and only 90 eyes (7%) had moderate or severe ischemia. Consequently, the ETDRS recommended caution in applying their findings supporting focal/grid laser for clinically significant macular edema in eyes with extensive ischemia.[114] Among eyes with diabetic retinopathy with and without macular edema, decreased acuity significantly correlates with measures of increased ischemia, such as extent of foveal capillary loss ($r = 0.585$, $p = 0.0001$), size of FAZ ($r = 0.484$, $p = 0.0015$), and outline of FAZ ($r = 0.542$, $p = 0.0004$).[189] Several investigators report that DMI is associated with poor visual prognosis in the treatment of diabetic macular edema (DME) with laser even though reduction in edema can be achieved.[187,190–192] Similarly, coexistent DMI reduces the short-term beneficial visual effects of bevacizumab and triamcinolone acetonide treatment of DME.[81,135] The visual outcome of vitrectomy performed for a variety of indications is poorer in eyes with macular ischemia as well.[133,134,193] Unfortunately, it is often difficult to determine the primary cause of decreased vision when multiple potential causes are present (e.g., edema, ERM, traction, previous macular detachment, and RPE atrophy). Thus, macular ischemia may be a more significant cause of limited vision in diabetes than is commonly recognized.

In the case of concomitant macular edema and ischemia, it may be useful to determine the degree to which ischemia accounts for decreased vision. If there is no reasonable hope for improvement in vision due to the presence of macular ischemia, laser may be deferred.[191] A trial of intravitreal triamcinolone acetonide for rapid resolution of macular edema may be of use to this end.[194] When presented with the scenario of combined macular edema/ischemia, a recent survey of the American Society of Retinal Specialists (ASRS) showed that almost one-half of 309 respondents indicated they would offer laser treatment among other treatment modalities, including anti-VEGF therapy, steroids, and vitrectomy.[195] This wide spectrum of suggested treatment options underscores the difficulty encountered in managing this clinical presentation.

8.6 Controversies and Conundrums

There are a number of issues of contention regarding diabetic macular ischemia. For example, what role does macular ischemia play in the development of diabetic macular edema? Diabetic macular edema is generally attributed to a breakdown of the blood–ocular barrier. This vasogenic edema results in extracellular accumulation of serous fluid.[196] Others have proposed cytotoxic edema as an additional causative mechanism for DME. Cytotoxic edema may initially manifest as intracellular edema induced by hyperglycemia or hypoxia.[196–199] Retinal hypoxia exacerbated by nocturnal hypotension or high altitude may induce macular edema as evidenced by reversibility upon resolution of the aggravating factor.[198,200,201] The two proposed types of macular edema may not be mutually exclusive. The same factors (ischemia/hypoxia) that presumably induce intracellular edema by a cytotoxic mechanism may also initiate extracellular vasogenic edema through the induction of VEGF.[202]

In eyes with clinically significant macular edema and ischemia, is it safe to treat microaneurysms that line the foveal avascular zone? The ETDRS research group advised against treating microaneurysms bordering capillary dropout near the fovea so as to avoid further capillary closure.[188] This advice appears to have been anecdotal. There is no hard evidence that current focal treatment will exacerbate ischemia. A separate issue is whether the patient might become aware of a scotoma from parafoveal photocoagulation. Further study is needed, but this treatment approach is not proscribed by high-level evidence at this time.

Does the value added by DMI interpretation in clinical care justify the use of fluorescein angiography (FA)? Certainly, the role of FA has decreased with the widespread availability of non-invasive optical coherence tomography (OCT). OCT has proved useful in the management of diabetic macular edema, preretinal membranes, and vitreomacular traction syndromes.[132,142,143,145,163,203,204] Isolated macular ischemia is also identifiable as retinal thinning and loss of retinal structure.[141] The adjunctive use of fluorescein angiography may particularly be helpful in advanced proliferative diabetic retinopathy complicated by macular edema and/or preretinal membranes. In these clinical scenarios the identification of extensive capillary dropout on fluorescein angiography may lead the ophthalmologist away from aggressive treatment aimed at recovery of central vision. However, routine use of fluorescein angiography screening for diabetic macular ischemia appears unnecessary.

What is the role of the choroid in diabetic macular ischemia? Evidence supports recent theories of an ischemic penumbra in diabetic retinopathy, wherein there is preservation of hypoxic retina in a paravascular distribution in the peripheral retina due to the diffusion of oxygen from the larger caliber radial vessels.[68] The persistent release of VEGF from the hypoxic retina may perpetuate the neovascular response in PDR. The release of VEGF also protects retinal capillary endothelial cells from apoptosis and subsequent capillary closure.[55,205,206] Similarly, the choroidal circulation may play a role in the development of capillary dropout in diabetic retinopathy. The choroid supplies oxygen to the outer retina up to the inner nuclear layer.[207] Therefore, the neurosensory retina in the FAZ derives its blood supply from the choroid.[126] Conceivably, the choroidal circulation may offer relative protection against ischemic neurosensory apoptosis from diabetic retinopathy. The general preponderance of retinal capillary occlusion in the peripheral retina as opposed to the posterior pole is consistent with the greater choroidal blood flow in the posterior pole compared with the periphery.[183,186,208,209] If choroidal perfusion becomes impaired, the retina might be more susceptible to ischemic damage from retinal capillary basement membrane thickening. Indeed, there is evidence of a relationship between decreased choroidal blood volume and flow in eyes with more advanced diabetic retinopathy.[210–215] It is interesting to note that choroidal blood flow increases in the macula following panretinal photocoagulation, suggesting a possible secondary beneficial effect on macular perfusion.[216,217] Pentoxyphylline also improves choroidal blood flow in diabetic retinopathy.[218]

8.7 Summary of Key Points

- Diabetic macular ischemia (DMI) is caused by complex interactions of the cellular and noncellular constituents of the vascular wall, the intraluminal blood, and the extraluminal neurosensory retina resulting in nonperfused acellular capillaries and neurosensory cellular apoptosis.
- Macular ischemia can be detected early in diabetic retinopathy and becomes increasingly apparent with advancing stages of severity of diabetic retinopathy.
- DMI is suspected clinically by fundoscopy in areas of "featureless" retina surrounded by typical diabetic microangiopathy. Fluorescein angiography demonstrates the hallmark non-filling of macular capillaries, enlargement and irregularity of the foveal avascular zone (FAZ), and increased perifoveal intercapillary area (PIA). Optical coherence tomography reveals neurosensory macular thinning.
- The magnitude of DMI correlates with visual acuity in diabetic retinopathy with or without macular edema. Consequently, eyes with DMI respond poorly to treatment for concomitant vitreoretinal pathology such as diabetic macular edema, preretinal membrane, and traction macular detachment.
- The FAZ area is a reliable measure of DMI and is recommended for use in clinical studies. Currently, there is no convincing evidence for the need of routine measurements of the FAZ area in clinical practice.

8.8 Future Directions

Prevention of diabetes or prevention of diabetic retinopathy through optimal management of diabetes is an ideal goal. An improved understanding of the autoimmune mechanisms of type 1 diabetes mellitus may eliminate this form of diabetes.[219,220] Unfortunately, epidemic obesity makes the likelihood of elimination of type 2 diabetes an elusive goal in the foreseeable future.[221] However, since the published reports of the DCCT and UKPDS, others have reported decreased prevalence of diabetic retinopathy due to improved metabolic control. In 2003, Henricsson reported a prevalence of diabetic retinopathy of 39% in type 1 diabetes mellitus of 10 years duration in Sweden compared with 63% prevalence in the DCCT.[222] The WESDR also demonstrated a decrease in annual prevalence in the latter part of the 25-year follow-up of eyes with type 1 diabetes.[223] More progress may be anticipated with further improvement in diabetes management.

There is a need for standardization in the method of assessing DMI for uniformity among studies of diabetic retinopathy. The ETDRS method of DMI assessment was detailed, but cumbersome, and has been used in few subsequent studies.[85,132] Various measures commonly studied include FAZ perimeter, FAZ area, and perifoveal intercapillary area (PIA). There is need for general agreement on methods of measurement and on categories of severity in order to assist with comparison among studies. Furthermore, a practical method of assessing DMI would be useful for clinicians, especially if such measurement is found to be pertinent to patient care.

There is a very practical need for improvement in interpretation of optical coherence tomography. Although isolated DMI is associated with macular thinning, coexisting macular pathology may confound OCT interpretation.[141] Diabetic macular edema, preretinal membrane, and vitreomacular traction may cause thickening of the retina despite the presence of ischemia.[141] In addition, retinal thickening is often interpreted as representing retinal edema, regardless of cause. However, as an example, the clinical management of retina thickening from DME is clearly different from that of preretinal membrane.

Research is needed to better understand the correlation of DMI and visual function. Among the many measures that have been evaluated, which ones correlate best with visual acuity and/or visual function? Many studies examine the foveal avascular zone without regard to the potential significance of increased perifoveal intercapillary area.[2,13,84,133,185,224] The practical application of this research might be the proscription of surgery for preretinal membrane or traction retinal detachment if specific criteria are met for severity of DMI. Similarly, an eye with DME may not be capable of improvement in vision if profound ischemia is present. Thus, observation would be in order in such a case rather than protracted treatment.

References

1. Fluorescein angiographic risk factors for progression of diabetic retinopathy. 0TDRS report number 13. Early treatment diabetic retinopathy study research group. *Ophthalmology*. 1991;98:834–40.
2. Conrath J, Giorgi R, Ridings B, Raccah D. Metabolic factors and the foveal avascular zone of the retina in diabetes mellitus. *Diabetes Metab*. 2005;31:465–470.
3. Ashton N. Arteriolar involvement in diabetic retinopathy. *Br J Ophthalmol*. 1953;37:282–292.
4. Garner A. Histopathology of diabetic retinopathy in man. *Eye*. 1993;7(Pt 2):250–253.
5. Cogan DG, Toussant D, Kuwabara T. Retinal vascular patterns. IV. Diabetic retinopathy. *Arch Ophthalmol*. 1961;66:366–378.
6. Kuwabara T, Cogan DG. Retinal vascular patterns. VI. Mural cells of the retinal capillaries. *Arch Ophthalmol*. 1963;69:492–502.
7. Bresnick GH, Engerman R, Davis MD, et al. Patterns of ischemia in diabetic retinopathy. *Trans Sect Ophthalmol Am Acad Ophthalmol Otolaryngol*. 1976;81:OP694–OP709.
8. Classification of diabetic retinopathy from fluorescein angiograms. ETDRS report number 11. Early treatment diabetic retinopathy study research group. *Ophthalmology*. 1991;98:807–822.
9. Kohner EM, Henkind P. Correlation of fluorescein angiogram and retinal digest in diabetic retinopathy. *Am J Ophthalmol*. 1970;69:403–414.
10. UK Prospective Diabetes Study Group. Tight blood pressure control and risk of macrovascular and microvascular complications in type 2 diabetes: UKPDS 38. *BMJ*. 1998;317:703–713.
11. UK Prospective Diabetes Study (UKPDS) Group. Intensive blood-glucose control with sulphonylureas or insulin compared with conventional treatment and risk of complications in patients with type 2 diabetes (UKPDS 33). *Lancet*. 1998;352:837–853.

12. The Diabetes Control and Complications Trial Research Group. The effect of intensive diabetes treatment on the progression of diabetic retinopathy in insulin-dependent diabetes mellitus. *Arch Ophthalmol.* 1995;113:36–51.
13. Conrath J, Giorgi R, Raccah D, Ridings B. Foveal avascular zone in diabetic retinopathy: quantitative vs. qualitative assessment3. *Eye.* 2005;19:322–326.
14. Golubovic-Arsovska M. Correlation of diabetic maculopathy and level of diabetic retinopathy. *Prilozi.* 2006;27:139–150.
15. Klein R, Klein BE, Moss SE, et al. The Wisconsin epidemiologic study of diabetic retinopathy. II. Prevalence and risk of diabetic retinopathy when age at diagnosis is less than 30 years. *Arch Ophthalmol.* 1984; 102:520–526.
16. Klein R, Klein BE, Moss SE, et al. The Wisconsin epidemiologic study of diabetic retinopathy. III. Prevalence and risk of diabetic retinopathy when age at diagnosis is 30 or more years. *Arch Ophthalmol.* 1984;102:527–532.
17. Golubovic-Arsovska M. Correlation of diabetic maculopathy and level of diabetic retinopathy. *Prilozi.* 2006;27: 139–150.
18. Flynn HW, Jr., Chew EY, Simons BD, et al. Pars plana vitrectomy in the early treatment diabetic retinopathy study. ETDRS report number 17. The early treatment diabetic retinopathy study research group. *Ophthalmology.* 1992;99:1351–1357.
19. Tsilibary EC. Microvascular basement membranes in diabetes mellitus. *J Pathol.* 2003;200:537–546.
20. Ljubimov AV, Burgeson RE, Butkowski RJ, et al. Basement membrane abnormalities in human eyes with diabetic retinopathy. *J Histochem Cytochem.* 1996;44: 1469–1479.
21. Frank RN. Aldose reductase activity and basement membrane thickening. *Metabolism.* 1986;35:35–40.
22. Kuiper EJ, Hughes JM, Van Geest RJ, et al. Effect of VEGF-A on expression of profibrotic growth factor and extracellular matrix genes in the retina. *Invest Ophthalmol Vis Sci.* 2007;48:4267–4276.
23. Arjamaa O, Nikinmaa M. Oxygen-dependent diseases in the retina: role of hypoxia-inducible factors. *Exp Eye Res.* 2006;83:473–483.
24. Gardiner TA, Anderson HR, Stitt AW. Inhibition of advanced glycation end-products protects against retinal capillary basement membrane expansion during long-term diabetes. *J Pathol.* 2003;201:328–333.
25. Ferrara N. Vascular endothelial growth factor: basic science and clinical progress. *Endocr Rev.* 2004;25: 581–611.
26. Glaser BM, Kalebic T, Garbisa S, et al. Degradation of basement membrane components by vascular endothelial cells: role in neovascularization. *Ciba Found Symp.* 1983;100:150–162.
27. Williamson JR, Kilo C. Basement-membrane thickening and diabetic microangiopathy. *Diabetes.* 1976;25: 925–927.
28. Zarbin MA. Age-related macular degeneration: review of pathogenesis. *Eur J Ophthalmol.* 1998;8:199–206.
29. Wayland H. Permeability characteristics of microvascular walls. *Biorheology.* 1984;21:107–120.
30. Shepro D, Morel NM. Pericyte physiology. *FASEB J.* 1993;7:1031–1038.
31. Matsugi T, Chen Q, Anderson DR. Contractile responses of cultured bovine retinal pericytes to angiotensin II. *Arch Ophthalmol.* 1997;115:1281–1285.
32. Butryn RK, Ruan H, Hull CM, Frank RN. Vasoactive agonists do not change the caliber of retinal capillaries of the rat. *Microvasc Res.* 1995;50:80–93.
33. Nachman RL, Rafii S. Platelets, petechiae, and preservation of the vascular wall. *N Engl J Med.* 2008;359: 1261–1270.
34. Mizutani M, Kern TS, Lorenzi M. Accelerated death of retinal microvascular cells in human and experimental diabetic retinopathy. *J Clin Invest.* 1996;97:2883–2890.
35. Pfister F, Feng Y, von Hagen F, et al. Pericyte migration: a novel mechanism of pericyte loss in experimental diabetic retinopathy. *Diabetes.* 2008;57:2495–2502.
36. Beltramo E, Buttiglieri S, Pomero F, et al. A study of capillary pericyte viability on extracellular matrix produced by endothelial cells in high glucose. *Diabetologia.* 2003;46:409–415.
37. Li W, Yanoff M, Liu X, Ye X. Retinal capillary pericyte apoptosis in early human diabetic retinopathy. *Chin Med J (Engl).* 1997;110:659–663.
38. Hammes HP, Lin J, Renner O, et al. Pericytes and the pathogenesis of diabetic retinopathy. *Diabetes.* 2002;51: 3107–3112.
39. Nayak RC, Lynch K, Gustavsson C, et al. Circulating antipericyte autoantibodies: a novel modifier of risk of progression of diabetic retinopathy? *Retina.* 2007;27: 211–215.
40. Nayak RC, Agardh E, Kwok MG, et al. Albuminuria and hypertension are independently associated with circulating antipericyte autoantibodies in type 2 diabetic patients. *Metabolism.* 2005;54:188–193.
41. Attawia MA, Nayak RC. Circulating antipericyte autoantibodies in diabetic retinopathy. *Retina.* 1999; 19:390–400.
42. El-Osta A, Brasacchio D, Yao D, et al. Transient high glucose causes persistent epigenetic changes and altered gene expression during subsequent normoglycemia. *J Exp Med.* 2008;205:2409–2417.
43. Brownlee M, Cerami A. The biochemistry of the complications of diabetes mellitus. *Annu Rev Biochem.* 1981;50: 385–432.
44. Brownlee M, Vlassara H, Cerami A. Nonenzymatic glycosylation and the pathogenesis of diabetic complications. *Ann Intern Med.* 1984;101:527–537.
45. Tesfamariam B. Free radicals in diabetic endothelial cell dysfunction. *Free Radic Biol Med.* 1994;16: 383–391.
46. Kuroki M, Voest EE, Amano S, et al. Reactive oxygen intermediates increase vascular endothelial growth factor expression in vitro and in vivo. *J Clin Invest.* 1996;98:1667–1675.
47. Du Y, Smith MA, Miller CM, Kern TS. Diabetes-induced nitrative stress in the retina, and correction by aminoguanidine. *J Neurochem.* 2002;80:771–779.
48. Adamis AP. Is diabetic retinopathy an inflammatory disease? *Br J Ophthalmol.* 2002;86:363–365.

49. Gabbay KH. The sorbitol pathway and the complications of diabetes. *N Engl J Med*. 1973;288:831–836.
50. Xia P, Inoguchi T, Kern TS, et al. Characterization of the mechanism for the chronic activation of diacylglycerol-protein kinase C pathway in diabetes and hypergalactosemia. *Diabetes*. 1994;43:1122–1129.
51. Grant MB, Afzal A, Spoerri P, et al. The role of growth factors in the pathogenesis of diabetic retinopathy. *Expert Opin Invest Drugs*. 2004;13:1275–1293.
52. Aiello LP. The potential role of PKC beta in diabetic retinopathy and macular edema. *Surv Ophthalmol*. 2002;47(Suppl 2):S263–S269.
53. Aiello LP, Wong JS. Role of vascular endothelial growth factor in diabetic vascular complications. *Kidney Int Suppl*. 2000;77:S113–S119.
54. Deinum J, Chaturvedi N. The Renin-Angiotensin system and vascular disease in diabetes. *Semin Vasc Med*. 2002;2:149–156.
55. Stellmach V, Crawford SE, Zhou W, Bouck N. Prevention of ischemia-induced retinopathy by the natural ocular antiangiogenic agent pigment epithelium-derived factor. *Proc Natl Acad Sci USA*. 2001;98:2593–2597.
56. Gupta K, Kshirsagar S, Li W, et al. VEGF prevents apoptosis of human microvascular endothelial cells via opposing effects on MAPK/ERK and SAPK/JNK signaling. *Exp Cell Res*. 1999;247:495–504.
57. Chibber R, Ben-Mahmud BM, Chibber S, Kohner EM. Leukocytes in diabetic retinopathy. *Curr Diabetes Rev*. 2007;3:3–14.
58. De La Cruz JP, Moreno A, Guerrero A, de la Cuesta FS. Antiplatelet effects of prostacyclin and nitric oxide in patients with type I diabetes and ischemic or edematous retinopathy. *Platelets*. 2001;12:210–217.
59. Joussen AM, Poulaki V, Mitsiades N, et al. Nonsteroidal anti-inflammatory drugs prevent early diabetic retinopathy via TNF-alpha suppression. *FASEB J*. 2002;16: 438–440.
60. Joussen AM, Murata T, Tsujikawa A, et al. Leukocyte-mediated endothelial cell injury and death in the diabetic retina. *Am J Pathol*. 2001;158:147–152.
61. Giusti C, Schiaffini R, Brufani C, et al. Coagulation pathways and diabetic retinopathy: abnormal modulation in a selected group of insulin dependent diabetic patients. *Br J Ophthalmol*. 2000;84:591–595.
62. McMillan DE. Development of vascular complications in diabetes. *Vasc Med*. 1997;2:132–142.
63. Nishijima K, Kiryu J, Tsujikawa A, et al. Platelets adhering to the vascular wall mediate postischemic leukocyte-endothelial cell interactions in retinal microcirculation. *Invest Ophthalmol Vis Sci*. 2004;45:977–984.
64. Yamashiro K, Tsujikawa A, Ishida S, et al. Platelets accumulate in the diabetic retinal vasculature following endothelial death and suppress blood-retinal barrier breakdown. *Am J Pathol*. 2003;163:253–259.
65. Wilson SH, Ljubimov AV, Morla AO, et al. Fibronectin fragments promote human retinal endothelial cell adhesion and proliferation and ERK activation through alpha5beta1 integrin and PI 3-kinase. *Invest Ophthalmol Vis Sci*. 2003;44:1704–1715.
66. Hofman P, van Blijswijk BC, Gaillard PJ, et al. Endothelial cell hypertrophy induced by vascular endothelial growth factor in the retina: new insights into the pathogenesis of capillary nonperfusion. *Arch Ophthalmol*. 2001;119:861–866.
67. Boeri D, Maiello M, Lorenzi M. Increased prevalence of microthromboses in retinal capillaries of diabetic individuals. *Diabetes*. 2001;50:1432–1439.
68. McLeod D. A chronic grey matter penumbra, lateral microvascular intussusception and venous peduncular avulsion underlie diabetic vitreous haemorrhage. *Br J Ophthalmol*. 2007;91:677–689.
69. Barouch FC, Miyamoto K, Allport JR, et al. Integrin-mediated neutrophil adhesion and retinal leukostasis in diabetes. *Invest Ophthalmol Vis Sci*. 2000;41:1153–1158.
70. Ogura Y. In vivo evaluation of leukocyte dynamics in the retinal and choroidal circulation. *Jpn J Ophthalmol*. 2000;44:322–323.
71. Lutty GA, Cao J, McLeod DS. Relationship of polymorphonuclear leukocytes to capillary dropout in the human diabetic choroid. *Am J Pathol*. 1997;151:707–714.
72. Bek T. Glial cell involvement in vascular occlusion of diabetic retinopathy. *Acta Ophthalmol Scand*. 1997;75: 239–243.
73. Vinores SA, Youssri AI, Luna JD, et al. Upregulation of vascular endothelial growth factor in ischemic and non-ischemic human and experimental retinal disease. *Histol Histopathol*. 1997;12:99–109.
74. Petrovic MG, Korosec P, Kosnik M, et al. Local and genetic determinants of vascular endothelial growth factor expression in advanced proliferative diabetic retinopathy. *Mol Vis*. 2008;14:1382–1387.
75. Endo M, Yanagisawa K, Tsuchida K, et al. Increased levels of vascular endothelial growth factor and advanced glycation end products in aqueous humor of patients with diabetic retinopathy. *Horm Metab Res*. 2001;33:317–322.
76. Deissler H, Deissler H, Lang S, Lang GE. VEGF-induced effects on proliferation, migration and tight junctions are restored by ranibizumab (Lucentis) in microvascular retinal endothelial cells. *Br J Ophthalmol*. 2008;92:839–843.
77. Nguyen QD, Tatlipinar S, Shah SM, et al. Vascular endothelial growth factor is a critical stimulus for diabetic macular edema. *Am J Ophthalmol*. 2006;142: 961–969.
78. Lange J, Yafai Y, Reichenbach A, et al. Regulation of pigment epithelium-derived factor production and release by retinal glial (Mueller) cells under hypoxia. *Invest Ophthalmol Vis Sci*. 2008;49:5161–5167.
79. Ramsay WJ, Ramsay RC, Purple RL, Knobloch WH. Involutional diabetic retinopathy. *Am J Ophthalmol*. 1977;84:851–858.
80. Nishijima K, Ng YS, Zhong L, et al. Vascular endothelial growth factor-A is a survival factor for retinal neurons and a critical neuroprotectant during the adaptive response to ischemic injury. *Am J Pathol*. 2007;171:53–67.
81. Chung EJ, Roh MI, Kwon OW, Koh HJ. Effects of macular ischemia on the outcome of intravitreal bevacizumab therapy for diabetic macular edema. *Retina*. 2008;28:957–963.

82. Chen E, Hsu J, Park CH. Acute visual acuity loss following intravitreal bevacizumab for diabetic macular edema. *Ophthalmic Surg Lasers Imaging*. 2009;40: 68–70.
83. McDonald HR. Diagnostic and therapeutic challenges. *Retina*. 2009;28:1357–1360.
84. Kook D, Wolf A, Kreutzer T, et al. Long-term effect of intravitreal bevacizumab (avastin) in patients with chronic diffuse diabetic macular edema. *Retina*. 2008;28:1053–1060.
85. Bonini-Filho M, Costa RA, Calucci D, et al. Intravitreal Bevacizumab for diabetic macular edema associated with severe capillary loss: one-year results of a pilot study. *Am J Ophthalmol*. 2009; 147:1022–30.
86. Neubauer AS, Kook D, Haritoglou C, et al. Bevacizumab and retinal ischemia. *Ophthalmology*. 2007;114: 2096.
87. Avery RL. Regression of retinal and iris neovascularization after intravitreal bevacizumab (Avastin) treatment. *Retina*. 2006;26:352–354.
88. Gardner TW, Antonetti DA, Barber AJ, et al. Diabetic retinopathy: more than meets the eye. *Surv Ophthalmol*. 2002;47(Suppl 2):S253–S262.
89. Fletcher EL, Phipps JA, Ward MM, et al. Neuronal and glial cell abnormality as predictors of progression of diabetic retinopathy. *Curr Pharm Des*. 2007;13: 2699–2712.
90. Tzekov R, Arden GB. The electroretinogram in diabetic retinopathy. *Surv Ophthalmol*. 1999;44:53–60.
91. Yoshida A, Kojima M, Ogasawara H, Ishiko S. Oscillatory potentials and permeability of the blood-retinal barrier in noninsulin-dependent diabetic patients without retinopathy. *Ophthalmology*. 1991;98:1266–1271.
92. Li Q, Zemel E, Miller B, Perlman I. Early retinal damage in experimental diabetes: electroretinographical and morphological observations. *Exp Eye Res*. 2002;74:615–625.
93. Shimada Y, Li Y, Bearse MA Jr, et al. Assessment of early retinal changes in diabetes using a new multifocal ERG protocol. *Br J Ophthalmol*. 2001;85: 414–419.
94. Ewing FM, Deary IJ, Strachan MW, Frier BM. Seeing beyond retinopathy in diabetes: electrophysiological and psychophysical abnormalities and alterations in vision. *Endocr Rev*. 1998;19:462–476.
95. Barton FB, Fong DS, Knatterud GL. Classification of Farnsworth-Munsell 100-hue test results in the early treatment diabetic retinopathy study. *Am J Ophthalmol*. 2004;138:119–124.
96. Ong GL, Ripley LG, Newsom RS, Casswell AG. Assessment of colour vision as a screening test for sight threatening diabetic retinopathy before loss of vision. *Br J Ophthalmol*. 2003;87:747–752.
97. Han Y, Adams AJ, Bearse MA Jr, Schneck ME. Multifocal electroretinogram and short-wavelength automated perimetry measures in diabetic eyes with little or no retinopathy. *Arch Ophthalmol*. 2004;122: 1809–1815.
98. Arden GB, Wolf JE, Tsang Y. Does dark adaptation exacerbate diabetic retinopathy? Evidence and a linking hypothesis. *Vision Res*. 1998;38:1723–1729.
99. Kaneko M, Sugawara T, Tazawa Y. Electrical responses from the inner retina of rats with streptozotocin-induced early diabetes mellitus. *Nippon Ganka Gakkai Zasshi*. 2000;104:775–778.
100. Klemp K, Larsen M, Sander B, et al. Effect of short-term hyperglycemia on multifocal electroretinogram in diabetic patients without retinopathy. *Invest Ophthalmol Vis Sci*. 2004;45:3812–19.
101. Lonneville YH, Ozdek SC, Onol M, et al. The effect of blood glucose regulation on retinal nerve fiber layer thickness in diabetic patients. *Ophthalmologica*. 2003;217:347–350.
102. Zheng L, Gong B, Hatala DA, Kern TS. Retinal ischemia and reperfusion causes capillary degeneration: similarities to diabetes. *Invest Ophthalmol Vis Sci*. 2007;48:361–367.
103. Chavakis E, Dimmeler S. Regulation of endothelial cell survival and apoptosis during angiogenesis. *Arterioscler Thromb Vasc Biol*. 2002;22:887–893.
104. Amin RH, Frank RN, Kennedy A, et al. Vascular endothelial growth factor is present in glial cells of the retina and optic nerve of human subjects with nonproliferative diabetic retinopathy. *Invest Ophthalmol Vis Sci*. 1997;38:36–47.
105. Jin KL, Mao XO, Greenberg DA. Vascular endothelial growth factor: direct neuroprotective effect in in vitro ischemia. *Proc Natl Acad Sci USA*. 2000;97:10242–10247.
106. Pulido JE, Pulido JS, Erie JC, et al. A role for excitatory amino acids in diabetic eye disease. *Exp Diabetes Res*. 2007;2007:36150.
107. Hardy P, Beauchamp M, Sennlaub F, et al. New insights into the retinal circulation: inflammatory lipid mediators in ischemic retinopathy. *Prostaglandins Leukot Essent Fatty Acids*. 2005;72:301–325.
108. Nao-i N, Fukiyama J, Sawada A. Retinitis pigmentosa with recurrent vitreous hemorrhage. *Acta Ophthalmol Scand*. 1996;74:509–512.
109. Catalani E, Cervia D, Martini D, et al. Changes in neuronal response to ischemia in retinas with genetic alterations of somatostatin receptor expression. *Eur J Neurosci*. 2007;25:1447–1459.
110. Mali RS, Cheng M, Chintala SK. Plasminogen activators promote excitotoxicity-induced retinal damage. *FASEB J*. 2005;19:1280–1289.
111. Puro DG. Diabetes-induced dysfunction of retinal Muller cells. *Trans Am Ophthalmol Soc*. 2002;100: 339–352.
112. Fong DS, Strauber SF, Aiello LP, et al. Comparison of the modified early treatment diabetic retinopathy study and mild macular grid laser photocoagulation strategies for diabetic macular edema. *Arch Ophthalmol*. 2007; 125:469–480.
113. Arend O, Wolf S, Jung F, et al. Retinal microcirculation in patients with diabetes mellitus: dynamic and morphological analysis of perifoveal capillary network. *Br J Ophthalmol*. 1991;75:514–518.
114. Focal photocoagulation treatment of diabetic macular edema. Relationship of treatment effect to fluorescein angiographic and other retinal characteristics at baseline: ETDRS report no. 19. early treatment diabetic

retinopathy study research group. *Arch Ophthalmol.* 1995;113:1144–1155.
115. Mansour AM, Schachat A, Bodiford G, Haymond R. Foveal avascular zone in diabetes mellitus. *Retina.* 1993;13:125–128.
116. Sander B, Larsen M, Engler C, et al. Early changes in diabetic retinopathy: capillary loss and blood-retina barrier permeability in relation to metabolic control. *Acta Ophthalmol (Copenh).* 1994;72:553–559.
117. Scott IU, Amirikia A, Flynn HW, Jr. Improved retinal capillary perfusion following treatment of severe proliferative diabetic retinopathy. *Ophthalmic Surg Lasers.* 2000;31:148–150.
118. Takahashi K, Kishi S, Muraoka K, Shimizu K. Reperfusion of occluded capillary beds in diabetic retinopathy. *Am J Ophthalmol.* 1998;126:791–797.
119. Kohner EM. The evolution and natural history of diabetic retinopathy. *Int Ophthalmol Clin.* 1978;18:1–16.
120. de B, I, Kestenbaum B, Rue TC, et al. Insulin therapy, hyperglycemia, and hypertension in type 1 diabetes mellitus. *Arch Intern Med.* 2008;168:1867–1873.
121. Li HY, Wei JN, Sung FC, Chuang LM. Higher rate of obesity and hypertension in adolescents with type 2 diabetes than in those with type 1 diabetes. *Diabetes Care.* 2006;29:2326.
122. Eppens MC, Craig ME, Cusumano J, et al. Prevalence of diabetes complications in adolescents with type 2 compared with type 1 diabetes. *Diabetes Care.* 2006;29:1300–1306.
123. Grading diabetic retinopathy from stereoscopic color fundus photographs–an extension of the modified Airlie House classification. ETDRS report number 10. early treatment diabetic retinopathy study research group. *Ophthalmology.* 1991;98:786–806.
124. Bresnick GH, de Venecia G, Myers FL, et al. Retinal ischemia in diabetic retinopathy. *Arch Ophthalmol.* 1975;93:1300–1310.
125. Goldbaum MH. Retinal depression sign indicating a small retinal infarct. *Am J Ophthalmol.* 1978;86:45–55.
126. Bresnick GH, Condit R, Syrjala S, et al. Abnormalities of the foveal avascular zone in diabetic retinopathy. *Arch Ophthalmol.* 1984;102:1286–1293.
127. Bligard E, de Venesia G, Wallow I, et al. Aging changes of the parafoveal vasculature. *Invest Ophthalmol Vis Sci.* 1982;22(suppl):8.
128. Laatikainen L, Larinkari J. Capillary-free area of the fovea with advancing age. *Invest Ophthalmol Vis Sci.* 1977;16:1154–1157.
129. Arend O, Wolf S, Harris A, Reim M. The relationship of macular microcirculation to visual acuity in diabetic patients. *Arch Ophthalmol.* 1995;113:610–614.
130. Parodi MB, Visintin F, Della RP, Ravalico G. Foveal avascular zone in macular branch retinal vein occlusion. *Int Ophthalmol.* 1995;19:25–28.
131. Bradley A, Applegate RA, Zeffren BS, van Heuven WA. Psychophysical measurement of the size and shape of the human foveal avascular zone. *Ophthalmic Physiol Opt.* 1992;12:18–23.
132. Goebel W, Kretzchmar-Gross T. Retinal thickness in diabetic retinopathy: a study using optical coherence tomography (OCT). *Retina.* 2002;22:759–767.
133. Mason JO, III, Colagross CT, Haleman T, et al. Visual outcome and risk factors for light perception and no light perception vision after vitrectomy for diabetic retinopathy. *Am J Ophthalmol.* 2005;140:231–235.
134. Pendergast SD, Hassan TS, Williams GA, et al. Vitrectomy for diffuse diabetic macular edema associated with a taut premacular posterior hyaloid. *Am J Ophthalmol.* 2000;130:178–186.
135. Jonas JB, Martus P, Degenring RF, et al. Predictive factors for visual acuity after intravitreal triamcinolone treatment for diabetic macular edema. *Arch Ophthalmol.* 2005;123:1338–1343.
136. Wilkinson CP, Ferris FL, III, Klein RE, et al. Proposed international clinical diabetic retinopathy and diabetic macular edema disease severity scales. *Ophthalmology.* 2003;110:1677–1682.
137. McDonald HR, Williams GA, Scott IU, et al. Laser scanning imaging for macular disease: a report by the American academy of ophthalmology. *Ophthalmology.* 2007;114:1221–1228.
138. Nilsson M, von WG, Wanger P, Martin L. Early detection of macular changes in patients with diabetes using Rarebit Fovea Test and optical coherence tomography. *Br J Ophthalmol.* 2007;91:1596–1598.
139. Biallosterski C, van Velthoven ME, Michels RP, et al. Decreased optical coherence tomography-measured pericentral retinal thickness in patients with diabetes mellitus type 1 with minimal diabetic retinopathy. *Br J Ophthalmol.* 2007;91:1135–1138.
140. Oshitari T, Hanawa K, chi-Usami E. Changes of macular and RNFL thicknesses measured by Stratus OCT in patients with early stage diabetes. *Eye.* 2009;23:884–889.
141. Unoki N, Nishijima K, Sakamoto A, et al. Retinal sensitivity loss and structural disturbance in areas of capillary nonperfusion of eyes with diabetic retinopathy. *Am J Ophthalmol.* 2007;144:755–760.
142. Lang GE. Optical coherence tomography findings in diabetic retinopathy. *Dev Ophthalmol.* 2007;39:31–47.
143. Gupta P, Sadun AA, Sebag J. Multifocal retinal contraction in macular pucker analyzed by combined optical coherence tomography/scanning laser ophthalmoscopy. *Retina.* 2008;28:447–452.
144. Brasil OF, Smith SD, Galor A, et al. Predictive factors for short-term visual outcome after intravitreal triamcinolone acetonide injection for diabetic macular oedema: an optical coherence tomography study. *Br J Ophthalmol.* 2007;91:761–765.
145. Soliman W, Sander B, Jorgensen TM. Enhanced optical coherence patterns of diabetic macular oedema and their correlation with the pathophysiology. *Acta Ophthalmol Scand.* 2007;85:613–617.
146. Sakata K, Funatsu H, Harino S, et al. Relationship between macular microcirculation and progression of diabetic macular edema. *Ophthalmology.* 2006;113:1385–1391.
147. Bengtsson B, Heijl A, Agardh E. Visual fields correlate better than visual acuity to severity of diabetic retinopathy. *Diabetologia.* 2005;48:2494–2500.
148. Pahor D. Reduction of retinal light sensitivity in diabetic patients. *Klin Monatsbl Augenheilkd.* 2003;220: 868–872.

149. Realini T, Lai MQ, Barber L. Impact of diabetes on glaucoma screening using frequency-doubling perimetry. *Ophthalmology*. 2004;111:2133–2136.
150. Verrotti A, Lobefalo L, Altobelli E, et al. Static perimetry and diabetic retinopathy: a long-term follow-up. *Acta Diabetol*. 2001;38:99–105.
151. Racette L, Sample PA. Short-wavelength automated perimetry. *Ophthalmol Clin North Am*. 2003;16:227-vii.
152. Bengtsson B, Hellgren KJ, Agardh E. Test-retest variability for standard automated perimetry and short-wavelength automated perimetry in diabetic patients. *Acta Ophthalmol*. 2008;86:170–176.
153. Federman JL, Lloyd J. Automated static perimetry to evaluate diabetic retinopathy. *Trans Am Ophthalmol Soc*. 1984;82:358–370.
154. Pahor D. Automated static perimetry as a screening method for evaluation of retinal perfusion in diabetic retinopathy. *Int Ophthalmol*. 1997;21:305–309.
155. Remky A, Arend O, Hendricks S. Short-wavelength automated perimetry and capillary density in early diabetic maculopathy. *Invest Ophthalmol Vis Sci*. 2000;41:274–281.
156. Agardh E, Stjernquist H, Heijl A, Bengtsson B. Visual acuity and perimetry as measures of visual function in diabetic macular oedema. *Diabetologia*. 2006;49: 200–206.
157. Rohrschneider K, Bultmann S, Springer C. Use of fundus perimetry (microperimetry) to quantify macular sensitivity. *Prog Retin Eye Res*. 2008;27:536–548.
158. Takahashi H, Goto T, Shoji T, et al. Diabetes-associated retinal nerve fiber damage evaluated with scanning laser polarimetry. *Am J Ophthalmol*. 2006;142:88–94.
159. Lopes de Faria JM, Russ H, Costa VP. Retinal nerve fibre layer loss in patients with type 1 diabetes mellitus without retinopathy. *Br J Ophthalmol*. 2002;86:725–728.
160. Apaydin KC, Akar Y, Akar ME, et al. Menstrual cycle dependent changes in blue-on-yellow visual field analysis of young diabetic women with severe nonproliferative diabetic retinopathy. *Clin Experiment Ophthalmol*. 2004;32:265–269.
161. Fortune B, Schneck ME, Adams AJ. Multifocal electroretinogram delays reveal local retinal dysfunction in early diabetic retinopathy. *Invest Ophthalmol Vis Sci*. 1999;40:2638–2651.
162. Bronson-Castain KW, Bearse MA, Jr., Han Y, et al. Association between multifocal ERG implicit time delays and adaptation in patients with diabetes. *Invest Ophthalmol Vis Sci*. 2007;48:5250–5256.
163. Holm K, Larsson J, Lovestam-Adrian M. In diabetic retinopathy, foveal thickness of 300 mm seems to correlate with functionally significant loss of vision. *Doc Ophthalmol*. 2007;114:117–124.
164. Weiner A, Christopoulos VA, Gussler CH, et al. Foveal cone function in nonproliferative diabetic retinopathy and macular edema. *Invest Ophthalmol Vis Sci*. 1997;38:1443–1449.
165. Barton FB, Fong DS, Knatterud GL. Classification of Farnsworth-Munsell 100-hue test results in the early treatment diabetic retinopathy study. *Am J Ophthalmol*. 2004;138:119–124.
166. Barton FB, Fong DS, Knatterud GL. Classification of Farnsworth-Munsell 100-hue test results in the early treatment diabetic retinopathy study. *Am J Ophthalmol*. 2004;138:119–124.
167. Mortlock KE, Chiti Z, Drasdo N, et al. Silent substitution S-cone electroretinogram in subjects with diabetes mellitus. *Ophthalmic Physiol Opt*. 2005;25:392–399.
168. Cho NC, Poulsen GL, Ver Hoeve JN, Nork TM. Selective loss of S-cones in diabetic retinopathy. *Arch Ophthalmol*. 2000;118:1393–1400.
169. Barton FB, Fong DS, Knatterud GL. Classification of Farnsworth-Munsell 100-hue test results in the early treatment diabetic retinopathy study. *Am J Ophthalmol*. 2004;138:119–124.
170. Fong DS, Barton FB, Bresnick GH. Impaired color vision associated with diabetic retinopathy: early treatment diabetic retinopathy study report no. 15. *Am J Ophthalmol*. 1999;128:612–617.
171. Tregear SJ, Knowles PJ, Ripley LG, Casswell AG. Chromatic-contrast threshold impairment in diabetes. *Eye*. 1997;11(Pt 4):537–546.
172. Findl O, Dallinger S, Rami B, et al. Ocular haemodynamics and colour contrast sensitivity in patients with type 1 diabetes. *Br J Ophthalmol*. 2000;84:493–498.
173. Arend O, Remky A, Evans D, et al. Contrast sensitivity loss is coupled with capillary dropout in patients with diabetes. *Invest Ophthalmol Vis Sci*. 1997;38:1819–1824.
174. Talwar D, Sharma N, Pai A, et al. Contrast sensitivity following focal laser photocoagulation in clinically significant macular oedema due to diabetic retinopathy. *Clin Exp Ophthalmol*. 2001;29:17–21.
175. Verrotti A, Lobefalo L, Petitti MT, et al. Relationship between contrast sensitivity and metabolic control in diabetics with and without retinopathy. *Ann Med*. 1998;30:369–374.
176. Harris A, Arend O, Danis RP, et al. Hyperoxia improves contrast sensitivity in early diabetic retinopathy. *Br J Ophthalmol*. 1996;80:209–213.
177. Rimmer T, Fallon TJ, Kohner EM. Long-term follow-up of retinal blood flow in diabetes using the blue light entoptic phenomenon. *Br J Ophthalmol*. 1989;73:1–5.
178. Yap M, Gilchrist J, Weatherill J. Psychophysical measurement of the foveal avascular zone. *Ophthalmic Physiol Opt*. 1987;7:405–410.
179. Sinclair SH. Macular retinal capillary hemodynamics in diabetic patients. *Ophthalmology*. 1991;98:1580–1586.
180. Smith RT, Lee CM, Charles HC, et al. Quantification of diabetic macular edema. *Arch Ophthalmol*. 1987;105:218–222.
181. Fong DS, Ferris FL, III, Davis MD, Chew EY. Causes of severe visual loss in the early treatment diabetic retinopathy study: ETDRS report no. 24. Early treatment diabetic retinopathy study research group. *Am J Ophthalmol*. 1999;127:137–141.
182. Helbig H. Surgery for diabetic retinopathy. *Ophthalmologica*. 2007;221:103–111.
183. Shimizu K, Kobayashi Y, Muraoka K. Midperipheral fundus involvement in diabetic retinopathy. *Ophthalmology*. 1981;88:601–612.

184. Shukla D, Kolluru CM, Singh J, et al. Macular ischaemia as a marker for nephropathy in diabetic retinopathy. *Indian J Ophthalmol.* 2004;52:205–210.
185. Espiritu RB, Sy GT. Fluorescein angiographically evident diabetic maculopathy. *Clin Hemorheol Microcirc.* 2003;29:357–365.
186. Niki T, Muraoka K, Shimizu K. Distribution of capillary nonperfusion in early-stage diabetic retinopathy. *Ophthalmology.* 1984;91:1431–1439.
187. Ticho U, Patz A. The role of capillary perfusion in the management of diabetic macular edema. *Am J Ophthalmol.* 1973;76:880–886.
188. Photocoagulation for diabetic macular edema. Early treatment diabetic retinopathy study report number 1. Early treatment diabetic retinopathy study research group. *Arch Ophthalmol.* 1985;103:1796–1806.
189. Sakata K, Funatsu H, Harino S, et al. Relationship of macular microcirculation and retinal thickness with visual acuity in diabetic macular edema. *Ophthalmology.* 2007;114:2061–2069.
190. Cruess AF, Williams JC, Willan AR. Argon green and krypton red laser treatment of diabetic macular edema. *Can J Ophthalmol* 1988;23:262–266.
191. Gardner TW, Eller AW, Friberg TR. Reduction of severe macular edema in eyes with poor vision after panretinal photocoagulation for proliferative diabetic retinopathy. *Graefe's Arch Clin Exp Ophthalmol.* 1991;229:323–328.
192. Olk RJ, Akduman L. Minimal intensity diode laser (810 nanometer) photocoagulation (MIP) for diffuse diabetic macular edema (DDME). *Semin Ophthalmol.* 2001;16:25–30.
193. Gastaud P, Negre F, Leguay JM. Surgical treatment of serous detachments of the macular neuroepithelium in diabetics. *J Fr Ophthalmol.* 1997;20:741–748.
194. Cunningham MA, Edelman JL, Kaushal S. Intravitreal steroids for macular edema: the past, the present, and the future. *Surv Ophthalmol.* 2008;53:139–149.
195. Mittra RA and Pollack JS, ASRS PAT Survey. http://www.asrs.org/services/pat_survey/reports/report.php? 2008. Accessed November 15, 2008.
196. Lobo C, Bernardes R, Faria dA, Jr., Cunha-Vaz JG. Novel imaging techniques for diabetic macular edema. *Doc Ophthalmol.* 1999;97:341–347.
197. Lobo CL, Bernardes RC, Cunha-Vaz JG. Alterations of the blood-retinal barrier and retinal thickness in preclinical retinopathy in subjects with type 2 diabetes. *Arch Ophthalmol.* 2000;118:1364–1369.
198. Hayreh SS. Role of retinal hypoxia in diabetic macular edema: a new concept. *Graefe's Arch Clin Exp Ophthalmol.* 2008;246:353–361.
199. Blair NP, Shahidi M, Lai WW, Zelkha R. Correlation between microaneurysms and retinal thickness in diabetic macular edema. *Retina.* 2008;28:1097–1103.
200. Averous K, Erginay A, Timsit J, et al. Resolution of diabetic macular oedema following high altitude exercise. *Acta Ophthalmol Scand.* 2006;84:830–831.
201. Daniele S, Daniele C. Aggravation of laser-treated diabetic cystoid macular edema after prolonged flight: a case report. *Aviat Space Environ Med.* 1995;66:440–442.
202. Lee M, Choi D, Choi MJ, et al. Hypoxia-inducible gene expression system using the erythropoietin enhancer and 3'-untranslated region for the VEGF gene therapy. *J Control Release.* 2006;115:113–119.
203. Browning DJ, Glassman AR, Aiello LP, et al. Relationship between optical coherence tomography-measured central retinal thickness and visual acuity in diabetic macular edema. *Ophthalmology.* 2007;114:525–536.
204. Srinivasan VJ, Wojtkowski M, Witkin AJ, et al. High-definition and 3-dimensional imaging of macular pathologies with high-speed ultrahigh-resolution optical coherence tomography. *Ophthalmology.* 2006; 113:2054e1–14.
205. Lu M, Adamis AP. Vascular endothelial growth factor gene regulation and action in diabetic retinopathy. *Ophthalmol Clin North Am.* 2002;15:69–79.
206. El-Remessy AB, Bartoli M, Platt DH, et al. Oxidative stress inactivates VEGF survival signaling in retinal endothelial cells via PI 3-kinase tyrosine nitration. *J Cell Sci.* 2005;118:243–252.
207. Ring HG, Fujino T. Observations on the anatomy and pathology of the choroidal vasculature. *Arch Ophthalmol.* 1967;78:431–444.
208. Alm A, Bill A. Ocular and optic nerve blood flow at normal and increased intraocular pressures in monkeys (Macaca irus): a study with radioactively labelled microspheres including flow determinations in brain and some other tissues. *Exp Eye Res.* 1973;15:15–29.
209. Yoneya S, Tso MO. Angioarchitecture of the human choroid. *Arch Ophthalmol.* 1987;105:681–687.
210. Schocket LS, Brucker AJ, Niknam RM, et al. Foveolar choroidal hemodynamics in proliferative diabetic retinopathy. *Int Ophthalmol.* 2004;25:89–94.
211. Nagaoka T, Kitaya N, Sugawara R, et al. Alteration of choroidal circulation in the foveal region in patients with type 2 diabetes. *Br J Ophthalmol.* 2004;88:1060–1063.
212. Shiragami C, Shiraga F, Matsuo T, et al. Risk factors for diabetic choroidopathy in patients with diabetic retinopathy. *Graefe's Arch Clin Exp Ophthalmol.* 2002;240:436–442.
213. Dimitrova G, Kato S, Tamaki Y, et al. Choroidal circulation in diabetic patients. *Eye.* 2001;15:602–607.
214. Langham ME, Grebe R, Hopkins S, et al. Choroidal blood flow in diabetic retinopathy. *Exp Eye Res.* 1991;52:167–173.
215. Fryczkowski AW, Hodes BL, Walker J. Diabetic choroidal and iris vasculature scanning electron microscopy findings. *Int Ophthalmol.* 1989;13:269–279.
216. Takahashi A, Nagaoka T, Sato E, Yoshida A. Effect of panretinal photocoagulation on choroidal circulation in the foveal region in patients with severe diabetic retinopathy. *Br J Ophthalmol.* 2008;92:1369–1373.
217. Augsten R, Konigsdorffer E, Schweitzer D, Strobel J. Nonproliferative diabetic retinopathy-reflection spectra of the macula before and after laser photocoagulation. *Ophthalmologica.* 1998;212:105–111.
218. Sebag J, Tang M, Brown S, et al. Effects of pentoxifylline on choroidal blood flow in nonproliferative diabetic retinopathy. *Angiology.* 1994;45:429–433.

219. Li L, Yi Z, Tisch R, Wang B. Immunotherapy of type 1 diabetes. *Arch Immunol Ther Exp (Warsz)*. 2008;56: 227–236.
220. Eldor R, Kassem S, Raz I. Immune modulation in type 1 diabetes mellitus using DiaPep277: a short review and update of recent clinical trial results. *Diabetes Metab Res Rev*. 2009;25:316–20.
221. Ogden CL, Carroll MD, Curtin LR, et al. Prevalence of overweight and obesity in the United States, 1999–2004. *JAMA*. 2006;295:1549–1555.
222. Henricsson M, Nystrom L, Blohme G, et al. The incidence of retinopathy 10 years after diagnosis in young adult people with diabetes: results from the nationwide population-based Diabetes Incidence Study in Sweden (DISS). *Diabetes Care*. 2003;26: 349–354.
223. Klein R, Knudtson MD, Lee KE, et al. The Wisconsin epidemiologic study of diabetic retinopathy: XXII the twenty-five-year progression of retinopathy in persons with type 1 diabetes. *Ophthalmology*. 2008;115:1859–1868.
224. Figueroa MS, Contreras I, Noval S. Surgical and anatomical outcomes of pars plana vitrectomy for diffuse nontractional diabetic macular edema. *Retina*. 2008; 28:420–426.

Chapter 9
Treatment of Proliferative Diabetic Retinopathy

Scott E. Pautler

9.1 Introduction

Proliferative diabetic retinopathy (PDR) is an advanced stage of diabetic microangiopathy in which extensive retinal capillary occlusion results in the growth of preretinal fibrovascular tissue. The pathogenesis is not well understood. Underlying pathophysiologic changes in diabetic retinopathy include abnormal shunting of glucose via the aldose reductase pathway, formation of advanced glycation end-products, activation of protein kinase-C beta isoform, induction of vascular endothelial growth factor (VEGF), oxidative damage, and inflammation.[1–5] Pathological anatomic changes evolve with abnormal thickening of capillary basement membrane, loss of pericytes, breakdown of the blood–retinal barrier, changes in microvascular caliber, microaneurysm formation, endothelial cell loss associated with capillary occlusion, and neovascularization within the retina (intraretinal microvascular abnormalities) and in the preretinal space with varying degrees of preretinal fibrosis. PDR may cause loss of vision from edema, ischemia, intraocular hemorrhage, premacular membranes, vitreomacular traction, traction retinal detachment, traction–rhegmatogenous retinal detachment, and neovascular glaucoma.[6]

Advanced glycation end-product formation and metabolic memory: Metabolic memory is a term used to describe the phenomenon of the delayed effect of changzes in metabolic control on the microcirculation. Improved metabolic control reported in the Diabetes Control and Complications Trial was associated with a delayed beneficial effect on the incidence and progression of diabetic retinopathy.[7,8] Similarly, after loss of strict control of hyperglycemia, a continued protective effect persists for years.[9,10] There is a molecular mechanism that may offer an explanation. Hyperglycemia is associated with non-enzymatic glycation of proteins, termed as advanced glycation end-products (AGE). Glycation of the proteins in retinal capillary basement membrane is implicated as playing a role in diabetic retinopathy.[1,11] As the turnover of structural proteins is slow, these advanced glycation end-products (AGEs) have been implicated as a cause of metabolic memory.[12]

Neovascularization (NV) is a distinctive ocular manifestation of diabetes mellitus and develops as a result of retinal ischemia/hypoxia in diabetic retinopathy.[13–15] NV grows from the surface of the retina at the posterior border of retinal capillary nonperfusion, from the surface of the disk, and from

S.E. Pautler (✉)
Department of Ophthalmology, University Community Hospital, University of South Florida, Tampa, FL 33607, USA
e-mail: pautlers@aol.com

D.J. Browning (ed.), *Diabetic Retinopathy*, DOI 10.1007/978-0-387-85900-2_9,

anterior sites (iris, ciliary body, and anterior retina) in eyes with increasing degrees of ischemia.[13,16,17] Retinal neovascularization generally arises from retinal veins or postcapillary venules near sites of arteriovenous crossing or venous branching.[18,19] The distribution of retinal NV follows a C-shaped extramacular distribution, sparing the temporal raphe.[13,18,19] Neovascularization of the disk (NVD) is associated with extensive retinal nonperfusion.[13,17] Presumably, NVD occurs as VEGF and other growth factors migrate from peripheral ischemic retina to the disk by way of vitreopapillary drainage.[13,15] The neovascular tissue grows within the outer cortical vitreous and may induce overlying secondary vitreous degeneration.[20–23] With time the vascular nature of the NV is associated with fibrous tissue proliferation, likely mediated by agents other than VEGF, such as connective tissue growth factor.[24–26] Initial contraction of the fibrous tissue may lead to retinal striae and retinal dragging.[27–30] Further vitreous traction may lead to retinal detachment with or without retinal breaks.[31,32] Release of angiogenic growth factors from hypoxic retina continues until neurosensory cell death occurs (in the very late stages of natural history or following photocoagulation) after which neovascular involution occurs.[13,33] The fibrous tissue remains and vitreous traction may continue to progress.[18,21,34] The clinical presentation of proliferative diabetic retinopathy includes a wide spectrum of disease due to variability in the relative developmental stages of vascular and fibrous proliferation.

An important factor affecting the presentation of PDR is the status of the vitreous. The vitreous undergoes a number of pathological changes in diabetes, including an increase in the number of collagen crosslinks and an increase in glycation end-products.[35] These changes contribute to premature degeneration and liquefaction of the vitreous in diabetes.[36] In the absence of a posterior vitreous detachment, the cortical vitreous provides a scaffold on which preretinal neovascularization proliferates.[22] With continued neovascular growth, extensive areas of fibrovascular proliferation create firm attachment between the retina and the vitreous cortex.[18] This is a common presentation in type 1 and early-onset type 2 diabetes mellitus as PDR develops in the environment of an intact vitreous body. The presentation of PDR in an older individual differs in large part due to the degree of vitreous degeneration and posterior separation.[37,38] If incomplete PVD is present, NV may grow anteriorly from the site of attachment (e.g., the disk) within the elevated posterior vitreous cortex, but it does not create further extension of fibrovascular plaques on the surface of the retina. In the presence of complete PVD, clinically important neovascularization does not usually develop.[37,39] However, anterior ocular neovascularization may become manifest (e.g., NV involving the anterior retina, ciliary body, and iris).[40]

Iris neovascularization (rubeosis) may occur in advanced stages of diabetic retinopathy and threatens pain and blindness from neovascular glaucoma.[41,42] Rubeosis frequently begins at the superior pupillary border of the iris and trabeculum due to convection currents in the anterior chamber, which in a head-up posture results in an upward flow of aqueous over the surface of the iris.[43,44] Rubeosis progresses more slowly in phakic than aphakic eyes, likely due to the effect of the crystalline lens as a barrier to the diffusion of neovascular growth factors into the anterior chamber.[45–47] The vitreous possesses inhibitors of NV and may also be a physical barrier to vasoproliferative factors that give relative protection against NV developing in the anterior segment.[13,48] This explains the increased incidence of neovascularization of the iris and other anterior structures following vitrectomy and lensectomy, especially in eyes with under-treated or untreated PDR.[13,40,47,49] The reader is referred to Chapter 1 for extensive review of the pathophysiology of diabetic retinopathy.

Why Is Neovascularization Rare After Isolated Central and Branch Retinal Artery Occlusions?

Retinal neovascularization is well described in branch retinal vein occlusion, sickle retinopathy, and diabetic retinopathy, but not in isolated retinal artery occlusion.[18,50,51] The explanation may lie with the difference in the rate of onset and magnitude of ischemia. The slow onset and chronic nature of ischemia induced by diabetic retinopathy result in the development of hypoxic retina, which allows time for the induction of neovascular growth factors.[18] Acute retinal artery occlusion causes abrupt cell death preventing the induction of vascular growth factors in the retina.[13,18] In addition, subsequent reperfusion of an occluded retinal artery may also protect against neovascular sequelae.[18]

Diabetes mellitus is a leading cause of blindness. The complications of neovascularization and macular edema are the most common causes of vision loss in diabetic retinopathy.[52] The relatively high prevalence of blindness from diabetes is related to the expanding epidemic of obesity and diabetes.[53] About two-thirds of adult Americans are overweight or obese.[54] Almost 11% of the US population (23.5 million persons) over the age of 20 years has diabetes. An additional 57 million have pre-diabetes.[55] Although there is high-level evidence that the incidence and progression of diabetic retinopathy may be reduced by intensive control of blood glucose and blood pressure,[7,56,57] sustaining strict diabetes management regimens is difficult.[9,10] Furthermore, routine eye examinations for early detection of retinopathy fall short of recommended guidelines.[58,59] Thus, diabetic retinopathy is common. About 40% of diabetics 40 years of age or older have diabetic retinopathy, and 8% have vision-threatening retinopathy.[60] The average annual progression to proliferative diabetic retinopathy is 1–4% and the cumulative 25-year progression to PDR is 42% among patients with type 1 diabetes mellitus.[61,62] The number of persons with diabetic retinopathy is expected to triple by 2050 to 17.7 million.[63] The reader is referred to Chapter 3 for additional information regarding the epidemiology of PDR. Given the high prevalence of diabetes and associated retinopathy, appropriate treatment is of paramount importance in preventing blindness.

This chapter focuses on the clinical management of proliferative diabetic retinopathy. The intent is to present a rational approach to problems encountered in the treatment of PDR by incorporating relevant information gleaned from research since the seminal publications of the Diabetic Retinopathy Study (DRS) group, the Early Treatment Diabetic Retinopathy Study (ETDRS) group, and the Diabetic Retinopathy Vitrectomy Study (DRVS) group. Tables 9.1, 9.2, and 9.3 summarize the salient findings from these studies relevant to proliferative diabetic retinopathy. Additional information from the literature is presented to assist in the process of deciding from among myriad treatment possibilities in order to minimize risk and maximize the benefits of intervention. Also included is a brief discussion of current studies which may lead to potential therapies in the future.

9.2 Laser Photocoagulation

Retinal photocoagulation for diabetic retinopathy has evolved since the initial reports by Meyer-Schwickerath using the xenon-arc photocoagulator.[64] Technological advances have provided more suitable tools with which the ophthalmologist can treat the retina with more precision and control. In addition, improved understanding of diabetic retinopathy through the work of the Diabetic Retinopathy Study (DRS) led to the routine use of scatter laser treatment (panretinal photocoagulation) of the hypoxic peripheral retina to induce involution of neovascularization in eyes with high-risk PDR.[65,66] Further refinements were made with the Early Treatment Diabetic Retinopathy Study (ETDRS) with regard to the indications and application of photocoagulation.[67,68] Both the ETDRS and the Diabetic Retinopathy Vitrectomy Study (DRVS) provided high-level evidence in support of vitrectomy for complications of PDR.[69–74] Although there have been no large-scale, randomized, controlled, multi-center studies of treatment for PDR since these studies, there has been significant progress. Panretinal photocoagulation (PRP) reduces the 5-year risk of blindness by 90%.[58] Improved metabolic control not only is associated with decreased progression of diabetic retinopathy but may also improve response to PRP.[75]

Table 9.1 Summary of the Diabetic Retinopathy Study (DRS) reports

DRS #1 (1976)[65]

Preliminary report of effects of photocoagulation therapy

Eligibility requirements

1. Both eyes with severe NPDR or at least one eye with PDR
2. Visual acuity $\geq$ 20/100

Treatment and follow-up

1. One eye promptly treated with argon or xenon photocoagulation
2. Scatter laser plus direct treatment of non-elevated NVE (argon-treated eyes also underwent direct treatment of NVD and elevated NVE)
3. 1727 patients treated (858 argon and 869 xenon)
4. Followed every 4 months
5. End point: <5/200 on two or more consecutive visits (severe visual loss-SVL)

Results at 2-year follow-up analysis

1. 57% reduction of SVL between treated and untreated eyes (9.4% untreated eyes vs. 4.1% treated eyes)
2. No difference in benefit between argon and xenon photocoagulation
3. Small loss of vision measured 4 months post-treatment (recovered at 2-year analysis in argon group only)
4. Reduced visual field score in xenon-treated eyes only

Protocol change

1. Consider treating fellow eye if possess high-risk characteristics
2. Direct treatment of NVD and elevated NVE was made optional

DRS #2 (1978)[66]

Coined the term “high-risk characteristics” (HRC)

1. Disk neovascularization (NVD) > standard photograph 10A
2. Vitreous hemorrhage with any NVD or NVE > ½ disk area

At 1-year analysis of treated eyes, no NV was present in 78.8% of NPDR eyes compared with 21.2% of eyes with moderate-to-severe NVD at baseline

Summary

1. Prompt PRP recommended for eyes with HRC
2. Call for ETDRS to study prompt vs. deferred PRP for eyes < HRC

DRS #10 (1985)[760]

Natural history: 2-year follow-up data

The presence and extent of NVD was the strongest predictor of SVL

The second strongest predictor was extent of retinal hemorrhage/microaneurysm

DRS #11 (1987)[761]

Photocoagulation reduces the risk of intraocular hypertension, apparently by preventing neovascular glaucoma

DRS #12 (1987)[762]

Risk factors for decrease in vision measured 6 weeks following PRP

1. Pre-existing macular edema
2. Intensity of PRP

Recommendations

1. Focal laser of macular edema before PRP
2. Divide PRP into multiple sessions and decrease intensity of burns

DRS #13 (1989)[763]

Risk factors for SVL despite PRP during 5 years after randomization

1. Increasing NVD (most important factor)
2. Increasing retinal hemorrhages/microaneurysms
3. Increasing retinal elevation (detachment)
4. Increasing proteinuria
5. Increasing hyperglycemia
6. Decreasing treatment density

Note: Treatment density was identified as an independent predictor of visual outcome supporting the practice of repeating PRP if initial treatment does not reduce or stabilize PDR

Table 9.2 Summary of the Early Treatment Diabetic Retinopathy Study (ETDRS) reports for PDR

ETDRS #3 (1987)[68]

Technique for photocoagulation of PDR

- Scatter (PRP): 500 μ (Goldmann) moderately intense burns
- Local: confluent treatment of flat NVE
- Details described in chapter

ETDRS #8 (1991)[764] and ETDRS #20 (1995)[765]

Effects of aspirin treatment (ASA 650 mg/day) on diabetic retinopathy

1. No clinically important beneficial or harmful effects in eyes with mild-to-severe NPDR or early PDR
2. No prevention of development of high-risk PDR or risk of visual loss
3. No increased risk of vitreous hemorrhage
4. No effect on severity or duration of vitreous hemorrhage

ETDRS #12 (1991)[100]

Fundus photographic risk factors for progression of diabetic retinopathy

1. Severity of intraretinal microvascular abnormalities
2. Severity of retinal hemorrhages/microaneurysms
3. Severity of venous beading
4. NOT soft exudates (cotton–wool spots)

ETDRS #13 (1991)[630]

Fluorescein angiographic (FA) risk factors for progression of diabetic retinopathy

1. Fluorescein leakage (particularly, diffuse)
2. Capillary loss and dilation
3. Arteriolar abnormalities (e.g., focal narrowing, pruning, staining)
4. FA risk factors offer increased power to predict progression of DR, but do not offer clinically important information over clinical exam and color photography

ETDRS #17 (1992)[69]

Pars plana vitrectomy in the ETDRS

1. 208 eyes (5.6%) of 3711 enrolled in ETDRS
2. Diabetes mellitus type: 51.9% type 1, 35.1% mixed, and 13% type 2
3. Preoperative PRP initiated in 88% of eyes (>1200 burns in 69%)
4. Primary indication: vitreous hemorrhage (53.9%), retinal detachment (46.1%)
5. Preoperative vision: 66.7% $\leq$ 5/200, 6.2% > 20/100
6. Postoperative vision (1-year): 20.2% < 5/200, 47.6% $\geq$ 20/100, and 24% $\geq$ 20/40
7. Note: endolaser became available early in ETDRS (1983)

ETDRS #18 (1998)[102]

Risk factors for high-risk PDR and severe visual loss[a] (SVL)

Baseline risk factors for high-risk PDR

1. Higher glycosylated hemoglobin
2. History of diabetic neuropathy
3. Lower hematocrit
4. Elevated triglycerides
5. Lower serum albumen
6. Type 1 diabetes

Baseline risk factors for severe visual loss

1. Development of high-risk PDR
2. Decreased visual acuity at baseline

Baseline risk factors for SVL before reaching high-risk PDR

1. Decreased visual acuity (or increased extent of macular edema)
2. Female gender
3. Type 2 diabetes

ETDRS #21 (1995)[766]

Transient decrease in accommodative amplitude of 1/3 diopter measured at the 4-month exam following scatter photocoagulation ($P < 0.001$)

Table 9.2 (continued)

ETDRS #24 (1999)[615]
Causes of severe visual loss in the ETDRS
Persistent severe visual loss was rare due to PRP/vitrectomy
149 eyes of 127 persons (3711 persons in ETDRS)
Causes of severe visual loss (decreasing order of frequency)

1. Vitreous/preretinal hemorrhage (despite vitrectomy) 61 eyes (41%) Of the 61 eyes, 17 eyes with RD (27.9%) and 3 eyes with NVG (4.9%)
2. Macular edema
3. Macular pigmentary change (e.g., past edema or RD)
4. Retinal detachment
5. Narrow or opaque arteries (i.e., ischemia)

Risk factors for persistent severe visual loss[b]

1. Elevated glycosylated hemoglobin
2. Elevated cholesterol

[a]<5/200 measured on two consecutive visits 4 months apart
[b]<5/200 without improvement on follow-up examinations

Table 9.3 Summary of the Diabetic Retinopathy Vitrectomy Study (DRVS) reports

DRVS #1 (1985)[70]
Two-year course of visual acuity in severe PDR with conventional management
744 eyes followed with conventional management
Risk factors for decreased vision: (45% SVL in eyes with NV > 4 disk areas and Va ≤ 20/60 at baseline)
Vitrectomy required (25%) in eyes with TRD involving center of macula or severe, nonclearing VH (1-year duration)

DRVS #2 (1985)[71]
Early Vitrectomy for severe vitreous hemorrhage (VH) in diabetic retinopathy
616 eyes with severe VH (≤5/200) randomized: early vs. 1-year deferral for Vtx
Visual acuity ≥20/40 at 2-year follow-up
  Total group: 25% early group vs. 15% deferral group ($P = 0.01$)
  Subgroup (type 1 DM): 36% early group vs. 12% deferral ($P = 0.0001$)
  Subgroup (type 2 DM): 16% early group vs. 18% deferral
The evidence of a difference in response by type of DM was of borderline significance
Conclusion: Early vitrectomy for acute, severe vitreous hemorrhage hastens return of vision and is especially significant for patients with type 1 diabetes mellitus

DRVS #3 (1988)[72]
Early vitrectomy for severe PDR with useful vision
370 eyes with advanced, active PDR (≥20/400): early vtx vs. conventional
Visual acuity ≥20/400 at 4-year follow-up
  Early vitrectomy group: 44%
  Conventional management group: 28%
The advantages of early vitrectomy increased with increasing severity of NV

DRVS #4 (1988)[73]
Clinical application of DRVS #3 (examples)

DRVS #5 (1990)[74]
Early vitrectomy for severe vitreous hemorrhage in DR. Four-year results
616 eyes described in DRVS #2 with extended follow-up
The proportion of eyes ≥20/40 was higher in early vtx group than deferral group
Up to the 18-month visit, the early group had higher rate of NLP
Eyes with severe VH in patients with type 1 DM benefit from early vitrectomy

DM = diabetes mellitus, DR = diabetic retinopathy, vtx = vitrectomy, NLP = no light perception, SVL = severe visual loss (<5/200 on two or more consecutive 4-month visits)

Theories on the mechanism of action of PRP have expanded and may not be mutually exclusive. During the process of DRS, the researchers came to an agreement on the value of peripheral scatter treatment as a means in which to ablate ischemic retina presumably to decrease the stimulus for neovascular growth.[68] Since then, vascular endothelial growth factor (VEGF) has been identified as playing a major role in the development of PDR.[76] PRP laser appears to decrease VEGF production and induces the release of angiostatin, a potent inhibitor of neovascularization in the retina and vitreous.[77–79] A great number of other agents are undoubtedly involved and there appears to be an alteration in the complex balance and interaction of growth factors (e.g., angiopoietin,[80,81] cortistatin,[82] insulin-like growth factor-1,[83] basic fibroblast growth factor,[4] platelet-derived growth factor,[4] endothelin-1,[84] transforming growth factor beta-1,[85] connective tissue growth factor,[86] growth hormone[87]) and inhibitors (e.g., pigment epithelium-derived factor,[88–90] soluble vascular endothelial growth factor receptor-1,[91] somatostatin,[4] endostatin,[92] angiostatin,[79] thrombospondin[4]) that result in tissue proliferation in PDR.[4,93]

Panretinal photocoagulation may also allow an influx of oxygen from the choroid into the ischemic retina by thinning the retina and focally diminishing oxygen consumption by outer retinal mitochondria.[94] The oxygen tension in the preretinal vitreous cavity is greater over areas of retina treated by PRP than over untreated areas in diabetic eyes.[95] Consequently, there is a reduction of blood flow in major retinal vessels and decreased venous dilatation following peripheral scatter laser photocoagulation for PDR.[96,97]

The physical effect of retinal photocoagulation is a result of the absorption of light energy not only by pigment, primarily melanin in the retinal pigment epithelium, but also by hemoglobin. Light energy is thereby transformed into heat energy, which is conducted into the neurosensory retina. The amount of laser energy required to achieve the desired degree of photocoagulation is dependent on the concentration of laser energy delivered to the retina through the media of the eye. Retinal whitening becomes visible as the retina coagulates and the intensity of the whitening relates to the depth of heat penetration into the retina. Very intense whitening of the retina indicates full thickness retinal photocoagulation, regardless of the laser wavelength used.[75,98]

9.2.1 Indications

The current indications for laser treatment of PDR are based on the recommendations from the prospective, randomized, controlled trials carried out by the Diabetic Retinopathy Study group and the Early Treatment Diabetic Retinopathy Study group. The DRS identified the clinical features of eyes with proliferative diabetic retinopathy at high risk for visual loss and termed this group as high-risk proliferative diabetic retinopathy (HR-PDR), which included eye with either (1) neovascularization of the disk (NVD) equal to or greater than standard photograph 10A or (2) preretinal or vitreous hemorrhage associated with NVD $<$ standard photograph 10A or NVE $\geq 1/2$ disk area.[65,66,99] Figure 9.1 shows standard photograph 10A. The risk of severe visual loss in eyes with HR-PDR was shown to be reduced by greater than 50% over a

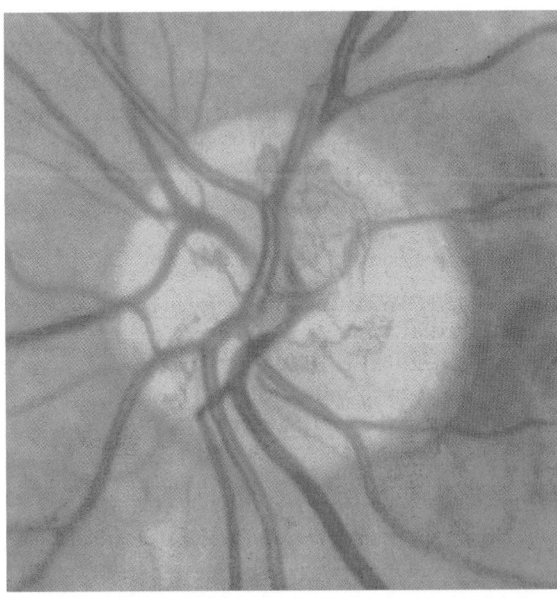

Fig. 9.1 ETDRS standard photo 10A. NVD (NV on or within one disk diameter of the disk border) of approximately one-quarter to one-third disk area[67] (reproduced with permission from the Early Treatment Diabetic Retinopathy Study Research Group. All rights reserved)

2-year period with the application of peripheral scatter laser photocoagulation, now commonly referred to as panretinal photocoagulation (PRP).[65,99] Despite clear benefit from PRP, the 4-year rate of severe visual loss (visual acuity less than 5/200, measured at two or more consecutive visits) in eyes with high-risk PDR was 20.4%.[67] It is important to note that the DRS included cases with HR-PDR of varying degrees of severity, not just new-onset HR-PDR.

The ETDRS was designed to compare the effect of early vs. delayed PRP in earlier stages of diabetic retinopathy in an effort to further decrease the risk of visual loss. The 5-year rate of severe visual loss in the ETDRS was 2.6 and 3.7% in the early treatment and delayed deferral group, respectively.[67] The ETDRS adopted from the DRS the definition of severe nonproliferative diabetic retinopathy (S-NPDR) and high-risk proliferative diabetic retinopathy and expanded the diabetic retinopathy severity scale.[67,100]

Regarding the treatment of mild-to-moderate NPDR, the ETDRS recommended against PRP as the risk of severe visual loss in this group was low and there was adverse risk of moderate visual loss following treatment. This recommendation was made with the provision that these patients could be followed for progression.[67]

The ETDRS recommendations for the treatment of severe nonproliferative diabetic retinopathy (S-NPDR) and early proliferative diabetic retinopathy (E-PDR) with scatter laser (PRP) were less definite.[67] The ETDRS definition of S-NPDR in Table 9.4 refers to ETDRS photographic fields (Fig. 9.2), to standard photo 2A (Fig. 9.3), and to standard photo 8A (Fig. 9.4). Early PDR was defined as new vessels present, but less than high-risk PDR. The ETDRS made a recommendation to "consider" PRP in eyes with severe nonproliferative diabetic retinopathy and early proliferative

Table 9.4 ETDRS definition of severe nonproliferative diabetic retinopathy

Either of two definitions below
1. Any three of the following findings
a. Soft exudates in at least two fields[a]
b. Venous beading in at least two fields[a]
c. Intraretinal microvascular abnormalities in at least two fields[a]
d. Hemorrhages and microaneurysms ≥ standard photo 2A Present in at least one field[a]
2. Intraretinal microvascular abnormalities (IRMA) in all four fields[a] and IRMA severity ≥ standard photo 8A in at least two fields[a]

[a]30° photographic fields 4–7 (shown in Fig. 9.2)
Standard photograph 2A is shown in Fig. 9.3
Standard photograph 8A is shown in Fig. 9.4

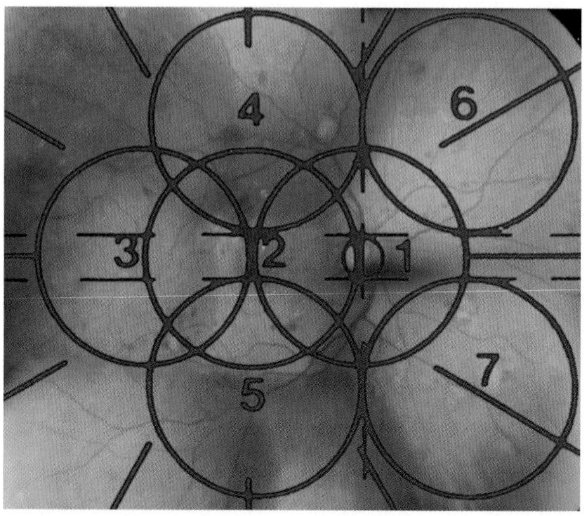

Fig. 9.2 ETDRS diagram for right eye showing 30° photographic fields. Fields 4–7 are used for grading severe nonproliferative diabetic retinopathy (the ETDRS diagram was reproduced with permission from Ophthalmology.[628] Copyright © 1991 American Academy of Ophthalmology. All rights reserved)

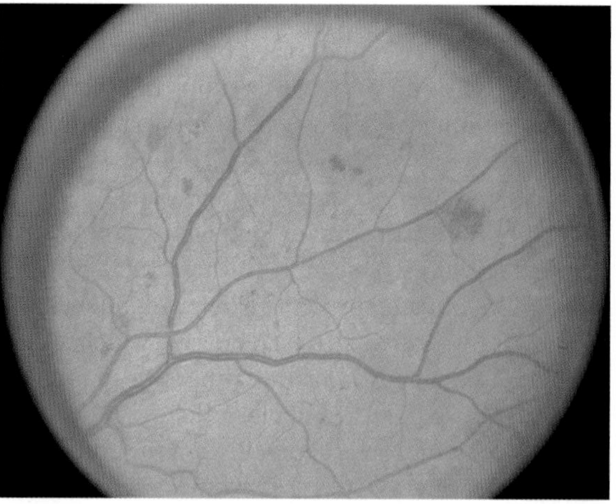

Fig. 9.3 ETDRS standard photograph 2A demonstrating moderate hemorrhages and microaneurysms (reproduced with permission from the Early Treatment Diabetic Retinopathy Study Research Group. All rights reserved)

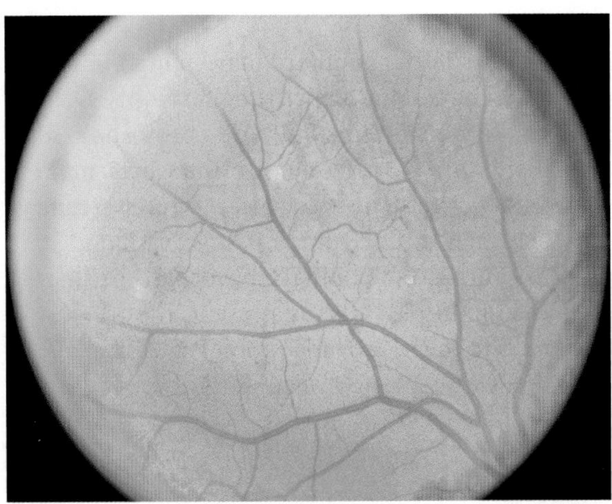

Fig. 9.4 ETDRS standard photograph 8A demonstrating IRMA severity (reproduced with permission from the Early Treatment Diabetic Retinopathy Study Research Group. All rights reserved)

Table 9.5 Proposed factors promoting decision to treat S-NPDR and E-PDR

1. Bilateral diabetic retinopathy approaching high-risk PDR
2. Poor compliance with follow-up visits
3. Poor metabolic control
4. Type 1 diabetes mellitus (especially, if poorly controlled)
5. Presence of diabetic macular edema
6. Presence of iris neovascularization
7. Pregnancy
8. Recent, rapid improvement in metabolic control
9. Previous severe visual loss in fellow eye from PDR
10. Total NVE area greater than two disk areas

diabetic retinopathy.[67] This cautious wording may have led physicians away from treating this group of eyes. There are, however, some issues that may compel a decision to treat. For example, the ETDRS used somewhat stronger wording in favor of treating at least one eye when both eyes are approaching HR-PDR by stating that it "seems particularly appropriate." They logically considered the potential difficulty in urgently treating both eyes if they simultaneously developed HR-PDR at a later date. The 5-year risk of developing HR-PDR is greater than 70% in this cohort.[67]

There are other factors that might reasonably influence the clinician to offer PRP in eyes with S-NPDR or E-PDR. Such factors include situations in which an eye may be at increased risk of progression or poor outcome (Table 9.5).[101] Patients who are unable to adhere to appropriate follow-up examinations are at increased risk of progressing to HR-PDR without being detected and treated in a timely fashion.[67] In ETDRS report #17, there was a higher risk to progress to vitrectomy in eyes of patients with type 1 diabetes mellitus with poor metabolic control.[69] In addition, the ETDRS and DRVS described a disproportionate percentage of patients with type 1 diabetes mellitus with very severe PDR consistent with other studies suggesting this group of eyes is at increased risk of progression.[70,102] Eyes with diabetic macular edema are at increased risk of both severe visual loss and vitrectomy and these eyes might be treated with PRP after appropriate management of edema.[67] Findings of neovascularization of the iris (NVI) or neovascular glaucoma (NVG) portend a poor prognosis.[67,103] Such eyes may not present with high-risk PDR, especially if there is a posterior vitreous detachment.[38,39] Patients with recent improvement in diabetes management with a rapid decrease in hemoglobin A1c may experience an "early worsening" in retinopathy before long-term stabilization.[8] Therefore, documented progression to S-NPDR or E-PDR in this situation may be an indication for PRP. Similarly, worsening of diabetic retinopathy is well described in pregnancy.[104–106] Other factors in favor or treatment include the previous severe loss of vision from diabetic retinopathy in the fellow eye and, possibly, family history of poor outcome from diabetic retinopathy.[107] In the ETDRS there were few eyes with NVE greater than two disk areas in extent to provide significant data.[67] These eyes with more extensive NVE might be reasonably considered for PRP as they appear to be at increased risk of severe visual loss.[70]

Alternatively, there are factors that may influence the physician to observe S-NPDR and E-PDR. For example, observation may be preferable in cases with laser-induced complications in the fellow eye, patient preference after counseling, good metabolic control, no DME, asymptomatic eye, low-risk fellow eye, and in cases without documentation of progression (e.g., the initial visit).

Iris neovascularization or pupillary vascular tufts? Vascular tufts of the pupillary margin are uncommon, unilateral or bilateral, capillary hamartomas with an estimated prevalence ranging from 0.0015 to 3.5% in the general population.[108–114] They may be solitary or multiple and are best visualized with fluorescein angiography.[110,115] Although most patients are asymptomatic, some present in adulthood with spontaneous hyphema.[108,110,115] There is no consistent association with systemic disease with the possible exception of diabetes.[114,115] The tufts differ from rubeosis in that they appear as elevated vascular loops adjacent to the pupillary ruff at the pupillary border, sometimes associated with fine radial vessels on the iris.[108,115,116] When multiple tufts are present, they do not form a vascular network.[116] The tufts do not visibly extend into the iris stroma or angle.[110] In an eye with diabetic retinopathy, proper management is dependent on making a distinction between iris neovascularization and pupillary vascular tufts (Fig. 9.5).

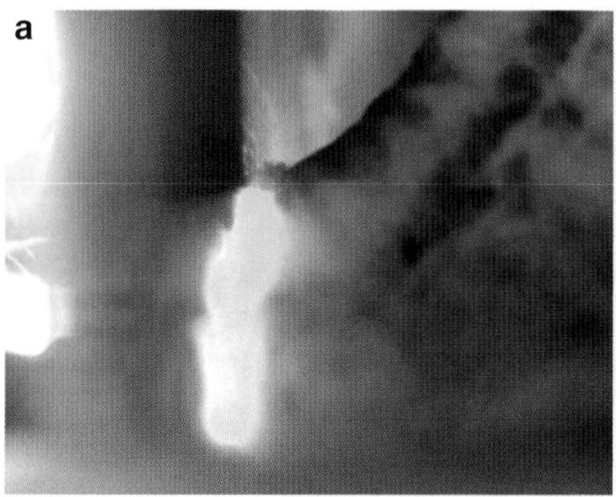

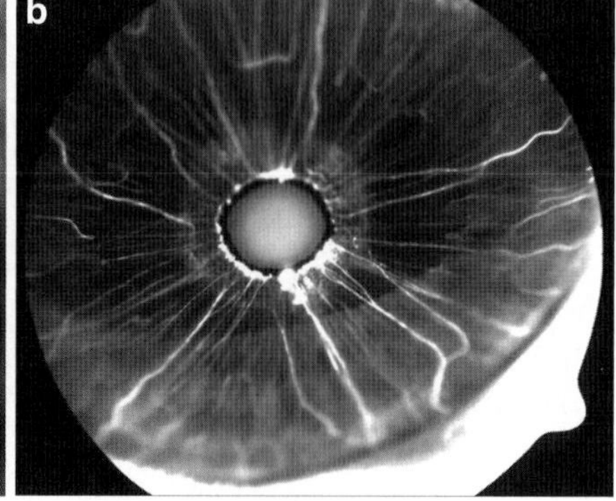

Fig. 9.5 Elevated iris pupillary vascular tuft (microhemangioma) demonstrated by slitlamp photograph (**a**). The Iris fluorescein angiogram reveals numerous hyperfluorescent vascular tufts at pupillary margin (**b**) (reprinted with permission from Bakke et al.[114] Copyright © 2006 Wiley-Blackwell. All rights reserved)

A unique subset of patients may present with "end-stage" or "burned-out" proliferative diabetic retinopathy (Fig. 9.6). These eyes may have extensive fibrous proliferation with or without traction retinal detachment (TRD) in the absence of a significant vascular component to the preretinal tissue.[117,118] In these cases the neovascularization has undergone spontaneous involution. Therefore, the value of PRP is debatable. As vitreous traction may continue in the absence of active NV, PRP may be helpful in creating chorioretinal adhesions to decrease the likelihood of progressive TRD.[20,24–26,34,119,120] However, there may be concern that inflammation associated with PRP may stimulate fibrous tissue contraction. This issue has not been studied adequately for definitive recommendations.

9.2.2 PRP Technique

The application of panretinal photocoagulation continues to evolve in an effort to maximize the benefits and minimize the risks of treatment. The ETDRS technique of applying scatter laser in PDR was proven effective.[67,68] The following is a detailed review of this technique and a discussion of considerations for modification based on new information and technology.

Prior to initiating PRP, consideration is given to pain management in order to ensure patient satisfaction and continuity of care. Peribulbar and retrobulbar anesthesia are equally effective for pain control and were used optionally in the ETDRS.[68,121] There appears to be little benefit of oral medications (benzodiazepines, acetaminophen, nonsteroidal

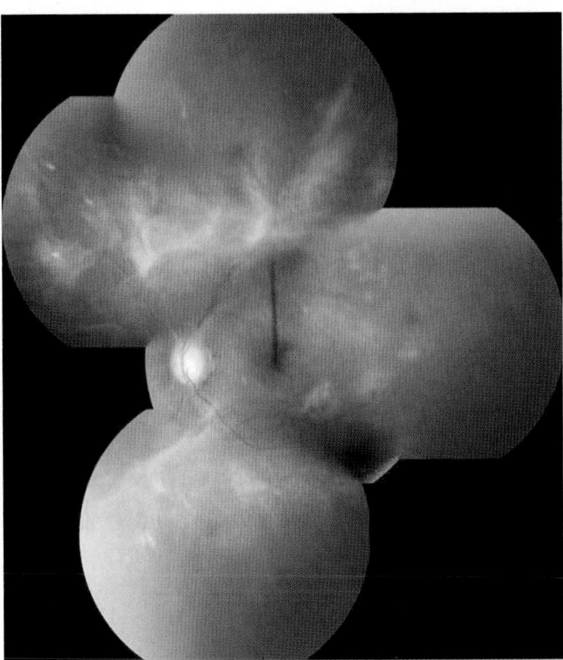

Fig. 9.6 Fundus photographic montage showing "burned-out" proliferative diabetic retinopathy with extensive preretinal fibrous proliferation and spontaneous regression of neovascularization in the absence of photocoagulation

anti-inflammatory drugs), intramuscular injections (ketorolac), or topical anti-inflammatory drops (ketorolac) for control of pain, but these agents may be helpful in selected patients (e.g., prelaser benzodiazepines for anxiety).[122–127] There is evidence to support the use of subtenons anesthesia, which may be safer and administered with less discomfort than retrobulbar anesthesia.[128] Avoiding laser emission in the red end of the spectrum minimizes discomfort.[129,130] The use of laser applications of short duration (e.g., 0.01–0.05 s) reduces pain.[131–133] With these changes in laser parameters, topical anesthesia is often satisfactory and eliminates the risks of injection anesthesia.[134,135]

Slitlamp delivery of laser is standard in the office setting, but binocular indirect ophthalmoscopic (BIO) laser delivery may offer advantages where physical handicaps prevent proper positioning at the slitlamp.[136,137] Additionally, scleral depression provides excellent access to the far peripheral retina, especially in eyes with poor visualization through cataract, intraocular lens, posterior capsular opacity, and vitreous hemorrhage.[136,138] However, a relatively smaller laser spot size is created on the retina when scleral depression is employed and this may result in hyperintense treatment.[139] Low-volume retrobulbar block may allow for the retention of ocular motility to aid in treatment, while providing patient comfort.[140]

Contact lens selection for laser treatment in the ETDRS included the Goldmann, the McLean, and the Rodenstock contact lenses, though the Goldmann three-mirror contact lens was most widely used.[68] Newer, wide-angle contact lenses have become popular since the ETDRS as they provide ease, efficiency, and speed of use.[141] Methylcellulose, sodium hyaluronate, and other viscous coupling agents are commonly used, but may cause more corneal epithelial trauma than non-viscous agents such as normal saline.[142] In eyes with severe diabetic corneal neuropathy and epitheliopathy, the use of a bandage contact lens may provide protection against epithelial trauma.[143]

Initially, argon blue-green laser was used in the ETDRS, but green-only and krypton red lasers were allowed when they became available.[68] Green-only laser offers advantages over the blue-green laser as there is less scatter of laser light, less absorption by xanthophyll pigments in the treated eye, and less potential laser-induced color vision complications in the eyes of the treating physician.[144,145] Krypton red laser appears equally effective in comparison with argon blue-green laser and has been popularized for its improved penetration through cataract and vitreous hemorrhage.[130,146,147] However, laser light of longer wavelengths penetrate deeper into the choroid, increasing the risk of pain and choroidal hemorrhage.[129,130] Regardless of laser selection, there may be reason for concern regarding laser light flashback into the eyes of the ophthalmologist when laser is performed soon after fluorescein angiography.[148] In an additional note of caution, unintentional inner retinal photocoagulation may result from laser photocoagulation after staining of the internal limiting membrane with indocyanine green.[149]

The intensity of the laser burn was described in the ETDRS as "moderately intense white burns that do not spread to become appreciably larger than 500 µm."[68] Care must be taken in reducing the laser power in the peripheral retina where less energy is required to cause retinal whitening.[150] In addition, a careful approach is necessary in eyes with pale fundi. Although greater laser energy may be required due to decreased concentration of melanin, these eyes provide less contrast in which to appreciate laser-induced whitening.[151] Thus, a relatively less intense burn may be a suitable goal. Intense laser treatment causes more prominent visual field defects than mild-to-moderate whitening.[152]

Supported by preliminary studies, less intense burns are often the current goal in an effort to decrease pain with treatment and to reduce the side effects of PRP.[128,129,131,152,153] The Diabetic Retinopathy Clinical Research Network protocol called for mild-to-medium white burns.[154] Pushing the limits of decreasing the laser-whitening effect on the retina, diode subthreshold micropulse laser employs short bursts of laser to produce subvisible laser applications limiting the conduction of heat from the retinal pigment epithelium to the retina in an effort to minimize side effects of treatment.[155] Randomized controlled trials are needed to compare these strategies with ETDRS protocol.

To achieve a desired intensity the treating ophthalmologist may make adjustments in several laser parameters. The laser spot size and duration are first selected after which the power is adjusted to reach the desired goal of retinal whitening.[68] The ETDRS protocol called for a setting of 500 μm for the diameter of the laser spot using a Goldmann lens. This setting was adjusted to 250–300 μm when using the Rodenstock lens to achieve a similar effect without changing the number of burns required for a complete initial treatment. However, calculations suggest that a photocoagulator spot size setting of 383 μm using a Rodenstock panfundoscopic lens might more closely approximate the retinal photocoagulative effect of a spot setting of 500 μm while using a Goldmann lens (Table 9.6).[156–158] In the ETDRS, allowance was made for adjusting to a smaller spot size to reach the desired intensity in eyes with opaque media (cataract or vitreous hemorrhage).[68] The spot size may also be reduced to allow for better pain control.[128,132] When using smaller spot sizes, a greater number of burns are needed to treat a comparable area of the retina. As the area of the laser spot is proportional to the square of the radius, four times as many spots may be needed if the spot size is reduced by 50%. Another concern with the use of a smaller laser spot size is the risk of creating a hyperintense burn resulting in the rupture of Bruch's membrane and hemorrhage.[159]

The laser flash duration in the ETDRS was 0.1 s, but longer duration was allowed if needed to reach the intensity goal as needed in eyes with opaque media.[68] Alternatively, the flash duration may be shortened in an effort to decrease pain with treatment.[128] Laser flashes with shorter duration (0.01–0.05 s) are less painful than longer duration (0.1 s) controlling for end point laser intensity.[131,132] Flash duration also correlates with breadth and depth of the zone of coagulation. Longer pulse duration is associated with greater conductive spread of retinal photocoagulation, likely accounting for pain and possibly accounting for therapeutic benefit.[132] Burns longer than 0.1 s duration may increase the risk of traction retinal detachment following treatment for PDR.[160] Shorter pulse duration is associated with increased risk of chorioretinal hemorrhage.[161,162] This risk may be mitigated by increasing the laser spot size.[161]

The goal of spacing of laser burns in the retina in the ETDRS was to aim for a final appearance of burn separation (after expansion of the burn) of one-half burn diameter. Therefore, laser burns could be placed from one-half to one burn diameter apart to reach this target (Fig. 9.7).[68] As laser scars may expand over time, this pattern may result in confluent atrophy from laser with attendant loss of visual field (Fig. 9.8).[163,164] Although this adverse effect may call for a change in the pattern density of

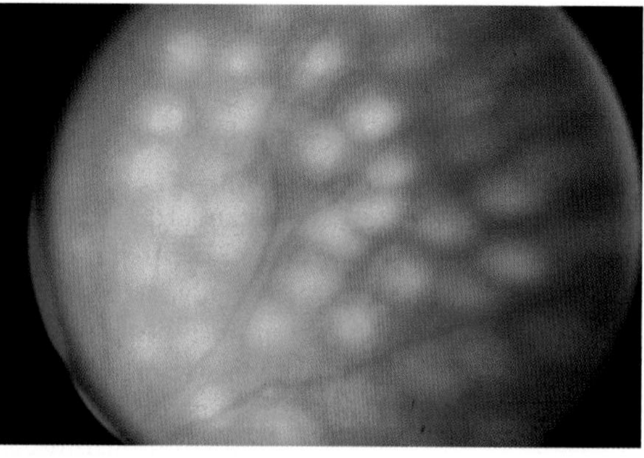

Fig. 9.7 Immediate post-laser appearance of retina following ETDRS-style PRP

Table 9.6 Comparison of fundus contact lenses for PRP laser

Name of lens	Field of view (degrees) static/dynamic	Magnification factor view through lens	Spot size magnification factor	Laser photocoagulator setting equivalent to 500 micron Goldmann	Number of burns = ETDRS PRP[a] with laser settings as shownbelow: 500	200	100
O-I Mainster (standard)	90/121	0.96	1.05	514	1,693	10,580	42,318
O-I Reichel Mainster 1X	102/133	0.95	1.05	514	1,693	10,580	42,318
O-I Goldmann 3-mirror (Karickhoff)	36/140	0.93	1.08	500	1,600	10,000	40,000
O-I Mainster High Mag	75/88	0.80	1.25	432	1,194	7,465	29,860
Rodenstock Panfundoscope	84% greater than Goldmann	0.71	1.41	383	939	5,867	23,468
Volk TransEquator	110/132	0.70	1.44	375	900	5,625	22,500
O-I Mainster Wide Field	118/127	0.68	1.50	360	829	5,184	20,736
Kreiger	8% greater than Goldmann	0.66	1.53	353	797	4,983	19,931
O-I Mainster PRP 165	165/180	0.51	1.96	276	486	3,036	12,145
Volk Quadr Aspheric	120/144	0.51	1.97	274	481	3,005	12,022
O-I Reichel-Mainster 2X	117/142	0.50	2.00	270	467	2,916	11,664
O-I ProRetina 120 PB	120/136	0.50	2.00	270	467	2,916	11,664
Volk SuperQuad 160 (Volk H–R Wide Field)	160/165	0.50	2.00	270	467	2,916	11,664
Volk Equator Plus	114/137	0.44	2.27	238	362	2,264	9,054

O-I Ocular Instruments

[a]1600 burns using 500 μm laser setting with a Goldmann contact lens (assuming fixed pulse duration)

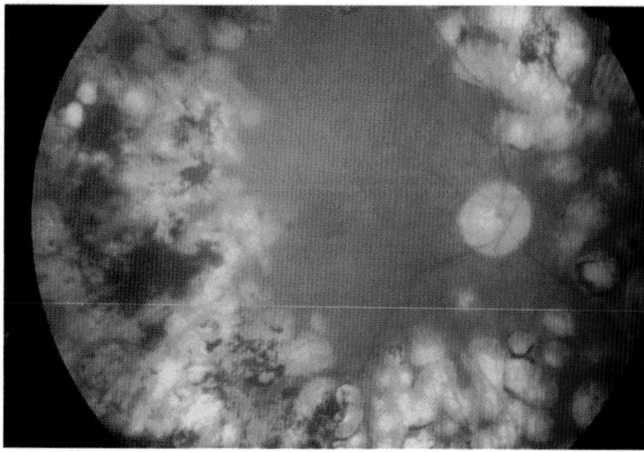

Fig. 9.8 Confluent areas of chorioretinal atrophy and scarring following panretinal photocoagulation (Fig. 9.7 shows the same eye immediately following laser treatment)

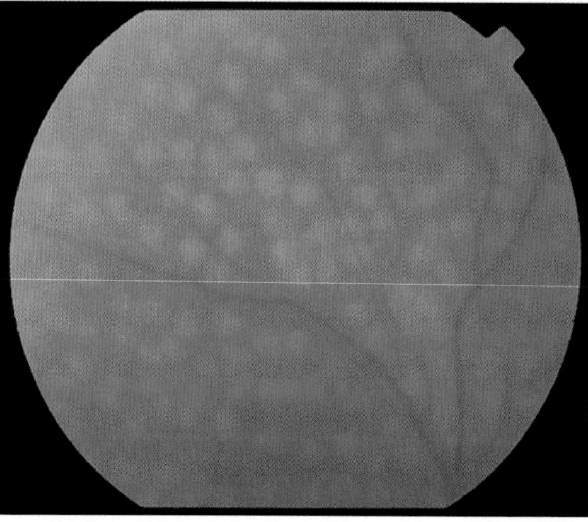

Fig. 9.9 Mild-to-moderate white PRP burns consistent with the Diabetic Retinopathy Clinical Research Network protocol

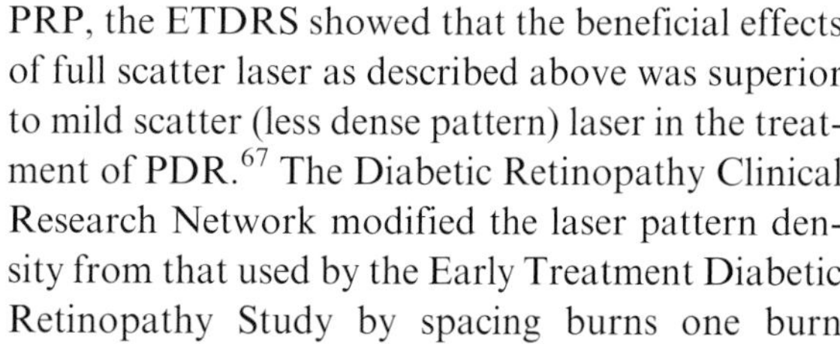

PRP, the ETDRS showed that the beneficial effects of full scatter laser as described above was superior to mild scatter (less dense pattern) laser in the treatment of PDR.[67] The Diabetic Retinopathy Clinical Research Network modified the laser pattern density from that used by the Early Treatment Diabetic Retinopathy Study by spacing burns one burn diameter apart without aiming for a final burn separation of one-half burn diameter after expansion (Fig. 9.9).[154]

The Pattern Scan Laser Photocoagulator (PASCAL®)

The pattern scan laser photocoagulator offers the convenience and efficiency of placing multiple laser burns with a single pedal depression. This frequency-doubled Nd:YAG diode laser delivers 532 nm laser pulses of sufficiently short duration so as to permit the delivery of multiple retinal burns in less than 650 ms. Predetermined patterns of square arrays (2 × 2, 3 × 3, 4 × 4, and 5 × 5) and triple-burn-width arcs (18 burns) may be applied to perform PRP. Test spots may be used to adjust the laser power during treatment for desired intensity of photocoagulation.[165]

The location within the retina for the placement of scatter laser was also well defined in the ETDRS. The posterior extent of scatter laser was described as forming an oval around the macula and including the disk "defined by a line passing two disk diameters above, temporal to, and below the center of the macula and 500 μm from the nasal one-half of the disk margin." The anterior extent of scatter laser reaches "to or beyond the equator" avoiding direct treatment of major vessels, preretinal hemorrhage, and chorioretinal scars (to avoid rupturing Bruch's membrane).[68] Since the ETDRS publications, several studies emphasize the importance of treating the retina well anterior to the equator, especially in severe cases, to reduce the risk of anterior neovascularization and associated complications.[166–169] Recent insights also suggest the utility of applying laser in a pattern on each side of the medium-sized, radiating, midperipheral retinal vessels as the hypoxic retinal tissue mantle in this paravascular area appears to a persistent source of neovascular cytokines.[18]

The Ischemic Penumbra

The concept of an ischemic penumbra in diabetic retinopathy is borrowed from our understanding of cerebrovascular accidents in which there is a core of infarcted tissue surrounded by a mantle of hypoxic tissue (the penumbra). In ischemic diabetic retinopathy there are areas of viable, hypoxic retinal tissue adjacent to patches of capillary nonperfusion. These zones of hypoxic retina may be an important source of production of vasoproliferative factors, such as VEGF. Furthermore, attention to treating these zones may prove to be a useful method of controlling neovascularization. One well-recognized mantle of hypoxic retina is along the posterior border of midperipheral capillary dropout. More recently, McLeod presented cogent reasoning for the existence of a paravascular hypoxic penumbra involving the midperipheral radiating retinal vessels.[18] Oxygen may diffuse into the surrounding retina from these major vessels providing for survival despite oligemia from surrounding retinal acapillarity. Indeed, increased VEGF production has been detected in this perivascular distribution.[170] This concept may offer further explanation for the frequent sparing of the far peripheral retina from early capillary occlusion in diabetic retinopathy.[17,171] The thin peripheral retina receives much of its oxygen from the choroid, which may offer relative protection against apoptosis in the face of retinal capillary insufficiency. Perhaps a similar mechanism underlies the apparent protective effect of high myopia and advanced glaucoma on the progression of diabetic retinopathy.[13,18,172,173]

With some exceptions the ETDRS required direct, confluent treatment (200–1000 μm, 0.1–0.5 s, moderately intense whitening) of small, flat areas of NVE (not more than 2 disk areas, i.e., circle of 1.5 disk diameter) avoiding treatment closer than 500–1000 μm from the center of the macula. The base of elevated NVE was treated confluently as well. Although direct photocoagulation may be currently less popular for the purpose of regression of NV, there may be a role for treating NVE to create an adhesion in order to reduce the risk of retinal detachment from future vitreous/membrane contraction.[119,174] Photocoagulation for PDR rarely involves the macula with the notable exception of treating ischemic areas temporal to the center of the macula in cases of active PDR despite standard PRP.[67] In addition, avoiding direct treatment over the long posterior ciliary nerve minimizes pain and reduces the risk of parasympathetic denervation of iris and ciliary body.[175]

As PRP is frequently completed in two or more sessions, a decision is made as to which areas of the retina need treatment first. The order of treatment in the ETDRS was optional for the ophthalmologist. Then as now, the most urgent areas of the retina were treated first. If vitreous hemorrhage threatens to gravitate inferiorly, treatment is begun in the inferior quadrants. If macular edema is present, the nasal quadrants are treated first in order to minimize adverse effects on visual acuity. When treating the temporal quadrants, initial treatment beginning posteriorly around the macula may help lessen the chance of inadvertent macular photocoagulation.[68]

Treatment anterior to the equator was optional in the ETDRS, but there are compelling reasons to routinely treat well anterior to the equator.[17,171] Standard panretinal photocoagulation applied posterior to the equator may cause severe visual field loss rendering the patient unable to drive an automobile.[164] A prospective randomized trial showed that anterior PRP is as effective as standard PRP in causing involution of PDR with fewer complications of DME and less visual field loss.[176] In addition, anterior PRP reduces the risk for anterior hyaloidal neovascularization and retinal detachment following subsequent vitrectomy surgery.[18,119,166–168,174] Figure 9.10 shows an example of neovascular proliferation on the anterior border of PRP. The potential for anterior choroidal effusion with shallowing of anterior chamber following PRP anterior to the equator may be minimized by

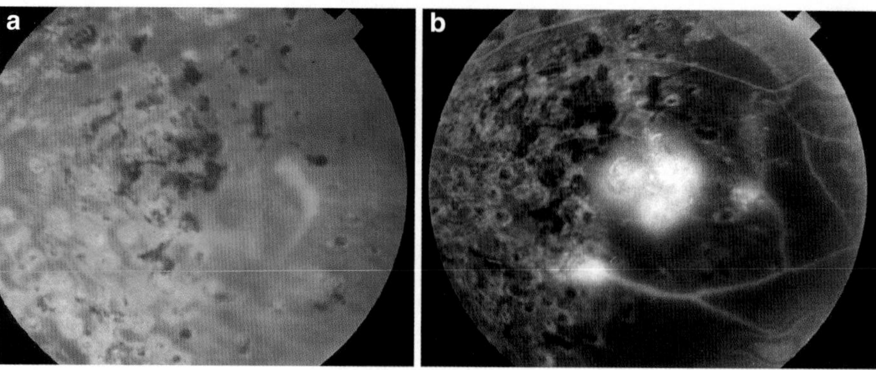

Fig. 9.10 Fundus photograph (**a**) and fluorescein angiogram (**b**) showing NVE anterior to previously placed PRP

avoiding excessive laser intensity and by dividing the treatment into multiple sessions, especially in hyperopic eyes.[177]

The ETDRS protocol specified the details regarding the duration of a laser session, the number of sessions, the time between sessions, and the definition of completion of PRP. The number of laser burns per session did not exceed 900 in order to avoid complications from excessive treatment.[68] However, when urgent treatment completion is needed, exceeding this guideline is not proscribed in clinical practice.[178] Alternatively, fewer laser burns per session may be considered in a sensitive patient or when shallow anterior chamber angles threaten closure.[67]

The number of sessions to complete initial PRP was two or more in the ETDRS.[68] A randomized controlled trial showed that PRP may be completed in a single treatment without increased long-term adverse effects compared with divided sessions. Short-term side-effects did include serous choroidal and retinal detachment and angle closure.[178] Another more recent prospective trial by the DRCR.net demonstrated no major increased risk of macular edema in comparing single-session vs. four-session PRP in eyes with severe NPDR or early PDR without pretreatment diabetic macular edema.[154] Thus, there is latitude in deciding the number of sessions in which to complete PRP.

In the ETDRS, the time interval between treatment sessions was at least 2 weeks apart if total of two sessions were planned for completion of treatment. A separation of at least 4 days was required if three or more episodes were planned for complete initial PRP. Completion of initial PRP occurred within 5 weeks in the ETDRS.[68] A desire for rapid completion of initial PRP is considered in eyes with PDR at high risk for vitreous hemorrhage.[68] An increased interval between laser sessions is desirable in eyes with diabetic macular edema, especially if adjunctive therapy is not employed as described later in this chapter.[178,179]

The ETDRS protocol defined the completion of PRP in terms of total laser applications from all initial treatment sessions. Between 1200 and 1600 laser burns were required for initial PRP to be complete.[68] However, there may be situations in which less extensive laser may be satisfactory. For example, response to PRP can be rapid with dramatic resolution of NV within 3 weeks and these early responders tend to remain stable for at least 6 months.[180] As adverse effects from laser are directly related to number of laser burns, a predetermined number of burns may be imprudent in cases where NV resolves before completion of intended PRP.[67] An alternative strategy in this scenario may be to observe rather than continue treatment session after regression from high-risk PDR with reinstitution of treatment when worsening of NV is documented. Another factor to consider in deciding when to stop initial PRP is the status of the vitreous. PRP is known to precipitate posterior vitreous detachment, and if PVD were documented before completion of initial PRP, observation may be in order given the anticipated benign clinical course reported in eyes with PVD.[38,181,182] Alternatively, if vitrectomy surgery is planned in an eye with severe PDR, more extensive PRP appears to improve outcome.[49,183,184] Thus, although guidelines are helpful, a predetermined number of laser applications may not be a clinically relevant goal in the treatment of proliferative diabetic retinopathy.

During follow-up after the completion of initial PRP, retreatment was optional in the ETDRS.

Retreatment with scatter laser was indicated for the redevelopment of high-risk characteristics at which time a minimum of 500 scatter laser burns were given between previous laser scars, anterior to the equator, and the macula. Factors considered in the decision to retreat included the following: (1) change in NV since last treatment, (2) appearance of NV (caliber, degree of capillary network, extent of fibrous tissue), (3) frequency and extent of VH since last treatment, (4) extent of laser scars, and (5) extent of fibrous tissue/TRD. Additionally, ETDRS protocol recommended local confluent or scatter laser treatment to newly occurring small flat NVE.[68] Since the publications by the ETDRS, scatter laser of the macula is usually avoided to minimize visual side effects.[185] However, focal macular laser has been shown to reduce the rate of progression of PDR and scatter laser to ischemic temporal macula seems appropriate when active NV is present despite adequate peripheral retinal treatment.[67] In cases of recurrent vitreous hemorrhage, retreatment with laser reduces the rate of future VH.[186] The risk factors predictive of the need for retreatment include the presence of NVD and the severity of diabetes (e.g., younger age at onset of DM and short time from diagnosis of DM to development of high-risk characteristics).[187] Over the course of a year following initial PRP for proliferative diabetic retinopathy, retreatment may be anticipated in about a third of patients.[187]

There is disagreement on the issue of determining end point in the application of PRP. There are proponents of high-intensity, high-density photocoagulation and this pattern may be most appropriate for severe proliferative diabetic retinopathy as seen in some patients with severe PDR from type 1 diabetes.[188,189] However, both the benefits and the adverse effects of scatter laser are dose dependent.[67] Therefore, if vitreous traction rather than progressive NV growth is the primary cause of VH, vitrectomy surgery is more appropriate than exhaustive laser retreatment leading to peripheral retinal ablation.[20,164,189–191]

9.2.3 Complications

Complications of laser photocoagulation of PDR are important to identify, treat promptly, and prevent when possible.[185,192] A potentially serious anterior segment complication is corneal epithelial trauma.[142] Diabetic eyes are predisposed to abrasion due to poor adhesion of the epithelium to the basement membrane, which may relate to corneal neuropathy. Friction from the contact lens creates a shear force that overcomes the pathologic adhesion.[142] Rarely, severe thermal damage to the cornea may be caused by pigment, such as mascara, on the corneal surface during treatment.[193] Anterior segment breakdown of the blood–aqueous barrier may be more long lasting in eyes with darker color irides, but appears to be clinically insignificant.[194] Lenticular burns may occur in cataractous eyes treated with small-diameter, high-power, long-duration argon photocoagulation.[195] Posterior segment adverse effects due to breakdown of the blood–ocular barrier include macular edema, serous macular/retinal detachment, contraction of preretinal membranes, and choroidal detachment, which may lead to shallowing of the anterior chamber, transient myopia, and secondary glaucoma.[160,196–199] These complications were reported by the ETDRS and were found to be less common in eyes randomized to less extensive scatter laser.[67] In ETDRS protocol, PRP was not applied over fibrous tissue to minimize the risk of preretinal fibrous contraction and TRD.[67] Despite this precaution, vitrectomy surgery may be required for the treatment of traction retinal detachment following PRP.[120] Ciliochoroidal effusion is common after PRP and usually asymptomatic; however, it may cause angle closure in hyperopic eyes with shallow chambers (Fig. 9.11).[177,199] Treatment involves the use of topical and oral glaucoma medications and steroids. Iridotomy is not typically helpful in these cases.[200] Inadvertent direct photocoagulation of the macula may result in permanent scotoma and may be best prevented by following a strict regimen beginning with photocoagulation posteriorly and working anteriorly.[68] Rupture of Bruch's membrane with associated risk of hemorrhage and neovascularization secondary to laser photocoagulation is uncommon and appears to be related to highly intense, small spot-size burns, and the red spectrum of laser light.[201–206] Even without direct macular photocoagulation, multifocal ERG of the macula may show reduced amplitudes after PRP despite good acuity and lack of increase in thickening on OCT.[207] Inadvertent photocoagulation of the long posterior ciliary

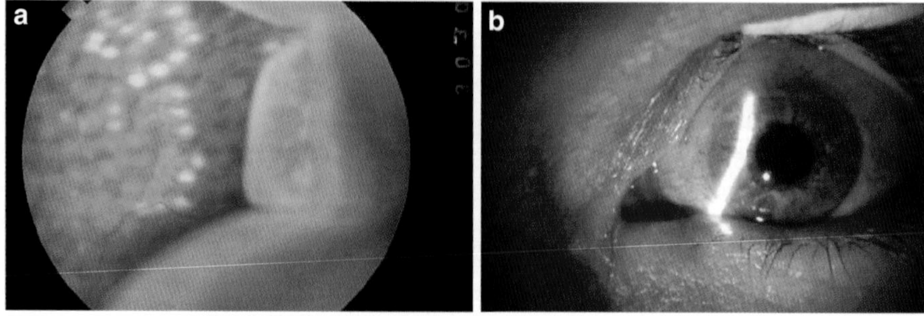

Fig. 9.11 Peripheral choroidal effusion (**a**) following PRP with secondary shallow chamber (**b**)

nerve may result in permanent mydriasis and loss of accommodation.[208] Profound visual field loss may be caused by high-density, high-intensity PRP.[67,152,164] Even with standard PRP visual complications may include decreased acuity, visual field, color vision, and contrast sensitivity.[185]

9.2.4 Outcome

The ETDRS demonstrated that immediate full scatter (PRP) decreased the rate of development of high-risk proliferative diabetic retinopathy by approximately 50% over a 2-year period.[67] Even in the group with poorest prognosis (severe nonproliferative diabetic retinopathy with macular edema) the 5-year rate of severe visual loss (<5/200) was only 6.5% with immediate PRP.[67] Risk factors for poor visual outcome include poor baseline vision, more severe PDR at baseline, and presence of DME. [67,187,209]

9.3 Intraocular Pharmacological Therapy

Subsequent to the completion of the ETDRS and DRVS, a number of pharmacological agents have been used with increasing frequency in an effort to improve outcome in the management of PDR.[210] In general, the risks of intravitreal injection include vitreous hemorrhage, endophthalmitis (0.02–0.87%), pseudo-endophthalmitis, and transient extreme elevation of intraocular pressure following injection.[211–215] Individual agents are discussed below with attendant benefits and risks.

Triamcinolone acetonide: Triamcinolone acetonide (TA) has anti-inflammatory, anti-angiogenic, and anti-fibrotic effects making it an appealing pharmacological choice to treat the complications of PDR and short-term adverse consequences of laser and vitrectomy.[211] Its mechanism of action in reducing neovascular proliferation may include lowering vascular endothelial growth factor (VEGF) and promotion of apoptosis of NV.[216,217] Corticosteroids stabilize the blood–retinal barrier and may protect the neurosensory retina against apoptosis.[211] Intravitreal triamcinolone acetonide (IVT) has been used in PDR to prevent or treat loss of vision from macular thickening and inflammation after panretinal laser and vitrectomy, as well as to treat serous macular detachment following PRP.[218–221] IVT appears to decrease early postoperative ciliary body thickening and anterior chamber angle narrowing after vitrectomy.[222] IVT induces regression of neovascularization of the retina and iris in PDR and NVG, respectively.[223–227] The aqueous half-life of 1.5 mg intravitreally injected TA is 18.6 days in the non-vitrectomized human eye and 3.2 days in the vitrectomized human eye, in which there is a greater probability of dispersion of TA throughout the vitreous cavity and into the anterior chamber.[228,229] Clinically, the duration of effect of a single intravitreal injection is 2–4 months for a 4 mg intravitreal injection and 6 months to 1.5 years for a 20–25 mg injection.[223,229] The particulate size of TA crystals varies from one preparation to another and this difference may account of variable rates of clearance and durations of action among commercially available preparations.[229] There is no significant evidence of therapeutic systemic levels of triamcinolone following IVT.[229] The benefits, however, must be weighed against the adverse effects of cataract (51%), ocular hypertension/glaucoma (21–53%), cytomegalovirus retinitis, reactivation of herpes simplex keratitis, central serous retinopathy, and others.[211,223,229–235] Additionally, concerns have been raised regarding the potential toxicity of triamcinolone acetonide or its preservative on the retina.[236–238] In one study of several, commercially produced preparations of TA using a rabbit model, there was no evidence of toxicity found with a commonly used preparation (Kenalog®).[239] Clinical reports to date suggest that triamcinolone acetonide is useful in select cases of PDR.[211] Readers are directed to Chapter 7 for discussion of triamcinolone acetonide in nonproliferative diabetic retinopathy.

Anti-VEGF Therapy: Intravitreal anti-VEGF drugs offer many advantages of triamcinolone acetonide without the steroid-associated risks of cataract and glaucoma.[240–243] By blocking the effect of vascular endothelial growth factor-A (VEGF-A), these drugs decrease vascular permeability and proliferation.[241,244,245] The most commonly used drug in this class is bevacizumab, which blocks all isoforms of VEGF-A.[246] The aqueous half-life of 1.5 mg intravitreally injected bevacizumab (IVB) is 9.82 days in the non-vitrectomized human eye and is similar to that of ranibizumab.[247] In general, impressive results of bevacizumab have been reported in treating macular edema, retinal neovascularization, neovascular glaucoma, and other complications of PDR.[241,248–250] IVB prior to PRP decreases the risk of post-laser foveal thickening and loss of acuity through its inhibition of the vasopermeability effect of VEGF.[251,252] In vitrectomized eyes the effect of IVB on improving diabetic macular edema is diminished.[253] In the short term, IVB induces regression of NV in active, progressive PDR.[242,254–259] However, due to limited duration of effect, they may be best used adjunctively with other modalities, such as laser and/or vitrectomy.[257,260,261] In eyes with PDR and dense vitreous hemorrhage, IVB may stabilize NV until spontaneous clearing of hemorrhage allows for PRP.[262,263] Some investigators have found that the preoperative injection of bevacizumab improves the ease of vitrectomy, especially in eyes with traction retinal detachment.[246,264] With regression of NV, membranes may be dissected from the retina more readily and intraoperative bleeding is reduced.[265] However, the optimal timing of the preoperative injection is uncertain. Injections less than 7 days prior to vitrectomy may allow for regression of NV and permit surgical intervention before adherent fibrous membranes develop.[266] Bevacizumab is also used adjunctively with laser/surgery for the management of neovascular glaucoma.[250,267,268] The rapid resolution of iris neovascularization may halt the progression of angle synechiae while retinal ablative therapy takes effect and may improve the outcome of glaucoma surgery by decreasing risk of intraoperative or postoperative hemorrhage.[242,248,267,269] IVB may also help prevent bleb failure.[270] Resolution of vitreomacular traction has been reported in a diabetic patient after ranizumab injection.[271] However, adverse effects of anti-VEGF injections for PDR include new-onset traction retinal detachment (approximate 2–5% incidence) occurring at a mean of 13 days following injection (range, 3–31 days).[212,254,255,272,273] Notable progression of pre-existing TRD may occur in approximately 18% of cases.[274] These complications may occur because of the unopposed action of connective tissue growth factors in PDR.[24,85,86] Similar rapid progression of fibrovascular traction with retinal detachment may occur following panretinal photocoagulation.[120] There is also concern that pan-VEGF inhibition may induce neurosensory apoptosis in ischemic conditions, such as PDR.[275] Of interest, however, is the finding of short-term improvement in peripheral retinal perfusion after a single IVB injection in a small series.[276] Currently, the use of IVB is widespread and further studies will help define the optimal role of anti-VEGF therapy.[6,210]

Hyaluronidase: Purified, preservative-free, ovine hyaluronidase has been shown to speed the clearance of vitreous hemorrhage to allow earlier treatment with PRP compared with sham injection in a randomized, controlled trial.[277–279] Its use may be limited by relative slow onset of action and dose-related iritis.[277] Nonetheless, this treatment option may be of special use for patients in whom the systemic risks of vitrectomy surgery and anesthesia are unacceptably high.

Pharmacologic vitreolysis: Pharmacologic vitreolysis offers improved ease of separation of vitreous from the retina.[280] Eyes with PDR and posterior vitreous detachment (PVD) follow a more favorable course than those without PVD.[38] Reports of small series described improved ease of surgery (no peeling or delamination required) and fewer complications (retinal tears) with vitrectomy aided by autologous plasmin enzyme.[281,282] Several pharmacological agents are under evaluation and are discussed later in this chapter. Interestingly, injection of SF6 has also been used to induce PVD to retard progression on PDR.[283] Further studies are needed to better define the role of pharmacologic vitreolysis in the treatment of PDR.

9.4 Vitreoretinal Surgery

Vitreoretinal surgery has an established role in the management of complications of diabetic retinopathy.[69,71,72] Vitrectomy was required in 208 eyes (5.6%) of 3711 patients enrolled in the ETDRS underscoring the lack of universal response of PDR to laser treatment.[69] Prior to the Diabetic Retinopathy Vitrectomy Study (DRVS), vitrectomy was reserved for dense nonclearing vitreous hemorrhage greater than 1-year duration and for traction retinal detachment involving the center of the macula. These conservative indications reflected the lack of experience with vitrectomy and the high rate of serious complications at that time.[71] Both the ETDRS and the DRVS were hindered by the lack of endophotocoagulation, which was not available until 1983.[71] With gains in experience and technology, the role of vitrectomy has expanded significantly since these important studies were published.

9.4.1 Indications

Following vitreous hemorrhage and traction retinal detachment are other less pressing indications for vitrectomy such as dense premacular hemorrhage, fibrovascular proliferation, and diabetic macular edema as well as conditions not specific to diabetes including macular pucker, vitreomacular traction, and macular hole. More severe conditions that are now approached include combined rhegmatogenous–traction retinal detachment, neovascular glaucoma, uncontrolled hemolytic/ghost cell glaucoma, anterior hyaloidal fibrovascular proliferation, and fibrinoid syndrome with retinal detachment.[284–286] The following sections define indications with management considerations and outcomes among these subgroups.

Vitreous hemorrhage: Although vitreous hemorrhage is a common indication for vitrectomy, surgery may be avoided in most eyes. Observation alone may result in improvement.[285] Bed rest with elevation of the head (with or without patching) may facilitate spontaneous resolution of vitreous hemorrhage.[287–289] Intravitreal injection of hyaluronidase hastens the clearing of vitreous hemorrhage.[278] When a portion of the retina can be visualized, panretinal photocoagulation is applied to induce regression of active neovascularization.[285] Krypton laser and long-wavelength diode laser systems penetrate vitreous hemorrhage with greater facility than argon laser and indirect ophthalmoscopic delivery systems may be more effective than slitlamp delivery.[285]

The DRVS demonstrated the benefit of early vitrectomy (1–4 months from onset) in severe vitreous hemorrhage (<5/200 vision) resulting in earlier recovery of vision and better visual outcome at 2 and 4 years, especially in type 1 diabetes mellitus. There was no significant increased risk of the severe complication of NLP vision with early vitrectomy, though it occurred sooner in the early-surgery group compared with the deferral group.[71] The DRVS enrolled 616 eyes with vision less than 5/200 due to severe vitreous hemorrhage with duration of less than 6 months. Eyes with VH present for at least 1 month were randomized to early vs. deferral of vitrectomy for 1 year. Recovery of vision of 20/100 or better by 3 months was more common in the early group (50%) compared with the deferral group (17%). The visual acuity at the 2-year follow-up was 20/40 or better in the early group was 25% compared with 15% in the deferral group ($P = 0.01$). The benefit was even greater in patients with type 1 diabetes mellitus (36% early group vs. 12% deferral group, $P = 0.0001$) compared with type 2 (16% early group vs. 18% deferral group). The benefit persisted at the 4-year follow-up visit and was most prominent in the type 1 patients, presumably due to the aggressive nature of PDR in these cases.[71] In a survey of the American Society of Retinal Specialists in 2008, the vast majority of 366 respondents routinely performed vitrectomy surgery between 1 and 3 months from onset of nonclearing vitreous hemorrhage.[210]

There are a number of issues to consider in evaluating the unimpressive results of early vitrectomy in type 2 patients. Poorer postoperative visual acuity may be a function of greater severity of maculopathy in type 2 patients compared with those with type 1 diabetes.[71] In addition, the DRVS did not report an analysis of the vitreous status in these eyes.[71] PVD is more common with age and is associated with better prognosis without intervention compared with eyes without PVD.[38,182] Therefore, in clinical decision making, the use of preoperative B-scan examinations may be helpful in stratifying this group of eyes. Eyes with more extensive vitreoretinal attachments may benefit from vitrectomy to a greater degree than those with more complete PVD. Another influential factor in determining the timing of vitrectomy for vitreous hemorrhage is the presence and degree of activity of iris rubeosis. Prompt vitrectomy is indicated to clear the media for the application of PRP in cases of progressive rubeosis and neovascular glaucoma.[285]

Subsequent to the DRVS, a retrospective study reviewed 353 eyes operated for diabetic vitreous hemorrhage and reported improved vision in 81% of cases. Final vision of 20/200 or better was achieved in 48% of operated eyes and 5/200 or better in 79%.[290] Favorable factors for good outcome were preoperative vision greater than 5/200, minimal cataract, no NVI/NVG, and PRP in at least one quadrant.[184] These data and others argue in favor of preparing for vitrectomy with augmentation of PRP laser when possible and applying endolaser at the time of surgery.[69,285] Postoperative vitreous hemorrhage is common and usually clears with observation; however, approximately 10% of cases require repeat vitrectomy or fluid–gas exchange.[285,291] In a retrospective study of 484 consecutive vitrectomy procedures for various complications of PDR, 4% of eyes required repeat vitrectomy for vitreous hemorrhage.[291]

Ghost cell glaucoma: Glaucoma may be encountered as a consequence of diabetic vitreous hemorrhage as degenerated red blood cells obstruct trabecular outflow resulting in elevated intraocular pressure.[292] This secondary open-angle glaucoma occurs most commonly in aphakic and/or vitrectomized eyes, as ghost cells do not penetrate the intact anterior hyaloid face.[290,293–296] Ghost cells are erythroclastic red blood cells that have become spherical, less pliable, and slower to clear from the eye. The indication for vitrectomy and anterior chamber lavage is uncontrolled intraocular pressure despite maximal medical therapy.[297] Response to surgery is generally favorable.[297]

Dense premacular (subhyaloid) hemorrhage: In PDR with intact vitreous, dense premacular hemorrhage may be trapped between the internal limiting membrane and the posterior hyaloid face resulting in acute, profound loss of visual acuity. The thick red hemorrhage is well circumscribed, usually round or oval in shape, and obscures all view of the underlying retina (Fig. 9.12). The natural history is not well defined as these cases were grouped with vitreous hemorrhage in the DRVS.[70,71] Most subhyaloid hemorrhages will clear without vitrectomy by spontaneously breaking through into the vitreous cavity.[284] However, dense nonclearing subhyaloid hemorrhages may be associated with fibrovascular proliferation, preretinal membrane formation, and traction macular detachment.[298] Vitrectomy surgery is used in these eyes to speed recovery of vision and decrease the risk of complications.[290,298,299] Although it is desirable to allow a few months time for the hemorrhage to clear, a further delay in surgery may make surgical dissection more difficult.[285]

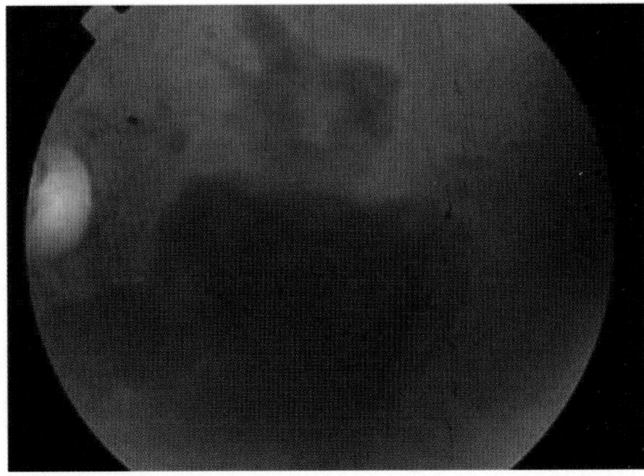

Fig. 9.12 Dense premacular hemorrhage trapped between the partially separated posterior cortical vitreous and the retina

Non-vitrectomy Management of Dense Premacular Hemorrhage

As a less invasive alternative to vitrectomy, laser (argon, krypton, or Nd:YAG) may be used to create an opening in the posterior hyaloid face to aid in the breakthrough of subhyaloid hemorrhage into the vitreous cavity.[300–304] However, laser membranotomy is not universally successful. In a retrospective study of 21 laser-treated eyes with hemorrhage from a variety of causes, the blood did not clear in five eyes (24%).[305] Furthermore, one eye developed a macular hole and one myopic eye developed retinal detachment.[305] Macular hole, however, has been reported to occur following subhyaloid premacular hemorrhage not treated with laser.[306,307] Laser membranotomy may be augmented with intravitreal tissue plasminogen activator (tPA).[300] Intravitreal gas (SF_6) injection can also resolve subhyaloid hemorrhage through the induction of a posterior vitreous detachment.[308] Intravitreal tPA alone or in combination with gas (C_3F_8 or SF_6) injection has been reported to be successful in small retrospective case series.[308–310]

Traction retinal detachment: Vitreoretinal traction is common in PDR as neovascular membranes grow within the cortical vitreous gel, create firm vitreoretinal adhesions, and contract over time.[28,285] Breakdown of the blood–ocular barrier contributes to vitreous contraction and subsequent traction retinal detachment (Fig. 9.13).[311] Traction macular detachment acutely involving or threatening the macula has become the most common indication for vitrectomy since the ETDRS and DRS.[285]

The DRVS described the course of extramacular traction retinal detachment (TRD) in the posterior pole over a 2-year period.[70] The study enrolled 290 eyes with vision ≥20/100 (or ≥20/400 due to

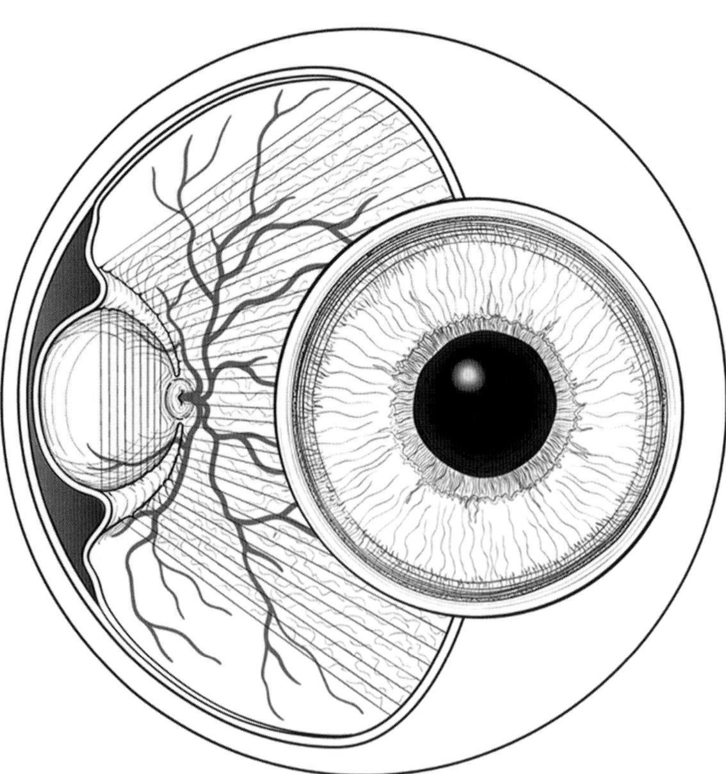

Fig. 9.13 Stylized illustration of traction retinal detachment involving the macula in PDR. Vitreous tractional forces are represented by multiple individual lines drawn along the posterior vitreous face

vitreous hemorrhage). At baseline the TRD measured at least four disk areas and extended within 30° from the center of the macula. Also included were TRD's less than four disk areas if the vitreoretinal adhesions causing the elevation were within 30° from the center of the macula and were associated with either active new vessels or recent vitreous hemorrhage. Photocoagulation was permitted at the discretion of the ophthalmologist. Two or more lines of vision were lost in 43% of eyes from baseline to the 2-year examination. Severe visual loss (<5/200 at two consecutive 4-month visits) increased from 0% at baseline to 15% at 1 year and 24% at 2 years. Subgroup analysis revealed poor prognosis in eyes with active NV (defined as NV containing visible blood) or recent vitreous hemorrhage (defined as red in color). Severe visual loss in eyes with and without these characteristics was 21–30% and 14%, respectively. Among eyes with active NV or recent vitreous hemorrhage, the extent of TRD was also a significant factor for severe visual loss: 21% for eyes with TRD less than four disk areas compared to 30% for eyes with TRD greater than four disk areas. The most common causes of severe visual loss included vitreous hemorrhage and retinal detachment. Of significance, only 35.2% of all eyes with TRD had PRP at the baseline examination. By the 2-year follow-up examination, 54.8% had not received PRP.[70] Currently, earlier intervention with PRP and vitrectomy offers an improved prognosis in these cases.[70,285]

The management of extramacular traction retinal detachments appears to be undergoing change. Traditionally, extramacular traction detachments were observed as the rate of progression into the macula (approximately 15% annual risk) was felt to be lower than the risk poor outcome with vitrectomy.[312] However, the anatomic results following vitrectomy have improved since earlier reports and the risk of loss of vision with vitrectomy has decreased.[274,313,314] Unfortunately, the functional results of vitrectomy surgery following the successful repair of macula-off traction retinal detachment remains disappointing (Table 9.7). Consequently, a number of researchers have called for vitrectomy surgery at an earlier stage, prior to severe visual loss from TRD.[274,315]

A number of retrospective studies of eyes operated for diabetic TRD are available for review, although direct comparison is not possible due to variability in the patient populations (Table 9.7). A variety of surgical techniques have been employed. Improving anatomic results have been apparent with the evolution of vitrectomy from removal of axial traction by core vitrectomy to sophisticated methods of relieving tangential traction by segmentation and delamination with membrane peeling relegated to a minor role in the management of minimally adherent membranes.[49,274,313,315–319] Reports over the past 20 years indicate visual improvement may be achieved in 60–75% of cases.[274,313,320–323] The final visual acuity results generally reveal a modest 20/200 or better in 47–57% of eyes, and 5/200 or better in 69–77%.[313,318,319,321,322,324,325] Successful anatomic reattachment of the macula is achieved in 81–100% of cases.[313,318,319,321,322,324,325] Favorable factors include age <50 years, preoperative PRP laser, preoperative vision >5/200, minimal cataract/vitreous hemorrhage, no NVI/NVG, less extensive retinal neovascularization, absence of iris neovascularization, macular detachment for less than 30 days, no need for lensectomy/gas tamponade, and no iatrogenic break.[49,69,325,326] The incidence of surgical complications appears to be greater in eyes undergoing vitrectomy for PDR with TRD compared with other indications in diabetic retinopathy.[326] The need for reoperation following vitrectomy for diabetic traction retinal detachment generally ranges from 24 to 47% (excluding laser and cataract extraction).[49,313,318,319]

Chronic TRD involving macula (>6 months duration) is managed conservatively.[69,71] In one study, macula-off TRD of greater than 1 month duration was associated with poor visual prognosis (<20/200, $P = 0.042$, univariate analysis).[325] In eyes with chronic macular detachment, the retina is atrophic beneath tightly adherent fibrovascular membranes, which lower the potential for successful surgery.[18,285]

Combined traction–rhegmatogenous retinal detachment: PDR may cause severe fibrovascular proliferation resulting in progressive traction and posterior retinal breaks.[327] The resultant retinal detachment appears different from TRD. Combined traction–rhegmatogenous retinal detachments (TRRD) appear convex and often extend anteriorly to the ora serata.[120] The retinal often

Table 9.7 Literature summary of vitrectomy for diabetic traction retinal detachment[a]

Source Year	N	Intervention	Outcome: Macula/Retina attached (%)	Outcome: ≥5/200 (%)	Outcome: ≥20/200 (%)	Comments
Tolentino[317] 1980	140	Vtx, seg/peel ± SBP/AFE, Lnx 4% no gas/silicone	74/NR	67	51	65% better, 18% same, 17% worse Reoperation: NR Phthisis: NR
Aaberg[315] 1981	125	Vtx, seg/peel/delam ± SBP/GFE, Lnx no silicone oil	≥91/91	NR	58	72% better, 11% same, 17% worse Reoperation: NR Phthisis: NR
Rice[767] 1983	197	Vtx, seg/peel SBP >35%, Lnx 47% 360cryo 37%, ± GFE no silicone oil	66/57	59	NR	57% better, 9% same, 35% worse Reoperation: 29% Phthisis: 9%
Thompson[49] 1987	360	Vtx, seg/peel SBP 22%, Lnx 29% 360cryo 32%, GFE 42% no silicone oil	71/69	64	NR	59% better, 41% same or worse Reoperation: 24% Phthisis: 11% included series from rice (above)
Williams[318] 1989	69	Vtx, en bloc delam SBP 17%, Lnx 7% GFE 51%, no silicone	88/83	71	NR	NR% better, NR% same, NR% worse re-operation: 47% (29% return to OR) Phthisis: 6%
Oldendoerp[321] 1989	100	Vtx, seg/peel SBP 39%, no Lnx GFE 65%, Silicone 9%	81/NR	77	47	71% better, 29% same or worse Reoperation: NR9% Pre-phthisis/phthisis: 18%
Han[319] 1994	30	Vtx, mod EB delam SBP 17%, Lnx 3% GFE 40%, no silicone	≥97/97	77	54	NR% better, NR% same, NR% worse Reoperation: 27% (7% in OR) Phthisis: none reported
Meier[324] 1997	28	Vtx, mod EB delam SBP 57%, Lnx 36% GFE 14%, Silicone 86%	86/79	NR	50	Silicone oil not removed Reoperation: NR Phthisis: NR
Steinmetz[313] 2002	67	Vtx, delam SBP 24%, Lnx 6% GFE 64%, Silicone 1%	100/93	70	57	72% better, 28% same or worse Reoperation: 33% Phthisis: 0%

[a]Included reports >100 cases prior to 1988, follow-up ≥6 months. Note: endolaser became available ca 1983.
NR = not reported, N = number of cases in reported series, Vtx = vitrectomy, seg = membrane segmentation, peel = membrane peeling, EB = en bloc, SBP = scleral buckle procedure, AFE = air–fluid exchange, GFE = gas–fluid exchange, Lnx = lensectomy, delam = membrane delamination, 360cryo = 360 degree peripheral retinal cryopexy

has hydration lines, white lines in the inner retina, which are diagnostic of a retinal break (Fig. 9.14).[285] Subretinal hemorrhage may be present.[328] There is usually a single, small, paravascular retinal break near posterior fibrovascular proliferation, often not identified until surgery.[120,317,329] Silicone oil tamponade is frequently used, especially in patients with poor vision in the fellow eye.[120,330] Silicone oil reduces the incidence of postoperative rubeosis and phthisis.[120,330] Early reports of retrospective consecutive series demonstrated retinal reattachment in 47–82% and improvement in vision in 20–53% of operated eyes with final visual acuity of 5/200 or better in 55–68% of all eyes operated.[32,317,329,331,332] With the availability of silicone oil, subsequent studies reported retinal

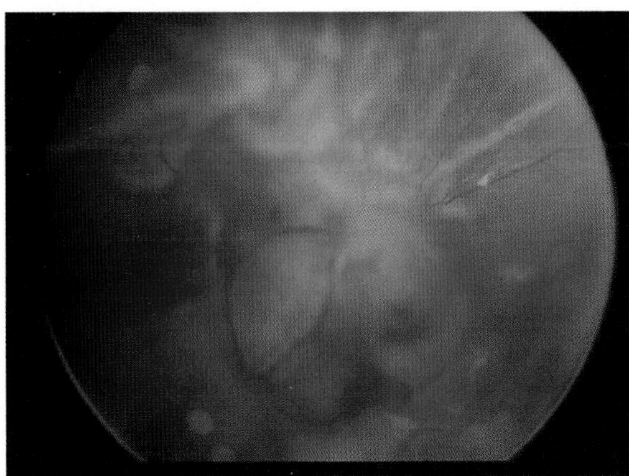

Fig. 9.14 Combined traction–rhegmatogenous retinal detachment from PDR. The fundus photograph shows the convex nature of the retinal detachment with hydration lines within the retina. Preretinal hemorrhage obscures the view of the macula

reattachment in 73–93% and an improvement in vision in 64–81% of eyes following vitrectomy with final visual acuity of 5/200 or better in 55–68% of all eyes operated (Table 9.8).[330,333–335] To achieve these results reoperation was required in 29–90% of eyes.[49,120,329,330,334] The incidence of phthisis decreased from 8 to 10% in early, large series to 0% with the use of silicone oil in later series.[49,120,329,330] Favorable factors for postoperative vision >5/200 include preoperative vision >5/200, no NVI, no macular involvement, and no iatrogenic break.[32,120]

Severe fibrovascular proliferation: The progressive proliferation of fibrovascular preretinal tissue may occur despite photocoagulation, especially in poorly controlled type 1 diabetes.[70] Without surgical intervention, severe fibrovascular proliferation (FVP) threatens profound loss of vision.[285] The DRVS reported the natural history study of 142 eyes with severe FVP (NV >4DA with elevation of the border of the NV from traction, but no significant VH or TRD) and showed the percentage of eyes that developed severe visual loss at the 2-year follow-up increased from 0 to 32%. A majority of eyes (52%) suffered a loss of acuity of two or more lines mostly within the first year. The percentage of eyes with good vision (≥20/40) decreased from 57 to 39%. Visual acuity at baseline was a significant negative risk factor; eyes with <20/40 vision at baseline deteriorated to <5/200 at 2 years in approximately 40% of cases. In interpreting this data, however, it should be noted that 73% of these eyes had no PRP at baseline, and by the 2-year follow-up, the percentage of eyes without any PRP was 35.9%.[336] Today, more aggressive application of PRP likely improves the outcome in this cohort.[69]

The DRVS developed the definition of "advanced, active, neovascular or fibrovascular proliferation" (AA-PDR) from a review of the natural history study referenced above. They randomized to early vitrectomy vs. conventional management 370 eyes with useful vision (≥20/400) and AA-PDR. At the 4-year follow-up exam, good vision (≥20/40) was present in 44% of eyes in the early vitrectomy group compared with 28% of the conventional group (observation until TRD involved the macular or nonclearing VH >6 months) ($P < 0.05$). There was no reported difference between the two groups regarding risk of poor vision from surgical intervention. The final rate of severe visual loss was similar in the two groups. The benefit of surgery tended to increase with increasing severity of neovascularization (borderline statistical significance). Significant favorable factors included better vision at baseline and preoperative PRP laser.

Thus, the DRVS recommended early vitrectomy for eyes with any one of the following characteristics diagnostic of AA-PDR: (1) severe new vessels and severe fibrous proliferations; (2) severe new vessels and red vitreous hemorrhage; or (3) moderate new vessels (standard photo 10A, Fig. 9.1), severe fibrous proliferation, and red vitreous hemorrhage. Severe new vessels were defined as (1) NVD equaling or exceeding standard photograph 10C (Fig. 9.15) or (2) NVE equaling or exceeding standard photograph 7 (Fig. 9.16) in at least one 30° photographic field or (3) total new vessels (NVD and all NVE) summed over all photographic fields estimated to equal or exceed four disk areas. The DRVS concluded that eyes most suitable for early vitrectomy were those with both severe fibrous proliferation and at least moderately severe NV despite extensive PRP or hemorrhage precluding such treatment.[69,337] Severe fibrous proliferations were defined as (1) fibrovascular proliferations on or within one disk diameter of the disk

Table 9.8 Literature summary of vitrectomy for diabetic traction–rhegmatogenous retinal detachment[a]

Source Year	N	Diagnosis	Intervention	Outcome: Macula/Retina attached (%)	Outcome: ≥5/200 (%)	Outcome: ≥20/200 (%)	Comments
Michels[331] 1978	10	TR–RD No VH	Vtx, Lnx SBP, cryo	NR	NR	NR	20% better, 40% same, 40% worse mixed case series limited data segregation Reoperation: NR, Phthisis: NR
Peyman[332] 1978	26	RD with VH or "vitreous retraction"	Vtx (vitrophage) limited details	NR	NR	NR	42% better, 46% same, 12% worse mixed case series/limited data Reoperation: NR, Phthisis: NR
Tolentino[317] 1980	34	TR–RD m-off 100%	Vtx, seg, min peel SBP 100%, AFX, Lnx	82/NR	68	29	47% better, 35% same, 18% worse mixed series/limited data Va ≥ 20/40 in 12% of eyes Reoperation: NR, Phthisis: NR
Rice[329] 1983	107	TR–RD m-off 89%	Vtx, seg, cryo/laser SBP/360cryo 58% AFX 100%, Lnx 60%	64/47	55	36	53% better, 6% same, 41% worse Va ≥ 20/40 in 10% of eyes Reoperation: 29%, Phthisis: 8%
Thompson[32] 1987	172	TR–RD m-off 87%	Vtx, seg, SBP 63% 360cryo 56%, A-GFE, Lnx 42%	≥52/52	56	±42	48% better, 7% same, 45% worse Va > 20/40 in 9% of eyes, 23% NLP Included Rice series (above) Reoperation: 32%, Phthisis: 10%
Sima[334] 1994	26	TR–RD m-off NR%	Vtx, seg, NR delam Lnx, SBP cryo/laser, SO 100%	NR/NR	NR	61	81% better, 19% same or worse mixed series/limited data SO removed in most eyes Reoperation: NR%, Phthisis: NR%
Douglas[330] 2003	22	TR–RD m-off 100%	Vtx, seg, delam en bloc, laser Lnx 100% (no IOL) SO 100%	91/91	68	55	64% better, 9% same, 27% worse 68% ≥ 20/400 Silicone removed 64% of eyes Reoperation: 64%, Phthisis: 0%
Yang[120] 2008	40	TR–RD m-off 100%	Vtx, Lnx, seg, peel, delam, SBP 100% 15% C3F8 42.5% SO 57.5%	93/93	55	48	70% better, 15% same, 15% worse Note: SO was not removed Reoperation: 90%, phthisis: 0%

[a]Retrospective case series with follow-up ≥ 6 months. Note: Endolaser became available ca 1983
N = number of cases in report, NR = not reported, TR–RD = combined traction–rhegmatogenous retinal detachment, VH = vitreous hemorrhage, m-off = macula-off (macular detachment), Vtx = vitrectomy, Lnx = lensectomy, IOL = intraocular lens, SBP = scleral buckle procedure, cryo = retinal cryopexy, 360cryo = 360° peripheral retinal cryopexy, seg = membrane segmentation, min = minimal, peel = membrane peeling, AFX = air–fluid exchange, A-GFX = air– or gas–fluid exchange, SO = silicone oil.

border (FVD) equaling or exceeding two disk areas, or (2) fibrous proliferations elsewhere (FVE) equaling or exceeding standard photograph 11 (Fig. 9.17) in at least one photographic field, or (3) total fibrous proliferations (FVD and FVE) equal to or exceeding four disk areas.

Others have reported favorable surgical results for severe fibrovascular proliferation as well. In retrospective series, stable or improved vision was reported in approximately 78% of cases. Final vision >5/200 was reported in 81–82% of operated eyes.[290] Favorable prognostic factors include young

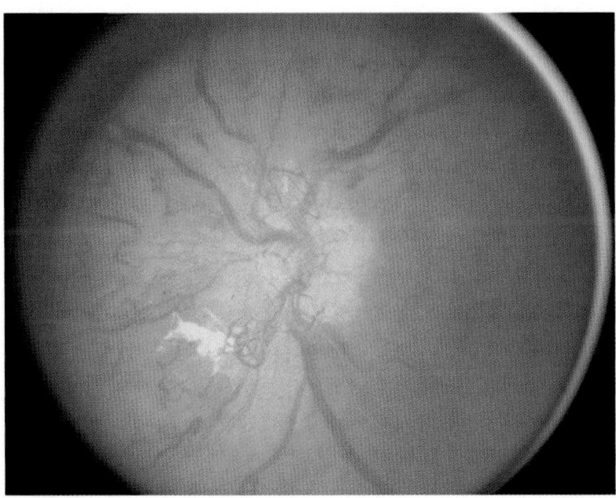

Fig. 9.15 Standard photograph 10C defining the lower limit of severe new vessels on or within one disk diameter of the disk (printed with permission from the Early Treatment Diabetic Retinopathy Study Research Group. All rights reserved)

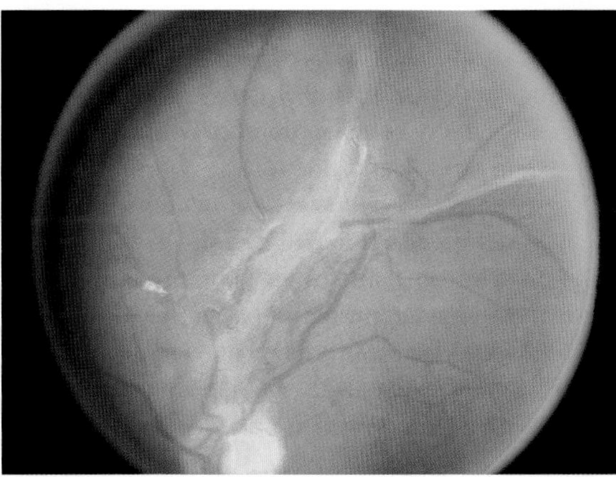

Fig. 9.17 Standard photograph 11 defining the lower limit of severe fibrous proliferation elsewhere (>1 disk diameter from the disk border) (printed with permission from the Early Treatment Diabetic Retinopathy Study Research Group. All rights reserved)

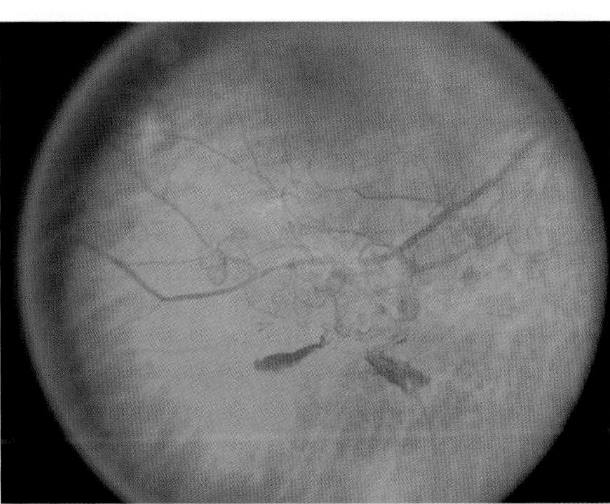

Fig. 9.16 Standard photograph 7 defining the lower limit of severe NVE (NV >1 disk diameter from disk border) (printed with permission from the Early Treatment Diabetic Retinopathy Study Research Group. All rights reserved)

age (<40 years), good preoperative vision (>5/200), no NVI, preoperative PRP, and no iatrogenic break at surgery.[183]

From the literature we conclude that these cases are best managed with extensive PRP laser prior to early vitrectomy, which is best undertaken prior to the development of extensive, strong vitreoretinal attachments.[285,338] As some eyes lose vision despite surgery, it is essential to counsel the patient regarding the benefits and risks of surgery vs. natural history. These issues are of particular importance in patients with relatively asymptomatic pathology.

Diabetic macular edema: The reader is referred to Chapter 7, which includes a discussion of vitrectomy for diabetic macular edema.

Postvitrectomy fibrinoid syndrome with retinal detachment: The syndrome of intraocular fibrin deposition following diabetic vitrectomy is discussed under the section on complications of vitrectomy surgery later in this chapter. Repeat vitrectomy surgery may be attempted in severe cases with secondary traction retinal detachment and neovascular glaucoma, but the prognosis is poor.[285] Adjunctive use of steroids and tissue plasminogen activator may improve success rate.[285,339–341]

Anterior hyaloidal fibrovascular proliferation (AHFVP): The growth of fibrovascular tissue on the anterior vitreous base in PDR is a severe complication following vitrectomy.[342,343] If progressive membranes cause retinal detachment, ciliary body detachment, or neovascular glaucoma, repeat vitrectomy surgery may be indicated.[285] The reader is referred to the subsequent section on complications of vitreoretinal surgery for further details.

A less rapidly progressive form of AHFVP has been described after cataract extraction in nonvitrectomized eyes. Risk factors included PDR, iris rubeosis, and ischemic anterior retina. Delayed onset was noted at an average of 12 months following cataract surgery and no progression was noted over an average 6-month follow-up. Vision was rarely affected and no complications of vitreous hemorrhage or traction detachment were reported.[343]

Vitreomacular interface pathology: Epiretinal membranes (ERM), macular hole, vitreomacular traction syndrome, and other vitreoretinal interface disorders are encountered in patients with or without diabetes. However, there may be unique features in the presentation, management, and outcome with vitrectomy in patients with diabetes mellitus.[344–347]

Epiretinal membranes in PDR may be vascular or avascular.[348,349] Below is a discussion of avascular, premacular, epiretinal membranes associated with diabetic retinopathy. Although pathogenesis of ERM in diabetic retinopathy shares some features with idiopathic ERM, the role of fibrogenic growth factors maybe greater in diabetic ERM.[25,26,350,351] In addition, the cellular and extracellular composition of ERM varies with underlying etiology.[352,353] The proliferative activity of diabetic ERM may be greater than the idiopathic variety.[354] In preparation for surgery, optical coherence tomography demonstrates the variable vitreoretinal relationships seen with diabetic ERM.[355] Diabetic ERM is more likely to have focal rather than global attachments to the macula compared to idiopathic ERM ($P = 0.007$).[356] Factors associated with visual improvement after membrane peeling in PDR include age and preoperative visual acuity.[348] Concomitant peeling of internal limiting membrane (ILM) may improve macular appearance on OCT[349] and improve visual outcome.[349,357] However, peeling of ILM in eyes with diabetic macular edema may rarely be associated with macular hole formation.[358,359]

In general, the presentation of macular holes in patients with diabetes may be similar to those without diabetes. The causative mechanism of macular hole appears to be tangential vitreous traction, although diabetic macular edema may play an additional causative role in diabetic retinopathy.[360,361] Macular holes may form in association with PDR alone (Fig. 9.18) or following bevacizumab injection, triamcinolone injection, or vitrectomy surgery with or without peeling of the ILM.[272,359,362,363] Complex vitreoretinal attachments may be

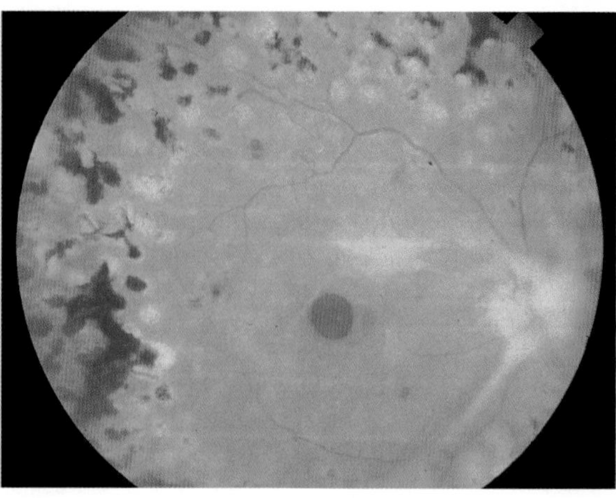

Fig. 9.18 Macular hole due to fibrous proliferation and contraction in PDR

encountered with fibrovascular proliferation at the macular hole, which may result in retinal detachment.[32,364,365] Peeling of ILM may be difficult and unnecessary for successful closure of macular hole in cases of moderate or high macular detachment.[364] The rate of successful closure of macular hole is 73–100% (Table 9.9).[344–347,360,362,364,366,367] The visual prognosis correlates negatively with poor preoperative visual acuity, increased degree of macular detachment, increased severity of diabetic retinopathy, and the presence of submacular hemorrhage.[344–346,346,347,364] Generally, there is only limited visual improvement following repair of macular hole associated with proliferative diabetic retinopathy. Spontaneous closure of macular hole with PDR may occur.[368]

Vitreomacular traction may present with complex vitreoretinal adhesions potentially requiring more extensive vitrectomy surgery than that required in non-diabetic patients (Fig. 9.19). The intact posterior hyaloid may be taut in cases of ERM and macular edema.[369–371] Progressive contraction of the intact cortical vitreous may result in traction retinoschisis.[372] Alternatively, tangential traction may result in macular heterotopia as a cause of decreased acuity, metamorphopsia, and diplopia.[27,30,369,373–378]

Controversial indications for vitrectomy: Vitreopapillary traction (VPT) is a relatively new and equivocal indication for diabetic vitrectomy with proponents in Europe.[183,379–381] VPT occurs as a result of anomalous posterior vitreous detachment.

Table 9.9 Literature summary of vitrectomy for macular hole with proliferative diabetic retinopathy[a]

Source Year	*N*	Diagnosis (*N*)	Intervention (*N*)	Follow-up (months)	Outcome (% closed)	Comments
Flynn[347] 1994	2	PDR s/p PRP (1) PDR (1)	Vtx, 16% C_3F_8 (2)	7–12	100%	Case 1: from 20/400 to 20/200 Case 2: from 20/400 to 20/300
Brazitikos[360] 1999	3	PDR (3) -with VH (1)	Vtx, no ILM peel (3) -"gas" (1) -20% SF_6 (2)	4–6	100%	Case 1: Va unreported Case 2: from 20/400 to 20/200 Case 3: from 20/50 to 20/40
Ghoraba[346] 2002	14	TR–RD (5) TRD (3), PMH (3) CME (3)	Vtx (14), -ILM peel (1) -SF_6 (3), SO (11)	3–19 (av 7.6)	73%	Limited improvement (≤20/100) 11/14 previously operated severe PDR
Kurihara[344] 2005	3	PDR s/p PRP (3)-regressed NV (3)	Vtx, ILM peel (3) -20% SF_6 (3)	NR	100%	Mean improvement in Va: two Snellen lines
Yan[367] 2007	12	DR unspecified	Vtx, ILM peel (12) -18% C_3F_8 (9) -SO (3)	3–24 (mean 6)	83%	Va "improved" in 83% cases
Yeh[364] 2008	23	TRD (17) TR–RD (6)	Vtx (23) -ILM peel (4)	NR	83%	ILM peeling may not be needed in cases with moderate to high macular detachment
Mason[366] 2008	6	TRD (6)	Vtx, ILM peel (6) -"gas" (6)	10 (mean)	100%	Mean pre-op Va: 20/250 Mean postop Va: 20/100
Kumagai[362] 2008	9	PDR (9) postop from previous Vtx	Vtx with SF_6 (9) - ILM peel (3)	59 (mean)	78%	Mean pre-op Va: 20/154 Mean postop Va: 20/125 better closure rate with ILM peeling

[a]Retrospective case series

NR = not reported, *N* = number of cases in series, PDR = proliferative diabetic retinopathy, PRP = panretinal photocoagulation, VH = vitreous hemorrhage, TR–RD = traction–rhegmatogenous retinal detachment, TRD = traction retinal detachment, PMH = premacular hemorrhage, CME = cystoid macular edema, NV = neovascularization, Vtx = pars plana vitrectomy, ILM = internal limiting membrane, SO = silicone oil, av = average, Va = visual acuity (Snellen)

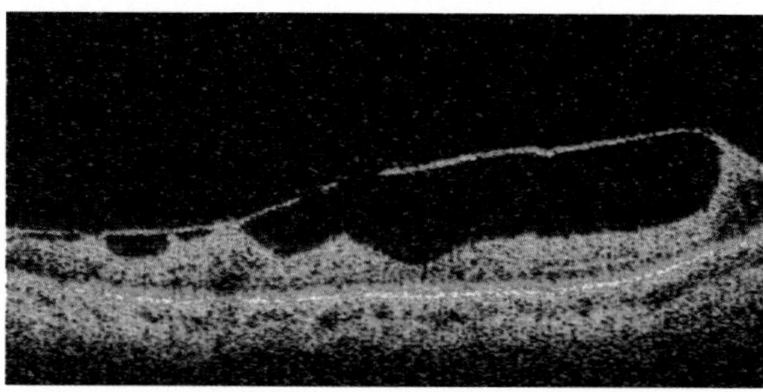

Fig. 9.19 Optical coherence tomograph of right eye (20/40) with established PDR demonstrating incomplete separation of vitreous with multiple vitreoretinal attachments

The macromolecular changes that result in vitreous gel liquefaction occur without concurrent separation of the posterior cortical vitreous from the surface of the optic disk.[382] The optic disk may appear elevated and hyperemic with blurred margins due to condensation of the overlying vitreous or due to traction on the disk and peripapillary retina.[383] Optical coherence tomography is useful to confirm the diagnosis.[384,385] Vitreopapillary traction has been described as an isolated phenomenon or in association with other pathology, including diabetic retinopathy. Among those cases without diabetic retinopathy, VPT may occur in young patients in whom myopia may induce vitreous liquefaction and mildly dyplastic optic disks may contribute to unusual vitreopapillary adherence.[386,387] Although most patients are asymptomatic despite the presence of intrapapillary and peripapillary hemorrhage,[386,387] gaze-evoked amaurosis may occur.[388] Generally, VPT remains stable with follow-up and does not require intervention.[386,387] However, macular exudates presenting as a stellate maculopathy may rarely develop in association with peripapillary traction detachment in VPT.[389] In older patients with involutional vitreous degeneration, persistent vitreopapillary adhesion of unknown cause may result in VPT. These patients usually present without symptoms and may be detected on fluorescein angiography with disk staining.[390,391] However, symptomatic vitreomacular traction and traction macular detachment may complicate VPT.[384,385] Ischemic central retinal vein occlusion has been reported to cause VPT; however, the report of three cases was complicated by coexisting diabetes, diabetic retinopathy, and severe premacular fibrous proliferation.[392] In diabetes mellitus, glycation of vitreous collagen and other secondary vitreous changes may play a role in VPT.[382,383] No functional abnormalities are reported with vitreopapillary traction unassociated with other complications of diabetic retinopathy.[393] A causative role of VPT has been suggested in eyes with coexistent symptomatic diabetic macular edema.[381] Supporting this notion is the report of an isolated case of spontaneous resolution of diabetic macular edema and disk edema following spontaneous posterior vitreous detachment in an eye with VPT and PDR.[394] Others have proposed early vitrectomy to prevent optic neuropathy secondary to VPT, though supportive data are limited at this time.[379,380] Although threatened axonal damage from VPT is proposed as an indication for vitrectomy, removal of the optic disk stalk in diabetic eyes may result in axonal loss as well.[395] There is limited evidence that isolated vitreopapillary traction affects visual function and that surgery improves outcome.[381] Vitreopapillary traction is often seen in association with other complications of proliferative diabetic retinopathy (e.g., traction retinal detachment), which provide a clearer indication for surgery.[183]

Subfoveal exudates are an uncommon indication for vitrectomy surgery. The reader is referred to Chapter 7 for discussion.

9.4.2 Preoperative Management

The surgical preparation of a patient with complications of PDR is complex. The presence of advanced diabetic retinopathy may be indicative of the presence of significant systemic microvascular and macrovascular disease. In addition, the nonretinal ocular complications of diabetes are protean and proper assessment is critical to successful surgery. Thus, the preoperative management may require extensive examination, counseling, and consultation.

General medical considerations: The exhaustive list of issues to be considered in the systemic management of the diabetic patient prior to surgery is beyond the scope of this chapter. Given the high cardiovascular risk of these patients, the ophthalmologist may elect to refer the patient for preoperative evaluation and clearance with the primary care physician, cardiologist, nephrologist, and/or endocrinologist.[396] Optimal preoperative control of blood glucose may offer protection against infection.[397] Clear instructions are given to the patient regarding adjustments of medications, especially those taken for blood glucose control. Antiplatelet and anticoagulant medications may be stopped at the discretion of the surgeon. Blood pressure medications should not be mistakenly discontinued by the patient and, indeed, the addition of a preoperative beta-blocker may be considered by the internist.[398] Included in preparation is a counseling session with the patient to review systemic risks of surgery and anesthesia.

Ocular considerations: Aside from evaluation of the retina, a number of important issues may necessitate management decisions prior to vitreoretinal surgery. Although preoperative antibacterial prophylaxis has not been proven effective in a randomized controlled trial, the preponderance of evidence suggests its effectiveness.[399] Topical antibiotics may be considered especially in specific instances when the risk of endophthalmitis may be increased (e.g., blepharitis or contralateral prosthesis).[399] Infectious lesions of the lid, adnexae, nasolacrimal duct, conjunctiva, and corneal are treated prior to surgery. Careful examination for exposure of a previously placed scleral buckle may necessitate removal prior to entering the eye. If the anterior chamber is shallow, prophylactic laser iridotomy may prevent angle closure postoperatively. The presence of iris rubeosis may necessitate prompt intervention with vitrectomy and strong consideration of preoperative PRP and/or intravitreal injection of bevacizumab or triamcinolone acetonide.[227,241,248] An assessment of lens clarity identifies the need for cataract extraction either before or during vitreous surgery. Identifying a silicone intraocular lens implant is important to raise the threshold for capsulotomy or use of silicone oil tamponade. Silicone oil firmly adheres to silicone IOL's leading to poor visualization of the retina during surgery and decreased visual acuity postoperatively.[400,401]

Preoperative vitreoretinal evaluation is critical. Careful examination of the vitreous by ophthalmoscopy, echography, and/or optical coherence tomography to define the configuration of vitreous attachments to the retina helps to plan the surgical approach (Fig. 9.20).[402–404] Preoperative electrophysiological testing (ERG and VEP) may be useful in predicting visual outcome in cases of media opacity, but the outcome may be contradictory and these tests are not routinely used clinically.[405] There is ample evidence to support the use of adequate PRP laser prior to surgery and special consideration may be given to anterior peripheral retinal coverage to reduce the risk of anterior hyaloidal neovascularization, especially in severe PDR in type 1 diabetes mellitus.[17,49,69,176,183,184,406,407]

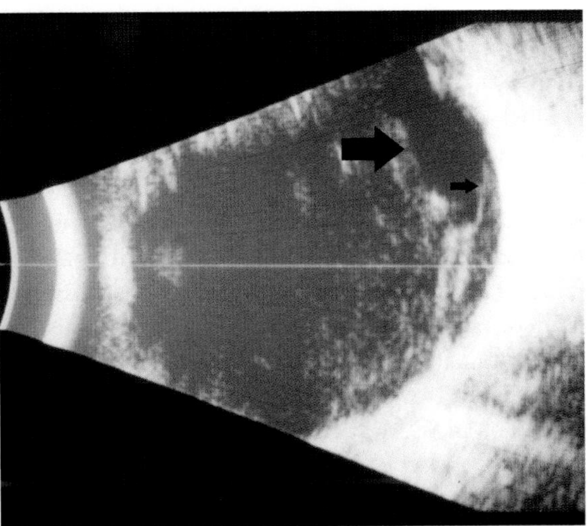

Fig. 9.20 Preoperative B-scan demonstrates vitreous hemorrhage and vitreoschisis. *Large arrow* shows inner wall of schisis cavity and *smaller arrow* shows taut outer wall with subhyaloid hemorrhage

As with all surgical procedures, the determination to operate is dependent on the outcome of counseling the patient and family regarding the risks, benefits, alternatives, and limitations of surgery. This complicated, decision-making process involves not only a working knowledge of the general medical and ocular pathology on the part of the physician but also the understanding of the impact of surgery by the patient. Finally, a mutual decision to proceed with surgery is made based on the needs and values of the patient. It may be helpful to provide written information for the patient to review after the office discussion.

9.4.3 Instrumentation

With increasing technological demands, the instrumentation available to the surgeon continues to grow. This section reviews general concepts regarding instrumentation with selected examples of specific tools that may be useful in the management of complicated situations.

Lens systems: There are a variety of lens systems used for negating the refractive power of the cornea to visualize the vitreous and retina. A variety of contact lenses are available for macular or peripheral retinal surgery. They may be self-stabilizing or may require centration and stabilization by a skilled assistant or with the use of sutured rings.[408] The plano-concave macular lenses offer excellent stereopsis and resolution.[409] Wide-angle lenses and prism lenses are also available for peripheral retinal surgery.[408] Biconcave contact lenses negate the refractive effects of intravitreal gas in the phakic eye.[410] The incidence of corneal epithelial defects is greater with contact lenses, especially irrigating contact lens systems.[411] This issue may be of particular significance in eyes having undergone LASIK surgery, after which displacement of the LASIK flap may occur at the time of vitrectomy.[412,413]

Non-contact lens systems are attached to the operating microscope and provide a wide field of view. Compared with contact lenses, non-contact lenses offer greater depth of field and better visualization through anterior media opacities (corneal haze, cataract), but lack fine stereropsis.[414] The wide-angle view of non-contact lenses may explain the reported lower incidence of postoperative retinal detachment.[415]

Vitrectomy systems: There are relative advantages and disadvantages to using vitrectomy instruments of varied caliber. Larger (20-gauge) instruments currently offer the greatest number supplementary instruments with which to work and provide excellent structural integrity with minimal instrument flex.[416] Smaller caliber instruments (23, 25 gauge, and smaller) rarely require suturing of the sclerotomy incision if angled entry incisions are created.[417] Therefore, they may provide less inflammation, less postoperative discomfort, and more rapid recovery.[418,419] There is a divided opinion on whether operating time is reduced.[418,419] Small-gauge vitrectomy surgery is more prone to postoperative hypotony and is less efficient at removing vitreous, especially dense vitreous hemorrhage.[416,420–422] Although there are exceptions, small-gauge instruments are especially suitable for less complicated vitrectomy procedures.[210,418] The choice of vitrectomy instrumentation is dependent on the surgeon's experience until evidence-based information becomes available.[423]

Illumination systems: Extensive options for illumination during vitrectomy are available. Hand-held illuminators permit the surgeon to direct the light source and include single-function illumination probes to multifunctional, illuminated picks, forceps, aspirators, coagulators, vitrectomy probes, and scissors.[313,424–426] Bimanual dissection is also made possible by the use of illuminators inserted into the sclera apart from or through working sclerotomies.[313,427,428] During peripheral dissection, illumination may be provided by co-axial illumination from the microscope with external scleral depression, from an illuminated contact lens, or from external application of the fiberoptic light probe on the sclera.

Membrane manipulators: Preretinal membranes may be removed with the use of tissue forceps, various picks, spatulas, scissors, soft-tipped cannulas, or with gentle suction by the vitrectomy probe or tissue manipulator.[429–431] Epiretinal membranes may be removed with a flexible intraocular rake.[432] Depending on their structure and relationship to surrounding tissues, membranes may be removed by a number of instruments at the discretion of the surgeon.

Membrane-cutting instruments: The vitrectomy probe functions well to cut membranes. Segmentation and isolation of individual islands of fibrovascular proliferation may be performed especially well with newer vitrectomy probes with the cutting port placed close to the end of the probe.[274] Vertical-cutting scissors do not push tissues away from the blades compared with horizontal-cutting scissors. However, horizontal scissors may be inserted more easily between the cortical vitreous and the retina for delamination. A variety of designs of scissors, blades, and spatulas have been described for cutting membranes.

Retinopexy instruments: Endodiathermy is commonly used to stop bleeding during surgery and is often used to mark retinal breaks for better visualization for photocoagulation after gas–fluid exchange. Laser may be applied to the retina by internal probes or by indirect ophthalmoscopic delivery. Endolaser allows for delicate placement of burns posteriorly. Indirect ophthalmoscopic delivery allows for ease of laser placement in the far periphery in phakic eyes avoiding the risk of lens trauma from the endolaser probe. With either method of laser delivery, scleral depression may be useful for peripheral treatment.

Internal tamponade: Various gases and liquids are used as instruments for internal tamponade of the retina. Perfluorocarbon liquid (perfluoro-*n*-octane) not only is used most commonly as a short-term intraoperative tamponade to reattach the retina but may also be used to separate lens fragments from the retina, to protect the retina against ultrasonic damage from the phacofragmentor, and to aid in membranes dissection.[433–437] Gases and silicone oils are frequently used for more prolonged retinal tamponade in cases of retinal detachment. Gases possess superior surface tension and dissolve during the postoperative course. Silicone oils remain in place as needed until surgical removal. The choice of gas vs. silicone depends on many factors including the location of retinal break(s), the presence of persistent tractional tissue, the presence of a crystalline lens, the need for air travel, and the patient's ability to position properly after surgery. Depending on the pathology, if very short-term tamponade is required, filtered air is used as it lasts for a few days at most. Longer tamponade is possible with SF6 (approximately 2 weeks) and C3F8 (approximately 6 weeks). However, the gas progressive dissolves in the vitreous fluids providing less tamponade as it disappears. Thus, gases work especially well for superior peripheral and posterior pathology and may be considered for inferior pathology if exceptional positioning is possible.[438]

Silicone oil is the agent of choice in severe cases if extended tamponade is required, if air travel is necessary, or if postoperative positioning is not possible.[439] In the United States 1,000 and 5,000 cs silicone oils are available, though elsewhere heavy silicone oil is used.[440,441] Silicone oil may be helpful to sequester neovascular growth factors in severe PDR with rubeosis and reduce the risk of hypotony/phthisis in eyes with complicated retinal detachment.[442,443]

Endoscopic surgery: When there is a need for excellent visualization of the ciliary body as in severe anterior hyaloidal fibrovascular proliferation, endoscopy provides a unique approach. Other indications include circumstances that may obscure the surgeon's view for standard pars plana vitrectomy including corneal opacity, hyphema, posterior capsular fibrosis, and profound miosis.[444] The endoscope is inserted through the pars plana providing direct, non-stereoscopic visualization of the vitreoretinal anatomy.

9.4.4 Techniques

A great variety of surgical techniques are available for the many challenges that face the vitreoretinal surgeon. The specific approach chosen for a given case is based on the ocular pathology as well as the surgeon's preference. Presented herein are selected techniques, which may be included in the armamentarium. However, successful surgery is dependent on an excellent understanding of the complex and variable relationships between the retina and the vitreous in diabetic retinopathy.[20,21,402]

Maintaining visibility: Excellent visibility is essential for the successful execution of delicate vitreoretinal surgical techniques. The tear film must be maintained to protect the corneal epithelium. The adjunctive use of carboxymethylcellulose (Genteal®) gel at surgery appears to promote corneal clarity superior to the use of hydoxypropylmethlycellulose (Goniosol®).[445] Corneal epithelial edema may obscure the surgeon's view and may be prevented by using non-contact lens systems and by avoiding prolonged elevation of intraocular pressure.[411,445] If epithelial edema does occur, corneal clarity may be recovered by carefully rolling a moist cotton-tipped applicator over the corneal surface to detergence the epithelium. In some cases, gentle debridement of the edematous epithelium may be necessary to operate safely.

Intraoperative pupillary mydriasis is essential. Instillation of preoperative mydriatic ophthalmic solutions may include combinations of phenylephrine 2.5%, tropicamide 1.0%, cyclopentolate 0.5–2.0%, scopolamine 0.25%, and atropine 1.0%. The addition of topical nonsteroidal anti-inflammatory eye drops promotes improved mydriasis for vitrectomy as in cataract surgery.[446,447] Epinephrine is frequently added to the infusion fluid to augment the effects of the preoperative regime.[448] Wide-angle viewing systems may provide satisfactory visualization in cases of pupillary miosis or mild-to-moderate cataract. Mechanical pupil expanders provide improved view when pharmacological agents fail to dilate the pupil adequately.[449,450] Posterior synechiae may require mechanical lysis, in which case the procoagulant effects of sodium hyaluronate may be helpful.[451] The management of cataract is discussed later in this chapter.

The vitrectomy infusion fluid: A variety of infusion solutions and additives are available for vitrectomy. BSS Plus® is a modified glutathione-bicarbonate-Ringer's solution aimed to provide the appropriate ions, buffers, and substrates for cellular metabolism, function, and structure.[452] In a randomized controlled trial, BSS Plus® produced less corneal edema on the first postoperative day following pars plana vitrectomy compared with lactated Ringer's solution.[453] One prospective study demonstrated a significant decrease in corneal endothelial cell loss following aphakic vitrectomy with BSS Plus® compared with lactated Ringer's solution.[454] Another prospective, randomized, masked clinical study comparing BSS Plus® with BSS showed no significant difference in endothelial cell loss following vitrectomy.[455] BSS Plus® produces less of a decrease in B-wave amplitude compared to normal saline or balanced salt solution.[456] In laboratory studies, BSS Plus® caused less retinal edema and less dysfunction of the retina pigment epithelium compared to normal saline and lactated Ringer's solution.[457,458] To promote mydriasis during vitrectomy, 0.3 cc epinephrine 1:1,000 may be added to the BSS Plus® infusion bottle. In diabetic vitrectomy, intraoperative opacification of the crystalline lens may be minimized by the addition of 3 cc $D_{50}W$ to the infusion bottle.[459]

The view of the retina may be obscured by condensation of water vapor on the posterior surface of a silicone intraocular lens implant. This occurs when the posterior capsule is open during intravitreal gas infusion. In some cases a viscoelastic liquid may be injected onto the back surface of the IOL. However, simple means for resolving the condensation involve warming the anterior segment. Methods include the application of a warming pad to the closed eye or using warm contact lens irrigating fluid.[460,461]

Occasionally, the surgical view is hindered by hemorrhage in the anterior vitreous adherent to the posterior capsule of the crystalline lens. Attempts to remove the blood by vitrectomy are fraught with risk of damage to the lens. An alternative technique involves the injection of balanced salt solution into the anterior chamber to hydrodissect the anterior hyaloid face from the posterior capsule allowing for safer removal of the hemorrhage by vitrectomy (Fig. 9.21). This technique is most effective in eyes of older patients and eyes with widely dilated pupils. A slow rate of injection may decrease the risk of posterior displacement of the lens–iris diaphragm, which may weaken the zonules.[462]

Retrohyaloid hemorrhage may hamper the view during vitrectomy. The blood in the subhyaloid space is often diffused with free-floating red blood cells, which may be liberated into the vitreous cavity as a "storm" when a large opening is made in the posterior hyaloid. To avoid this obstacle, a small opening in the posterior hyaloid is made through which retrohyaloid hemorrhage is removed.[463] Layered preretinal blood may obscure the view of membranes and can usually be removed with a soft-tipped cannula.[464] Drug-assisted techniques for removal of clotted preretinal blood are not in widespread use as they offer limited benefit and are associated with complications.[465–467]

Several techniques are available to stop active bleeding from the surface of the retina.[468] Brief elevation of intraocular pressure stops acute bleeding, but prolonged elevation may cause corneal edema and may threaten vascular compromise of ischemic neuroretinal tissues. Gentle pressure may be directly applied to the bleeding site with a soft-tipped cannula. Mild bipolar diathermy or laser may be used with care not to coagulate the retina or occlude a major vessel.[463] The use of bipolar cautery of vascular tissue before delamination is an effective prophylaxis.[469] Perfluorocarbon liquids provide local hemostatic tamponade to allow for application of laser or diathermy for hemostasis, and silicone oil or gas–fluid exchange may be used from prolonged effect.[434,468,470] Intravitreal thrombin significantly decreases bleeding time, but is associated with increased postoperative inflammation.[467]

Removal of fibrovascular membranes: The great number of techniques described to remove fibrovascular membranes from the surface of the retina is indicative of the difficulty in their management. Key to the successful removal of membranes is a complete understanding of vitreoretinal relationships.[402] Preoperative assessment with biomicroscopy, B-scan echography, and optical coherence tomography helps identify the degree of vitreous separation of the vitreous, areas of traction, and vitreoschisis.[402–404,471–473] Intraoperative reassessment is performed after core vitrectomy. If limited, focal, cortical vitreous attachments are encountered,

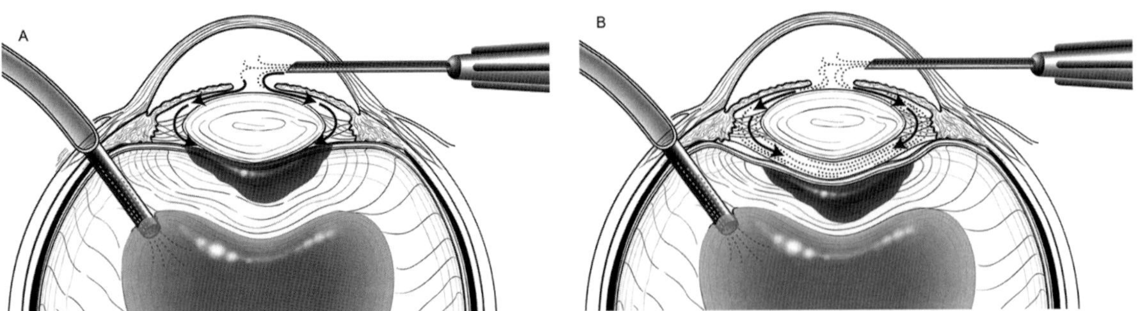

Fig. 9.21 The injection of infusion fluid into the anterior chamber (A) hydrodissects the anterior hyaloid from the posterior lens capsule (B) to facilitate removal of retrolenticular hemorrhage

minimally adherent membranes may be peeled from the surface of the retina. Care is taken to avoid tearing the retina and peeling is abandoned in favor of segmentation and delamination when resistance is met. More extensive proliferation of fibrovascular membranes occurs commonly with type 1 diabetes, in which the posterior cortical vitreous has not significantly separated from the retina.[69]

Essential to the successful removal of fibrovascular membranes is the accurate assessment of the posterior cortical vitreous. The detection of residual cortical vitreous may be facilitated by passing a soft-tipped cannula with gentle suction over the surface of the retina. The cannula will bend when it encounters cortical vitreous (Fig. 9.22 illustrates the "fish-strike" sign).[474] Triamcinolone acetonide (TA) or autologous blood injected onto the retina or oral fluorescein may be used to identify residual vitreous cortex as well.[475–477] TA may offer addition benefit in decreasing postoperative inflammation, decrease reproliferation of membranes, and reduce the rate of reoperation.[229]

The posterior cortical vitreous must be separated from the retina to facilitate dissection of fibrovascular plaques. Existing areas of focal posterior vitreous separation may occur at the edge of the disk, at the edge of elevated fibrovascular membranes, and overlying clotted blood adherent to the surface of the retina.[402,478] When there is minimal elevation of taut posterior hyaloid over the retina, an MVR blade may be used to incise the membrane. When there is no pre-existing separation of the posterior cortical vitreous from the retina, the use of a barbed MVR blade, pick, horizontal scissors, or vacuum-enabled instrument may achieve this goal (Fig. 9.23).[463] The separation of the cortical vitreous is extended from the fibrovascular plaque toward the periphery in an attempt to create a more favorable scenario.[479] This method is also effective when initiated in the midperipheral retina, preferably in an area of the retina previously treated with scatter laser, and away from fibrovascular proliferation to reduce the chance of bleeding or retinal tear.[463] The peripapillary area is another site in which to initiate dissection in an eye without pre-existing posterior vitreous separation and may be a preferred site in eyes with combined rhegmatogenous–traction retinal detachment.[120,402,478] Prepapillary tissue may be gently removed with forceps or left in place if tightly adherent. Nerve fiber axons have been identified in removed optic disk stalks, although no associated adverse visual outcome was noted.[395] An alternative method to separate cortical vitreous from the retina is by hydro-separation. In this technique, balanced salt solution is slowly injected through a small-gauge cannula (e.g., 38 gauge),

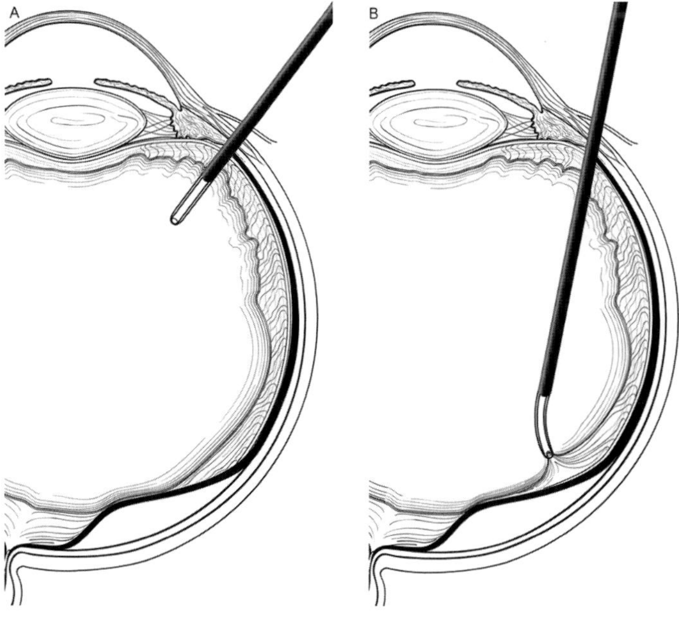

Fig. 9.22 (A) The "fish strike" sign. A soft-tipped cannula is passed over the surface of the retina under gentle aspiration. (B) When the silicone tip encounters residual outer cortical vitreous adherent to the retina, the tip suddenly bends similar to a fishing pole bending after a fish strike

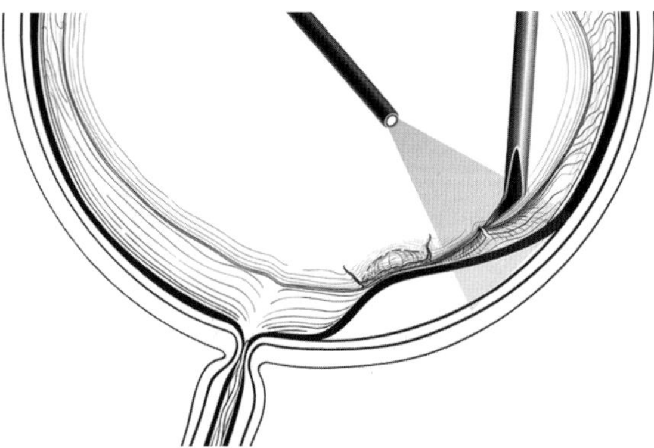

Fig. 9.23 A bent needle or barbed MVR blade may be used to engage the posterior cortical vitreous to induce separation of the vitreous from the retina

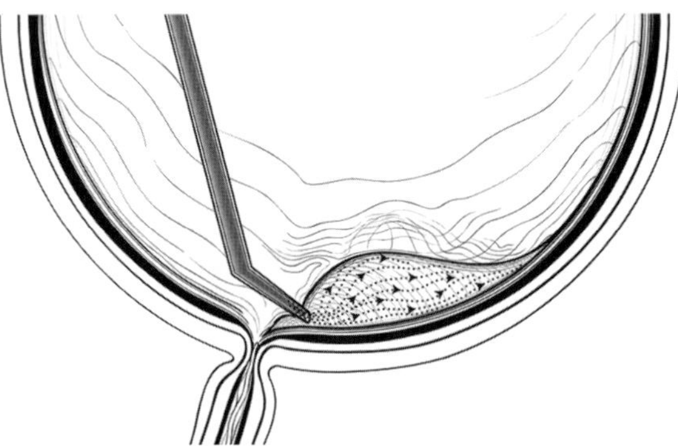

Fig. 9.24 Hydro-separation of cortical vitreous from the retina. A 38-gauge needle is inserted beneath the cortical vitreous and balanced salt solution is injected

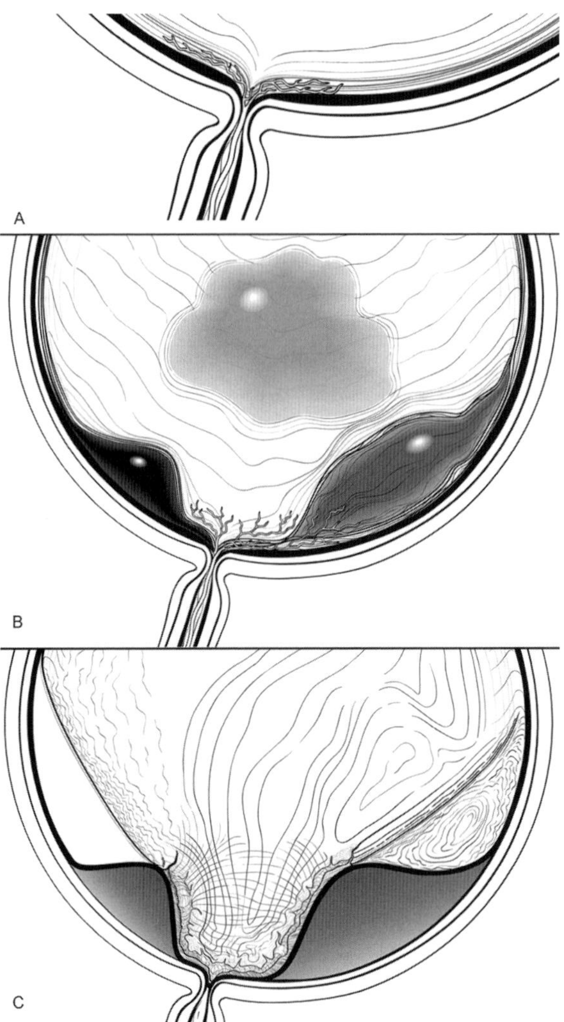

Fig. 9.25 Proposed evolution of vitreoschisis.[471] (**a**) Neovascularization develops from neuroretinal surface and grows into the posterior cortical vitreous. (**b**) Hemorrhage from neovascularization spreads into subhyaloid space and vitreous body and dissects between cortical vitreous lamellae creating hemorrhagic schisis cavity. (**c**) Contraction of the fibrovascular membrane and vitreous creates a traction retinal detachment with incomplete posterior vitreous detachment (*left* of disk) and with vitreoschisis (*right* of disk)

which is introduced into the subhyaloid space to elevate the cortical vitreous and minimize retinal traction (Fig. 9.24).[480]

Vitreoschisis is a splitting of the posterior cortical vitreous that may simulate focal posterior vitreous detachment. In this scenario a cavity may form within the cortical vitreous, possibly as a result of previous vitreous hemorrhage (Fig. 9.25).[471] Such bleeding within the cortical vitreous may arise from neovascularization, which is know to grow into the collagenous lamellae of the vitreous cortex.[23,471] The inner wall of the schisis cavity may condense to form a membrane between a fibrovascular plaque and the peripheral retina. Contraction of this membrane results in a traction retinal detachment.[471,473] If this membrane is falsely identified as the posterior hyaloid face, a difficult and incomplete dissection will result.[402,473] A barbed MVR blade may be used to elevate the outer wall of the schisis cavity to strip the cortical vitreous from the retina.[402,473] Horizontal scissors may also be used to identify and separate cortical vitreous by advancing the scissors along the edge of the fibrovascular membrane or along the slope of traction retinal detachment (Fig. 9.26).[481]

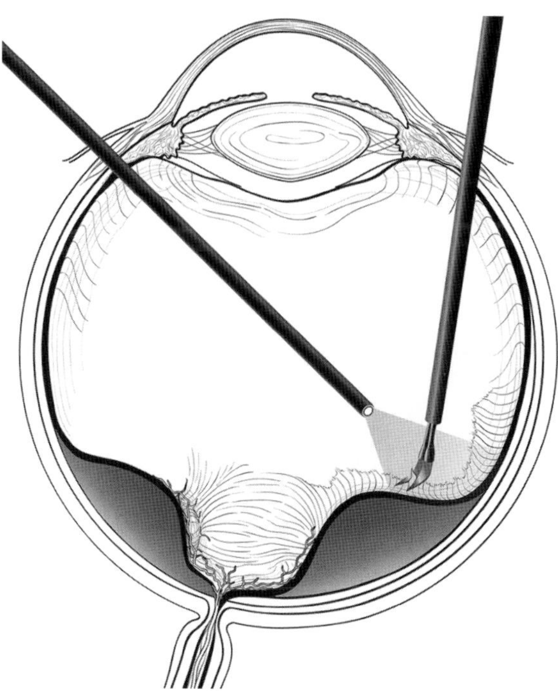

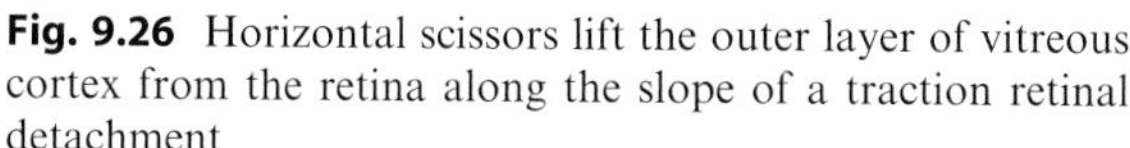

Fig. 9.26 Horizontal scissors lift the outer layer of vitreous cortex from the retina along the slope of a traction retinal detachment

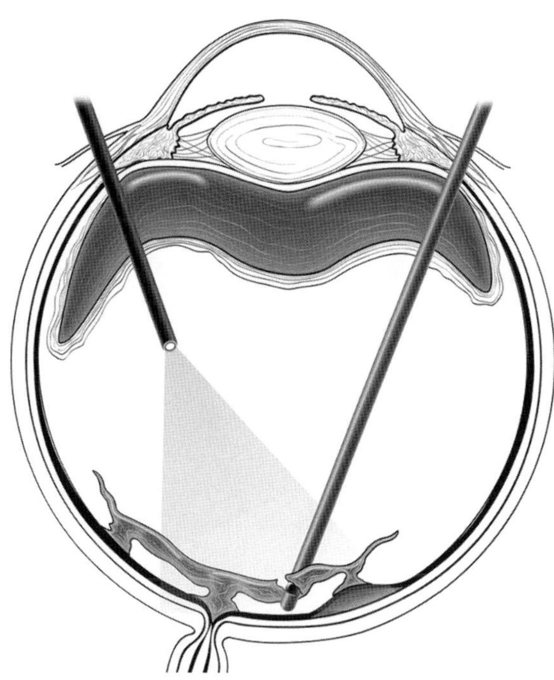

Fig. 9.27 Segmentation technique using the vitreous cutter to remove cortical vitreous traction between islands of fibrovascular proliferation

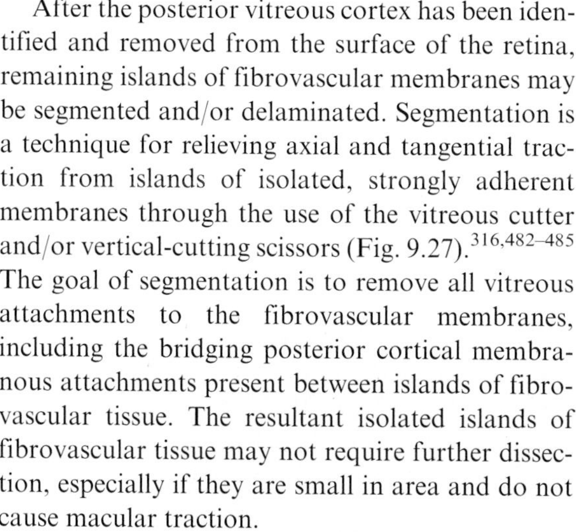

After the posterior vitreous cortex has been identified and removed from the surface of the retina, remaining islands of fibrovascular membranes may be segmented and/or delaminated. Segmentation is a technique for relieving axial and tangential traction from islands of isolated, strongly adherent membranes through the use of the vitreous cutter and/or vertical-cutting scissors (Fig. 9.27).[316,482–485] The goal of segmentation is to remove all vitreous attachments to the fibrovascular membranes, including the bridging posterior cortical membranous attachments present between islands of fibrovascular tissue. The resultant isolated islands of fibrovascular tissue may not require further dissection, especially if they are small in area and do not cause macular traction.

Delamination is a technique in which the posterior hyaloid is sharply dissected from the internal limiting membrane of the retina in areas of fibrovascular proliferation.[486] This may be accomplished uni-manually with the vitrectomy cutter or scissors.[274,482] Alternatively, in the "en bloc" technique, residual axial vitreous traction is used to elevate the fibrovascular membrane in order to facilitate sharp dissection with horizontal scissors (Fig. 9.28).[481] Additional elevation of the membranes may be achieved with the use of an accessory instrument such as an illuminated pick.[319]

In bimanual delamination of extensive fibrovascular plaques, an illuminated instrument is used in the nondominant hand to elevate the edge of the plaque while horizontal or vertical scissors sever the connections to the retina. Excellent visibility is essential by means of a bright light source along with various options of illuminated instruments and chandeliers. A forcep or tissue manipulator is used in the nondominant hand to stabilize and gently elevate the membrane, while horizontal- or vertical-cutting scissors perform delamination with the dominant hand (Fig. 9.29). The fibrovascular membrane/traction retinal detachment may be approached from the peripheral edge on the side of the surgeon's dominant hand or from the posterior edge by starting over the macula.[402,463] In difficult cases the membrane may be approached from both sides in an alternating fashion. Small cuts across focal areas of adherence allow for controlled

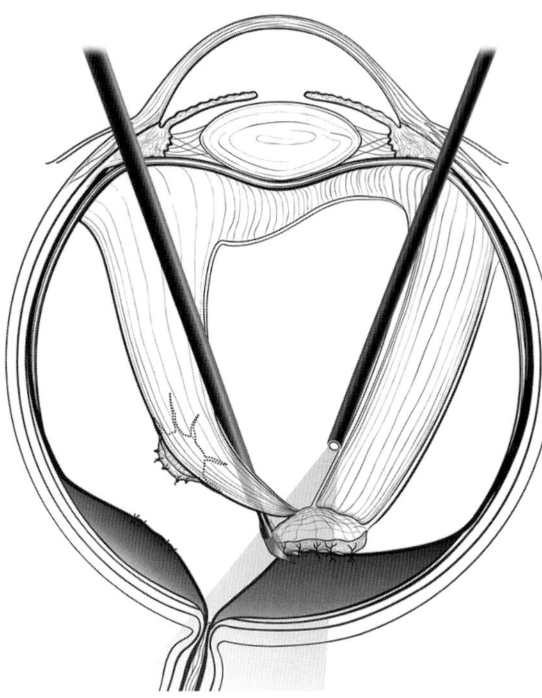

Fig. 9.28 "En bloc" delamination of fibrovascular membrane. Elevation of the membrane is provided by residual vitreous traction while horizontal scissors delaminate the fibrovascular plaque from the surface of the retina

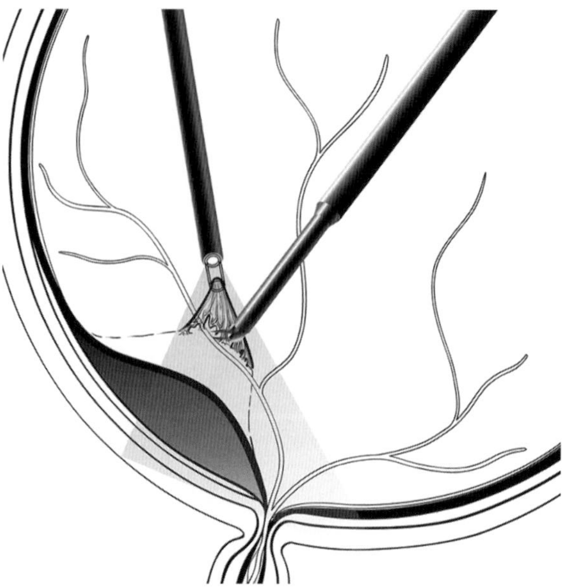

Fig. 9.29 Bimanual delamination of fibrovascular membrane. The tissue manipulator elevates the membrane from the retinal surface exposing focal peg-like adhesions that are cut with scissors

dissection and minimize the chance of creating retinal breaks. If breaks do occur, continued dissection is important to relieve all traction.[402,463] Perfluorocarbon liquid (perfluoro-*n*-octane) may be used to flatten the retina while the dissection continues.[319] At the conclusion of the case, retinal breaks are supported with internal tamponade with gas or silicone oil.

Broad fibrovascular plaques may be removed by a combination of delamination and segmentation. Careful dissection of the multiple peg-like adhesions gradually releases the plaque from the retina. This free edge may then be trimmed by vitrectomy to gain visualization for continued delamination. During dissection, new areas of separation are identified, which allow for segmentation of the plaque into smaller segments.[402,463] With care and persistence, the plaque can usually be removed (Fig. 9.30).

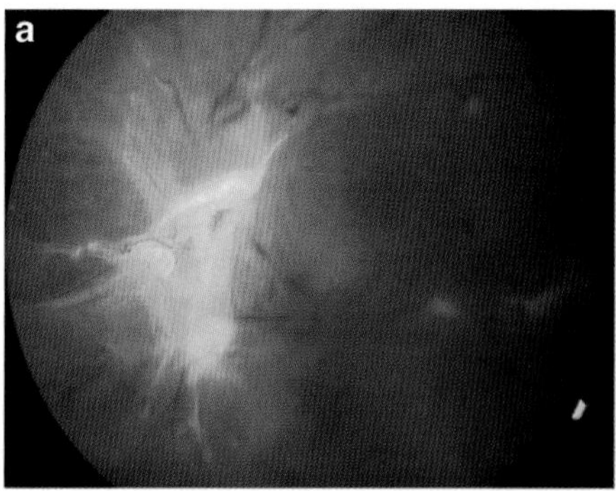

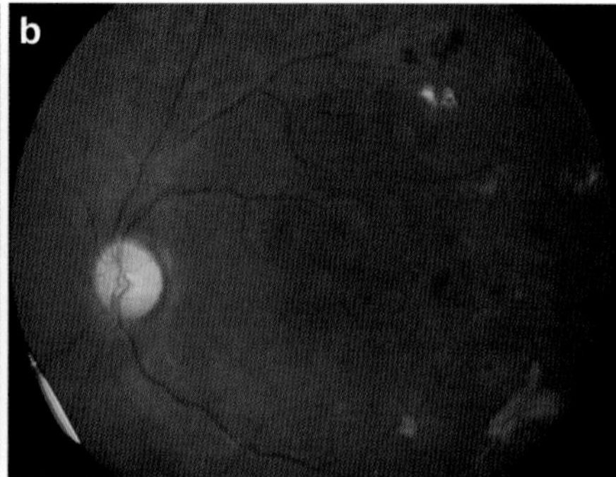

Fig. 9.30 (**a**) Fundus photograph of diabetic traction macular detachment with mild vitreous hemorrhage. (**b**) Postoperative fundus photograph showing attached macula. The residual islands of fibrous tissue were free of tangential and axial traction and, therefore, remained asymptomatic without contraction or hemorrhage

The Dissection of Fibrovascular Membranes: Persist or Capitulate?

There is limited information available in the literature to help make the determination when to stop the dissection of fibrovascular membranes. Ideally, the goal of vitrectomy is to remove all membranes in order to eliminate traction and reduce the rate of reproliferation and bleeding.[481] Certainly, there is a priority for the removal of fibrovascular membranes causing macular folds, traction, and detachment. Following the surgical dictum, "the greatest enemy of 'good' is 'better,'" some surgeons recommend limiting membrane removal to within four disk diameters from the center of the macula.[319] Extended dissection of chronic, extramacular, traction detachments may be more difficult due to strongly adherent membranes, may be more prone to iatrogenic retinal breaks, and may be less likely to improve visual function.[69,71,481,484] It may be preferable to approach some cases of chronic, extramacular, fibrovascular plaques with limited surgery aimed at removing axial and tangential vitreous traction and avoiding attempts at separating the tightly adherent membrane from the atrophic retina.[319] Past concerns[331] that residual islands of fibrovascular proliferation may cause future reproliferation and hemorrhage may be mitigated by improved contemporary management of the vitreoretinal interface (e.g., vitreoschisis)[471–473] and the improved availability and application of panretinal photocoagulation.[69] Ultimately, the extent of the fibrovascular dissection in a given case is determined by the relative ease of dissection of the fibrovascular membranes and potential benefits to be achieved.

Perfluorocarbon liquids may be used to assist membrane peeling or to flatten the retina for laser treatment.[434,487] Both perfluorocarbon liquids and sodium hyaluronate may be useful for separating the membranes from the retina. In a technique termed viscodissection, these liquids are injected with a cannula between the membrane and the retina to create further separation. Residual areas of retinal adhesion may then be more easily delaminated with scissors.[433,488,489] Furthermore, the procoagulant effects of sodium hyaluronate and other properties of perfluoro-*n*-octane may decrease bleeding.[451,470]

Fibrovascular proliferation located at the equator poses unique challenges. Due to the peripheral location, lensectomy may be required to improve access for bimanual dissection. When traction cannot be relieved by segmentation and delamination, additional techniques include scleral buckling with or without retinectomy.[169]

Anterior hyaloidal fibrovascular proliferation may require surgical dissection in advanced stages in which the addition of peripheral retinopexy is insufficient. Visualization is improved with scleral depression and placement of the fiberoptic light source externally on the sclera overlying the area of interest.[490,491] Severe peripheral fibrovascular proliferation may necessitate the use of relaxing retinotomy and silicone oil injection.[442,492] Endoscopic dissection has been described, but is not in widespread use.[444] Despite surgical intervention, prognosis is poor.[285]

Peeling internal limiting membrane: When deemed important to remove the internal limiting membrane (ILM) in diabetic vitrectomy, the techniques are identical to those used in non-diabetic eyes. Unaided peeling with picks and forceps is effective, but limited by poor visualization of the ILM.[493] Therefore, a number of agents may be used adjunctively including indocyanine green, trypan blue, triamcinolone acetonide, and perfluorocarbon liquids.[494–497] Whereas indocyanine green selectively stains the ILM, trypan blue stains both the ILM and preretinal membranes.[495,498] There are concerns regarding potential toxicity of vital stains.[499,500]

Intraoperative laser photocoagulation and cryoretinopexy: Not available in the operating room until 1983, laser photocoagulation plays a central role in diabetic vitrectomy to reduce the risk of neovascular complications and to prevent retinal detachment.[69,501] The effective use of laser requires that the retina be apposed to the retinal pigment epithelium. Internal tamponade may be required to achieve this goal.[434] The power of the laser is adjusted throughout the procedure depending on the distance of the endolaser probe to the retina and the clarity of the media. Although retinal whitening is the goal, hyperintense photocoagulation should be avoided.[130] Cryopexy causes more inflammation than laser, but is useful in treating peripheral retina (e.g., tears or ischemia) when laser treatment is not possible due to limited view (e.g., hemorrhage at vitreous base). The cryoprobe is placed on scleral surface while internal visualization by indirect ophthalmoscopy confirms the corresponding location of the anticipated cryopexy. Soon after retinal freezing is seen, the cryoprobe pedal is released to avoid excessive postoperative inflammation. The probe is held steady during the thawing process to avoid choroidal hemorrhage.[502] In a gas-filled eye, although the freezing effect may be faster in onset, the slow thaw may require the probe be held steady for a longer period of time. When the view of an area of retinal pathology is obscured (e.g., the inferior vitreous base in a phakic eye), a visible area of the retina is treated first and the time-to-freeze is noted. Then cryopexy may be applied to the obscured areas using the established time to freeze. If extensive areas are obscured from view, a pattern of cryopexy may be applied without the use of the binocular indirect ophthalmoscope. Instead, the cryoprobe is placed on the sclera under direct visualization to place an orderly grid pattern.

Retinal tamponade: Internal tamponade of the retina may be indicated for closing a retinal break or to control bleeding. The most common agents include air, SF6, C3F8, and silicone oil. Relative advantages and disadvantages of various agents are reviewed under the instruments section in this chapter. In most cases an air–fluid exchange is the first step in reattaching the retina after all membranes have been removed and hemostasis has been achieved. Diathermy is used to label all breaks to improve visualization after air–fluid exchange. A soft-tipped extrusion needle is passed through a break/retinotomy in the retina and as the subretinal fluid is drained either passively or actively, air infusion is started.[474] In a phakic eye, visualization is improved with the use of a biconcave contact lens or by shortening the distance between the two lenses in the non-contact system and lowering magnification.[463] The use of humidified air may avoid phakic lens opacity due to air infusion.[503] When the retina is flat, the cannula is held outside the break until the vitreous cavity is air filled. The break is then flattened by draining the remaining subretinal fluid. Additional membrane removal is needed if the retina does not flatten completely under air. Laser can then be applied as needed to surround the breaks and to treat PDR. If very short-term tamponade is needed, air may be sufficient. A rare problem encountered in an aphakic eye is collapse of the anterior chamber during air–fluid exchange. In some cases the anterior chamber spontaneously forms with face-down positioning during the postoperative course. However, at the time of surgery the anterior chamber may be reformed with a viscoelastic liquid, such as sodium hyaluronate. Postoperative face-down positioning may still be helpful and IOP is monitored.

If longer tamponade is desired, a non-expansile gas mixture with filtered air is prepared resulting in 18–20% SF_6 or 12–15% C_3F_8 in a 60 cc syringe. One method to perform air–gas exchange is to suture the supranasal sclerotomy and plug the remaining sclerotomy. The infusion tubing is clamped shut and the syringe with gas is attached so that gas infusion may be started when the infusion line is unclamped. A controlled, slow injection of gas is begun when the scleral plug is removed. Rapid injection may be associated with increased risk of visual field defects presumably due to retinal dessication.[504] After approximately 40 cc's of gas has slowly flushed out the air in the eye, the supratemporal sclerotomy is sutured while the assistant keeps the eye formed with gentle pressure on the plunger of the syringe. The final sclerotomy closure is most efficiently accomplished by using the same suture used to secure the infusion cannula. If self-sealed incisions are used, cannulas at each sclerotomy site are simply removed and a cotton-tipped applicator is applied for a few seconds to ensure closure. At the conclusion of the case, the intraocular pressure is measured and an adjustment in the amount of gas in the eye can be made using a 30-gauge needle through the pars plana. When intraocular gas is used, the anesthesiologist is asked to avoid using nitrous oxide as it may cause elevated intraocular pressure.[505]

If long-term complete internal tamponade is needed, silicone oil is injected into the eye after the air–fluid exchange. The supranasal sclerotomy is closed and a suture is placed, but not tied, at the supratemporal sclerotomy site. A high-pressure syringe filled with silicone oil is used with a short 18–20 gauge cannula inserted into the supratemporal sclerotomy. Silicone oil completely fills the eye and when it starts to back up into the infusion line, the air infusion pressure is dropped to 0 mmHg to facilitate the entry of silicone into infusion tubing. Enough silicone is allowed to enter the air infusion line to permit reflux back into the eye once the supratemporal sclerotomy is sutured and the air infusion pressure is set to 20 mmHg to normalize the intraocular pressure. When silicone ceases to move within the air infusion line, the infusion cannula is removed and immediately closed with the preplaced suture. When planning for the use of silicone oil in an eye with a silicone IOL, an effort is made to keep the posterior capsule intact to avoid contact between the two silicone products. In an aphakic eye an inferior iridectomy is necessary to prevent pupillary block glaucoma. A basal iridectomy is best performed prior to gas–fluid exchange and silicone injection. The tip of the vitrectomy probe is placed cutter-side up at the pupil. Remaining close to the posterior surface of the iris, the vitrectomy probe is gently directed toward the 6 o'clock position until it comes to rest in the ciliary sulcus. Very slight anterior movement of the instrument tip moves the iris forward and assures proper positioning. The vitrectomy cutter is activated on low suction and a basal iridectomy is created. Bleeding is a rare problem that can be managed by elevating IOP or by placing sodium hyaluronate into the anterior chamber.

Surgical management of neovascular glaucoma: The reader is referred to Chapter 11 for discussion.

Scleral buckle procedures: The reader is referred elsewhere on the techniques of scleral buckle placement.[506] In the absence of persistent peripheral retinal traction or peripheral retinal break, a scleral buckle is usually not necessary in diabetic vitrectomy.[402] Furthermore, the possibility of anterior segment ischemia from scleral buckling is best avoided in the diabetic eye.[507]

9.4.5 Postoperative Management

A number of postoperative concerns guide the care of the diabetic patient after vitrectomy surgery. Communication and coordination with the internist is important for optimal patient care.[508] Topical antibiotics and steroids are commonly prescribed to prevent infection and minimize inflammation. Pain control may not be an issue in straightforward cases with the use of smaller gauge instruments which do not require sutures or when conjunctival sutures knots are buried. Pain from corneal epithelial defects may be mild due to diabetic neuropathy. There in good evidence for the effectiveness of topical nonsteroidal anti-infammatory for controlling pain from traumatic corneal abrasions.[509] Patching does not appear to be helpful for control of pain.[510] The use of a therapeutic contact lens may improve comfort, but is not commonly employed.[511] With extensive surgery pain control may warrant narcotic analgesics. Anterior segment inflammation is mild when surgery is limited to the vitreous and retina, but is treated aggressively with steroids and cycloplegics to control pain and prevent complications. Unexpected inflammation prompts concern of endophthalmitis and may require vitreous culture and antibiotic injection. Intraocular pressure is monitored and normalized to prevent pain and visual field loss. The posterior segment is evaluated on routine examinations to give assurance of proper healing and to identify complications. Preoperative traction retinal detachment may take months to resolve following successful surgery and may be monitored with ocular coherence tomography.[512] Patient compliance is facilitated by the use of written instructions.[513]

Intravitreal gas: The need for postoperative positioning with intravitreal gas depends on the location of retinal breaks and may be facilitated with positioning pillows and tables. A sitting (head-up) position is needed to support the superior retina and face-down positioning is necessary to maximally support the posterior pole. Rarely, a patient may properly position the head to support the inferior retina.[438] Adhesion of the retina to the RPE occurs in 1–4 days after laser retinopexy.[514–516] Feathering of the crystalline lens may be minimized by face-down positioning to improve visualization of the retina in the postoperative course. Furthermore, an attempt is made to avoid prolonged face-up positioning as contact of gas with the crystalline lens promotes cataract formation. In a pseudophakic eye face-up positioning may cause iris capture, iridocorneal adhesion, or anterior synechiae. In an aphakic eye the anterior chamber may completely flatten.[517] A Medic Alert Bracelet is worn by the patient who is advised to avoid nitrous oxide and air travel until released by the retinal surgeon.[518,519]

If laser treatment is needed while a gas bubble is present, precautions may be required to avoid inadvertent retinal damage from the reflection of laser by the gas/fluid interface. Proposed methods of prevention include avoiding argon blue-green laser and efforts to minimize the angle of incidence of the laser beam with the gas–fluid interface.[520]

When using intravitreal gases, there is a potential for elevation of intraocular pressure. Topical antiglaucoma drops instilled at the conclusion of surgery may reduce the incidence of damaging elevation of IOP.[521,522] Topical and oral pressure lowering medication may be continued during the postoperative period as needed. If unacceptable IOP elevation occurs in the presence of a complete gas fill, a par plana tap may be necessary to remove gas and normalize the IOP.

Silicone oil: Postoperative positioning is less critical with a complete silicone oil fill and there are no restrictions to air travel or anesthesia. Intravitreal silicone interferes with diagnostic ultrasonography and axial length measurements for IOL calculations.[523,524] Early postoperative anterior chamber migration of silicone oil may be indicative of choroidal effusion or hemorrhage and is more common in the aphakic eye than in the phakic or pseudophakic eye with intact zonules. Delayed postoperative anterior migration of silicone oil may be indicative of proliferative vitreoretinopathy or closure of the inferior iridectomy.[525] Apart from the occasional need for early removal of silicone oil in response to complications, silicone oil is routinely removed for optimal return of vision and to prevent complications associated with extended retention of oil. Extraction of silicone is performed at the surgeon's discretion, usually in 3–6 months. Recurrent retinal detachment occurs in a minority of cases and appears independent of duration of silicone oil tamponade.[526,527] After removal of silicone oil, the incidence of entopically detected residual droplets of silicone oil does not appear to be influenced by air infusion at the time of silicone removal.[528] Removal of silicone is usually performed through a sclerotomy either actively or passively, but it may be removed through the anterior chamber combined with cataract surgery.[528,529] Silicone is typically removed as soon as the retina appears stable in order to prevent complications, but may be used for long-term tamponade in severe cases to prevent phthisis.[120,330,530,531]

9.4.6 Complications

Important complications of vitrectomy surgery include those associated with systemic disease and anesthesia. Untoward effects may be ocular or systemic in nature. The following is a review of ocular complications from the vitrectomy surgical procedure itself.

Conjunctival complications: Aside from the common findings of hemorrhage, edema, and inflammation from surgery, stitch abscess can progress to scleritis or endophthalmitis and may warrant continuing topical antibiotics until surface sutures have dissolved.[532] Burying suture knots may decrease suture exposure and improve comfort. Careful conjunctival closure helps prevent recession and exposure of glaucoma setons and scleral exoplants. Subconjunctival granuloma from silicone oil is prevented by complete closure of sclerotomies.[533]

Corneal complications: Corneal complications of vitreoretinal surgery may interfere with postoperative healing and compromise final visual return. Corneal epithelial defects are common during and after vitrectomy surgery in diabetics. Poor adhesion of the epithelium to the basement membrane and corneal neuropathy increases the susceptibility to damage.[142,534] Risk factors include duration of surgery and the use of an irrigating surgical contact lens.[534] The need for intentional surgical debridement of the epithelium may be minimized by avoiding prolonged elevation of intraocular pressure during surgery. The tendency for delayed re-epithelialization and potential for infection complicates the postoperative recovery. The prompt identification and management of dellen formation due to elevation/edema of limbal conjunctiva may prevent serious complications.[535] Treatment with lubricants improves comfort and antibiotic prophylaxis may prevent ulcerative keratitis. Particular care must be taken to preserve corneal epithelial integrity in post-LASIK eyes to prevent flap displacement.[536] Corneal endothelial trauma may manifest with chronic long-term complications following vitrectomy. Causes of damage to the endothelium include contact with irrigating fluids, gas, silicone oil, and other vitreous substitutes and agents used for tamponade.[534] Therefore, preventive efforts are aimed at preserving a barrier between the vitreous and the anterior chamber (the crystalline lens, lens implant, or lens capsule). Removal of silicone and perfluorocarbon liquids from the anterior chamber reduces the risk of corneal decompensation.[534] Corneal astigmatism from sclerotomy incisions is usually transient and may be minimized by avoiding an excessively tight sclerotomy closure or with self-sealed, small-gauge incisions.[537] The reader is referred to Chapter 12 for further discussion.

Scleral complications: Proper management of the sclerotomy site is important in preventing scleral complications. Postoperative wound leaks due to incomplete closure of a sclerotomy incision may be transient and inconsequential. However, complications include conjunctival bleb, choroidal effusion, and endophthalmitis.[420,538,539] Infectious scleritis is a rare, but serious complication.[540] Fibroplasia at the scleral incision site may lead to fibrous ingrowth and contribute to the development of anterior hyaloidal fibrovascular proliferation.[541] Unknown is the significance of wound closure, but persistent VEGF production from ischemic retina appears critical.[542] Additional internal complications related to the sclerotomy include vitreous traction causing retinal tears, retinal detachment, and vitreous hemorrhage.[541] With repeated vitrectomy procedures, scleral thinning at a previous sclerotomy site may necessitate the use of new sites for sclerotomy to avoid difficulty with closure. Severe scleral thinning that requires a tectonic graft is rare.[543]

Iritis and hyphema: Postoperative iritis is usually mild following vitreoretinal surgery. Significant pain and marked cellular and fibrin response is unusual and prompts consideration of infectious endophthalmitis. Pseudo-endophthalmitis may present when triamcinolone is used at surgery regardless of the phakic status of the eye. The triamcinolone crystals may form a pseudohypopyon, which is not usually associated with pain or significant fibrin. The chalk-white appearance of the particles of varying size points toward the correct diagnosis.[544]

Intraoperative hyphema may occur especially with rubeosis and is controlled by elevating the IOP or with sodium hyaluronate.[451] The preoperative discontinuation of anticoagulants may reduce the incidence of hyphema in high-risk cases. Postoperative hyphema is rare and may require testing for sickle hemoglobinopathy and requires strict attention to IOP control.[545]

Fibrinoid syndrome associated with postvitrectomy retinal detachment: The deposition of fibrin strands in the anterior chamber and vitreous may occur following vitrectomy for severe PDR. Fibrin strands may be seen initially on the surface of the retina and in the anterior chamber, potentially causing pupillary block glaucoma.[339] A gelatinous mass forms in the vitreous cavity and subsequent contraction results in traction retinal detachment, rubeosis, and neovascular glaucoma.[341] Fibrinoid syndrome causing retinal detachment is reported following approximately 5% of diabetic vitrectomy procedures with mixed indications.[341,341] Milder forms of postoperative fibrin deposition are more common. Postoperative fibrin in the anterior chamber without retinal detachment is reported in 10–22% of combined vitrectomy–phacoemulsification–IOL (VPI).[546,547] Fibrinous inflammatory reaction is a proposed cause of an increased incidence of posterior capsular fibrosis in this cohort.[548] Postoperative fibrin is seen significantly more frequently after combined VPI when the indication for vitrectomy is diabetic retinopathy compared to non-diabetic VPI in some retrospective series[549] and not in others.[550] In these combined procedures, the method of cataract extraction appears to influence the incidence of fibrin formation. The rate is higher with extracapsular extraction (80%)[551] and lower with pars plana lensectomy.[552] Risk factors of fibrinoid syndrome with retinal detachment include poorly controlled type 1 diabetes; previous surgery for diabetic retinal detachment; and surgical risk factors of extensive surgery including scleral buckling, membrane dissection, extensive PRP/cryopexy, and lensectomy.[285,341,547] Approximately one-third of affected eyes respond to high-dose systemic and topical steroids.[341] Prompt resolution of fibrin is reported with intracameral injection of tissue plasminogen activator (tPA).[339,340,553] However, postinjection intraocular bleeding is common as in subsequent recurrence of the fibrinoid syndrome.[553] Therefore, repeat injections of tPA may be needed.[554] Prognosis is poor in severe cases in which vitrectomy surgery has been attempted.[284,285] Prevention of fibrin formation with intravitreal steroids performed at the time of the initial surgery may be considered in high-risk cases.[555]

Iris/trabecular complications: Intraoperative iris manipulation is avoided to minimize postoperative iritis. However, inferior iridotomy is required in some cases (refer to section on silicone oil complications). Postoperative ocular hypertension may result from a number of causes including corticosteroid use, hyphema or diffuse blood, ghost cells, neovascularization, expansile gas, silicone oil, or suprachoroidal hemorrhage. In addition, pupillary block glaucoma may be precipitated by ciliary body edema/anterior choroidal effusion from laser/inflammation from surgery.[197] Treatment is directed at the underlying cause.

Rubeosis and neovascular glaucoma (NVG) portend very poor prognosis. In the ETDRS 74% of such eyes lost light perception.[69] The incidence of new-onset NVG has been reported to be approximately 0.9–14% after vitrectomy/laser surgery with best results reported with the use of intraoperative augmentation of anterior peripheral scatter laser.[40,69,314,334,556] Factors that may be related to reduced risk of NVG include retention of the crystalline lens, scatter laser photocoagulation (PRP), and postoperative retinal attachment. However, the significance of lens removal as a risk factor appears to be decreased with the use of PRP.[40,47,49,69,314,557,558] The new onset of rubeosis following vitrectomy raises the suspicion of anterior hyaloidal fibrovascular proliferation or retinal detachment.[342,559]

Anterior hyaloidal fibrovascular proliferation (AHFVP): The spectrum of presentation of AHFVP includes the growth of neovascular tissue from the retina or sclerotomy sites onto the vitreous base, anterior retina, ciliary body, lens capsule, and/or iris following vitrectomy for severe PDR.[342] Patients may present with vitreous hemorrhage, rubeosis, peripheral retinal tractional detachment, and/or hypotony.[342] Diagnosis may be confirmed with high-resolution ultrasound biomicroscopy of the peripheral retina and ciliary body (Fig. 9.31).[560,561]

Risk factors for AHFVP appear to include male gender, type 1 diabetes, severe retinal ischemia/neovascularization, and previous vitreous surgery with placement of a scleral buckle.[342] Inadequate PRP may allow for the postoperative progression of neovascularization, especially anteriorly in the vitreous base. The origin of the anterior neovascularization may be the retina or the sclerotomy sites.[407,562,563] Dilated external scleral vessels at the sclerotomy site suggest fibrovascular ingrowth.[166,407,561] However, fibrovascular ingrowth may be present in the absence of dilated external vessels.[541] Peripheral retinal photocoagulation or cryopexy with or without treatment of sclerotomy sites may be useful with consideration of anterior dissection in very severe cases in which fibrovascular membranes are associated with traction detachment.[166,167,407] Dissection of membranes, lensectomy, retinectomy, scleral buckling, confluent laser/cryopexy, and silicone oil may be required.[342] As the membranes are highly vascularized, preoperative intravitreal bevacizumab may be useful for short-term regression.[240] As treatment is often difficult and unsuccessful, efforts toward prevention and early detection are important.[285] In eyes at risk for AHFVP, consideration may be given to the application of extensive PRP with anterior extension to the ora serrata.

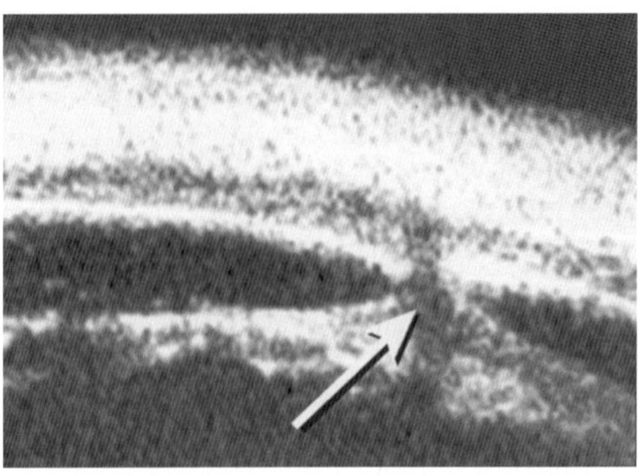

Fig. 9.31 Ultrasound biomicroscopic image of fibrovascular ingrowth. Soft tissue lesion with hyporeflective vascular core adherent to vitreous (reproduced with permission from *Ophthalmology*.[561])

Lens complications: Cataract is a well-recognized complication of vitrectomy.[564,565] However, visually significant cataracts may be less common following diabetic vitrectomy, compared with vitrectomy for macular pucker and macular hole. In eyes with clear lenses preoperatively, the 2-year cumulative rate of cataract extraction is 15, 53, and 66% for diabetic retinopathy, macular pucker, and macular hole, respectively.[564] Many factors may play a causative role including light exposure from the operating room equipment, direct trauma from vitrectomy instruments, loss of antioxidant properties of formed vitreous, the irrigation fluid, and retinal tamponade.[564–566] Efforts at prevention include minimizing microscope light exposure and duration of surgery, avoiding direct instrument contact with the lens, and the use of supplemental 50% dextrose in the infusion fluid.[459] Cataract surgery may be performed before, during, or after vitrectomy depending on the severity of the cataract and the status of the retina. If the cataract is mild, it is usually retained unless severe PDR requires extensive anterior dissection.[407] Refer to Chapter 10 and the Section 9.6.1 later in this chapter for further discussion.

Endophthalmitis: The incidence of endophthalmitis following vitrectomy is low, but remains potentially devastating.[544] Recent data suggest that there is no significant difference in the occurrence of endophthalmitis (0.03–0.23%) between 20- and 25-gauge instruments.[567,568] Others have previously reported a higher incidence in smaller gauge (25 and 23 gauge) vitrectomy presumably due to inadequate closure of self-sealed sclerotomy incisions.[569,570] Aside from being a common indication for vitrectomy, poorly controlled diabetes may be an independent risk factor for endophthalmitis and poor outcome.[397,571,572] Preoperative antibiotic prophylaxis, lid hygiene, improvement of blood glucose levels, and sterile technique are common prevention tactics.[573] A high index of suspicion and low threshold to culture the intraocular fluids leads to early diagnosis and treatment with intravitreal antibiotics such as vancomycin and ceftazidime.[570] Outcome is dependent on the infecting organism and early diagnosis/treatment.[574]

Phototoxicity: Light from the microscope or the internal light source must be kept to a minimum and directed away from the macula whenever possible. Phototoxicity appears related to light intensity and duration of exposure.[575] Halothane anesthesia may offer protection against retinal phototoxicity.[576] There appears to be no increased risk with multiple-illumination systems compared with singular endoillumination.[577]

Postoperative vitreous hemorrhage: Vitreous hemorrhage may be present immediately following vitrectomy surgery or may occur postoperatively. The incidence of vitreous hemorrhage following vitrectomy for proliferative diabetic retinopathy covers a wide range (12–79%), likely reflecting the varied indications for surgery.[578,579] Persistent hemorrhage immediately following vitrectomy may be due to the release of blood from the peripheral vitreous skirt, especially in phakic eyes in which anterior vitrectomy is limited.[579] Bleeding may also occur from vascular membranes transected at surgery, persistent vitreoretinal traction, or active neovascularization.[342,579] Residual traction posteriorly has been described with vitreoschisis, whereby the vitreous falsely appears to be separated from the retina at the time of vitrectomy surgery.[471–473] If all cortical vitreous is not removed from the retina during vitrectomy, postoperative vitreous hemorrhage may occur from tangential traction.[580] Anterior hyaloidal fibrovascular proliferation is a well-recognized cause of recurrent postoperative vitreous hemorrhage and is discussed above. All-cause incidence of postoperative hemorrhage appears to be reduced by intraoperative PRP, regardless of the amount of preoperative PRP laser present.[406] The use of intravitreal gas at the conclusion of vitrectomy is of undetermined value in decreasing the incidence of postoperative vitreous hemorrhage.[579,581] The combined use of preoperative bevacizumab with postoperative gas tamponade may yield better results.[582]

Management of postoperative vitreous hemorrhage involves an initial period of observation. Echography is employed to monitor the retina for detachment. Elevation of IOP may complicate vitreous hemorrhage and may hasten intervention in medically uncontrollable cases.[292,296] Gas–fluid exchange or fluid–fluid exchange with or without tissue plasminogen activator may clear the hemorrhage to restore vision and to allow for further evaluation of the underlying cause of bleeding and for the addition of laser/cryopexy, if indicated.[578,583,584] However, repeat vitrectomy is often employed for the treatment of persistent traction or anterior hyaloidal fibrovascular proliferation.[342,578,579]

Retinal detachment: The incidence of retinal detachment (RD) after vitrectomy largely depends on the severity of preoperative PDR. It was reported in 4.3% of eyes operated primarily for vitreous hemorrhage and 4–8% of eyes with mixed complications of PDR.[291,314,334,585] The DRVS studied 616 eyes and 12.3% in the early vitrectomy group developed RD compared to 18.8% in the deferral group.[71] In eyes with extensive PRP, observation of asymptomatic peripheral retinal detachment may be an option.[119] However, when postvitrectomy rhegmatogenous retinal detachment (RRD) requires additional surgery for repair, outcome may be poor. In a large retrospective review ($n = 484$) of consecutive vitrectomy cases for complications of PDR, 18 eyes developed RRD and 10 (56% of the 18 eyes) progressed to NLP vision despite additional surgery.[291]

Gas-related complications: Intravitreal gas increases the risk of cataract formation and elevation of IOP.[295,586,587] Gas–lens contact may interfere with lens metabolism.[588,589] Diabetic eyes may be at increased risk of developing gas-related cataracts.[590] Therefore, appropriate posturing may be helpful in minimizing the risk of cataract formation. Intraocular pressure (IOP) elevation may be due to expansion of gas and/or shallowing of anterior chamber angle.[295,591] Factors that promote gas expansion include C_3F_8 mixtures exceeding 12–14%, SF_6 mixtures exceeding 20%, postoperative air travel, mountain travel, and nitrous oxide anesthesia.[402,519,592–594] Elevated IOP due to expanding gas often requires vitreous tap. Forward movement of the iris with shallowing or flattening of the anterior chamber may be caused by intravitreal gas.[590,591] It may result in pupillary capture of an intraocular lens.[595] If the vitreous cavity is less than 100% gas filled, the anterior chamber may deepen with face-down positioning alone, obviating the need for gas removal. However, reformation of the anterior chamber with gas or sodium hyaluronate may be needed if face-down positioning fails to deepen the chamber and early synechiae are suspected.[595] Anterior chamber migration of gas may result in corneal decompensation due to endothelial cell damage.[590,596] This problem is most common in an aphakic eye and may be prevented by retaining the lens, the lens implant, or the posterior capsule.

Silicone-related complications: An extensive list of complications have been reported in association with silicone oil, including cataract, glaucoma, and keratopathy.[597] Cataract is common following vitrectomy with silicone oil and was reported to occur in 64% of 265 eyes by 6 months. The incidence of cataract is expected to increase with time following surgery.[440] The reader is referred to the section later in this chapter on management of cataract and PDR as well as Chapter 10.

The most common cause of corneal complications from silicone oil involves anterior chamber migration of oil, which is usually prevented by an intact lens, a posterior chamber lens implant, or inferior peripheral iridectomy. Extensive contact of silicone oil with the corneal endothelium over time results in corneal edema and band keratopathy and is best avoided by removal of silicone oil as soon as the retina is stable.[598]

Glaucoma may develop via open-angle or closed-angle mechanisms. Intraocular pressure elevation was reported in 3% of 1196 eyes with silicone oil studied prospectively.[440] The most common mechanism of glaucoma is blockage of the trabecular meshwork due to emulsification of silicone oil.[599] The incidence of emulsification increases with duration of intraocular silicone oil retention.[530] In addition, mechanical energy from phacoemulsification, phacofragmentation, and high-speed vitrectomy probes appears to cause emulsification.[600] Prevention of glaucoma by early removal of silicone oil is ideal. Once open-angle glaucoma develops, the IOP is normalized with topical or surgical therapy and stabilization may occur with removal of intravitreal silicone oil and anterior chamber lavage to remove emulsified silicone oil droplets.

Pupillary block glaucoma from silicone oil is avoided with inferior peripheral iridotomy in the aphakic eye. However, continued postoperative patency may be problematic and require the use of steroids and Nd:YAG iridotomy.[525,601] Iridotomy is usually not needed in phakic eyes or in eyes with posterior chamber lens implants, but may be performed by Nd:YAG laser postoperatively as needed for pupillary seclusion from synechiae or functional pupillary block.[602]

Silicone oil may interact adversely with lens implants. Adherence of silicone oil to a silicone intraocular lens may affect the visual outcome by altering the posterior refractive surface. An intact posterior capsule helps separate the two silicone products. If contact is unavoidable, the silicone may be mechanically removed in some cases.[603] More frequently, an IOL exchange restores vision in symptomatic patients who have the potential for improvement.

Silicone may migrate from the vitreal cavity to extraocular sites. Subconjunctival and orbital migration of silicone oil may occur through glaucoma drainage devices.[604,605] Placement of the tube inferiorly in the anterior chamber and avoiding anterior migration of silicone may prevent this complication. A rare, but serious complication of silicone oil seen in ocular hypertensive eyes is dissection of silicone oil from the eye into the brain.[606,607] Glaucomatous optic neuropathy may be requisite.[608] Therefore, removal of silicone oil or evisceration/enucleation should be considered in a sightless, silicone-filled eye with elevated IOP even in the absence of pain.

Hypotony/phthisis: The DRVS reported the incidence of enucleation/phthisis/retrobulbar alcohol injection to be 12.3% in the early vitrectomy group compared with 9.1% in the deferral group.[71] The most common causes of hypotony/phthisis include late effects of persistent retinal detachment, anterior hyaloidal fibrovascular proliferation, and end-stage neovascular glaucoma.[321,342,559] Management is directed at cosmesis and pain control and may require topical medication, alcohol block, enucleation/evisceration, or scleral shell.[609]

Sympathetic ophthalmia: The potentially blinding complication of sympathetic ophthalmia is a rare complication of vitreoretinal surgery.[610] Present findings include anterior chamber and vitreal inflammatory cells with variable posterior segment changes.[611] The DRVS reported sympathetic ophthalmia in 1% of early vitrectomy group as opposed to 0.3% in the deferral group.[71] These rates are higher than the expected incidence of 0.01–0.06% following vitrectomy surgery.[612] The potential of blindness from sympathetic ophthalmia underscores the importance of avoiding multiple surgeries in eyes with very poor prognosis.[612,613] For those patients who do undergo vitrectomy, careful postoperative evaluation of the fellow eye is critical to diagnose sympathetic ophthalmia. With early detection and appropriate treatment, a good prognosis may be expected.[614]

Macular hole: Vitrectomy has rarely been associated with macular hole, both with and without ILM peeling.[358,360,362] This finding is not surprising given the strong vitreoretinal adherence in diabetic retinopathy.[18] The presence of diabetic macular edema may be a risk factor for the development of macular hole.[358,360] Management is discussed under the heading of vitrectomy indications.

9.4.7 General Outcome

Vitrectomy surgery generally improves the quality of life in diabetic patients, though the results are largely dependent on the underlying retinal pathology.[615,616] Improved vision-related quality of life and visual function after vitrectomy depends on improvement in visual acuity and contrast sensitivity in both the better-seeing eye and the worse-seeing eye.[616] Visual acuity outcomes with vitrectomy have been reported earlier in this chapter as they relate to specific indications for surgery. There is an overall 67–86% rate of visual improvement after vitrectomy for various complications of diabetic retinopathy.[285,326] The overall 2-year visual acuity results reported by the ETDRS (early vitrectomy group) and the DRVS are comparable: 24.5–28% were 20/40 or better, 17.1–20% were <20/40 to 20/100, 18.9–19.3% were <20/100 to 20/400, 3.6–8.0% were <20/400 to 5/200, and 24.7–36% were <5/200.[69,71] Over the 9-year study period of the ETDRS, 2% of 7411 eyes suffered severe visual loss (<5/200). These eyes were enrolled with mild-to-severe NPDR and early PDR. The low rate of severe visual loss was attributed to close follow-up and timely laser/vitrectomy intervention. Risk factors for severe visual loss were high mean hemoglobin A1c and elevated cholesterol.[615]

A more recent, retrospective review of 340 eyes operated for a variety of complications of diabetic retinopathy showed an 86% incidence of improvement in vision. A final postoperative visual acuity of 20/40 or better was achieved in 60% of eyes.[326]

Other studies correlated postoperative vision inversely with severity of PDR. For example, better final vision was present in eyes with vitreous hemorrhage or good preoperative vision and worse outcome in eyes with retinal detachment.[290] Preoperative risk factors for severe visual loss included pre-op vision <5/200, cataract, NVI/NVG, and retinal detachment.[285,617] Intraoperative risk factors included the use of gas for internal tamponade and creation of iatrogenic retinal break.[617] The long-term outcome after vitrectomy is good for up to 10 years in eyes with good vision and attached retina at the 6-month visit.[69,618–620]

9.5 Follow-Up Considerations in PDR

Evaluation and management of proliferative diabetic retinopathy over the course of time requires extensive consideration of systemic and ocular factors and the appropriate use of diagnostic testing. Systemic factors include assessment of blood glucose and blood pressure status, extraocular diabetic complications, cardiovascular health, renal function, serum lipid levels, fluid retention, psychological status, pregnancy, medications, and visual needs. Complete routine ocular examination is of paramount importance.

Follow-up interval: The interval between office visits will be determined by the aforementioned factors. Daily to weekly visits are warranted in severe PDR with active neovascularization, e.g., neovascular glaucoma. Monthly to quarterly visits are reasonable as PDR stabilizes. After PRP is complete and NV has regressed, annual visits may be considered for metabolically stable patients.

Pregnancy is associated with progression of PDR. Follow-up examination each trimester or more often is recommended to detect and treat PDR. Diabetic retinopathy tends to stabilize after pregnancy and no long-term severe adverse effects are reported in patients who become pregnant compared to those who do not. Factors for increased risk of progression during pregnancy include duration of diabetes, degree of metabolic control, extraocular complications of pregnancy, and severity of retinopathy at conception.[104,621,622]

Ocular factors that may increase the rate of progression and need for close follow-up include intraocular inflammation and cataract surgery.[623–627]

Refer to the Section 9.6.6 on conditions affecting the presentation of PDR.

Ancillary testing: Complete slitlamp examination with fundoscopy is the primary method of evaluation; however, ancillary testing may be useful in selected circumstances. Especially in patients who have difficulty in maintaining visual fixation, serial photography helps identify progression of diabetic retinopathy.[628] Fluorescein angiography is not required to initiate treatment of PDR, but may be helpful in difficult cases. For example, fluorescein angiography may confirm the presence of suspected new-onset neovascularization presenting with vitreous hemorrhage.[629,630] Fluorescein angiography may also help determine the cause of decreased vision by demonstrating macular capillary dropout.[629,631]

Optical coherence tomography (OCT) provides useful information in the management of diabetic retinopathy. OCT demonstrates retinal thinning in macular ischemia/atrophy, cystic spaces in macular edema, retinal thickening and surface irregularity with preretinal membrane, and retinal elevation in cases of vitreoretinal traction.[371,390,632–635] Difficulty remains in determining the relative significance of these changes as they relate to visual function, especially in eyes with multiple pathological changes.

Visual field examination by perimetry may be considered in evaluating for driver safety. Although visual acuity may be acceptable, visual field may be compromised to an unsafe degree for driving in patients with advanced PDR.[636]

9.6 Case Management: Decision-Making in Complicated Cases

9.6.1 Cataract and PDR

The coexistence of cataract and PDR is common and requires special consideration.[637] Chapter 10 reviews this issue for diabetic retinopathy in general. This section identifies specific issues as they relate to proliferative disease. Although cataract may interfere with visual function and evaluation of the retina, only rarely does cataract interfere with laser placement, especially with the availability of long wavelength (red) laser.[146,147] When cataract extraction is indicated, the timing of surgery depends on the activity of the PDR.

Optional strategies depend on the relative severity of the cataract and PDR, as well as the presence of macular edema. The visual prognosis is guarded in this group of eyes.[624,638] In general, PDR is treated with PRP before cataract surgery, but laser may be given by indirect ophthalmoscopic delivery at the time of cataract surgery or at the slitlamp promptly after surgery.[639] There is limited information on the optimal sequence of PRP and cataract extraction with regard to the risk of loss of acuity and macular edema.[640] Results of cataract surgery with untreated PDR are poor and fraught with progression of PDR and early post-cataract laser may be difficult due to pain, inflammation, corneal edema, and wound concerns.[641–643] However, in a small randomized trial, PRP after cataract extraction was associated with reduced loss of acuity ($P = 0.012$) and less macular edema ($P = 0.033$) 12 months after surgery compared with the fellow eye that underwent PRP before cataract extraction.[640] If PRP is indicated, but not possible due to poor view through cataract, triamcinolone acetonide or anti-VEGF agents may be injected for short-term stabilization for cataract surgery until laser can be applied postoperatively.[218,260,261] These same agents may be helpful in the short-term management of macular edema exacerbated by cataract surgery.[219,644] Intraocular VEGF and other cytokine levels are elevated following diabetic cataract surgery.[645] Poor metabolic control is associated with an increased risk of progression of diabetic retinopathy after cataract surgery.[646] However, efforts to improve short-term worsening of diabetic retinopathy and maculopathy by rapid improvement in glycolic control prior to cataract extraction appear to be ineffective, if not harmful.[647]

If vitrectomy surgery is indicated, cataract surgery before or during vitrectomy lowers the rate of repeat vitrectomy compared to phakic vitrectomy, possibly due to improved access to the peripheral retina in the non-phakic eye.[314,330,648,649] Sequential cataract surgery followed by vitrectomy has the disadvantage of two separate visits to the operating suite, but may diminish the inflammation and complications seen with combined surgery.[650] Sequential surgeries may be facilitated by the use of triamcinolone acetonide and anti-VEGF injection as noted above.

Cataract extraction at the time of vitrectomy may speed the recovery of vision in selected cases.[314,651] Extracapsular cataract extraction or phacoemulsification with posterior chamber lens implantation may be combined with vitrectomy surgery.[652] However, there appears to be an increased rate of intraoperative lens capsular tears and zonulysis as well as postoperative inflammation, posterior synechiae formation, and posterior capsular fibrosis.[314,548,650,653] A poor red reflex in eyes with vitreous hemorrhage makes cataract surgery more challenging.[314] Combined procedures with extracapsular cataract extraction appear to create more inflammation than with phacoemulsification.[551] Aggressive management of inflammation is needed with consideration for the use of triamcinolone injection, which may also help control the increased incidence of macular edema.[654–656] Combined phacoemulsification/vitrectomy may be especially suitable in a patient presenting with cataract and indications for diabetic vitrectomy in the presence of poor vision in the fellow eye.[314]

Combined vitrectomy with pars plana lensectomy is another alternative. This approach involves less anterior segment manipulation and, therefore, may cause less anterior chamber inflammation. The anterior capsule may be retained for the placement of a ciliary sulcus lens implant at the time of vitrectomy or subsequently.[657–660] This approach has been reported to be successful in highly complicated cases with combined traction–rhegmatogenous retinal detachment requiring silicone oil injection.[330] Limited data show no definitive advantage of pars plana lensectomy compared with trans-corneal phacoemulsification.[661,662] However, there may be less anterior chamber inflammation and fibrin deposition associated with pars plana lensectomy.[552]

Cataract surgery performed on an elective basis after vitrectomy generally produces improved vision. However, capsular tears and zonulysis complicate surgery in approximately 10% of cases, increasing the risk of posterior dislocation of lens fragments or lens implant.[650,663]

Regardless of the relative timing of cataract and vitrectomy surgery, complications may occur. Postoperative anterior capsular contraction occurs more often in eyes with diabetic retinopathy and may result in traction on the ciliary body with hypotony and ciliary effusion.[664,665] With appropriate use of PRP, the risk of rubeosis and neovascular glaucoma is minimized. The ETDRS reported NVI/NVG in

6% of eyes after cataract extraction.[69,666] Small retrospective studies report similar low incidence of NVI/NVG, the risk of which correlates directly with the severity of PDR and indirectly with the amount of PRP.[69,667,668] With meticulous attention to completing PRP including the anterior periphery, the incidence of NVI/NVG may be decreased to less than 1%.[314] Finally, the risk of retinal detachment of approximately 5% following diabetic vitrectomy appears to be unaffected by the addition of cataract extraction.[314,585]

In the ETDRS, the visual outcome is related directly to the severity of diabetic retinopathy. Two hundred and seventy eyes were studied prospectively. One-year after cataract surgery, 55% of eyes with advanced diabetic retinopathy (severe NPDR or worse) experienced improved vision. The distribution of visual acuities in this group was as follows: 25% >20/40, 42% >20/100, and 22% 5/200 or worse.[666] Others estimate that patients with PDR are 30 times less likely to achieve 20/40 or better vision compared with diabetic patients without retinopathy. Compounding the problem is evidence that some patients with advanced PDR who undergo phacoemulsification may not experience improved visual function despite improvement in measured visual acuity.[669]

The effect of cataract surgery on progression of diabetic retinopathy is uncertain. The ETDRS showed a trend of borderline significance toward short-term worsening of diabetic retinopathy. The study showed no long-term increased prevalence of diabetic macular edema, but the study was not designed to detect an early increase in macular edema or an increase in severity of edema in the long term.[666] Others have provided conflicting evidence of progression of diabetic retinopathy after cataract surgery (for further discussion the reader is referred to Chapter 10).

9.6.2 Dense Vitreous Hemorrhage and Untreated PDR

The presence of dense vitreous hemorrhage in an eye with untreated PDR not only causes acute severe loss of vision but also places the eye in a category at high risk for potential persistent visual loss.[65,66,102] There are several options to reach the goal of clearing the vitreous hemorrhage and applying PRP. Elevation of the head at night or patching with strict bed rest may help clear the hemorrhage for office-based PRP.[287] Anti-VEGF agents may be injected to cause short-term involution of neovascularization while waiting for hemorrhage to clear.[210,263] Purified ovine hyaluronidase has been shown to speed the resolution of vitreous hemorrhage.[277–279] The status of the vitreous may play a role in the decision to intervene with vitrectomy. If a complete PVD is present, observation may be preferable to vitrectomy, especially if the fellow eye has good vision.[38,74] If severe PDR is suspected based on the history of type 1 diabetes, iris neovascularization, or extensive vitreoretinal traction seen on B-scan, early vitrectomy is indicated.[69,74] Previtrectomy intravitreal injection of bevacizumab may be considered prior to surgery in these high-risk cases.[248] On the other hand, the echographic finding of tractional retinal detachment may argue against anti-VEGF therapy.[273] If vitrectomy is necessary, even partial preoperative PRP may improve outcome.[184]

9.6.3 Untreated PDR with Diabetic Macular Edema

The presence of diabetic macular edema in eyes with PDR is indicative of increased severity of retinopathy with increased risk of retinopathy progression and severe visual loss compared to eyes with the same stage of retinopathy without edema. Panretinal photocoagulation (PRP) is useful to prevent profound loss of vision in PDR, but may increase macular edema and decrease visual acuity in a dose-related fashion.[67] For eyes with high-risk PDR, the ETDRS recommended macular focal/grid laser for clinically significant macular edema (CSME) at the initial session with the option of starting PRP for PDR in the nasal quadrants during the same session. PRP in the temporal quadrants was deferred for at least 2 weeks.[68] The ETDRS cautioned against delaying PRP for high-risk PDR with CSME. For eyes approaching, but not reaching high-risk PDR, the peripheral scatter treatment was not started until the edema had resolved after which "mild scatter" (lower density, fewer burns) treatment was applied. Retreatment in these eyes was only given if progression in retinopathy was documented. This treatment plan was shown to reduce the rate of severe visual loss compared to deferral of treatment.[67]

Small studies show that intravitreal triamcinolone decreases macular thickening and prevents worsening of vision after PRP.[221,670–674] A small, randomized, controlled, clinical trial demonstrated a significant benefit of triamcinolone acetonide in preventing decreased vision and increased macular edema following PRP and focal laser for eyes with PDR and CSME.[221] The benefits of this treatment must be balanced by the risks including cataract, glaucoma, and endophthalmitis.[211] An alternative to prophylactic treatment is rescue treatment with triamcinolone acetonide after PRP treatment if macular edema worsens with decreased vision. However, triamcinolone acetonide may be considered primarily as an adjunct to macular focal laser in the treatment of diabetic macular edema.[233] Anti-VEGF agents may be considered for a similar adjunctive role in the management of these difficult cases.[241] This topic is also discussed in Chapter 7.

9.6.4 PDR with Severe Fibrovascular Proliferation/Traction Retinal Detachment

There is an established role for early vitrectomy in the management of severe fibrovascular proliferation (FVP) and traction retinal detachment (TRD).[72] Panretinal photocoagulation improves outcome despite potential short-term risks.[17,49,69,176,183,184,406,407] Open to question is the role of anti-VEGF therapy. Although some have reported beneficial results with bevacizumab in these cases, there is anecdotal evidence of progression of TRD with anti-VEGF injection.[243,272,273] Until further research allows for risk stratification, bevacizumab should be used with caution. In cases of severe traction detachment with or without rubeosis, silicone oil tamponade may be useful for prolonged tamponade and for sequestration of fibrovascular growth factors until laser treatment has taken effect.[442]

9.6.5 PDR with Neovascular Glaucoma

Panretinal photocoagulation and peripheral retinal cryopexy play a key role in the management of active new vessel growth in neovascular glaucoma (NVG).[285,675] Extensive PRP is needed to treat the widespread areas of capillary dropout in these cases.[17] Indeed, prevention of NVG with appropriate timing and extent of PRP is preferable to treating established NVG.[69] New to the armamentarium are the anti-VEGF agents, which cause dramatic short-term resolution of neovascularization.[248–250,267,269,270] Their role may be best suited to minimize progression of angle neovascularization and secondary synechiae formation while peripheral laser/cryopexy takes effect.[210] Retinal detachment is associated with rubeosis and repair of the detachment may induce regression of the rubeosis.[676] Retinal tamponade with silicone oil is useful in these cases.[442]

When significant anterior synechiae block the trabecular meshwork, intervention is directed at destruction of the ciliary body to decrease aqueous production or at providing alternative routes for aqueous drainage. Surgery may lower IOP, but visual prognosis is grim.[69] Many surgical procedures are available to lower IOP, some of which are employed by the vitreoretinal surgeon. The reader is referred to Chapter 11 for further discussion.

9.6.6 Conditions Altering the Clinical Course of PDR

"Early worsening" with improved metabolic control: The primary issue in managing rapid worsening of diabetic retinopathy is identifying conditions in which rapid worsening might occur and initiating prompt treatment with PRP. Although improved metabolic control is associated with improved long-term outcome, "early worsening" was described in patients assigned to tight control in the Diabetes Control and Complications Trial.[8] The effect of early worsening of diabetic retinopathy was reversed by 18 months and did not result in serious visual loss.[6] Successful pancreas transplant surgery leads to improved control with the potential for short-term worsening of retinopathy.[677–681]

Pregnancy: There is an increased short-term risk of progression of diabetic retinopathy with pregnancy. The increased risk may continue for up to 1 year, but no long-term adverse effects of pregnancy were reported by the Diabetes Control and Complications Trial.[106] Additional factors that may increase the risk of progression in pregnancy include duration of diabetes (>10–15 years), poor glycemic control, hypertension, and the presence of moderate–to-severe NPDR at baseline.[105,682] Therefore, prompt PRP is indicated in pregnant patients with severe NPDR or early PDR.[69]

Carotid atherosclerosis: Atherosclerosis of the carotid artery may affect retinal vascular perfusion by embolization or stenosis.[683] Emboli may be liberated from an atherosclerotic plaque and occlude the central retinal artery or a branch retinal arteriole. In the presence of diabetic retinopathy, this added ischemic insult may precipitate neovascularization (Fig. 9.32).[50,684–687] Alternatively, if profound neurosensory apoptosis results from central retinal artery occlusion prior to the onset of diabetic retinopathy, there may be a protective effect against progression of diabetic retinopathy (Fig. 9.33).

There are conflicting reports regarding the effect of carotid stenosis on diabetic retinopathy. Most recent reports indicate carotid stenosis is associated with ipsilateral worsening of diabetic retinopathy.[173,688–691] However, relative ipsilateral sparing from diabetic retinopathy has also been described.[692–696] A possible explanation for these conflicting reports is presented in the Box. Systemic evaluation of patients presenting with asymmetric diabetic retinopathy may include non-invasive carotid Doppler ultrasonography. However, only a minority of patients with asymmetric diabetic retinopathy test positive for significant carotid occlusive disease.[690]

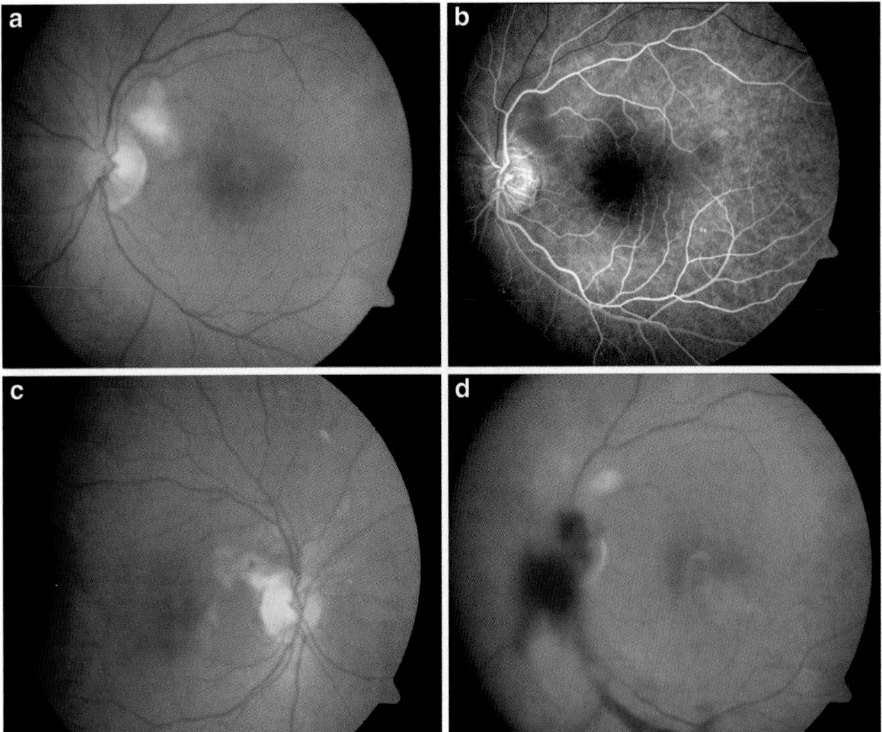

Fig. 9.32 Apparent asymmetric diabetic retinopathy. Ischemic retinal whitening superior to left disk (**a**) due to branch retinal artery occlusion with symptomatic inferior visual field loss. Mild NPDR is seen on fluorescein angiogram (**b**) along with delayed circulation time in superior hemispheric retinal vasculature. Several months later, the patient returned with further loss of vision OS due to vitreous hemorrhage from disk neovascularization (**d**). The right eye had mild NPDR (**c**). Note: photographic artifacts are seen centrally in macula OS and near disk OD

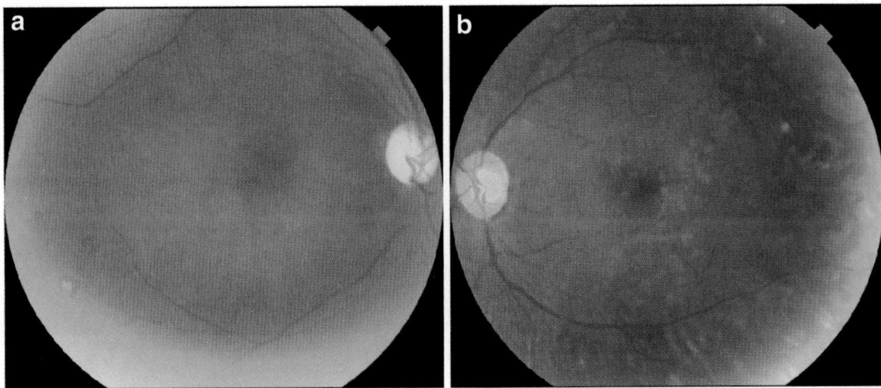

Fig. 9.33 Asymmetric diabetic retinopathy. Right eye (**a**) suffered from profound loss of vision many years ago due to central retinal artery occlusion with resultant pale disk and attenuated arterioles. Subsequently, less severe retinopathy developed in the right eye compared with the left eye (**b**), which had progressed to high-risk PDR requiring panretinal photocoagulation

Why are there conflicting reports regarding the effect of carotid stenosis on the severity of diabetic retinopathy? One explanation for this discrepancy may involve differences in time of onset and relative severity of the two pathologies. For example, if moderate carotid stenosis occurs before the onset of diabetic retinopathy, an ipsilateral decrease in the severity of diabetic retinopathy may be expected on the basis of protection against the known adverse effects of hypertension on diabetic retinopathy.[56,697,698] Conceivably, the degree of carotid stenosis may not be severe enough to cause venous stasis retinopathy. Conversely, if significant diabetic retinopathy is present prior to severe carotid occlusion, the added ischemic insult might precipitate a progression of the retinopathy ipsilateral to the carotid stenosis. Additional confusion may result from the similarity of venous stasis retinopathy to diabetic retinopathy. Venous stasis retinopathy, an uncommon manifestation of severe carotid stenosis, may cause blot hemorrhages and microaneurysms, but the findings tend to be ipsilateral to the stenotic artery and show midperipheral predominance.[699]

Neovascular glaucoma in diabetes may be caused by PDR or ocular ischemic syndrome (OIS). Findings suggestive of OIS as the primary cause include an unexpected low intraocular pressure and ipsilateral bright-light amaurosis, both likely due to poor ocular perfusion.[700–703] Revascularization of the occluded carotid artery may result in improved vision. However, complications may be encountered with improvement in perfusion. For example, an abrupt increase in intraocular pressure may occur following carotid surgery if extensive posterior synechiae are present.[691,701,704] Rarely, diabetic macular edema becomes manifest after endarterectomy.[705]

Miscellaneous ocular and systemic conditions: A variety of ocular conditions may affect PDR. Conditions associated with extensive destruction or thinning of the retina provide protection against the development of PDR. They include high myopia, previous central retinal artery occlusion (Fig. 9.33), advanced glaucoma (Fig. 9.34), optic atrophy, rod–cone degeneration, and extensive chorioretinal scarring from trauma or past inflammation.[13,172,173,706] Asteroid hyalosis may increase the risk of developing PDR, probably due to the associated lower prevalence of posterior vitreous detachment.[38,173]

Ocular inflammation generally appears to accelerate diabetic retinopathy in conditions such as anterior uveitis, posterior uveitis, surgery, and endophthalmitis.[623,625–627,643,707] A possible link is the common elevation of cellular fibronectin and adrenomedullin

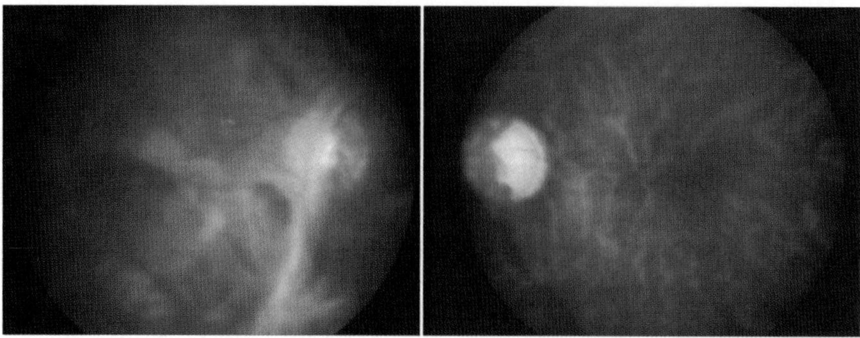

Fig. 9.34 Asymmetric diabetic retinopathy due to glaucoma with milder retinopathy in the eye with more advanced optic neuropathy/ganglion cell loss

in both uveitis and diabetic retinopathy.[708,709] There are exceptions to the notion of acceleration of diabetic retinopathy with uveitis that may be explained on the basis of severe retinal damage precluding the development of diabetic retinopathy.[710] In other cases there is no clear explanation for an apparent protective effect of uveitis on diabetic retinopathy.[627,711] The possible additive effect of vascular occlusions reported in HIV and autoimmune-mediated disease is unknown and requires further study.[712–715]

The coexistence of hemoglobinopathy and diabetes may affect the retinal presentation. Sickle retinopathy is uncommon in sickle trait unless diabetic retinopathy is present; conversely, the presence of sickle trait does not appear to affect the severity of diabetic retinopathy.[716,717] Hemoglobin SC disease appears to have no additive effect on diabetic retinopathy.[718] Thalassemia may delay the onset and decrease the severity of diabetic retinopathy.[719]

Medications: Medications may adversely affect diabetic retinopathy. Erythropoietin, used to treat anemia in end-stage renal disease, is a potent ischemia-induced angiogenic factor and may cause acceleration of PDR independent of VEGF.[720–723] However, benefit from erythropoietin has also been reported presumably due to decreased tissue hypoxia with improved hemoglobin level.[724,725] Uncertain are the effects of statins, which may be associated with elevated VEGF levels.[726]

9.7 Summary of Key Points

- Panretinal photocoagulation (PRP) is indicated for the treatment of high-risk proliferative diabetic retinopathy (HR-PDR) and eyes approaching HR-PDR (severe nonproliferative diabetic retinopathy and early proliferative diabetic retinopathy) that are at high risk for progression or for poor outcome.
- Trends in the modification of PRP as described by the ETDRS include aiming for a mild-to-moderate white burn, using shorter burn duration (0.03–0.05 s) for improved comfort, using 200 μm spot size with a wide-angle laser lens (such as the Volk H-R Wide Field, Volk SuperQuad 160, or the Ocular Instruments Mainster PRP 165), and anticipating the application of 3,000 total burns for retinal coverage equivalent to panretinal photocoagulation as described by the ETDRS.
- In severe PDR (commonly seen in type 1 diabetes mellitus, especially if poorly controlled), adequate PRP both anterior and posterior to the equator is important to improve the response to vitrectomy and reduce the risk of anterior neovascular complications/severe visual loss.
- Intravitreal injection of triamcinolone acetonide and bevacizumab offers valuable short-term benefits in the management of proliferative diabetic retinopathy, especially in complicated cases with combined HR-PDR/macular edema and neovascular glaucoma.
- Indications for vitrectomy include vitreous hemorrhage (final visual result is dependent on the status of the macula), traction retinal detachment (best results if vitrectomy is performed soon after macular involvement or when macula is threatened), combined traction–rhegmatogenous retinal detachment (vitrectomy with silicone oil tamponade yields fairly good results), severe fibrovascular proliferation (important to apply

extensive PRP prior to vitrectomy, if possible), postvitrectomy fibrinoid syndrome (best managed with adjunctive medication), anterior hyaloidal fibrovascular proliferation (poor prognosis, therefore best prevented with appropriate anterior retinopexy in high-risk eyes), and various presentations of vitreomacular interface pathology (preretinal membrane, vitreomacular traction syndrome, and macular hole).

- Vitrectomy techniques have evolved with improved instrumentation and understanding of vitreoretinal pathology in PDR. The recognition of vitreoschisis is of paramount importance in approaching complicated cases of fibrovascular proliferation with bimanual delamination.
- Complications of treatment of PDR can be minimized by recognition of important risk factors and by making appropriate modifications in the treatment plan.

9.8 Future Directions

There are a multitude of future directions to explore for improved management of proliferative diabetic retinopathy. Improved patient education and the management of the obstacles to care are of paramount importance.[727,728] Aside from managing blood glucose and blood pressure, studies to find other treatable coexisting abnormalities that exacerbate diabetic retinopathy may include serum lipids and anemia.[102,729]

Future therapy may include blocking metabolic pathways that translate hyperglycemia into physiological and structural abnormalities. Further research to block the polyol pathway may include improved aldose reductase inhibitors.[730] Promising reports offer hope for the benefit of blocking protein kinase-C with ruboxistaurin or other agents.[731,732] Renewed attempts to block the formation of advanced glycation end-products (AGE) or the receptors of AGE (RAGE) are warranted.[733–735] The renin–angiotensin system through its effector molecule, angiotensin II, plays a role in the generation of reactive oxygen species, inflammation, thrombosis, and angiogenesis.[12,736–739] Given the positive reports from the Diabetic Retinopathy Candesartan Trial, further research is in order.[740,741]

Other agents under study include somatostatin analogues (e.g., octreotide), which inhibit growth hormone secretion with subsequent suppression of insulin-like growth factor-1 and have direct antiproliferative and apoptotic effects on neovascular endothelial cells.[742,743] Rosiglitazone and related drugs may delay the onset of PDR.[744] Atorvastatin improves vascular resistance, reduces serum AGE levels, and inhibits AGE signaling to inflammation in diabetes.[12,745] Animal models suggest a role of cyclooxygenase-2 inhibitors to minimize inflammation in diabetic retinopathy.[746]

An extensive list of angiogenic factors, anti-angiogenic factors, cytokines, and other molecules likely play a role in various stages of diabetic retinopathy and are incompletely understood. For example, growth factors suspected to play a role include vascular endothelial growth factor[76] (VEGF), angiopoietin,[80,81] cortistatin,[82] insulin-like growth factor-1,[83] basic fibroblast growth factor,[4] platelet-derived growth factor,[4] endothelin-1,[84] transforming growth factor beta-1,[85] connective tissue growth factor,[86] and growth hormone.[87] Inhibitors under evaluation include pigment epithelium-derived factor,[88–90] soluble vascular endothelial growth factor receptor-1,[91] somatostatin,[4] endostatin,[92,92] angiostatin,[79] and thrombospondin.[4] Many more factors have been described and countless others are yet to be discovered. There is a complex balance of these factors that is not well understood making the successful micromanipulation of this environment a daunting prospect.[4,93]

Gene therapy for the treatment of diabetic retinopathy is in its infancy.[747] The identification of gene polymorphisms associated with retinopathy may provide the possibility for individualized drug therapy or future gene therapy.[748,749] Lentivirus-mediated expression of angiostatin has been used in a murine model to inhibit neovascularization in proliferative retinopathy.[750] Enthusiasm is restrained pending further research and evaluation of potential adverse effects.

Improvements in the application of laser photocoagulation may improve benefits and limit adverse effects. Shorter duration laser burns provide improved comfort and do not affect the inner retinal layers to the extent of conventional lasers.[155,751,752] However, the relative efficacy of less extensive photocoagulation is unknown. Randomized, controlled trials are needed for accurate comparison to the results obtained with ETDRS-style treatment.

As the benefits of vitrectomy include the removal of the cortical vitreous scaffold on which fibrovascular tissue proliferates, less invasive procedures are under development to achieve this goal. Therapeutic intravitreal injections may create a posterior vitreous detachment (PVD), which is associated with a more benign clinical course in diabetic retinopathy.[38,280] Various agents used to create PVD include hyaluronidase, urokinase, urea, plasminogen, autologous plasmin enzyme, microplasmin, and SF6 gas.[283] These agents may be helpful to facilitate the removal of fibrovascular membranes in surgery in some cases and obviate the need for vitrectomy in others. This approach alone does not address the underlying hypoxic stimulus for neovascularization. Thus, the need for photocoagulation would be expected to prevent anterior segment complications of PDR.

Techniques and technology continues to push the limits of vitrectomy surgery. Membrane removal remains the most technically challenging part of surgery and pharmacological vitreolysis may be used adjunctively with surgery as noted above.[281,282] Alternatively, precise tractionless cutting of membranes with or without cautery appears possible with the pulsed electron avalanche knife.[753,754] Improvements in instrument stiffness and functionality will undoubtedly promote the popularity of small-gauge vitrectomy and level-1 evidence-based research is needed for comparison with conventional 20-gauge vitrectomy.[210,423]

In the effort to prevent blindness from proliferative diabetic retinopathy, prevention is superior to treatment. Currently, the most accessible method of future prevention of PDR is the early detection and treatment of severe and very severe nonproliferative diabetic retinopathy.[630] Routine screening examinations leading to appropriate treatment have been shown to improve visual outcome.[755,756] Efforts aimed toward the prevention and treatment of obesity reduce the incidence of type 2 diabetes mellitus. Improved understanding of the autoimmune nature of type 1 diabetes may lead to a potential cure.[757] Continued progress toward improving metabolic control in diabetes of all types further will reduce the incidence of microvascular complications.[758,759]

References

1. Yamagishi S, Ueda S, Matsui T, et al. Role of advanced glycation end products (AGEs) and oxidative stress in diabetic retinopathy. *Curr Pharm Des*. 2008;14:962–968.
2. Lorenzi M. The polyol pathway as a mechanism for diabetic retinopathy: attractive, elusive, and resilient. *Exp Diabetes Res*. 2007;2007:61038.
3. Das EN, King GL. The role of protein kinase C activation and the vascular complications of diabetes. *Pharmacol Res*. 2007;55:498–510.
4. Simo R, Carrasco E, Garcia-Ramirez M, Hernandez C. Angiogenic and antiangiogenic factors in proliferative diabetic retinopathy. *Curr Diabetes Rev*. 2006;2:71–98.
5. Mitamura Y, Harada C, Harada T. Role of cytokines and trophic factors in the pathogenesis of diabetic retinopathy. *Curr Diabetes Rev*. 2005;1:73–81.
6. Mohamed Q, Gillies MC, Wong TY. Management of diabetic retinopathy: a systematic review. *JAMA*. 2007; 298:902–916.
7. The Diabetes Control and Complications Trial Research Group. The effect of intensive treatment of diabetes on the development and progression of long-term complications in insulin-dependent diabetes mellitus. *N Engl J Med*. 1993;329:977–986.
8. The Diabetes Control and Complications Trial. The effect of intensive diabetes treatment on the progression of diabetic retinopathy in insulin-dependent diabetes mellitus. *Arch Ophthalmol*. 1995;113:36–51.
9. Retinopathy and nephropathy in patients with type 1 diabetes four years after a trial of intensive therapy. *Am J Ophthalmol*. 2000;129:704–705.
10. Holman RR, Paul SK, Bethel MA, et al. 10-year follow-up of intensive glucose control in type 2 diabetes. *N Engl J Med*. 2008;359:1577–1589.
11. Gardiner TA, Anderson HR, Stitt AW. Inhibition of advanced glycation end-products protects against retinal capillary basement membrane expansion during long-term diabetes. *J Pathol*. 2003;201:328–333.
12. Yamagishi S, Matsui T, Nakamura K. Blockade of the advanced glycation end products (AGEs) and their receptor (RAGE) system is a possible mechanism for sustained beneficial effects of multifactorial intervention on mortality in type 2 diabetes. *Med Hypotheses*. 2008;71:749–751.
13. Henkind P. Ocular neovascularization. The Krill memorial lecture. *Am J Ophthalmol*. 1978;85:287–301.
14. Tsilibary EC. Microvascular basement membranes in diabetes mellitus. *J Pathol*. 2003;200:537–546.
15. Vinores SA, Youssri AI, Luna JD, et al. Upregulation of vascular endothelial growth factor in ischemic and non-ischemic human and experimental retinal disease. *Histol Histopathol*. 1997;12:99–109.
16. Niki T, Muraoka K, Shimizu K. Distribution of capillary nonperfusion in early-stage diabetic retinopathy. *Ophthalmology*. 1984;91:1431–1439.
17. Shimizu K, Kobayashi Y, Muraoka K. Midperipheral fundus involvement in diabetic retinopathy. *Ophthalmology*. 1981;88:601–612.

18. McLeod D. A chronic grey matter penumbra, lateral microvascular intussusception and venous peduncular avulsion underlie diabetic vitreous haemorrhage. *Br J Ophthalmol.* 2007;91:677–689.
19. Taylor E, Dobree JH. Proliferative diabetic retinopathy. Site and size of initial lesions. *Br J Ophthalmol.* 1970;54: 11–18.
20. Davis MD. Vitreous contraction in proliferative diabetic retinopathy. *Arch Ophthalmol.* 1965;74:741–751.
21. Kroll P, Rodrigues EB, Hoerle S. Pathogenesis and classification of proliferative diabetic vitreoretinopathy. *Ophthalmologica.* 2007;221:78–94.
22. Foos RY, Kreiger AE, Nofsinger K. Pathologic study following vitrectomy for proliferative diabetic retinopathy. *Retina.* 1985;5:101–106.
23. Faulborn J, Bowald S. Microproliferations in proliferative diabetic retinopathy and their relationship to the vitreous: corresponding light and electron microscopic studies. *Graefes Arch Clin Exp Ophthalmol.* 1985;223: 130–138.
24. Kuiper EJ, Van Nieuwenhoven FA, de Smet MD, et al. The angio-fibrotic switch of VEGF and CTGF in proliferative diabetic retinopathy. *PLoS ONE.* 2008; 3:e2675.
25. bu El-Asrar AM, Van den Steen PE, Al-Amro SA, et al. Expression of angiogenic and fibrogenic factors in proliferative vitreoretinal disorders. *Int Ophthalmol.* 2007; 27:11–22.
26. Kuiper EJ, de Smet MD, van Meurs JC, et al. Association of connective tissue growth factor with fibrosis in vitreoretinal disorders in the human eye. *Arch Ophthalmol.* 2006;124:1457–1462.
27. Michael JC, de Venecia G, Bresnick GH. Macular heterotopia in proliferative diabetic retinopathy. *Arch Ophthalmol.* 1994;112:1455–1459.
28. Walshe R, Esser P, Wiedemann P, Heimann K. Proliferative retinal diseases: myofibroblasts cause chronic vitreoretinal traction. *Br J Ophthalmol.* 1992;76:550–552.
29. Wallow IH, Greaser ML, Stevens TS. Actin filaments in diabetic fibrovascular preretinal membrane. *Arch Ophthalmol.* 1981;99:2175–2181.
30. Bresnick GH, Haight B, de Venecia G. Retinal wrinkling and macular heterotopia in diabetic retinopathy. *Arch Ophthalmol.* 1979;97:1890–1895.
31. McMeel JW. Diabetic retinopathy: fibrotic proliferation and retinal detachment. *Trans Am Ophthalmol Soc.* 1971; 69:440–493.
32. Thompson JT, de Bustros S, Michels RG, Rice TA. Results and prognostic factors in vitrectomy for diabetic traction-rhegmatogenous retinal detachment. *Arch Ophthalmol.* 1987;105:503–507.
33. Spranger J, Mohlig M, Osterhoff M, et al. Retinal photocoagulation does not influence intraocular levels of IGF-I, IGF-II and IGF-BP3 in proliferative diabetic retinopathy-evidence for combined treatment of PDR with somatostatin analogues and retinal photocoagulation? *Horm Metab Res.* 2001;33:312–316.
34. Dubey AK, Nagpal PN, Chawla S, Dubey B. A proposed new classification for diabetic retinopathy: the concept of primary and secondary vitreopathy. *Indian J Ophthalmol.* 2008;56:23–29.
35. Sebag J, Buckingham B, Charles MA, Reiser K. Biochemical abnormalities in vitreous of humans with proliferative diabetic retinopathy. *Arch Ophthalmol.* 1992; 110:1472–1476.
36. Sebag J. Abnormalities of human vitreous structure in diabetes. *Graefes Arch Clin Exp Ophthalmol.* 1993;231:257–260.
37. Shiraya T, Kato S, Fukushima H, Tanabe T. A case of diabetic retinopathy with both retinal neovascularization and complete posterior vitreous detachment. *Eur J Ophthalmol.* 2006;16:644–646.
38. Ono R, Kakehashi A, Yamagami H, et al. Prospective assessment of proliferative diabetic retinopathy with observations of posterior vitreous detachment. *Int Ophthalmol.* 2005;26:15–19.
39. Akiba J, Arzabe CW, Trempe CL. Posterior vitreous detachment and neovascularization in diabetic retinopathy. *Ophthalmology.* 1990;97:889–891.
40. Helbig H, Kellner U, Bornfeld N, Foerster MH. Rubeosis iridis after vitrectomy for diabetic retinopathy. *Graefes Arch Clin Exp Ophthalmol.* 1998;236:730–733.
41. Hayreh SS. Neovascular glaucoma. *Prog Retin Eye Res.* 2007;26:470–485.
42. Brown GC, Magargal LE, Schachat A, Shah H. Neovascular glaucoma. Etiologic considerations. *Ophthalmology.* 1984;91:315–320.
43. Heys JJ, Barocas VH. A boussinesq model of natural convection in the human eye and the formation of Krukenberg's spindle. *Ann Biomed Eng.* 2002;30:392–401.
44. Verdaguer J, le Clercq N, Holuigue J, Musalem R. Nonproliferative diabetic retinopathy with significant capillary nonperfusion. *Graefes Arch Clin Exp Ophthalmol.* 1987;225:157–159.
45. Blankenship GW. The lens influence on diabetic vitrectomy results. Report of a prospective randomized study. *Arch Ophthalmol.* 1980;98:2196–2198.
46. Sadiq SA, Chatterjee A, Vernon SA. Progression of diabetic retinopathy and rubeotic glaucoma following cataract surgery. *Eye.* 1995;9(Pt 6):728–738.
47. Blankenship G, Cortez R, Machemer R. The lens and pars plana vitrectomy for diabetic retinopathy complications. *Arch Ophthalmol.* 1979;97:1263–1267.
48. Preis I, Langer R, Brem H, Folkman J. Inhibition of neovascularization by an extract derived from vitreous. *Am J Ophthalmol.* 1977;84:323–328.
49. Thompson JT, de Bustros S, Michels RG, Rice TA. Results and prognostic factors in vitrectomy for diabetic traction retinal detachment of the macula. *Arch Ophthalmol.* 1987;105:497–502.
50. Jacobs NA, Trew DR. Occlusion of the central retinal artery and ocular neovascularisation: an indirect association? *Eye.* 1992;6(Pt 6):599–602.
51. Duker JS, Sivalingam A, Brown GC, Reber R. A prospective study of acute central retinal artery obstruction. The incidence of secondary ocular neovascularization. *Arch Ophthalmol.* 1991;109:339–342.
52. Klein BE. Overview of epidemiologic studies of diabetic retinopathy. *Ophthalmic Epidemiol.* 2007;14: 179–183.
53. Cheung N, Wong TY. Obesity and eye diseases. *Surv Ophthalmol.* 2007;52:180–195.

54. Ogden CL, Carroll MD, Curtin LR, et al. Prevalence of overweight and obesity in the United States, 1999–2004. *JAMA*. 2006;295:1549–1555.
55. National diabetes fact sheet, 2007. www.cdc.gov/diabetes/pubs/pdf/ndfs_2007.pdf. Accessed November 3. 2008.
56. Matthews DR, Stratton IM, Aldington SJ, et al. Risks of progression of retinopathy and vision loss related to tight blood pressure control in type 2 diabetes mellitus: UKPDS 69. *Arch Ophthalmol*. 2004;122:1631–1640.
57. UK Prospective Diabetes Study Group. Tight blood pressure control and risk of macrovascular and microvascular complications in type 2 diabetes: UKPDS 38. *BMJ*. 1998;317:703–713.
58. Lang GE. Laser treatment of diabetic retinopathy. *Dev Ophthalmol*. 2007;39:48–68.
59. American Diabetes Association. Diabetic retinopathy. *Diabetes Care*. 1998;21:157–159.
60. Kempen JH, O'Colmain BJ, Leske MC, et al. The prevalence of diabetic retinopathy among adults in the United States. *Arch Ophthalmol*. 2004;122:552–563.
61. Klein R, Klein BEK. Visual disorders in diabetes. In: Harris MI, Cowie CC, Stern MP, et al, eds. *Diabetes in America*. Bethesda, MD: US Public Health Service; 1995:293–338.
62. Klein R, Knudtson MD, Lee KE, et al. The Wisconsin Epidemiologic Study of Diabetic Retinopathy: XXII the twenty-five-year progression of retinopathy in persons with type 1 diabetes. *Ophthalmology*. 2008;115:1859–1868.
63. Bloomgarden ZT. Diabetic retinopathy. *Diabetes Care*. 2008;31:1080–1083.
64. Meyer-Schwickerath G. Light-coagulation. *Buech Augenarzt*. 1959;33:1.
65. Preliminary report on effects of photocoagulation therapy. The Diabetic Retinopathy Study Research Group. *Am J Ophthalmol*. 1976;81:383–396.
66. Photocoagulation treatment of proliferative diabetic retinopathy: the second report of diabetic retinopathy study findings. *Ophthalmology*. 1978;85:82–106.
67. Early Treatment Diabetic Retinopathy Study Research Group. Early photocoagulation for diabetic retinopathy. ETDRS report number 9. *Ophthalmology*. 1991;98:766–785.
68. The Early Treatment Diabetic Retinopathy Study Research Group. Techniques for scatter and local photocoagulation treatment of diabetic retinopathy: Early Treatment Diabetic Retinopathy Study Report no. 3. *Int Ophthalmol Clin*. 1987;27:254–264.
69. Flynn HW, Jr, Chew EY, Simons BD, et al. Pars plana vitrectomy in the Early Treatment Diabetic Retinopathy Study. ETDRS report number 17. The Early Treatment Diabetic Retinopathy Study Research Group. *Ophthalmology*. 1992;99:1351–1357.
70. Diabetic Retinopathy Vitrectomy Study (DRVS) report #1. Two-year course of visual acuity in severe proliferative diabetic retinopathy with conventional management. *Ophthalmology*. 1985;92:492–502.
71. The Diabetic Retinopathy Vitrectomy Study Research Group. Early vitrectomy for severe vitreous hemorrhage in diabetic retinopathy. Two-year results of a randomized trial. Diabetic Retinopathy Vitrectomy Study report 2. *Arch Ophthalmol*. 1985;103:1644–1652.
72. The Diabetic Retinopathy Vitrectomy Study Research Group. Early vitrectomy for severe proliferative diabetic retinopathy in eyes with useful vision. Results of a randomized trial–Diabetic Retinopathy Vitrectomy Study Report 3. *Ophthalmology*. 1988;95:1307–1320.
73. The Diabetic Retinopathy Vitrectomy Study Research Group. Early vitrectomy for severe proliferative diabetic retinopathy in eyes with useful vision. Clinical application of results of a randomized trial–Diabetic Retinopathy Vitrectomy Study Report 4. *Ophthalmology*. 1988;95:1321–1334.
74. Diabetic Retinopathy Vitrectomy Study. Early vitrectomy for severe vitreous hemorrhage in diabetic retinopathy. Four-year results of a randomized trial: Diabetic Retinopathy Vitrectomy Study Report 5. *Arch Ophthalmol*. 1990;108:958–964.
75. Kotoula MG, Koukoulis GN, Zintzaras E, et al. Metabolic control of diabetes is associated with an improved response of diabetic retinopathy to panretinal photocoagulation. *Diabetes Care*. 2005;28:2454–2457.
76. Aiello LP, Wong JS. Role of vascular endothelial growth factor in diabetic vascular complications. *Kidney Int Suppl*. 2000;77:S113–S119.
77. Boulton M, Foreman D, Williams G, McLeod D. VEGF localisation in diabetic retinopathy. *Br J Ophthalmol*. 1998;82:561–568.
78. Aiello LP, Avery RL, Arrigg PG, et al. Vascular endothelial growth factor in ocular fluid of patients with diabetic retinopathy and other retinal disorders. *N Engl J Med*. 1994;331:1480–1487.
79. Spranger J, Hammes HP, Preissner KT, et al. Release of the angiogenesis inhibitor angiostatin in patients with proliferative diabetic retinopathy: association with retinal photocoagulation. *Diabetologia*. 2000;43:1404–1407.
80. Patel JI, Hykin PG, Gregor ZJ, et al. Angiopoietin concentrations in diabetic retinopathy. *Br J Ophthalmol*. 2005;89:480–483.
81. Watanabe D, Suzuma K, Suzuma I, et al. Vitreous levels of angiopoietin 2 and vascular endothelial growth factor in patients with proliferative diabetic retinopathy. *Am J Ophthalmol*. 2005;139:476–481.
82. Hernandez C, Carrasco E, Casamitjana R, et al. Somatostatin molecular variants in the vitreous fluid: a comparative study between diabetic patients with proliferative diabetic retinopathy and nondiabetic control subjects. *Diabetes Care*. 2005;28:1941–1947.
83. Inokuchi N, Ikeda T, Imamura Y, et al. Vitreous levels of insulin-like growth factor-I in patients with proliferative diabetic retinopathy. *Curr Eye Res*. 2001;23:368–371.
84. bu El-Asrar AM, Struyf S, Kangave D, et al. Chemokines in proliferative diabetic retinopathy and proliferative vitreoretinopathy. *Eur Cytokine Netw*. 2006;17:155–165.
85. Khan ZA, Chan BM, Uniyal S, et al. EDB fibronectin and angiogenesis – a novel mechanistic pathway. *Angiogenesis*. 2005;8:183–196.
86. Hinton DR, Spee C, He S, et al. Accumulation of NH2-terminal fragment of connective tissue growth factor in the vitreous of patients with proliferative diabetic retinopathy. *Diabetes Care*. 2004;27:758–764.
87. Wilkinson-Berka JL, Wraight C, Werther G. The role of growth hormone, insulin-like growth factor and

somatostatin in diabetic retinopathy. *Curr Med Chem.* 2006;13:3307–3317.

88. Yamagishi S, Matsui T, Nakamura K, et al. Pigment epithelium-derived factor (PEDF) prevents diabetes- or advanced glycation end products (AGE)-elicited retinal leukostasis. *Microvasc Res.* 2006;72:86–90.
89. Spranger J, Osterhoff M, Reimann M, et al. Loss of the antiangiogenic pigment epithelium-derived factor in patients with angiogenic eye disease. *Diabetes.* 2001; 50:2641–2645.
90. Stellmach V, Crawford SE, Zhou W, Bouck N. Prevention of ischemia-induced retinopathy by the natural ocular antiangiogenic agent pigment epithelium-derived factor. *Proc Natl Acad Sci* USA. 2001;98: 2593–2597.
91. Matsunaga N, Chikaraishi Y, Izuta H, et al. Role of Soluble Vascular Endothelial Growth Factor Receptor-1 in the Vitreous in Proliferative Diabetic Retinopathy. *Ophthalmology.* 2008;115:1916–1922.
92. Noma H, Funatsu H, Yamashita H, et al. Regulation of angiogenesis in diabetic retinopathy: possible balance between vascular endothelial growth factor and endostatin. *Arch Ophthalmol.* 2002;120:1075–1080.
93. Patel JI, Tombran-Tink J, Hykin PG, et al. Vitreous and aqueous concentrations of proangiogenic, antiangiogenic factors and other cytokines in diabetic retinopathy patients with macular edema: implications for structural differences in macular profiles. *Exp Eye Res.* 2006;82:798–806.
94. Stefansson E. The therapeutic effects of retinal laser treatment and vitrectomy. A theory based on oxygen and vascular physiology. *Acta Ophthalmol Scand.* 2001; 79:435–440.
95. Stefansson E, Machemer R, de Juan E Jr, et al. Retinal oxygenation and laser treatment in patients with diabetic retinopathy. *Am J Ophthalmol.* 1992;113:36–38.
96. Fujio N, Feke GT, Goger DG, McMeel JW. Regional retinal blood flow reduction following half fundus photocoagulation treatment. *Br J Ophthalmol.* 1994; 78:335–338.
97. Remky A, Arend O, Beausencourt E, et al. [Retinal vessels before and after photocoagulation in diabetic retinopathy. Determining the diameter using digitized color fundus slides]. *Klin Monatsbl Augenheilkd.* 1996; 209:79–83.
98. Brooks HL, Jr, Eagle RC, Jr, Schroeder RP, et al. Clinicopathologic study of organic dye. Laser in the human fundus. *Ophthalmology.* 1989;96:822–834.
99. The Diabetic Retinopathy Study Research Group. Four risk factors for severe visual loss in diabetic retinopathy. The third report from the Diabetic Retinopathy Study. The Diabetic Retinopathy Study Research Group. *Arch Ophthalmol.* 1979;97:654–655.
100. Early Treatment Diabetic Retinopathy Study Research Group. Fundus photographic risk factors for progression of diabetic retinopathy. ETDRS report number 12. Early Treatment Diabetic Retinopathy Study Research Group. *Ophthalmology.* 1991;98:823–833.
101. The Diabetic Retinopathy Study Research Group. Indications for photocoagulation treatment of diabetic retinopathy: Diabetic Retinopathy Study Report no. 14. The Diabetic Retinopathy Study Research Group. *Int Ophthalmol Clin.* 1987;27:239–253.
102. Davis MD, Fisher MR, Gangnon RE, et al. Risk factors for high-risk proliferative diabetic retinopathy and severe visual loss: Early Treatment Diabetic Retinopathy Study Report #18. *Invest Ophthalmol Vis Sci.* 1998; 39:233–252.
103. Jacobson DR, Murphy RP, Rosenthal AR. The treatment of angle neovascularization with panretinal photocoagulation. *Ophthalmology.* 1979;86:1270–1277.
104. Kaaja R, Loukovaara S. Progression of retinopathy in type 1 diabetic women during pregnancy. *Curr Diabetes Rev.* 2007;3:85–93.
105. Temple RC, Aldridge VA, Sampson MJ, et al. Impact of pregnancy on the progression of diabetic retinopathy in Type 1 diabetes. *Diabet Med.* 2001;18:573–577.
106. Effect of pregnancy on microvascular complications in the diabetes control and complications trial. The Diabetes Control and Complications Trial Research Group. *Diabetes Care.* 2000;23:1084–1091.
107. Clustering of long-term complications in families with diabetes in the diabetes control and complications trial. The Diabetes Control and Complications Trial Research Group. *Diabetes.* 1997;46:1829–1839.
108. Sellman A. Hyphaema from microhaemangiomas. *Acta Ophthalmol* (Copenh). 1972;50:58–61.
109. Rosen E, Lyons D. Microhemangiomas at the pupillary border demonstrated by fluorescein photography. *Am J Ophthalmol.* 1969;67:846–853.
110. Hagen AP, Williams GA. Argon laser treatment of a bleeding iris vascular tuft. *Am J Ophthalmol.* 1986;101:379–380.
111. Welch RB. Spontaneous anterior chamber hemorrhage from the iris: a unique cinematographic documentation. *Trans Am Ophthalmol Soc.* 1980;78:132–147.
112. Blanksma LJ, Hooijmans JM. Vascular tufts of the pupillary border causing a spontaneous hyphaema. *Ophthalmologica.* 1979;178:297–302.
113. Meades KV, Francis IC, Kappagoda MB, Filipic M. Light microscopic and electron microscopic histopathology of an iris microhaemangioma. *Br J Ophthalmol.* 1986;70:290–294.
114. Bakke EF, Drolsum L. Iris microhaemangiomas and idiopathic juxtafoveolar retinal telangiectasis. *Acta Ophthalmol Scand.* 2006;84:818–822.
115. Podolsky MM, Srinivasan BD. Spontaneous hyphema secondary to vascular tuft of pupillary margin of the iris. *Arch Ophthalmol.* 1979;97:301–302.
116. Cobb B. Vascular tufts at the pupillary margin: a preliminary report on 44 patients. *Trans Ophthalmol Soc UK.* 1969;88:211–221.
117. Ramsay WJ, Ramsay RC, Purple RL, Knobloch WH. Involutional diabetic retinopathy. *Am J Ophthalmol.* 1977;84:851–858.
118. Freyler H. Combined vitrectomy and scleral resection in the therapy of massive epiretinal fibrous membranes due to diabetic retinopathy. *Graefes Arch Clin Exp Ophthalmol.* 1986;224:60–61.
119. Hudson HL, Chong LP, Frambach DA, et al. Encircling panretinal laser photocoagulation may prevent macular detachment after vitrectomy for proliferative diabetic retinopathy. *Int Ophthalmol.* 1994;18:101–104.

120. Yang CM, Su PY, Yeh PT, Chen MS. Combined rhegmatogenous and traction retinal detachment in proliferative diabetic retinopathy: clinical manifestations and surgical outcome. *Can J Ophthalmol.* 2008;43:192–198.
121. Alhassan MB, Kyari F, Ejere HO. Peribulbar versus retrobulbar anaesthesia for cataract surgery. *Cochrane Database Syst Rev.* 2008; (3):CD004083.
122. Wu WC, Hsu KH, Chen TL, et al. Interventions for relieving pain associated with panretinal photocoagulation: a prospective randomized trial. *Eye.* 2006;20:712–719.
123. Weinberger D, Ron Y, Lichter H, et al. Analgesic effect of topical sodium diclofenac 0.1% drops during retinal laser photocoagulation. *Br J Ophthalmol.* 2000;84: 135–137.
124. Esgin H, Samut HS. Topical ketorolac 0.5% for ocular pain relief during scatter laser photocoagulation with 532 nm green laser. *J Ocul Pharmacol Ther.* 2006;22: 460–464.
125. Vaideanu D, Taylor P, McAndrew P, et al. Double masked randomised controlled trial to assess the effectiveness of paracetamol in reducing pain in panretinal photocoagulation. *Br J Ophthalmol.* 2006;90:713–717.
126. Trento M, Tomelini M, Lattanzio R, et al. Perception of, and anxiety levels induced by, laser treatment in patients with sight-threatening diabetic retinopathy. A multicentre study. *Diabet Med.* 2006;23:1106–1109.
127. Duggan M, Dowd N, O'Mara D, et al. Benzodiazepine premedication may attenuate the stress response in daycase anesthesia: a pilot study. *Can J Anaesth.* 2002;49: 932–935.
128. Richardson C, Waterman H. Pain relief during panretinal photocoagulation for diabetic retinopathy: a national survey. *Eye.* 2009.
129. Seiberth V, Schatanek S, Alexandridis E. Panretinal photocoagulation in diabetic retinopathy: argon versus dye laser coagulation. *Graefes Arch Clin Exp Ophthalmol.* 1993;231:318–322.
130. Singerman LJ. Red krypton laser therapy of macular and retinal vascular diseases. *Retina.* 1982;2:15–28.
131. Al-Hussainy S, Dodson PM, Gibson JM. Pain response and follow-up of patients undergoing panretinal laser photocoagulation with reduced exposure times. *Eye.* 2008;22:96–99.
132. Mainster MA. Decreasing retinal photocoagulation damage: principles and techniques. *Semin Ophthalmol.* 1999;14:200–209.
133. Blumenkranz MS, Yellachich D, Andersen DE, et al. Semiautomated patterned scanning laser for retinal photocoagulation. *Retina.* 2006;26:370–376.
134. Biswell R. Retrobulbar and peribulbar regional anesthesia. *Ophthalmology.* 2002;109:1954.
135. Rodriguez-Coleman H, Spaide R. Ocular complications of needle perforations during retrobulbar and peribulbar injections. *Ophthalmol Clin North Am.* 2001;14:573–579.
136. Gurelik G, Coney JM, Zakov ZN. Binocular indirect panretinal laser photocoagulation for the treatment of proliferative diabetic retinopathy. *Ophthalmic Surg Lasers Imaging.* 2004;35:94–102.
137. Mizuno K. Binocular indirect argon laser photocoagulator. *Br J Ophthalmol.* 1981;65:425–428.
138. Heyworth P, Gregor Z. Broad laser indentation surface for retinal laser photocoagulation using indirect ophthalmoscopic delivery. *Arch Ophthalmol.* 1997; 115:280–281.
139. Benner JD, Huang M, Morse LS, et al. Comparison of photocoagulation with the argon, krypton, and diode laser indirect ophthalmoscopes in rabbit eyes. *Ophthalmology.* 1992;99:1554–1563.
140. Cuthbertson FM, Newsom RS, Wainwright AC. Kinetic anaesthesia for laser surgery. *Eye.* 2005;19: 1205–1207.
141. Blankenship GW. Panretinal laser photocoagulation with wide-angle fundus contact lens. *Ann Ophthalmol.* 1982;14:362–363.
142. Dogru M, Kaderli B, Gelisken O, et al. Ocular surface changes with applanation contact lens and coupling fluid use after argon laser photocoagulation in noninsulin-dependent diabetes mellitus. *Am J Ophthalmol.* 2004;138:381–388.
143. Arentsen JJ, Tasman W. Using a bandage contact lens to prevent recurrent corneal erosion during photocoagulation in patients with diabetes. *Am J Ophthalmol.* 1981;92:714–716.
144. Canning CR, Strong N, Berninger TA, Arden GB. Colour contrast sensitivity changes caused by peripheral retinal laser photocoagulation. *Eye.* 1991;5(Pt 3):348–351.
145. Berninger TA, Canning C, Strong N, et al. [Color vision disturbance in laser operators and patients: comparison of argon and dye lasers]. *Klin Monatsbl Augenheilkd.* 1990;197:494–497.
146. Blankenship GW, Gerke E, Batlle JF. Red krypton and blue-green argon laser diabetic panretinal photocoagulation. *Graefes Arch Clin Exp Ophthalmol.* 1989;227: 364–368.
147. The Krypton Argon Regression Neovascularization Study. Randomized comparison of krypton versus argon scatter photocoagulation for diabetic disc neovascularization. The Krypton Argon Regression Neovascularization Study report number 1. *Ophthalmology.* 1993;100:1655–1664.
148. Bujak MC, Mandelcorn MS, Parker JA. Light flashbacks during retinal laser photocoagulation following fluorescein angiography. *Ophthalmic Surg Lasers Imaging.* 2007;38:491–496.
149. Benz MS, Smiddy WE. Increased diode laser uptake in inner retinal layers after indocyanine green staining of the internal limiting membrane. *Ophthalmic Surg Lasers Imaging.* 2003;34:64–67.
150. Johnson RN, Irvine AR, Wood IS. Histopathology of krypton red laser panretinal photocoagulation. A clinicopathologic correlation. *Arch Ophthalmol.* 1987; 105:235–238.
151. Castillejos-Rios D, Devenyi R, Moffat K, Yu E. Dye yellow vs. argon green laser in panretinal photocoagulation for proliferative diabetic retinopathy: a comparison of minimum power requirements. *Can J Ophthalmol.* 1992;27:243–244.
152. Seiberth V, Alexandridis E. Function of the diabetic retina after panretinal argon laser photocoagulation. Influence of the intensity of the coagulation spots. *Ophthalmologica.* 1991;202:10–17.

153. Bandello F, Brancato R, Menchini U, et al. Light panretinal photocoagulation (LPRP) versus classic panretinal photocoagulation (CPRP) in proliferative diabetic retinopathy. *Semin Ophthalmol.* 2001;16:12–18.
154. Observational study of the development of diabetic macular edema following panretinal (scatter) photocoagulation given in 1 or 4 settings. Diabetic Retinopathy Clinical Research Network. *Arch Ophthalmol.* 2009;127:132–140.
155. Luttrull JK, Musch DC, Spink CA. Subthreshold diode micropulse panretinal photocoagulation for proliferative diabetic retinopathy. *Eye.* 2008;22:607–612.
156. Mainster MA, Crossman JL, Erickson PJ, Heacock GL. Retinal laser lenses: magnification, spot size, and field of view. *Br J Ophthalmol.* 1990;74:177–179.
157. http://www.volk.com/UserFiles/File/volkcatalogmay2008.pdf. Accessed January 21, 2009.
158. http://www.ocular-instruments.com/html/section_2/argon_diode.asp. Accessed January 21, 2009.
159. Obana A, Lorenz B, Gassler A, Birngruber R. The therapeutic range of chorioretinal photocoagulation with diode and argon lasers: an experimental comparison. *Lasers Light Ophthalmol.* 2009;4:147–156.
160. Wade EC, Blankenship GW. The effect of short versus long exposure times of argon laser panretinal photocoagulation on proliferative diabetic retinopathy. *Graefes Arch Clin Exp Ophthalmol.* 1990;228:226–231.
161. Jain A, Blumenkranz MS, Paulus Y, et al. Effect of pulse duration on size and character of the lesion in retinal photocoagulation. *Arch Ophthalmol.* 2008;126:78–85.
162. Birngruber R, Gabel VP, Hillenkamp F. Fundus reflectometry: a step towards optimization of the retina photocoagulation. *Mod Probl Ophthalmol.* 1977;18:383–390.
163. Morgan CM, Schatz H. Atrophic creep of the retinal pigment epithelium after focal macular photocoagulation. *Ophthalmology.* 1989;96:96–103.
164. Davies N. Altering the pattern of panretinal photocoagulation: could the visual field for driving be preserved? *Eye.* 1999;13(Pt 4):531–536.
165. http://www.optimedica.com/Pascal-Method/. Accessed February 1, 2009.
166. Yeh PT, Yang CM, Yang CH, Huang JS. Cryotherapy of the anterior retina and sclerotomy sites in diabetic vitrectomy to prevent recurrent vitreous hemorrhage: an ultrasound biomicroscopy study. *Ophthalmology.* 2005;112:2095–2102.
167. Neely KA, Scroggs MW, McCuen BW. Peripheral retinal cryotherapy for postvitrectomy diabetic vitreous hemorrhage in phakic eyes. *Am J Ophthalmol.* 1998;126:82–90.
168. Mosier MA, Del PE, Gheewala SM. Anterior retinal cryotherapy in diabetic vitreous hemorrhage. *Am J Ophthalmol.* 1985;100:440–444.
169. Han DP, Pulido JS, Mieler WF, Johnson MW. Vitrectomy for proliferative diabetic retinopathy with severe equatorial fibrovascular proliferation. *Am J Ophthalmol.* 1995;119:563–570.
170. Pe'er J, Folberg R, Itin A, et al. Upregulated expression of vascular endothelial growth factor in proliferative diabetic retinopathy. *Br J Ophthalmol.* 1996;80:241–245.
171. Niki T, Muraoka K, Shimizu K. Distribution of capillary nonperfusion in early-stage diabetic retinopathy. *Ophthalmology.* 1984;91:1431–1439.
172. Sultanov MI, Gadzhiev RV. [The characteristics of the course of diabetic retinopathy in myopia]. *Vestn Oftalmol.* 1990;106:49–51.
173. Dogru M, Inoue M, Nakamura M, Yamamoto M. Modifying factors related to asymmetric diabetic retinopathy. *Eye.* 1998;12(Pt 6):929–933.
174. Schmidt D. Macular-threatening traction detachment of the retina in diabetic proliferative retinopathy, treated by laser. *Int Ophthalmol.* 1997;21:99–106.
175. Kaufman PL. Parasympathetic denervation of the ciliary muscle following retinal photocoagulation. *Trans Am Ophthalmol Soc.* 1990;88:513–553.
176. Blankenship GW. A clinical comparison of central and peripheral argon laser panretinal photocoagulation for proliferative diabetic retinopathy. *Ophthalmology.* 1988;95:170–177.
177. Gentile RC, Stegman Z, Liebmann JM, et al. Risk factors for ciliochoroidal effusion after panretinal photocoagulation. *Ophthalmology.* 1996;103:827–832.
178. Doft BH, Blankenship GW. Single versus multiple treatment sessions of argon laser panretinal photocoagulation for proliferative diabetic retinopathy. *Ophthalmology.* 1982;89:772–779.
179. Shimura M, Yasuda K, Nakazawa T, et al. Quantifying alterations of macular thickness before and after panretinal photocoagulation in patients with severe diabetic retinopathy and good vision. *Ophthalmology.* 2003;110:2386–2394.
180. Doft BH, Blankenship G. Retinopathy risk factor regression after laser panretinal photocoagulation for proliferative diabetic retinopathy. *Ophthalmology.* 1984;91:1453–1457.
181. Sebag J, Buzney SM, Belyea DA, et al. Posterior vitreous detachment following panretinal laser photocoagulation. *Graefes Arch Clin Exp Ophthalmol.* 1990;228:5–8.
182. Jalkh A, Takahashi M, Topilow HW, et al. Prognostic value of vitreous findings in diabetic retinopathy. *Arch Ophthalmol.* 1982;100:432–434.
183. de Bustros S, Thompson JT, Michels RG, Rice TA. Vitrectomy for progressive proliferative diabetic retinopathy. *Arch Ophthalmol.* 1987;105:196–199.
184. Thompson JT, de Bustros S, Michels RG, Rice TA. Results and prognostic factors in vitrectomy for diabetic vitreous hemorrhage. *Arch Ophthalmol.* 1987;105:191–195.
185. Fong DS, Girach A, Boney A. Visual side effects of successful scatter laser photocoagulation surgery for proliferative diabetic retinopathy: a literature review. *Retina.* 2007;27:816–824.
186. Kleinmann G, Hauser D, Schechtman E, et al. Vitreous hemorrhage in diabetic eyes previously treated with panretinal photocoagulation. *Int Ophthalmol.* 2008;28:29–34.
187. Kaiser RS, Maguire MG, Grunwald JE, et al. One-year outcomes of panretinal photocoagulation in proliferative diabetic retinopathy. *Am J Ophthalmol.* 2000;129:178–185.

188. Vine AK. The efficacy of additional argon laser photocoagulation for persistent, severe proliferative diabetic retinopathy. *Ophthalmology*. 1985;92:1532–1537.
189. Aylward GW, Pearson RV, Jagger JD, Hamilton AM. Extensive argon laser photocoagulation in the treatment of proliferative diabetic retinopathy. *Br J Ophthalmol*. 1989;73:197–201.
190. Davis MD. Vitreous contraction in proliferative diabetic retinopathy. *Arch Ophthalmol*. 1965;74:741–751.
191. Shea M. Early vitrectomy in proliferative diabetic retinopathy. *Arch Ophthalmol*. 1983;101:1204–1205.
192. Neubauer AS, Ulbig MW. Laser treatment in diabetic retinopathy. *Ophthalmologica*. 2007;221:95–102.
193. Keithahn MA, Gross RH, Mannis MJ, et al. Corneal perforation associated with argon laser photocoagulation for a retinal tear. *Am J Ophthalmol*. 1997;123:125–127.
194. Moriarty AP, Spalton DJ, Shilling JS, et al. Breakdown of the blood-aqueous barrier after argon laser panretinal photocoagulation for proliferative diabetic retinopathy. *Ophthalmology*. 1996;103:833–838.
195. Bloom SM, Mahl CF, Schiller SB. Lenticular burns following argon panretinal photocoagulation. *Br J Ophthalmol*. 1992;76:630–631.
196. Larsson LI, Nuija E. Increased permeability of the blood-aqueous barrier after panretinal photocoagulation for proliferative diabetic retinopathy. *Acta Ophthalmol Scand*. 2001;79:414–416.
197. Pierro L, Azzolini C, Brancato R, et al. Ultrasound biomicroscopic evaluation of ciliochoroidal effusion after laser treatment. *Ophthalmologica*. 1999;213:281–285.
198. Lerner BC, Lakhanpal V, Schocket SS. Transient myopia and accommodative paresis following retinal cryotherapy and panretinal photocoagulation. *Am J Ophthalmol*. 1984;97:704–708.
199. Yuki T, Kimura Y, Nanbu S, et al. Ciliary body and choroidal detachment after laser photocoagulation for diabetic retinopathy. A high-frequency ultrasound study. *Ophthalmology*. 1997;104:1259–1264.
200. Congdon NG, Friedman DS. Angle-closure glaucoma: impact, etiology, diagnosis, and treatment. *Curr Opin Ophthalmol*. 2003;14:70–73.
201. Haupert CL, Grossniklaus HE, Sharara N, et al. Optimal laser power to rupture Bruch's membrane and the retinal vein in the pig. *Ophthalmic Surg Lasers Imaging*. 2003;34:122–127.
202. Vijayasekaran S, Yu DY, McAllister I, et al. Optimal conditions required for the creation of an iatrogenic chorioretinal venous anastomosis in the dog using argon green laser photocoagulation. *Curr Eye Res*. 1995;14:63–70.
203. Orth DH, Flood TP, Packo KH. Iatrogenic choroidal neovascularization after krypton red laser photocoagulation. *Ophthalmic Surg*. 1989;20:273–277.
204. Thomas EL, Apple DJ, Swartz M, Kavka-Van ND. Histopathology and ultrastructure of krypton and argon laser lesions in a human retina-choroid. *Retina*. 1984;4:22–39.
205. Peyman GA, Li M, Yoneya S, et al. Fundus photocoagulation with the argon and krypton lasers: a comparative study. *Ophthalmic Surg*. 1981;12:481–490.
206. Galinos SO, McMeel JW, Trempe CL, Schepens CL. Chorioretinal anastomoses after argon laser photocoagulation. *Am J Ophthalmol*. 1976;82:241–245.
207. Lovestam-Adrian M, Andreasson S, Ponjavic V. Macular function assessed with mfERG before and after panretinal photocoagulation in patients with proliferative diabetic retinopathy. *Doc Ophthalmol*. 2004;109:115–121.
208. Patel JI, Jenkins L, Benjamin L, Webber S. Dilated pupils and loss of accommodation following diode panretinal photocoagulation with sub-tenon local anaesthetic in four cases. *Eye*. 2002;16:628–632.
209. Dogru M, Nakamura M, Inoue M, Yamamoto M. Long-term visual outcome in proliferative diabetic retinopathy patients after panretinal photocoagulation. *Jpn J Ophthalmol*. 1999;43:217–224.
210. Mittra RA and Pollack JS. ASRS PAT Survey. http://www.asrs.org/services/pat_survey/reports/report.php? 2008. Accessed November 15, 2008.
211. Cunningham MA, Edelman JL, Kaushal S. Intravitreal steroids for macular edema: the past, the present, and the future. *Surv Ophthalmol*. 2008;53:139–149.
212. Shima C, Sakaguchi H, Gomi F, et al. Complications in patients after intravitreal injection of bevacizumab. *Acta Ophthalmol*. 2008;86:372–376.
213. Hollands H, Wong J, Bruen R, et al. Short-term intraocular pressure changes after intravitreal injection of bevacizumab. *Can J Ophthalmol*. 2007;42:807–811.
214. Wu L, Martinez-Castellanos MA, Quiroz-Mercado H, et al. Twelve-month safety of intravitreal injections of bevacizumab (Avastin(R)): results of the Pan-American Collaborative Retina Study Group (PACORES). *Graefes Arch Clin Exp Ophthalmol*. 2008;246:81–87.
215. Fintak DR, Shah GK, Blinder KJ, et al. Incidence of endophthalmitis related to intravitreal injection of bevacizumab and ranibizumab. *Retina*. 2008;28:1395–1399.
216. Brooks HL, Jr, Caballero S Jr, Newell CK, et al. Vitreous levels of vascular endothelial growth factor and stromal-derived factor 1 in patients with diabetic retinopathy and cystoid macular edema before and after intraocular injection of triamcinolone. *Arch Ophthalmol*. 2004;122:1801–1807.
217. Spandau UH, Vom HF, Hammes HP, Jonas JB. Effect of intravitreal triamcinolone acetonide on retinal apoptosis in experimental retinal neovascularization. *Graefes Arch Clin Exp Ophthalmol*. 2008;246:1069–1070.
218. Bandello F, Polito A, Pognuz DR, et al. Triamcinolone as adjunctive treatment to laser panretinal photocoagulation for proliferative diabetic retinopathy. *Arch Ophthalmol*. 2006;124:643–650.
219. Shimura M, Yasuda K, Shiono T. Posterior sub-Tenon's capsule injection of triamcinolone acetonide prevents panretinal photocoagulation-induced visual dysfunction in patients with severe diabetic retinopathy and good vision. *Ophthalmology*. 2006;113:381–387.
220. Gharbiya M, Grandinetti F, Balacco GC. Intravitreal triamcinolone for macular detachment following panretinal photocoagulation. *Eye*. 2005;19:818–820.
221. Maia OO, Jr, Takahashi BS, Costa RA, et al. Combined Laser and Intravitreal Triamcinolone for Proliferative Diabetic Retinopathy and Macular Edema: one-year results of a randomized clinical trial. *Am J Ophthalmol*. 2008;147:291–297.

222. Lee GH, Ahn JK, Park YG. Intravitreal triamcinolone reduces the morphologic changes of ciliary body after pars plana vitrectomy for retinal vascular diseases. *Am J Ophthalmol*. 2008;145:1037–1044.
223. Jonas JB. Intravitreal triamcinolone acetonide for diabetic retinopathy. *Dev Ophthalmol*. 2007;39:96–110.
224. Jonas JB. Intravitreal triamcinolone acetonide: a change in a paradigm. *Ophthalmic Res*. 2006;38:218–245.
225. Jonas JB, Sofker A. Intravitreal triamcinolone acetonide for cataract surgery with iris neovascularization. *J Cataract Refract Surg*. 2002;28:2040–2041.
226. Jonas JB, Kreissig I, Degenring RF. Neovascular glaucoma treated by intravitreal triamcinolone acetonide. *Acta Ophthalmol Scand*. 2003;81:540–541.
227. Jonas JB, Hayler JK, Sofker A, Panda-Jonas S. Regression of neovascular iris vessels by intravitreal injection of crystalline cortisone. *J Glaucoma*. 2001;10: 284–287.
228. Beer PM, Bakri SJ, Singh RJ, et al. Intraocular concentration and pharmacokinetics of triamcinolone acetonide after a single intravitreal injection. *Ophthalmology*. 2003;110:681–668.
229. Jermak CM, Dellacroce JT, Heffez J, Peyman GA. Triamcinolone acetonide in ocular therapeutics. *Surv Ophthalmol*. 2007;52:503–522.
230. Shtein RM, Stahl RM, Saxe SJ, Mian SI. Herpes simplex keratitis after intravitreal triamcinolone acetonide. *Cornea*. 2007;26:641–642.
231. Saidel MA, Berreen J, Margolis TP. Cytomegalovirus retinitis after intravitreous triamcinolone in an immunocompetent patient. *Am J Ophthalmol*. 2005;140: 1141–1143.
232. Imasawa M, Ohshiro T, Gotoh T, et al. Central serous chorioretinopathy following vitrectomy with intravitreal triamcinolone acetonide for diabetic macular oedema. *Acta Ophthalmol Scand*. 2005;83:132–133.
233. Diabetic Retinopathy Clinical Research Network. A randomized trial comparing intravitreal triamcinolone acetonide and focal/grid photocoagulation for diabetic macular edema. *Ophthalmology*. 2008;115:1447–1449.
234. Jonas JB, Degenring RF, Kreissig I, et al. Intraocular pressure elevation after intravitreal triamcinolone acetonide injection. *Ophthalmology*. 2005;112:593–598.
235. Smithen LM, Ober MD, Maranan L, Spaide RF. Intravitreal triamcinolone acetonide and intraocular pressure. *Am J Ophthalmol*. 2004;138:740–743.
236. Schulze-Dobold C, Weber M. Loss of visual function after repeated intravitreal injections of triamcinolone acetonide in refractory uveitic macular oedema. *Int Ophthalmol*. 2008.
237. Luke M, Januschowski K, Beutel J, et al. The effects of triamcinolone crystals on retinal function in a model of isolated perfused vertebrate retina. *Exp Eye Res*. 2008; 87:22–29.
238. Lang Y, Zemel E, Miller B, Perlman I. Retinal toxicity of intravitreal kenalog in albino rabbits. *Retina*. 2007; 27:778–788.
239. Hida T, Chandler D, Arena JE, Machemer R. Experimental and clinical observations of the intraocular toxicity of commercial corticosteroid preparations. *Am J Ophthalmol*. 1986;101:190–195.
240. Eren E, Kucukerdonmez C, Yilmaz G, Akova YA. Regression of neovascular posterior capsule vessels by intravitreal bevacizumab. *J Cataract Refract Surg*. 2007; 33:1113–1115.
241. Schwartz SG, Flynn HW, Jr. Pharmacotherapies for diabetic retinopathy: present and future. *Exp Diabetes Res*. 2007;2007:52487.
242. Avery RL, Pearlman J, Pieramici DJ, et al. Intravitreal bevacizumab (Avastin) in the treatment of proliferative diabetic retinopathy. *Ophthalmology*. 2006;113: 1695–1615.
243. Quiroz-Mercado H, Ustariz-Gonzalez O, Martinez-Castellanos MA, et al. Our experience after 1765 intravitreal injections of bevacizumab: the importance of being part of a developing story. *Semin Ophthalmol*. 2007;22:109–125.
244. Sawada O, Kawamura H, Kakinoki M, et al. Vascular endothelial growth factor in aqueous humor before and after intravitreal injection of bevacizumab in eyes with diabetic retinopathy. *Arch Ophthalmol*. 2007;125: 1363–1366.
245. Ferrara N. Vascular endothelial growth factor: basic science and clinical progress. *Endocr Rev*. 2004;25:581–611.
246. Yeoh J, Williams C, Allen P, et al. Avastin as an adjunct to vitrectomy in the management of severe proliferative diabetic retinopathy: a prospective case series. *Clin Experiment Ophthalmol*. 2008;36:449–454.
247. Krohne TU, Eter N, Holz FG, Meyer CH. Intraocular pharmacokinetics of bevacizumab after a single intravitreal injection in humans. *Am J Ophthalmol*. 2008;146: 508–512.
248. Grisanti S, Biester S, Peters S, et al. Intracameral bevacizumab for iris rubeosis. *Am J Ophthalmol*. 2006;142: 158–160.
249. Wakabayashi T, Oshima Y, Sakaguchi H, et al. Intravitreal bevacizumab to treat iris neovascularization and neovascular glaucoma secondary to ischemic retinal diseases in 41 consecutive cases. *Ophthalmology*. 2008; 115:1571–1580.
250. Oshima Y, Sakaguchi H, Gomi F, Tano Y. Regression of iris neovascularization after intravitreal injection of bevacizumab in patients with proliferative diabetic retinopathy. *Am J Ophthalmol*. 2006;142:155–158.
251. Deissler HL, Lang GE. [In vitro studies on the mechanism of action of VEGF and its inhibitors]. *Klin Monatsbl Augenheilkd*. 2008;225:623–628.
252. Mason JO, III, Yunker JJ, Vail R, McGwin G, Jr. Intravitreal bevacizumab (Avastin) prevention of panretinal photocoagulation-induced complications in patients with severe proliferative diabetic retinopathy. *Retina*. 2008;28:1319–1324.
253. Yanyali A, Aytug B, Horozoglu F, Nohutcu AF. Bevacizumab (Avastin) for diabetic macular edema in previously vitrectomized eyes. *Am J Ophthalmol*. 2007;144:124–126.
254. Moradian S, Ahmadieh H, Malihi M, et al. Intravitreal bevacizumab in active progressive proliferative diabetic retinopathy. *Graefes Arch Clin Exp Ophthalmol*. 2008;246:1699–1705.
255. Arevalo JF, Wu L, Sanchez JG, et al. Intravitreal bevacizumab (avastin) for proliferative diabetic retinopathy: 6-months follow-up. *Eye*. 2007;23:117–123.

256. Jorge R, Costa RA, Calucci D, et al. Intravitreal bevacizumab (Avastin) for persistent new vessels in diabetic retinopathy (IBEPE study). *Retina.* 2006;26: 1006–1013.
257. Mason JO, III, Nixon PA, White MF. Intravitreal injection of bevacizumab (Avastin) as adjunctive treatment of proliferative diabetic retinopathy. *Am J Ophthalmol.* 2006;142:685–688.
258. Friedlander SM, Welch RM. Vanishing disc neovascularization following intravitreal bevacizumab (avastin) injection. *Arch Ophthalmol.* 2006;124:1365.
259. Bakri SJ, Donaldson MJ, Link TP. Rapid regression of disc neovascularization in a patient with proliferative diabetic retinopathy following adjunctive intravitreal bevacizumab. *Eye.* 2006;20:1474–1475.
260. Tonello M, Costa RA, Almeida FP, et al. Panretinal photocoagulation versus PRP plus intravitreal bevacizumab for high-risk proliferative diabetic retinopathy (IBeHi study). *Acta Ophthalmol.* 2008;86:385–389.
261. Mirshahi A, Roohipoor R, Lashay A, et al. Bevacizumab-augmented retinal laser photocoagulation in proliferative diabetic retinopathy: a randomized double-masked clinical trial. *Eur J Ophthalmol.* 2008;18:263–269.
262. Minnella AM, Savastano CM, Ziccardi L, et al. Intravitreal bevacizumab (Avastin) in proliferative diabetic retinopathy. *Acta Ophthalmol.* 2008;86:683–687.
263. Spaide RF, Fisher YL. Intravitreal bevacizumab (Avastin) treatment of proliferative diabetic retinopathy complicated by vitreous hemorrhage. *Retina.* 2006;26: 275–278.
264. Chen E, Park CH. Use of intravitreal bevacizumab as a preoperative adjunct for tractional retinal detachment repair in severe proliferative diabetic retinopathy. *Retina.* 2006;26:699–700.
265. Rizzo S, Genovesi-Ebert F, Di Bartolo E, et al. Injection of intravitreal bevacizumab (Avastin) as a preoperative adjunct before vitrectomy surgery in the treatment of severe proliferative diabetic retinopathy (PDR). *Graefes Arch Clin Exp Ophthalmol.* 2008;246:837–842.
266. Ishikawa K, Honda S, Tsukahara Y, Negi A. Preferable use of intravitreal bevacizumab as a pretreatment of vitrectomy for severe proliferative diabetic retinopathy. *Eye.* 2007;23:108–111.
267. Beutel J, Peters S, Luke M, et al. Bevacizumab as adjuvant for neovascular glaucoma. *Acta Ophthalmol.* 2008.
268. Silva PJ, Jorge R, Alves CR, et al. Short-term results of intravitreal bevacizumab (Avastin) on anterior segment neovascularization in neovascular glaucoma. *Acta Ophthalmol Scand.* 2006;84:556–557.
269. Sothornwit N. Intravitreal bevacizumab for ahmed glaucoma valve implantation in neovascular glaucoma: a case report. *J Med Assoc Thai.* 2008;91(Suppl 1): S162–S165.
270. Ichhpujani P, Ramasubramanian A, Kaushik S, Pandav SS. Bevacizumab in glaucoma: a review. *Can J Ophthalmol.* 2007;42:812–815.
271. Rouvas A, Petrou P, Ladas I, et al. Spontaneous resolution of vitreomacular traction following ranibizumab (Lucentis) injection. *Eur J Ophthalmol.* 2008;18:301–303.
272. Mitamura Y, Ogata K, Oshitari T, et al. Retinal detachment with macular hole following intravitreal bevacizumab in patient with severe proliferative diabetic retinopathy. *Br J Ophthalmol.* 2008;92:717–718.
273. Arevalo JF, Maia M, Flynn HW, Jr, et al. Tractional retinal detachment following intravitreal bevacizumab (Avastin) in patients with severe proliferative diabetic retinopathy. *Br J Ophthalmol.* 2008;92:213–216.
274. Oshima Y, Shima C, Wakabayashi T, et al. Microincision vitrectomy surgery and intravitreal bevacizumab as a surgical adjunct to treat diabetic traction retinal detachment. *Ophthalmology.* 2009;116:927–938.
275. Nishijima K, Ng YS, Zhong L, et al. Vascular endothelial growth factor-A is a survival factor for retinal neurons and a critical neuroprotectant during the adaptive response to ischemic injury. *Am J Pathol.* 2007;171:53–67.
276. Neubauer AS, Kook D, Haritoglou C, et al. Bevacizumab and retinal ischemia. *Ophthalmology.* 2007;114:2096.
277. Kuppermann BD, Thomas EL, de Smet MD, Grillone LR. Safety results of two phase III trials of an intravitreous injection of highly purified ovine hyaluronidase (Vitrase) for the management of vitreous hemorrhage. *Am J Ophthalmol.* 2005;140:585–597.
278. Kuppermann BD, Thomas EL, de Smet MD, Grillone LR. Pooled efficacy results from two multinational randomized controlled clinical trials of a single intravitreous injection of highly purified ovine hyaluronidase (Vitrase) for the management of vitreous hemorrhage. *Am J Ophthalmol.* 2005;140:573–584.
279. Bhavsar A, Grillone L, McNamara T, et al. Predicting response of vitreous hemorrhage and outcome of photocoagulation after intravitreous injection of highly purified ovine hyaluronidase in patients with diabetes. *Invest Ophthalmol Vis Sci.* 2008;49:4219–4225.
280. Gandorfer A. Pharmacologic vitreolysis. *Dev Ophthalmol.* 2007;39:149–156.
281. Hirata A, Takano A, Inomata Y, et al. Plasmin-assisted vitrectomy for management of proliferative membrane in proliferative diabetic retinopathy: a pilot study. *Retina.* 2007;27:1074–1078.
282. Williams JG, Trese MT, Williams GA, Hartzer MK. Autologous plasmin enzyme in the surgical management of diabetic retinopathy. *Ophthalmology.* 2001; 108:1902–1905.
283. Ochoa-Contreras D, sol-Coronado L, Buitrago ME, et al. Induced posterior vitreous detachment by intravitreal sulfur hexafluoride (SF6) injection in patients with nonproliferative diabetic retinopathy. *Acta Ophthalmol Scand.* 2000;78:687–688.
284. Aaberg TM, Abrams GW. Changing indications and techniques for vitrectomy in management of complications of diabetic retinopathy. *Ophthalmology.* 1987;94:775–779.
285. Ho T, Smiddy WE, Flynn HW, Jr. Vitrectomy in the management of diabetic eye disease. *Surv Ophthalmol.* 1992;37:190–202.
286. Joussen AM, Joeres S. Benefits and limitations in vitreoretinal surgery for proliferative diabetic retinopathy and macular edema. *Dev Ophthalmol.* 2007;39:69–87.
287. Wilkinson CP. What ever happened to bilateral patching? *Retina.* 2005;25:393–394.
288. Seelenfreund MH, Sternberg I, Hirsch I, Silverstone BZ. Retinal tears with total vitreous hemorrhage. *Am J Ophthalmol.* 1983;95:659–662.

289. Lincoff H, Stopa M, Kreissig I. Ambulatory binocular occlusion. *Retina*. 2004;24:246–253.
290. Thompson JT, de Bustros S, Michels RG, et al. Results of vitrectomy for proliferative diabetic retinopathy. *Ophthalmology*. 1986;93:1571–1574.
291. Brown GC, Tasman WS, Benson WE, et al. Reoperation following diabetic vitrectomy. *Arch Ophthalmol*. 1992;110:506–510.
292. Campbell DG, Simmons RJ, Grant WM. Ghost cells as a cause of glaucoma. *Am J Ophthalmol*. 1976;81:441–450.
293. Campbell DG, Simmons RJ, Tolentino FI, McMeel JW. Glaucoma occurring after closed vitrectomy. *Am J Ophthalmol*. 1977;83:63–69.
294. Ghartey KN, Tolentino FI, Freeman HM, et al. Closed vitreous surgery. XVII. Results and complications of pars plana vitrectomy. *Arch Ophthalmol*. 1980;98:1248–1252.
295. Han DP, Lewis H, Lambrou FH, Jr, et al. Mechanisms of intraocular pressure elevation after pars plana vitrectomy. *Ophthalmology*. 1989;96:1357–1362.
296. Campbell DG, Essigmann EM. Hemolytic ghost cell glaucoma. Further studies. *Arch Ophthalmol*. 1979;97: 2141–2146.
297. Singh H, Grand MG. Treatment of blood-induced glaucoma by trans pars plana vitrectomy. *Retina*. 1981;1:255–257.
298. Ramsay RC, Knobloch WH, Cantrill HL. Timing of vitrectomy for active proliferative diabetic retinopathy. *Ophthalmology*. 1986;93:283–289.
299. O'Hanley GP, Canny CL. Diabetic dense premacular hemorrhage. A possible indication for prompt vitrectomy. *Ophthalmology*. 1985;92:507–511.
300. Chung J, Park YH, Lee YC. The effect of Nd:YAG laser membranotomy and intravitreal tissue plasminogen activator with gas on massive diabetic premacular hemorrhage. *Ophthalmic Surg Lasers Imaging*. 2008;39:114–120.
301. Rennie CA, Newman DK, Snead MP, Flanagan DW. Nd:YAG laser treatment for premacular subhyaloid haemorrhage. *Eye*. 2001;15:519–524.
302. Chen YJ, Kou HK. Krypton laser membranotomy in the treatment of dense premacular hemorrhage. *Can J Ophthalmol*. 2004;39:761–766.
303. Khairallah M, Ladjimi A, Messaoud R, et al. Retinal venous macroaneurysm associated with premacular hemorrhage. *Ophthalmic Surg Lasers*. 1999;30:226–228.
304. Raymond LA. Neodymium:YAG laser treatment for hemorrhages under the internal limiting membrane and posterior hyaloid face in the macula. *Ophthalmology*. 1995;102:406–411.
305. Ulbig MW, Mangouritsas G, Rothbacher HH, et al. Long-term results after drainage of premacular subhyaloid hemorrhage into the vitreous with a pulsed Nd:YAG laser. *Arch Ophthalmol*. 1998;116:1465–1469.
306. Foos RY. Subhyaloid hemorrhage illustrating a mechanism of macular hole formation. *Arch Ophthalmol*. 1992;110:598.
307. Nork TM, Gioia VM, Hobson RR, Kessel RH. Subhyaloid hemorrhage illustrating a mechanism of macular hole formation. *Arch Ophthalmol*. 1991;109:884–885.
308. Park SW, Seo MS. Subhyaloid hemorrhage treated with SF6 gas injection. *Ophthalmic Surg Lasers Imaging*. 2004;35:335–337.
309. Conway MD, Peyman GA, Recasens M. Intravitreal tPA and SF6 promote clearing of premacular subhyaloid hemorrhages in shaken and battered baby syndrome. *Ophthalmic Surg Lasers*. 1999;30:435–441.
310. Chung J, Kim MH, Chung SM, Chang KY. The effect of tissue plasminogen activator on premacular hemorrhage. *Ophthalmic Surg Lasers*. 2001;32:7–12.
311. Ryan SJ. Traction retinal detachment. XLIX Edward Jackson Memorial Lecture. *Am J Ophthalmol*. 1993; 115:1–20.
312. Charles S, Flinn CE. The natural history of diabetic extramacular traction retinal detachment. *Arch Ophthalmol*. 1981;99:66–68.
313. Steinmetz RL, Grizzard WS, Hammer ME. Vitrectomy for diabetic traction retinal detachment using the multiport illumination system. *Ophthalmology*. 2002;109: 2303–2307.
314. Lahey JM, Francis RR, Kearney JJ. Combining phacoemulsification with pars plana vitrectomy in patients with proliferative diabetic retinopathy: a series of 223 cases. *Ophthalmology*. 2003;110:1335–1339.
315. Aaberg TM. Pars plana vitrectomy for diabetic traction retinal detachment. *Ophthalmology*. 1981;88:639–642.
316. Machemer R. Vitrectomy in diabetic retinopathy; removal of preretinal proliferations. *Trans Sect Ophthalmol Am Acad Ophthalmol Otolaryngol*. 1975;79: OP394–OP395.
317. Tolentino FI, Freeman HM, Tolentino FL. Closed vitrectomy in the management of diabetic traction retinal detachment. *Ophthalmology*. 1980;87:1078–1089.
318. Williams DF, Williams GA, Hartz A, et al. Results of vitrectomy for diabetic traction retinal detachments using the en bloc excision technique. *Ophthalmology*. 1989;96:752–758.
319. Han DP, Murphy ML, Mieler WF. A modified en bloc excision technique during vitrectomy for diabetic traction retinal detachment. Results and complications. *Ophthalmology*. 1994;101:803–808.
320. Nakae R, Saito Y, Nishikawa N, et al. [Results of vitrectomy for diabetic traction retinal detachment involving the macula; a comparison of six-month and three-year postoperative findings]. *Nippon Ganka Gakkai Zasshi*. 1989;93:271–275.
321. Oldendoerp J, Spitznas M. Factors influencing the results of vitreous surgery in diabetic retinopathy. I. Iris rubeosis and/or active neovascularization at the fundus. *Graefes Arch Clin Exp Ophthalmol*. 1989;227: 1–8.
322. Wu WC, Lin JC. The experience to use a modified en bloc excision technique in vitrectomy for diabetic traction retinal detachment. *Kaohsiung J Med Sci*. 1999;15: 461–467.
323. Altan T, Acar N, Kapran Z, et al. Transconjunctival 25-gauge sutureless vitrectomy and silicone oil injection in diabetic traction retinal detachment. *Retina*. 2008;28: 1201–1206.
324. Meier P, Wiedemann P. Vitrectomy for traction macular detachment in diabetic retinopathy. *Graefes Arch Clin Exp Ophthalmol*. 1997;235:569–574.
325. La Heij EC, Tecim S, Kessels AG, et al. Clinical variables and their relation to visual outcome after

vitrectomy in eyes with diabetic retinal traction detachment. *Graefes Arch Clin Exp Ophthalmol.* 2004;242:210–217.
326. Oda H, Konno K, Mitsui K, et al. [Recent outcomes of vitreous surgery for diabetic retinopathy]. *Nippon Ganka Gakkai Zasshi.* 2005;109:603–612.
327. Kakehashi A, Trempe CL, Fujio N, et al. Retinal breaks in diabetic retinopathy: vitreoretinal relationships. *Ophthalmic Surg.* 1994;25:695–699.
328. Morse LS, Chapman CB, Eliott D, et al. Subretinal hemorrhages in proliferative diabetic retinopathy. *Retina.* 1997;17:87–93.
329. Rice TA, Michels RG, Rice EF. Vitrectomy for diabetic rhegmatogenous retinal detachment. *Am J Ophthalmol.* 1983;95:34–44.
330. Douglas MJ, Scott IU, Flynn HW, Jr. Pars plana lensectomy, pars plana vitrectomy, and silicone oil tamponade as initial management of cataract and combined traction/rhegmatogenous retinal detachment involving the macula associated with severe proliferative diabetic retinopathy. *Ophthalmic Surg Lasers Imaging.* 2003;34:270–278.
331. Michels RG. Vitrectomy for complications of diabetic retinopathy. *Arch Ophthalmol.* 1978;96:237–246.
332. Peyman GA, Huamonte FU, Goldberg MF, et al. Four hundred consecutive pars plana vitrectomies with the vitrophage. *Arch Ophthalmol.* 1978;96:45–50.
333. Thompson JT, de BS, Michels RG, Rice TA. Results and prognostic factors in vitrectomy for diabetic traction-rhegmatogenous retinal detachment. *Arch Ophthalmol.* 1987;105:503–507.
334. Sima P, Zoran T. Long-term results of vitreous surgery for proliferative diabetic retinopathy. *Doc Ophthalmol.* 1994;87:223–232.
335. Stoffelns BM, Dick B. [Pars-plana vitrectomy in diabetic traction retinal detachments with holes]. *Klin Monatsbl Augenheilkd.* 2000;216:286–289.
336. Ho T, Smiddy WE, Flynn HW, Jr. Vitrectomy in the management of diabetic eye disease. *Surv Ophthalmol.* 1992;37:190–202.
337. Case reports to accompany Early Treatment Diabetic Retinopathy Study Reports 3 and 4. The Early Treatment Diabetic Retinopathy Study Research Group. *Int Ophthalmol Clin.* 1987;27:273–333.
338. Favard C, Guyot-Argenton C, Assouline M, et al. Full panretinal photocoagulation and early vitrectomy improve prognosis of florid diabetic retinopathy. *Ophthalmology.* 1996;103:561–574.
339. Jaffe GJ, Lewis H, Han DP, et al. Treatment of postvitrectomy fibrin pupillary block with tissue plasminogen activator. *Am J Ophthalmol.* 1989;108:170–175.
340. Williams GA, Lambrou FH, Jaffe GA, et al. Treatment of postvitrectomy fibrin formation with intraocular tissue plasminogen activator. *Arch Ophthalmol.* 1988;106:1055–1058.
341. Sebestyen JG. Fibrinoid syndrome: a severe complication of vitrectomy surgery in diabetics. *Ann Ophthalmol.* 1982;14:853–856.
342. Lewis H, Abrams GW, Williams GA. Anterior hyaloidal fibrovascular proliferation after diabetic vitrectomy. *Am J Ophthalmol.* 1987;104:607–613.
343. Ulbig MR, Hykin PG, Foss AJ, et al. Anterior hyaloidal fibrovascular proliferation after extracapsular cataract extraction in diabetic eyes. *Am J Ophthalmol.* 1993;115:321–326.
344. Kurihara T, Noda K, Ishida S, Inoue M. Pars plana vitrectomy with internal limiting membrane removal for macular hole associated with proliferative diabetic retinopathy. *Graefes Arch Clin Exp Ophthalmol.* 2005;243:724–726.
345. Cooper BA, Shah GK, Sheidow TG, et al. Outcome of macular hole surgery in diabetic patients with nonproliferative retinopathy. *Retina.* 2004;24:360–362.
346. Ghoraba H. Types of macular holes encountered during diabetic vitrectomy. *Retina.* 2002;22:176–182.
347. Flynn HW, Jr. Macular hole surgery in patients with proliferative diabetic retinopathy. *Arch Ophthalmol.* 1994;112:877–878.
348. Sakimoto S, Saito Y, Nakata K, et al. Surgical outcomes of epiretinal membrane removal after successful pars plana vitrectomy for retinal diseases. *Jpn J Ophthalmol.* 2008;52:227–230.
349. Chang PY, Yang CM, Yang CH, et al. Pars plana vitrectomy for diabetic fibrovascular proliferation with and without internal limiting membrane peeling. *Eye.* 2008;23:960–965.
350. Roldan-Pallares M, Rollin R, Martinez-Montero JC, et al. Immunoreactive endothelin-1 in the vitreous humor and epiretinal membranes of patients with proliferative diabetic retinopathy. *Retina.* 2007;27:222–235.
351. Hueber A, Wiedemann P, Esser P, Heimann K. Basic fibroblast growth factor mRNA, bFGF peptide and FGF receptor in epiretinal membranes of intraocular proliferative disorders (PVR and PDR). *Int Ophthalmol.* 1996;20:345–350.
352. Ioachim E, Stefaniotou M, Gorezis S, et al. Immunohistochemical study of extracellular matrix components in epiretinal membranes of vitreoproliferative retinopathy and proliferative diabetic retinopathy. *Eur J Ophthalmol.* 2005;15:384–391.
353. Clarkson JG, Green WR, Massof D. A histopathologic review of 168 cases of preretinal membrane 1977. *Retina.* 2005;25:1–17.
354. Heidenkummer HP, Kampik A, Petrovski B. Proliferative activity in epiretinal membranes. The use of the monoclonal antibody Ki-67 in proliferative vitreoretinal diseases. *Retina.* 1992;12:52–58.
355. Srinivasan VJ, Wojtkowski M, Witkin AJ, et al. High-definition and 3-dimensional imaging of macular pathologies with high-speed ultrahigh-resolution optical coherence tomography. *Ophthalmology.* 2006;113:2054–2014.
356. Mori K, Gehlbach PL, Sano A, et al. Comparison of epiretinal membranes of differing pathogenesis using optical coherence tomography. *Retina.* 2004;24:57–62.
357. Bovey EH, Uffer S, Achache F. Surgery for epimacular membrane: impact of retinal internal limiting membrane removal on functional outcome. *Retina.* 2004;24:728–735.
358. Yoon KC, Seo MS. Macular hole after peeling of the internal limiting membrane in diabetic macular edema. *Ophthalmic Surg Lasers Imaging.* 2003;34:478–479.

359. Grigorian R, Bhagat N, Lanzetta P, et al. Pars plana vitrectomy for refractory diabetic macular edema. *Semin Ophthalmol*. 2003;18:116–120.
360. Brazitikos PD, Stangos NT. Macular hole formation in diabetic retinopathy: the role of coexisting macular edema. *Doc Ophthalmol*. 1999;97:273–278.
361. Bruggemann A, Hoerauf H. [Atypical macular holes]. *Klin Monatsbl Augenheilkd*. 2008;225:281–285.
362. Kumagai K, Ogino N, Furukawa M, et al. Surgical outcomes for patients who develop macular holes after pars plana vitrectomy. *Am J Ophthalmol*. 2008;145: 1077–1080.
363. Lecleire-Collet A, Offret O, Gaucher D, et al. Full-thickness macular hole in a patient with diabetic cystoid macular oedema treated by intravitreal triamcinolone injections. *Acta Ophthalmol Scand*. 2007;85:795–798.
364. Yeh PT, Cheng CK, Chen MS, et al. Macular hole in proliferative diabetic retinopathy with fibrovascular proliferation. *Retina*. 2008;29:355–361.
365. Amemiya T, Yoshida H. Macular hole in diabetic maculopathy. *Ophthalmologica*. 1978;177:188–191.
366. Mason JO, Somaiya MD, White MF, Jr, Vail RS. Macular holes associated with diabetic tractional retinal detachments. *Ophthalmic Surg Lasers Imaging*. 2008;39:288–293.
367. Yan H, Cui J, Lu Y, et al. Vitrectomy for treatment of macular hole in diabetic retinopathy. *Ann Ophthalmol (Skokie)*. 2007;39:340–342.
368. Lee SN, Park KH, Song SJ. Spontaneous resolution of a full-thickness macular hole in proliferative diabetic retinopathy. *Jpn J Ophthalmol*. 2008;52:342–344.
369. Gandorfer A, Rohleder M, Grosselfinger S, et al. Epiretinal pathology of diffuse diabetic macular edema associated with vitreomacular traction. *Am J Ophthalmol*. 2005;139:638–652.
370. Basteau F, Mortemousque B, Aouizerate F. [Diffuse diabetic macular edema and vitreoretinal interface pathology: a study of seven cases (ten eyes)]. *J Fr Ophtalmol*. 2004;27:1109–1120.
371. Massin P, Duguid G, Erginay A, et al. Optical coherence tomography for evaluating diabetic macular edema before and after vitrectomy. *Am J Ophthalmol*. 2003;135:169–177.
372. Faulborn J, Ardjomand N. Tractional retinoschisis in proliferative diabetic retinopathy: a histopathological study. *Graefes Arch Clin Exp Ophthalmol*. 2000;238: 40–44.
373. Bresnick GH, Smith V, Pokorny J. Visual function abnormalities in macular heterotopia caused by proliferative diabetic retinopathy. *Am J Ophthalmol*. 1981; 92:85–102.
374. Muramatsu M, Yokoi M, Muramatsu A, et al. [Different outcome among eyes with proliferative diabetic retinopathy indicated for vitrectomy]. *Nippon Ganka Gakkai Zasshi*. 2006;110:950–960.
375. Sato Y, Shimada H, Aso S, Matsui M. Vitrectomy for diabetic macular heterotopia. *Ophthalmology*. 1994; 101:63–67.
376. Schroeder B, Krzizok T, Kaufmann H, Kroll P. [Disturbances of binocular vision in macular heterotopia]. *Klin Monatsbl Augenheilkd*. 1999;215:135–139.
377. Bixenman WW, Joffe L. Binocular diplopia associated with retinal wrinkling. *J Pediatr Ophthalmol Strabismus*. 1984;21:215–219.
378. Barton JJ. "Retinal diplopia" associated with macular wrinkling. *Neurology*. 2004;63:925–927.
379. Kroll P, Wiegand W, Schmidt J. Vitreopapillary traction in proliferative diabetic vitreoretinopathy [see comments]. *Br J Ophthalmol*. 1999;83:261–264.
380. Meyer CH, Schmidt JC, Mennel S, Kroll P. Functional and anatomical results of vitreopapillary traction after vitrectomy. *Acta Ophthalmol Scand*. 2007;85:221–222.
381. Karatas M, Ramirez JA, Ophir A. Diabetic vitreopapillary traction and macular oedema. *Eye*. 2005;19: 676–682.
382. Sebag J. Anomalous posterior vitreous detachment: a unifying concept in vitreo-retinal disease. *Graefes Arch Clin Exp Ophthalmol*. 2004;242:690–698.
383. Sebag J. Vitreopapillary traction as a cause of elevated optic nerve head. *Am J Ophthalmol*. 1999;128:261–262.
384. Aras C, Arici C, Akova N. Peripapillary serous retinal detachment preceding complete posterior vitreous detachment. *Graefes Arch Clin Exp Ophthalmol*. 2008; 246:927–929.
385. Hedges TR, III, Flattem NL, Bagga A. Vitreopapillary traction confirmed by optical coherence tomography. *Arch Ophthalmol*. 2006;124:279–281.
386. Katz B, Hoyt WF. Intrapapillary and peripapillary hemorrhage in young patients with incomplete posterior vitreous detachment. Signs of vitreopapillary traction. *Ophthalmology*. 1995;102:349–354.
387. Kokame GT, Yamamoto I, Kishi S, et al. Intrapapillary hemorrhage with adjacent peripapillary subretinal hemorrhage. *Ophthalmology*. 2004;111:926–930.
388. Katz B, Hoyt WF. Gaze-evoked amaurosis from vitreopapillary traction. *Am J Ophthalmol*. 2005;139:631–637.
389. Akura J, Ikeda T, Sato K, Ikeda N. Macular star associated with posterior hyaloid detachment. *Acta Ophthalmol Scand*. 2001;79:317–318.
390. Cabrera S, Katz A, Margalit E. Vitreopapillary traction: cost-effective diagnosis by optical coherence tomography. *Can J Ophthalmol*. 2006;41:763–765.
391. Bonnet M. [Papillary hyperfluorescence caused by traction of the vitreous body]. *J Fr Ophtalmol*. 1991;14:529–536.
392. Rumelt S, Karatas M, Pikkel J, et al. Optic disc traction syndrome associated with central retinal vein occlusion. *Arch Ophthalmol*. 2003;121:1093–1097.
393. Wisotsky BJ, Magat-Gordon CB, Puklin JE. Vitreopapillary traction as a cause of elevated optic nerve head. *Am J Ophthalmol*. 1998;126:137–139.
394. Saito Y, Ueki N, Hamanaka N, et al. Transient optic disc edema by vitreous traction in a quiescent eye with proliferative diabetic retinopathy mimicking diabetic papillopathy. *Retina*. 2005;25:83–84.
395. Pendergast SD, Martin DF, Proia AD, et al. Removal of optic disc stalks during diabetic vitrectomy. *Retina*. 1995;15:25–28.
396. Moitra VK, Meiler SE. The diabetic surgical patient. *Curr Opin Anaesthesiol*. 2006;19:339–345.
397. Gupta S, Koirala J, Khardori R, Khardori N. Infections in diabetes mellitus and hyperglycemia. *Infect Dis Clin North Am*. 2007;21:617–638, vii.

398. Auerbach AD, Goldman L. beta-Blockers and reduction of cardiac events in noncardiac surgery: clinical applications. *JAMA*. 2002;287:1445–1447.
399. Starr MB, Lally JM. Antimicrobial prophylaxis for ophthalmic surgery. *Surv Ophthalmol*. 1995;39:485–501.
400. Kusaka S, Kodama T, Ohashi Y. Condensation of silicone oil on the posterior surface of a silicone intraocular lens during vitrectomy. *Am J Ophthalmol*. 1996; 121:574–575.
401. Khawly JA, Lambert RJ, Jaffe GJ. Intraocular lens changes after short- and long-term exposure to intraocular silicone oil. An in vivo study. *Ophthalmology*. 1998;105:1227–1233.
402. Eliott D, Lee M, Abrams G. Proloferative diabetic retinopathy: principles and techniques of surgical treatment. In: Ryan SJ, Wilkinson C, eds. *Retina*. The Netherlands: Elsevier Mosby; 2006:2413–2449.
403. Iwasaki T, Miura M, Matsushima C, et al. Three-dimensional optical coherence tomography of proliferative diabetic retinopathy. *Br J Ophthalmol*. 2008;92:713.
404. Blankenship GW. Preoperative prognostic factors in diabetic pars plana vitrectomy. *Ophthalmology*. 1982; 89:1246–1249.
405. Tzekov R, Arden GB. The electroretinogram in diabetic retinopathy. *Surv Ophthalmol*. 1999;44:53–60.
406. Liggett PE, Lean JS, Barlow WE, Ryan SJ. Intraoperative argon endophotocoagulation for recurrent vitreous hemorrhage after vitrectomy for diabetic retinopathy. *Am J Ophthalmol*. 1987;103:146–149.
407. West JF, Gregor ZJ. Fibrovascular ingrowth and recurrent haemorrhage following diabetic vitrectomy. *Br J Ophthalmol*. 2000;84:822–825.
408. Chalam KV, Gupta SK, Agarwal S. Lightweight autoclavable wide-angle contact lens for vitreous surgery. *Ophthalmic Surg Lasers Imaging*. 2007;38:523–524.
409. Chalam KV, Shah VA. Two-piece, dual-purpose comprehensive contact lens for vitreous surgery. *Ophthalmic Res*. 2005;37:175–178.
410. Emi K, Oyagi T, Futamura H. [New biconcave prism contact lens for vitreous surgery in gas-filled eyes]. *Nippon Ganka Gakkai Zasshi*. 2005;109:400–405.
411. Virata SR, Kylstra JA, Singh HT. Corneal epithelial defects following vitrectomy surgery using hand-held, sew-on, and noncontact viewing lenses. *Retina*. 1999; 19:287–290.
412. Kuo IC, O'Brien TP, Haller JA, Jabbur NS. Complications of sequential keratorefractive and vitreoretinal surgery. *J Cataract Refract Surg*. 2006;32:2146–2148.
413. Tosi GM, Tilanus MA, Eggink C, Mittica V. Flap displacement during vitrectomy 24 months after laser in situ keratomileusis. *Retina*. 2005;25:1101–1103.
414. Senn P. [Practical experiences in conversion to the wide angle observation systems for vitreous surgery BIOM, SDI, VPF]. *Klin Monatsbl Augenheilkd*. 1991;198:480–481.
415. Virata SR, Kylstra JA. Postoperative complications following vitrectomy for proliferative diabetic retinopathy with sew-on and noncontact wide-angle viewing lenses. *Ophthalmic Surg Lasers*. 2001;32:193–197.
416. Hubschman JP, Gupta A, Bourla DH, et al. 20-, 23-, and 25-gauge vitreous cutters: performance and characteristics evaluation. *Retina*. 2008;28:249–257.
417. Taban M, Ventura AA, Sharma S, Kaiser PK. Dynamic evaluation of sutureless vitrectomy wounds: an optical coherence tomography and histopathology study. *Ophthalmology*. 2008;115:2221–2228.
418. Heimann H. [Primary 25- and 23-gauge vitrectomy in the treatment of rhegmatogenous retinal detachment–advancement of surgical technique or erroneous trend?]. *Klin Monatsbl Augenheilkd*. 2008;225:947–956.
419. Wimpissinger B, Kellner L, Brannath W, et al. 23-Gauge versus 20-gauge system for pars plana vitrectomy: a prospective randomised clinical trial. *Br J Ophthalmol*. 2008;92:1483–1487.
420. Byeon SH, Lew YJ, Kim M, Kwon OW. Wound leakage and hypotony after 25-gauge sutureless vitrectomy: factors affecting postoperative intraocular pressure. *Ophthalmic Surg Lasers Imaging*. 2008;39:94–99.
421. Sato T, Kusaka S, Oshima Y, Fujikado T. Analyses of cutting and aspirating properties of vitreous cutters with high-speed camera. *Retina*. 2008;28:749–754.
422. Shinoda H, Nakajima T, Shinoda K, et al. Jamming of 25-gauge instruments in the cannula during vitrectomy for vitreous haemorrhage. *Acta Ophthalmol*. 2008;86:160–164.
423. Williams GA. 25-, 23-, or 20-gauge instrumentation for vitreous surgery? *Eye*. 2008;22:1263–1266.
424. Horiguchi M, Kojima Y, Shimada Y. New system for fiberoptic-free bimanual vitreous surgery. *Arch Ophthalmol*. 2002;120:491–494.
425. Williams GA, Abrams GW, Mieler WF. Illuminated retinal picks for vitreous surgery. *Arch Ophthalmol*. 1989;107:1086.
426. Chalam KV, Shah GY, Agarwal S, Gupta SK. Illuminated curved 25-gauge vitrectomy probe for removal of subsclerotomy vitreous in vitreoretinal surgery. *Indian J Ophthalmol*. 2008;56:331–334.
427. Er H, Firat P. Posterior-segment surgeries with a two-port modified multiport illumination system. *Ophthalmologica*. 2008;222:145–148.
428. Oshima Y, Awh CC, Tano Y. Self-retaining 27-gauge transconjunctival chandelier endoillumination for panoramic viewing during vitreous surgery. *Am J Ophthalmol*. 2007;143:166–167.
429. Peyman GA, Lee KJ. New forceps for preretinal membrane removal. *Retina*. 1994;14:88–89.
430. Tolentino FA, Wu G. Diamond-dusted microspatula tips for vitreoretinal surgery. *Arch Ophthalmol*. 1987; 105:1732–1733.
431. Wafapoor H, Peyman GA. A new instrument (forceps/scissors) for preretinal membrane peeling, segmentation. *Arch Ophthalmol*. 1996;114:99.
432. Johnson TM, Glaser BM. Intraocular rake for removal of epiretinal membranes. *Am J Ophthalmol*. 2006;141: 381–383.
433. Arevalo JF. En bloc perfluorodissection for tractional retinal detachment in proliferative diabetic retinopathy. *Ophthalmology*. 2008;115:e21–e25.
434. Imamura Y, Minami M, Ueki M, et al. Use of perfluorocarbon liquid during vitrectomy for severe proliferative diabetic retinopathy. *Br J Ophthalmol*. 2003;87:563–566.
435. Ruiz-Moreno JM, Barile S, Montero JA. Phacoemulsification in the vitreous cavity for retained nuclear lens fragments. *Eur J Ophthalmol*. 2006;16:40–45.

436. Movshovich A, Berrocal M, Chang S. The protective properties of liquid perfluorocarbons in phacofragmentation of dislocated lenses. *Retina*. 1994;14:457–462.
437. Lewis H, Blumenkranz MS, Chang S. Treatment of dislocated crystalline lens and retinal detachment with perfluorocarbon liquids. *Retina*. 1992;12:299–304.
438. Chang TS, Pelzek CD, Nguyen RL, et al. Inverted pneumatic retinopexy: a method of treating retinal detachments associated with inferior retinal breaks. *Ophthalmology*. 2003;110:589–594.
439. Castellarin A, Grigorian R, Bhagat N, et al. Vitrectomy with silicone oil infusion in severe diabetic retinopathy. *Br J Ophthalmol*. 2003;87:318–321.
440. Azen SP, Scott IU, Flynn HW, Jr, et al. Silicone oil in the repair of complex retinal detachments. A prospective observational multicenter study. *Ophthalmology*. 1998;105:1587–1597.
441. Berker N, Batman C, Ozdamar Y, et al. Long-term outcomes of heavy silicone oil tamponade for complicated retinal detachment. *Eur J Ophthalmol*. 2007;17: 797–803.
442. Brourman ND, Blumenkranz MS, Cox MS, Trese MT. Silicone oil for the treatment of severe proliferative diabetic retinopathy. *Ophthalmology*. 1989;96:759–764.
443. Morse LS, McCuen BW. The use of silicone oil in uveitis and hypotony. *Retina*. 1991;11:399–404.
444. Ciardella AP, Fisher YL, Carvalho C, et al. Endoscopic vitreoretinal surgery for complicated proliferative diabetic retinopathy. *Retina*. 2001;21:20–27.
445. Garcia-Valenzuela E, Abdelsalam A, Eliott D, et al. Reduced need for corneal epithelial debridement during vitreo-retinal surgery using two different viscous surface lubricants. *Am J Ophthalmol*. 2003;136:1062–1066.
446. Kulshrestha MK, Rauz S, Goble RR, et al. The role of preoperative subconjunctival mydricaine and topical diclofenac sodium 0.1% in maintaining mydriasis during vitrectomy. *Retina*. 2000;20:46–51.
447. Mirshahi A, Djalilian A, Rafiee F, Namavari A. Topical administration of diclofenac (1%) in the prevention of miosis during vitrectomy. *Retina*. 2008;28:1215–1220.
448. Heyworth P, Bourke R, Moore C, et al. The systemic absorption of adrenaline from posterior segment infusion during vitreoretinal surgery. *Eye*. 1998;12(Pt 6): 949–952.
449. Graether JM. Graether pupil expander for managing the small pupil during surgery. *J Cataract Refract Surg*. 1996;22:530–535.
450. McCuen BW, Hickingbotham D, Tsai M, de Juan E Jr. Temporary iris fixation with a micro-iris retractor. *Arch Ophthalmol*. 1989;107:925–927.
451. Packer AJ, McCuen BW, Hutton WL, Ramsay RC. Procoagulant effects of intraocular sodium hyaluronate (Healon) after phakic diabetic vitrectomy. A prospective, randomized study. *Ophthalmology*. 1989;96:1491–1494.
452. Burke MJ, Parks MM, Calhoun JH, et al. Safety evaluation of BSS plus in pediatric intraocular surgery. *J Pediatr Ophthalmol Strabismus*. 1981;18:45–49.
453. Benson WE, Diamond JG, Tasman W. Intraocular irrigating solutions for pars plana vitrectomy. A prospective, randomized, double-blind study. *Arch Ophthalmol*. 1981;99:1013–1015.
454. Matsuda M, Tano Y, Edelhauser HF. Comparison of intraocular irrigating solutions used for pars plana vitrectomy and prevention of endothelial cell loss. *Jpn J Ophthalmol*. 1984;28:230–238.
455. Rosenfeld SI, Waltman SR, Olk RJ, Gordon M. Comparison of intraocular irrigating solutions in pars plana vitrectomy. *Ophthalmology*. 1986;93:109–115.
456. Moorhead LC, Redburn DA, Merritt J, Garcia CA. The effects of intravitreal irrigation during vitrectomy on the electroretinogram. *Am J Ophthalmol*. 1979;88: 239–245.
457. Saornil Alvarez MA, Pastor Jimeno JC. Role of the intraocular irrigating solutions in the pathogenesis of the postvitrectomy retinal edema. *Curr Eye Res*. 1987; 6:1369–1379.
458. Araie M, Kimura M. Intraocular irrigating solutions and barrier function of retinal pigment epithelium. *Br J Ophthalmol*. 1997;81:150–153.
459. Haimann MH, Abrams GW. Prevention of lens opacification during diabetic vitrectomy. *Ophthalmology*. 1984;91:116–121.
460. Browning DJ, Fraser CM. Clinical management of silicone intraocular lens condensation. *Am J Ophthalmol*. 2005;139:740–742.
461. Porter RG, Peters JD, Bourke RD. De-misting condensation on intraocular lenses. *Ophthalmology*. 2000;107: 778–782.
462. Ikeda T, Sato K, Katano T, Hayashi Y. Surgically induced detachment of the anterior hyaloid membrane from the posterior lens capsule. *Arch Ophthalmol*. 1999; 117:408–409.
463. Williamson T. *Diabetic Retinopathy and Other Vascular Disorders. Vitreoretinal Surgery*. New York: Springer; 2008:141–160.
464. Flynn HW, Lee WG, Parel JM. Design features and surgical use of a cannulated extrusion needle. *Graefes Arch Clin Exp Ophthalmol*. 1989;227:304–308.
465. Imamura Y, Kamei M, Minami M, et al. Heparin-assisted removal of clotting preretinal hemorrhage during vitrectomy for proliferative diabetic retinopathy. *Retina*. 2005;25:793–795.
466. Le MY, Korobelnik JF, Morel C, et al. TPA-assisted vitrectomy for proliferative diabetic retinopathy: results of a double-masked, multicenter trial. *Retina*. 1999;19: 378–382.
467. Thompson JT, Glaser BM, Michels RG, de Bustros S. The use of intravitreal thrombin to control hemorrhage during vitrectomy. *Ophthalmology*. 1986;93:279–282.
468. de Bustros S. Intraoperative control of hemorrhage in penetrating ocular injuries. *Retina*. 1990;10(Suppl 1): S55–S58.
469. Charles S, Chang S, McCuen BW. New techniques for hemostasis during diabetic vitrectomy. *Retina*. 2003;23:120–122.
470. Moreira Junior CA, Uscocovich CE, Moreira AT. Experimental studies with perfluoro-octane for hemostasis during vitreoretinal surgery. *Retina*. 1997;17:530–534.
471. Chu TG, Lopez PF, Cano MR, et al. Posterior vitreoschisis. An echographic finding in proliferative diabetic retinopathy. *Ophthalmology*. 1996;103: 315–322.

472. Kakehashi A, Schepens CL, de Sousa-Neto A, et al. Biomicroscopic findings of posterior vitreoschisis. *Ophthalmic Surg*. 1993;24:846–850.
473. Schwartz SD, Alexander R, Hiscott P, Gregor ZJ. Recognition of vitreoschisis in proliferative diabetic retinopathy. A useful landmark in vitrectomy for diabetic traction retinal detachment. *Ophthalmology*. 1996; 103:323–328.
474. Flynn HW, Jr, Davis JL, Parel JM, Lee WG. Applications of a cannulated extrusion needle during vitreoretinal microsurgery. *Retina*. 1988;8:42–49.
475. Sonoda KH, Sakamoto T, Enaida H, et al. Residual vitreous cortex after surgical posterior vitreous separation visualized by intravitreous triamcinolone acetonide. *Ophthalmology*. 2004;111:226–230.
476. Yao Y, Wang ZJ, Wei SH, et al. Oral sodium fluorescein to improve visualization of clear vitreous during vitrectomy for proliferative diabetic retinopathy. *Clin Experiment Ophthalmol*. 2007;35:824–827.
477. Schmidt JC, Chofflet J, Horle S, et al. Three simple approaches to visualize the transparent vitreous cortex during vitreoretinal surgery. *Dev Ophthalmol*. 2008;42: 35–42.
478. Kakehashi A. Total en bloc excision: a modified vitrectomy technique for proliferative diabetic retinopathy. *Am J Ophthalmol*. 2002;134:763–765.
479. Han DP, Abrams GW, Aaberg TM. Surgical excision of the attached posterior hyaloid. *Arch Ophthalmol*. 1988;106:998–1000.
480. Shinoda K, Inoue M, Katsura H, Ishida S. A new technique for separation of posterior vitreous in vitreous surgery. *Ophthalmic Surg Lasers*. 1999;30:588–590.
481. Abrams GW, Williams GA. "En bloc" excision of diabetic membranes. *Am J Ophthalmol*. 1987;103:302–308.
482. Cheema RA, Sengupta R. The 'suck-and-cut' bimanual technique for delamination of fibrovascular membranes in proliferative diabetic retinopathy. *Acta Ophthalmol Scand*. 2007;85:225.
483. Charles S. Vitrectomy for retinal detachment. *Trans Ophthalmol Soc* UK. 1980;100:542–549.
484. Michels RG. Vitreous surgery. London: CV Mosby; 1981:174–222.
485. Meredith TA, Kaplan HJ, Aaberg TM. Pars plana vitrectomy techniques for relief of epiretinal traction by membrane segmentation. *Am J Ophthalmol*. 1980; 89:408–413.
486. Charles S. *Vitreous Microsurgery*, 3rd edn. Baltimore, MD: Williams & Wilkins; 1987.
487. Maturi RK, Merrill PT, Lomeo MD, et al. Perfluoro-N-octane (PFO) in the repair of complicated retinal detachments due to severe proliferative diabetic retinopathy. *Ophthalmic Surg Lasers*. 1999;30:715–720.
488. Grigorian RA, Castellarin A, Bhagat N, et al. Use of viscodissection and silicone oil in vitrectomy for severe diabetic retinopathy. *Semin Ophthalmol*. 2003;18:121–126.
489. Grigorian RA, Castellarin A, Fegan R, et al. Epiretinal membrane removal in diabetic eyes: comparison of viscodissection with conventional methods of membrane peeling. *Br J Ophthalmol*. 2003;87:737–741.
490. Murray TG, Boldt HC, Lewis H, et al. A technique for facilitated visualization and dissection of the vitreous base, pars plana, and pars plicata. *Arch Ophthalmol*. 1991; 109:1458–1459.
491. Veckeneer M, Wong D. Visualising vitreous through modified trans-scleral illumination by maximising the Tyndall effect. *Br J Ophthalmol*. 2009;93:268–270.
492. Iverson DA, Ward TG, Blumenkranz MS. Indications and results of relaxing retinotomy. *Ophthalmology*. 1990; 97:1298–1304.
493. Brooks HL, Jr. Macular hole surgery with and without internal limiting membrane peeling. *Ophthalmology*. 2000;107:1939–1948.
494. Thompson JT. The effect of internal limiting membrane removal and indocyanine green on the success of macular hole surgery. *Trans Am Ophthalmol Soc*. 2007;105: 198–205.
495. Teba FA, Mohr A, Eckardt C, et al. Trypan blue staining in vitreoretinal surgery. *Ophthalmology*. 2003;110: 2409–2412.
496. Tognetto D, Zenoni S, Sanguinetti G, et al. Staining of the internal limiting membrane with intravitreal triamcinolone acetonide. *Retina*. 2005;25:462–467.
497. Brazitikos PD, Androudi S, Dimitrakos SA, Stangos NT. Removal of the internal limiting membrane under perfluorocarbon liquid to treat macular-hole-associated retinal detachment. *Am J Ophthalmol*. 2003; 135:894–896.
498. Gandorfer A, Messmer EM, Ulbig MW, Kampik A. Indocyanine green selectively stains the internal limiting membrane. *Am J Ophthalmol*. 2001;131:387–388.
499. Saeed MU, Heimann H. Atrophy of the retinal pigment epithelium following vitrectomy with trypan blue. *Int Ophthalmol*. 2008;29:239–241.
500. Stanescu-Segall D, Jackson TL. Vital staining with indocyanine green: a review of the clinical and experimental studies relating to safety. *Eye*. 2008;23:504–518.
501. Chaudhry NA, Lim ES, Saito Y, et al. Early vitrectomy and endolaser photocoagulation in patients with type I diabetes with severe vitreous hemorrhage. *Ophthalmology*. 1995;102:1164–1169.
502. Theodossiadis G, Chatzoulis D, Karantinos D, Maguritsas N. [Intraocular complications following Custodis-Lincoff operation]. *Arch Ophtalmol Rev Gen Ophtalmol*. 1975;35:627–638.
503. Harlan JB, Jr, Lee ET, Jensen PS, de Juan E Jr. Effect of humidity on posterior lens opacification during fluid-air exchange. *Arch Ophthalmol*. 1999;117:802–804.
504. Hirata A, Yonemura N, Hasumura T, et al. Effect of infusion air pressure on visual field defects after macular hole surgery. *Am J Ophthalmol*. 2000;130:611–616.
505. Hart RH, Vote BJ, Borthwick JH, et al. Loss of vision caused by expansion of intraocular perfluoropropane (C(3)F(8)) gas during nitrous oxide anesthesia. *Am J Ophthalmol*. 2002;134:761–763.
506. Williams G, Aaberg JT. Techniques of scleral buckling. In: Wilkinson C, Ryan S, eds. *Retina*. Los Angeles: Elsevier Mosby; 2006:2035–2070.
507. Lee BL, van Heuven WA. Hypopyon uveitis following panretinal photocoagulation. *Ophthalmic Surg Lasers*. 1997;28:505–507.
508. Hoogwerf BJ. Postoperative management of the diabetic patient. *Med Clin North Am*. 2001;85:1213–1228.

509. Alberti MM, Bouat CG, Allaire CM, Trinquand CJ. Combined indomethacin/gentamicin eyedrops to reduce pain after traumatic corneal abrasion. *Eur J Ophthalmol*. 2001;11:233–239.
510. Turner A, Rabiu M. Patching for corneal abrasion. *Cochrane Database Syst Rev*. 2006;(2):CD004764.
511. Vandorselaer T, Youssfi H, Caspers-Valu LE, et al. [Treatment of traumatic corneal abrasion with contact lens associated with topical nonsteroid anti-inflammatory agent (NSAID) and antibiotic: a safe, effective and comfortable solution]. *J Fr Ophtalmol*. 2001;24:1025–1033.
512. Barzideh N, Johnson TM. Subfoveal fluid resolves slowly after pars plana vitrectomy for tractional retinal detachment secondary to proliferative diabetic retinopathy. *Retina*. 2007;27:740–743.
513. Goeman DP, Douglass JA. Optimal management of asthma in elderly patients: strategies to improve adherence to recommended interventions. *Drugs Aging*. 2007;24:381–394.
514. Kain HL. Chorioretinal adhesion after argon laser photocoagulation. *Arch Ophthalmol*. 1984;102:612–615.
515. Yoon YH, Marmor MF. Rapid enhancement of retinal adhesion by laser photocoagulation. *Ophthalmology*. 1988;95:1385–1388.
516. Folk JC, Sneed SR, Folberg R, et al. Early retinal adhesion from laser photocoagulation. *Ophthalmology*. 1989;96:1523–1525.
517. Hilton GF, Tornambe PE, Brinton DA, et al. The complication of pneumatic retinopexy. *Trans Am Ophthalmol Soc*. 1990;88:191–207.
518. Mills MD, Devenyi RG, Lam WC, et al. An assessment of intraocular pressure rise in patients with gas-filled eyes during simulated air flight. *Ophthalmology*. 2001; 108:40–44.
519. Fu AD, McDonald HR, Eliott D, et al. Complications of general anesthesia using nitrous oxide in eyes with preexisting gas bubbles. *Retina*. 2002;22:569–574.
520. Whitacre MM, Mainster MA. Hazards of laser beam reflections in eyes containing gas. *Am J Ophthalmol*. 1990;110:33–38.
521. Mittra RA, Pollack JS, Dev S, et al. The use of topical aqueous suppressants in the prevention of postoperative intraocular pressure elevation after pars plana vitrectomy with long-acting gas tamponade. *Ophthalmology*. 2000;107:588–592.
522. Benz MS, Escalona-Benz EM, Murray TG, et al. Immediate postoperative use of a topical agent to prevent intraocular pressure elevation after pars plana vitrectomy with gas tamponade. *Arch Ophthalmol*. 2004;122:705–709.
523. Meldrum ML, Aaberg TM, Patel A, Davis J. Cataract extraction after silicone oil repair of retinal detachments due to necrotizing retinitis. *Arch Ophthalmol*. 1996;114:885–892.
524. Shugar JK, de Juan E Jr, McCuen BW, et al. Ultrasonic examination of the silicone-filled eye: theoretical and practical considerations. *Graefes Arch Clin Exp Ophthalmol*. 1986;224:361–367.
525. Madreperla SA, McCuen BW. Inferior peripheral iridectomy in patients receiving silicone oil. Rates of postoperative closure and effect on oil position. *Retina*. 1995;15:87–90.
526. Kampik A, Hoing C, Heidenkummer HP. Problems and timing in the removal of silicone oil. *Retina*. 1992;12:S11–S16.
527. Goezinne F, La Heij EC, Berendschot TT, et al. Risk factors for redetachment and worse visual outcome after silicone oil removal in eyes with complicated retinal detachment. *Eur J Ophthalmol*. 2007;17:627–637.
528. Dabil H, Akduman L, Olk RJ, Cakir B. Comparison of silicone oil removal with passive drainage alone versus passive drainage combined with air-fluid exchange. *Retina*. 2002;22:597–601.
529. Dada VK, Talwar D, Sharma N, et al. Phacoemulsification combined with silicone oil removal through a posterior capsulorhexis. *J Cataract Refract Surg*. 2001;27:1243–1247.
530. Lakits A, Nennadal T, Scholda C, et al. Chemical stability of silicone oil in the human eye after prolonged clinical use. *Ophthalmology*. 1999;106:1091–1100.
531. Shen YD, Yang CM. Extended silicone oil tamponade in primary vitrectomy for complex retinal detachment in proliferative diabetic retinopathy: a long-term follow-up study. *Eur J Ophthalmol*. 2007;17:954–960.
532. Stokes J, Wright M, Ramaesh K, et al. Necrotizing scleritis after intraocular surgery associated with the use of polyester nonabsorbable sutures. *J Cataract Refract Surg*. 2003;29:1827–1830.
533. Srinivasan S, Singh AK, Desai SP, et al. Foreign body episcleral granulomas complicating intravitreal silicone oil tamponade: a clinicopathological study. *Ophthalmology*. 2003;110:1837–1840.
534. Randleman JB, Hewitt SM, Song CD. Corneal and conjunctival changes after posterior segment surgery. *Ophthalmol Clin North Am*. 2004;17:513–520.
535. Insler MS, Tauber S, Packer A. Descemetocele formation in a patient with a postoperative corneal dellen. *Cornea*. 1989;8:129–130.
536. Sakurai E, Okuda M, Nozaki M, Ogura Y. Late-onset laser in situ keratomileusis (LASIK) flap dehiscence during retinal detachment surgery. *Am J Ophthalmol*. 2002;134:265–266.
537. Okamoto F, Okamoto C, Sakata N, et al. Changes in corneal topography after 25-gauge transconjunctival sutureless vitrectomy versus after 20-gauge standard vitrectomy. *Ophthalmology*. 2007;114:2138–2141.
538. Amato JE, Akduman L. Incidence of complications in 25-gauge transconjunctival sutureless vitrectomy based on the surgical indications. *Ophthalmic Surg Lasers Imaging*. 2007;38:100–102.
539. Gambrelle J, Kodjikian L, bi-Ayad N, et al. [Persistent unsealed sclerotomy after intravitreal injection of triamcinolone acetonide with a 30-gauge needle]. *J Fr Ophtalmol*. 2006;29:e22.
540. Feiz V, Redline DE. Infectious scleritis after pars plana vitrectomy because of methicillin-resistant Staphylococcus aureus resistant to fourth-generation fluoroquinolones. *Cornea*. 2007;26:238–240.
541. Kreiger AE. Wound complications in pars plana vitrectomy. *Retina*. 1993;13:335–344.
542. Itakura H, Kishi S, Kotajima N, Murakami M. Persistent secretion of vascular endothelial growth factor into the vitreous cavity in proliferative diabetic retinopathy after vitrectomy. *Ophthalmology*. 2004;111:1880–1884.

543. Chechelnitsky M, Mannis MJ, Chu TG. Scleromalacia after retinal detachment surgery. *Am J Ophthalmol.* 1995;119:803–804.
544. Roth DB, Flynn HW, Jr. Distinguishing between infectious and noninfectious endophthalmitis after intravitreal triamcinolone injection. *Am J Ophthalmol.* 2008; 146:346–347.
545. Walton W, Von HS, Grigorian R, Zarbin M. Management of traumatic hyphema. *Surv Ophthalmol.* 2002;47: 297–334.
546. Diolaiuti S, Senn P, Schmid MK, et al. Combined pars plana vitrectomy and phacoemulsification with intraocular lens implantation in severe proliferative diabetic retinopathy. *Ophthalmic Surg Lasers Imaging.* 2006;37: 468–474.
547. Honjo M, Ogura Y. Surgical results of pars plana vitrectomy combined with phacoemulsification and intraocular lens implantation for complications of proliferative diabetic retinopathy. *Ophthalmic Surg Lasers.* 1998;29:99–105.
548. Scharwey K, Pavlovic S, Jacobi KW. [Early posterior capsule fibrosis after combined cataract and vitreoretinal surgery with intraocular air/SF6 gas tamponade]. *Klin Monatsbl Augenheilkd.* 1998;212:149–153.
549. Mochizuki Y, Kubota T, Hata Y, et al. Surgical results of combined pars plana vitrectomy, phacoemulsification, and intraocular lens implantation. *Eur J Ophthalmol.* 2006;16:279–286.
550. Chung TY, Chung H, Lee JH. Combined surgery and sequential surgery comprising phacoemulsification, pars plana vitrectomy, and intraocular lens implantation: comparison of clinical outcomes. *J Cataract Refract Surg.* 2002;28:2001–2005.
551. Katsu Y, Ogino N, Kumagai E. [Posterior chamber lens implantation concurrent with vitrectomy for proliferative diabetic retinopathy]. *Nippon Ganka Gakkai Zasshi.* 1991;95:86–91.
552. Ariki G, Ogino N. [Postoperative anterior chamber inflammation after posterior chamber intraocular lens implantation concurrent with pars plana vitrectomy and lensectomy]. *Nippon Ganka Gakkai Zasshi.* 1992; 96:1300–1305.
553. Dabbs CK, Aaberg TM, Aguilar HE, et al. Complications of tissue plasminogen activator therapy after vitrectomy for diabetes. *Am J Ophthalmol.* 1990;110: 354–360.
554. Jaffe GJ, Abrams GW, Williams GA, Han DP. Tissue plasminogen activator for postvitrectomy fibrin formation. *Ophthalmology.* 1990;97:184–189.
555. Blankenship GW. Evaluation of a single intravitreal injection of dexamethasone phosphate in vitrectomy surgery for diabetic retinopathy complications. *Graefes Arch Clin Exp Ophthalmol.* 1991;229:62–65.
556. Kim YH, Suh Y, Yoo JS. Serum factors associated with neovascular glaucoma following vitrectomy for proliferative diabetic retinopathy. *Korean J Ophthalmol.* 2001;15:81–86.
557. Wand M, Madigan JC, Gaudio AR, Sorokanich S. Neovascular glaucoma following pars plana vitrectomy for complications of diabetic retinopathy. *Ophthalmic Surg.* 1990;21:113–118.
558. Rice TA, Michels RG, Maguire MG, Rice EF. The effect of lensectomy on the incidence of iris neovascularization and neovascular glaucoma after vitrectomy for diabetic retinopathy. *Am J Ophthalmol.* 1983;95:1–11.
559. Bopp S, Lucke K, Laqua H. Acute onset of rubeosis iridis after diabetic vitrectomy can indicate peripheral traction retinal detachment. *Ger J Ophthalmol.* 1992;1: 375–381.
560. Han DP, Lewandowski M, Mieler WF. Echographic diagnosis of anterior hyaloidal fibrovascular proliferation. *Arch Ophthalmol.* 1991;109:842–846.
561. Hershberger VS, Augsburger JJ, Hutchins RK, et al. Fibrovascular ingrowth at sclerotomy sites in vitrectomized diabetic eyes with recurrent vitreous hemorrhage: ultrasound biomicroscopy findings. *Ophthalmology.* 2004;111:1215–1221.
562. Sawa H, Ikeda T, Matsumoto Y, et al. Neovascularization from scleral wound as cause of vitreous rebleeding after vitrectomy for proliferative diabetic retinopathy. *Jpn J Ophthalmol.* 2000;44:154–160.
563. Lewis H, Abrams GW, Foos RY. Clinicopathologic findings in anterior hyaloidal fibrovascular proliferation after diabetic vitrectomy. *Am J Ophthalmol.* 1987; 104:614–618.
564. Smiddy WE, Feuer W. Incidence of cataract extraction after diabetic vitrectomy. *Retina.* 2004;24:574–581.
565. Panozzo G, Parolini B. Cataracts associated with posterior segment surgery. *Ophthalmol Clin North Am.* 2004;17:557–568, vi.
566. Rose RC, Richer SP, Bode AM. Ocular oxidants and antioxidant protection. *Proc Soc Exp Biol Med.* 1998;217:397–407.
567. Shimada H, Nakashizuka H, Hattori T, et al. Incidence of endophthalmitis after 20- and 25-gauge vitrectomy causes and prevention. *Ophthalmology.* 2008;115: 2215–2220.
568. Chen JK, Khurana RN, Nguyen QD, Do DV. The incidence of endophthalmitis following transconjunctival sutureless 25- vs 20-gauge vitrectomy. *Eye.* 2008;23:780–784.
569. Kunimoto DY, Kaiser RS. Incidence of endophthalmitis after 20- and 25-gauge vitrectomy. *Ophthalmology.* 2007;114:2133–2137.
570. Scott IU, Flynn HW, Jr, Dev S, et al. Endophthalmitis after 25-gauge and 20-gauge pars plana vitrectomy: incidence and outcomes. *Retina.* 2008;28:138–142.
571. Mino de Kaspar H, Shriver EM, Nguyen EV, et al. Risk factors for antibiotic-resistant conjunctival bacterial flora in patients undergoing intraocular surgery. *Graefes Arch Clin Exp Ophthalmol.* 2003;241:730–733.
572. Doft BH, Wisniewski SR, Kelsey SF, Fitzgerald SG. Diabetes and postoperative endophthalmitis in the endophthalmitis vitrectomy study. *Arch Ophthalmol.* 2001;119:650–656.
573. Bannerman TL, Rhoden DL, McAllister SK, et al. The source of coagulase-negative staphylococci in the Endophthalmitis Vitrectomy Study. A comparison of eyelid and intraocular isolates using pulsed-field gel electrophoresis. *Arch Ophthalmol.* 1997;115:357–361.
574. Microbiologic factors and visual outcome in the endophthalmitis vitrectomy study. *Am J Ophthalmol.* 1996;122:830–846.

575. Charles S. Illumination and phototoxicity issues in vitreoretinal surgery. *Retina*. 2008;28:1–4.
576. Keller C, Grimm C, Wenzel A, et al. Protective effect of halothane anesthesia on retinal light damage: inhibition of metabolic rhodopsin regeneration. *Invest Ophthalmol Vis Sci*. 2001;42:476–480.
577. Koch FH, Schmidt HP, Monks T, et al. The retinal irradiance and spectral properties of the multiport illumination system for vitreous surgery. *Am J Ophthalmol*. 1993;116:489–496.
578. Wu WC, Chang SM, Chen JY, Chang CW. Management of postvitrectomy diabetic vitreous hemorrhage with tissue plasminogen activator (t-PA) and volume homeostatic fluid-fluid exchanger. *J Ocul Pharmacol Ther*. 2001;17:363–371.
579. Yang CM, Yeh PT, Yang CH. Intravitreal long-acting gas in the prevention of early postoperative vitreous hemorrhage in diabetic vitrectomy. *Ophthalmology*. 2007;114:710–715.
580. Cheema RA, Mushtaq J, Cheema MA. Role of residual vitreous cortex removal in prevention of postoperative vitreous hemorrhage in diabetic vitrectomy. *Int Ophthalmol*. 2009.
581. Koutsandrea CN, Apostolopoulos MN, Chatzoulis DZ, et al. Hemostatic effects of SF6 after diabetic vitrectomy for vitreous hemorrhage. *Acta Ophthalmol Scand*. 2001;79:34–38.
582. Yang CM, Yeh PT, Yang CH, Chen MS. Bevacizumab pretreatment and long-acting gas infusion on vitreous clear-up after diabetic vitrectomy. *Am J Ophthalmol*. 2008;146:211–217.
583. Martin DF, McCuen BW. Efficacy of fluid-air exchange for postvitrectomy diabetic vitreous hemorrhage. *Am J Ophthalmol*. 1992;114:457–463.
584. Han DP, Murphy ML, Mieler WF, Abrams GW. Outpatient fluid-air exchange for severe postvitrectomy diabetic vitreous hemorrhage. Long-term results and complications. *Retina*. 1991;11:309–314.
585. Schrey S, Krepler K, Wedrich A. Incidence of rhegmatogenous retinal detachment after vitrectomy in eyes of diabetic patients. *Retina*. 2006;26:149–152.
586. Thompson JT. The role of patient age and intraocular gases in cataract progression following vitrectomy for macular holes and epiretinal membranes. *Trans Am Ophthalmol Soc*. 2003;101:485–498.
587. Novak MA, Rice TA, Michels RG, Auer C. The crystalline lens after vitrectomy for diabetic retinopathy. *Ophthalmology*. 1984;91:1480–1484.
588. Holekamp NM, Shui YB, Beebe D. Lower intraocular oxygen tension in diabetic patients: possible contribution to decreased incidence of nuclear sclerotic cataract. *Am J Ophthalmol*. 2006;141:1027–1032.
589. Hsuan JD, Brown NA, Bron AJ, et al. Posterior subcapsular and nuclear cataract after vitrectomy. *J Cataract Refract Surg*. 2001;27:437–444.
590. Sabates NR, Tolentino FI, Arroyo M, Freeman HM. The complications of perfluoropropane gas use in complex retinal detachments. *Retina*. 1996;16:7–12.
591. Konishi KI, Kondo H, Oshima K. Iridocorneal apposition after vitrectomy and gas injection. *Retina*. 2000;20:549–550.
592. Fang IM, Huang JS. Central retinal artery occlusion caused by expansion of intraocular gas at high altitude. *Am J Ophthalmol*. 2002;134:603–605.
593. Abrams GW, Edelhauser HF, Aaberg TM, Hamilton LH. Dynamics of intravitreal sulfur hexafluoride gas. *Invest Ophthalmol*. 1974;13:863–868.
594. Gandorfer A, Kampik A. [Expansion of intraocular gas due to reduced atmospheric pressure. Case report and review of the literature]. *Ophthalmologe*. 2000;97:367–370.
595. Rahman R, Rosen PH. Pupillary capture after combined management of cataract and vitreoretinal pathology. *J Cataract Refract Surg*. 2002;28:1607–1612.
596. Matsuda M, Tano Y, Inaba M, Manabe R. Corneal endothelial cell damage associated with intraocular gas tamponade during pars plana vitrectomy. *Jpn J Ophthalmol*. 1986;30:324–329.
597. Riedel KG, Gabel VP, Neubauer L, et al. Intravitreal silicone oil injection: complications and treatment of 415 consecutive patients. *Graefes Arch Clin Exp Ophthalmol*. 1990;228:19–23.
598. Yang CS, Chen KH, Hsu WM, Li YS. Cytotoxicity of silicone oil on cultivated human corneal endothelium. *Eye*. 2008;22:282–288.
599. Valone J, Jr, McCarthy M. Emulsified anterior chamber silicone oil and glaucoma. *Ophthalmology*. 1994;101:1908–1912.
600. Francis JH, Latkany PA, Rosenthal JL. Mechanical energy from intraocular instruments cause emulsification of silicone oil. *Br J Ophthalmol*. 2007;91:818–821.
601. Zalta AH, Boyle NS, Zalta AK. Silicone oil pupillary block: an exception to combined argon-Nd:YAG laser iridotomy success in angle-closure glaucoma. *Arch Ophthalmol*. 2007;125:883–888.
602. Jackson TL, Thiagarajan M, Murthy R, et al. Pupil block glaucoma in phakic and pseudophakic patients after vitrectomy with silicone oil injection. *Am J Ophthalmol*. 2001;132:414–416.
603. Kageyama T, Yaguchi S. Removing silicone oil droplets from the posterior surface of silicone intraocular lenses. *J Cataract Refract Surg*. 2000;26:957–959.
604. Friberg TR, Fanous MM. Migration of intravitreal silicone oil through a Baerveldt tube into the subconjunctival space. *Semin Ophthalmol*. 2004;19:107–108.
605. Nazemi PP, Chong LP, Varma R, Burnstine MA. Migration of intraocular silicone oil into the subconjunctival space and orbit through an Ahmed glaucoma valve. *Am J Ophthalmol*. 2001;132:929–931.
606. Fangtian D, Rongping D, Lin Z, Weihong Y. Migration of intraocular silicone into the cerebral ventricles. *Am J Ophthalmol*. 2005;140:156–158.
607. Eckle D, Kampik A, Hintschich C, et al. Visual field defect in association with chiasmal migration of intraocular silicone oil. *Br J Ophthalmol*. 2005;89:918–920.
608. Knecht P, Groscurth P, Ziegler U, et al. Is silicone oil optic neuropathy caused by high intraocular pressure alone? A semi-biological model. *Br J Ophthalmol*. 2007;91:1293–1295.
609. Cote RE, Haddad SE. Fitting a prosthesis over phthisis bulbi or discolored blind eyes. *Adv Ophthalmic Plast Reconstr Surg*. 1990;8:136–145.

610. Castiblanco CP, Adelman RA. Sympathetic ophthalmia. *Graefes Arch Clin Exp Ophthalmol*. 2008;247:289–302.
611. Pollack AL, McDonald HR, Ai E, et al. Sympathetic ophthalmia associated with pars plana vitrectomy without antecedent penetrating trauma. *Retina*. 2001;21: 146–154.
612. Gass JD. Sympathetic ophthalmia following vitrectomy. *Am J Ophthalmol*. 1982;93:552–558.
613. Jonas JB, Holbach LM, Schonherr U, Naumann GO. Sympathetic ophthalmia after three pars plana vitrectomies without prior ocular injury. *Retina*. 2000;20: 405–406.
614. Sisk RA, Davis JL, Dubovy SR, Smiddy WE. Sympathetic ophthalmia following vitrectomy for endophthalmitis after intravitreal bevacizumab. *Ocul Immunol Inflamm*. 2008;16:236–238.
615. Fong DS, Ferris FL, III, Davis MD, Chew EY. Causes of severe visual loss in the early treatment diabetic retinopathy study: ETDRS report no. 24. Early Treatment Diabetic Retinopathy Study Research Group. *Am J Ophthalmol*. 1999;127:137–141.
616. Okamoto F, Okamoto Y, Fukuda S, et al. Vision-related quality of life and visual function following vitrectomy for proliferative diabetic retinopathy. *Am J Ophthalmol*. 2008;145:1031–1036.
617. Thompson JT, Auer CL, de Bustros S, et al. Prognostic indicators of success and failure in vitrectomy for diabetic retinopathy. *Ophthalmology*. 1986;93:290–295.
618. Blankenship GW. Stability of pars plana vitrectomy results for diabetic retinopathy complications. A comparison of five-year and six-month postvitrectomy findings. *Arch Ophthalmol*. 1981;99:1009–1012.
619. Blankenship GW, Machemer R. Long-term diabetic vitrectomy results. Report of 10 year follow-up. *Ophthalmology*. 1985;92:503–506.
620. Rice TA, Michels RG. Long-term anatomic and functional results of vitrectomy for diabetic retinopathy. *Am J Ophthalmol*. 1980;90:297–303.
621. Kaaja R, Sjoberg L, Hellsted T, et al. Long-term effects of pregnancy on diabetic complications. *Diabet Med*. 1996;13:165–169.
622. Hellstedt T, Kaaja R, Teramo K, Immonen I. The effect of pregnancy on mild diabetic retinopathy. *Graefes Arch Clin Exp Ophthalmol*. 1997;235:437–441.
623. Dev S, Pulido JS, Tessler HH, et al. Progression of diabetic retinopathy after endophthalmitis. *Ophthalmology*. 1999;106:774–781.
624. Mittra RA, Borrillo JL, Dev S, et al. Retinopathy progression and visual outcomes after phacoemulsification in patients with diabetes mellitus. *Arch Ophthalmol*. 2000;118:912–917.
625. Tan CS, Yap EY. Rapid progression of diabetic retinopathy following endophthalmitis. *Eye*. 2004;18:1013–1015.
626. Knol JA, van KB, de Valk HW, Rothova A. Rapid progression of diabetic retinopathy in eyes with posterior uveitis. *Am J Ophthalmol*. 2006;141:409–412.
627. Murray DC, Sung VC, Headon MP. Asymmetric diabetic retinopathy associated with Fuch's heterochromic cyclitis. *Br J Ophthalmol*. 1999;83:988–989.
628. Early Treatment Diabetic Retinopathy Study Research Group. Grading diabetic retinopathy from stereoscopic color fundus photographs–an extension of the modified Airlie House classification. ETDRS report number 10. Early Treatment Diabetic Retinopathy Study Research Group. *Ophthalmology*. 1991;98:786–806.
629. Early Treatment Diabetic Retinopathy Study Research Group. Classification of diabetic retinopathy from fluorescein angiograms. ETDRS report number 11. Early Treatment Diabetic Retinopathy Study Research Group. *Ophthalmology*. 1991;98:807–822.
630. Early Treatment Diabetic Retinopathy Study Research Group. Fluorescein angiographic risk factors for progression of diabetic retinopathy. ETDRS report number 13. Early Treatment Diabetic Retinopathy Study Research Group. *Ophthalmology*. 1991;98:834–840.
631. Bresnick GH, Engerman R, Davis MD, et al. Patterns of ischemia in diabetic retinopathy. *Trans Sect Ophthalmol Am Acad Ophthalmol Otolaryngol*. 1976;81: OP694–OP709.
632. Michalewski J, Michalewska Z, Cisiecki S, Nawrocki J. Morphologically functional correlations of macular pathology connected with epiretinal membrane formation in spectral optical coherence tomography (SOCT). *Graefes Arch Clin Exp Ophthalmol*. 2007;245:1623–1631.
633. Biallosterski C, van Velthoven ME, Michels RP, et al. Decreased optical coherence tomography-measured pericentral retinal thickness in patients with diabetes mellitus type 1 with minimal diabetic retinopathy. *Br J Ophthalmol*. 2007;91:1135–1138.
634. Nilsson M, von Wendt G, Wanger P, Martin L. Early detection of macular changes in patients with diabetes using Rarebit Fovea Test and optical coherence tomography. *Br J Ophthalmol*. 2007;91:1596–1598.
635. Oshitari T, Hanawa K, chi-Usami E. Changes of macular and RNFL thicknesses measured by Stratus OCT in patients with early stage diabetes. *Eye*. 2008;23:884–889.
636. Barsam A, Laidlaw A. Visual fields in patients who have undergone vitrectomy for complications of diabetic retinopathy. A prospective study. *BMC Ophthalmol*. 2006;6:5.
637. Ederer F, Hiller R, Taylor HR. Senile lens changes and diabetes in two population studies. *Am J Ophthalmol*. 1981;91:381–395.
638. Mozaffarieh M, Heinzl H, Sacu S, Wedrich A. Clinical outcomes of phacoemulsification cataract surgery in diabetes patients: visual function (VF-14), visual acuity and patient satisfaction. *Acta Ophthalmol Scand*. 2005; 83:176–183.
639. Menchini U, Cappelli S, Virgili G. Cataract surgery and diabetic retinopathy. *Semin Ophthalmol*. 2003;18: 103–108.
640. Suto C, Hori S, Kato S. Management of type 2 diabetics requiring panretinal photocoagulation and cataract surgery. *J Cataract Refract Surg*. 2008;34:1001–1006.
641. West JA, Dowler JG, Hamilton AM, et al. Panretinal photocoagulation during cataract extraction in eyes with active proliferative diabetic eye disease. *Eye*. 1999;13(Pt 2):170–173.
642. Aiello LM, Wand M, Liang G. Neovascular glaucoma and vitreous hemorrhage following cataract surgery in patients with diabetes mellitus. *Ophthalmology*. 1983; 90:814–820.

643. Pollack A, Dotan S, Oliver M. Progression of diabetic retinopathy after cataract extraction. *Br J Ophthalmol.* 1991;75:547–551.
644. Munir WM, Pulido JS, Sharma MC, Buerk BM. Intravitreal triamcinolone for treatment of complicated proliferative diabetic retinopathy and proliferative vitreoretinopathy. *Can J Ophthalmol.* 2005;40:598–604.
645. Patel JI, Hykin PG, Cree IA. Diabetic cataract removal: postoperative progression of maculopathy–growth factor and clinical analysis. *Br J Ophthalmol.* 2006;90: 697–701.
646. Hauser D, Katz H, Pokroy R, et al. Occurrence and progression of diabetic retinopathy after phacoemulsification cataract surgery. *J Cataract Refract Surg.* 2004; 30:428–432.
647. Suto C, Hori S, Kato S, et al. Effect of perioperative glycemic control in progression of diabetic retinopathy and maculopathy. *Arch Ophthalmol.* 2006;124:38–45.
648. Bhatnagar P, Schiff WM, Barile GR. Diabetic vitrectomy: the influence of lens status upon surgical outcomes. *Curr Opin Ophthalmol.* 2008;19:243–247.
649. Schiff WM, Barile GR, Hwang JC, et al. Diabetic vitrectomy: influence of lens status upon anatomic and visual outcomes. *Ophthalmology.* 2007;114:544–550.
650. Treumer F, Bunse A, Rudolf M, Roider J. Pars plana vitrectomy, phacoemulsification and intraocular lens implantation. Comparison of clinical complications in a combined versus two-step surgical approach. *Graefes Arch Clin Exp Ophthalmol.* 2006;244:808–815.
651. Lahey JM, Francis RR, Kearney JJ, Cheung M. Combining phacoemulsification and vitrectomy in patients with proliferative diabetic retinopathy. *Curr Opin Ophthalmol.* 2004;15:192–196.
652. Benson WE, Brown GC. Combined extracapsular cataract extraction, posterior chamber lens implantation and pars plana vitrectomy. *Trans Pa Acad Ophthalmol Otolaryngol.* 1989;41:814–817.
653. Shinoda K, O'hira A, Ishida S, et al. Posterior synechia of the iris after combined pars plana vitrectomy, phacoemulsification, and intraocular lens implantation. *Jpn J Ophthalmol.* 2001;45:276–280.
654. Chalam KV, Malkani S, Shah VA. Intravitreal dexamethasone effectively reduces postoperative inflammation after vitreoretinal surgery. *Ophthalmic Surg Lasers Imaging.* 2003;34:188–192.
655. Kim SJ, Equi R, Bressler NM. Analysis of macular edema after cataract surgery in patients with diabetes using optical coherence tomography. *Ophthalmology.* 2007;114:881–889.
656. Kim SY, Yang J, Lee YC, Park YH. Effect of a single intraoperative sub-Tenon injection of triamcinolone acetonide on the progression of diabetic retinopathy and visual outcomes after cataract surgery. *J Cataract Refract Surg.* 2008;34:823–826.
657. Blankenship GW, Flynn HW, Jr, Kokame GT. Posterior chamber intraocular lens insertion during pars plana lensectomy and vitrectomy for complications of proliferative diabetic retinopathy. *Am J Ophthalmol.* 1989; 108:1–5.
658. Kokame GT, Flynn HW, Jr, Blankenship GW. Posterior chamber intraocular lens implantation during diabetic pars plana vitrectomy. *Ophthalmology.* 1989; 96:603–610.
659. Uchida H, Ogino N. [Pars plana lensectomy preserving a clear anterior capsule in vitreous surgery]. *Nippon Ganka Gakkai Zasshi.* 1991;95:1117–1123.
660. MacCumber MW, Packo KH, Civantos JM, Greenberg JB. Preservation of anterior capsule during vitrectomy and lensectomy for retinal detachment with proliferative vitreoretinopathy. *Ophthalmology.* 2002;109:329–333.
661. Romero P, Salvat M, Almena M, et al. [Combined surgery for lens extraction, vitrectomy, and implantation in the diabetic patient using phacoemulsification versus phacofragmentation]. *J Fr Ophtalmol.* 2006;29: 533–541.
662. Chaudhry NA, Cohen KA, Flynn HW, Jr, Murray TG. Combined pars plana vitrectomy and lens management in complex vitreoretinal disease. *Semin Ophthalmol.* 2003;18:132–141.
663. Pardo-Munoz A, Muriel-Herrero A, Abraira V, et al. Phacoemulsification in previously vitrectomized patients: an analysis of the surgical results in 100 eyes as well as the factors contributing to the cataract formation. *Eur J Ophthalmol.* 2006;16:52–59.
664. Salzmann J, Khaw PT, Laidlaw A. Choroidal effusions and hypotony caused by severe anterior lens capsule contraction after cataract surgery. *Am J Ophthalmol.* 2000;129:253–254.
665. Lanzl IM, Kopp C. Ciliary body detachment caused by capsule contraction. *J Cataract Refract Surg.* 1999;25: 1412–1414.
666. Chew EY, Benson WE, Remaley NA, et al. Results after lens extraction in patients with diabetic retinopathy: early treatment diabetic retinopathy study report number 25. *Arch Ophthalmol.* 1999;117:1600–1606.
667. Tseng HY, Wu WC, Hsu SY. Comparison of vitrectomy alone and combined vitrectomy, phacoemulsification and intraocular lens implantation for proliferative diabetic retinopathy. *Kaohsiung J Med Sci.* 2007;23: 339–343.
668. Kadonosono K, Matsumoto S, Uchio E, et al. Iris neovascularization after vitrectomy combined with phacoemulsification and intraocular lens implantation for proliferative diabetic retinopathy. *Ophthalmic Surg Lasers.* 2001;32:19–24.
669. Somaiya MD, Burns JD, Mintz R, et al. Factors affecting visual outcomes after small-incision phacoemulsification in diabetic patients. *J Cataract Refract Surg.* 2002;28:1364–1371.
670. Margolis R, Singh RP, Bhatnagar P, Kaiser PK. Intravitreal triamcinolone as adjunctive treatment to laser panretinal photocoagulation for concomitant proliferative diabetic retinopathy and clinically significant macular oedema. *Acta Ophthalmol.* 2008;86:105–110.
671. Choi KS, Chung JK, Lim SH. Laser photocoagulation combined with intravitreal triamcinolone acetonide injection in proliferative diabetic retinopathy with macular edema. *Korean J Ophthalmol.* 2007;21:11–17.
672. Kaderli B, Avci R, Gelisken O, Yucel AA. Intravitreal triamcinolone as an adjunct in the treatment of concomitant proliferative diabetic retinopathy and diffuse diabetic macular oedema. Combined IVTA and laser

treatment for PDR with CSMO. *Int Ophthalmol*. 2005; 26:207–214.
673. Zein WM, Noureddin BN, Jurdi FA, et al. Panretinal photocoagulation and intravitreal triamcinolone acetonide for the management of proliferative diabetic retinopathy with macular edema. *Retina*. 2006;26:137–142.
674. Zacks DN, Johnson MW. Combined intravitreal injection of triamcinolone acetonide and panretinal photocoagulation for concomitant diabetic macular edema and proliferative diabetic retinopathy. *Retina*. 2005; 25:135–140.
675. Ramsay RC, Cantrill HL, Knobloch WH. Cryoretinopexy for proliferative diabetic retinopathy. *Can J Ophthalmol*. 1982;17:17–20.
676. Scuderi JJ, Blumenkranz MS, Blankenship G. Regression of diabetic rubeosis iridis following successful surgical reattachment of the retina by vitrectomy. *Retina*. 1982;2:193–196.
677. Giannarelli R, Coppelli A, Sartini MS, et al. Pancreas transplant alone has beneficial effects on retinopathy in type 1 diabetic patients. *Diabetologia*. 2006;49:2977–2982.
678. Giannarelli R, Coppelli A, Sartini M, et al. Effects of pancreas-kidney transplantation on diabetic retinopathy. *Transpl Int*. 2005;18:619–622.
679. Koznarova R, Saudek F, Sosna T, et al. Beneficial effect of pancreas and kidney transplantation on advanced diabetic retinopathy. *Cell Transplant*. 2000;9:903–908.
680. Chow VC, Pai RP, Chapman JR, et al. Diabetic retinopathy after combined kidney-pancreas transplantation. *Clin Transplant*. 1999;13:356–362.
681. Schmidt D, Kirste G, Schrader W. Progressive proliferative diabetic retinopathy after transplantation of the pancreas. A case and a review of the topic. *Acta Ophthalmol (Copenh)*. 1994;72:743–751.
682. Rahman W, Rahman FZ, Yassin S, et al. Progression of retinopathy during pregnancy in type 1 diabetes mellitus. *Clin Experiment Ophthalmol*. 2007;35:231–236.
683. De Potter P, Zografos L. [Retinal artery occlusion: etiology and risk factors apropos of 151 cases]. *Klin Monatsbl Augenheilkd*. 1990;196:360–363.
684. Schafer S, Lang GE. [Iris neovascularization as a complication of central artery occlusion]. *Klin Monatsbl Augenheilkd*. 2005;222:343–345.
685. Meyer-Schwickerath R, Hagel A, Nahberger D, Gronemeyer U. [Ischemic or non-ischemic central artery occlusion. An explanation for the development or lack of development of neovascularization]. *Ophthalmologe*. 1994;91:293–297.
686. Vander JF, Brown GC, Benson WE. Iris neovascularization after central retinal artery obstruction despite previous panretinal photocoagulation for diabetic retinopathy. *Am J Ophthalmol*. 1990;109:464–468.
687. Duker JS, Brown GC. Neovascularization of the optic disc associated with obstruction of the central retinal artery. *Ophthalmology*. 1989;96:87–91.
688. Rowlands AG, Palimar P, Enevoldson TP. Ipsilateral proliferative diabetic retinopathy in carotid stenosis. *Eye*. 2001;15:110–111.
689. Murphy R, Wilson RM, Talbot JF. A case of ocular ischaemic syndrome in a young insulin dependent diabetic male. *Diabetes Res Clin Pract*. 1993;19:245–248.
690. Duker JS, Brown GC, Bosley TM, et al. Asymmetric proliferative diabetic retinopathy and carotid artery disease. *Ophthalmology*. 1990;97:869–874.
691. Ino-ue M, Azumi A, Kajiura-Tsukahara Y, Yamamoto M. Ocular ischemic syndrome in diabetic patients. *Jpn J Ophthalmol*. 1999;43:31–35.
692. Gay AJ, Rosenbaum AL. Retinal artery pressure in asymmetric diabetic retinopathy. *Arch Ophthalmol*. 1966;75:758–762.
693. Basu A, Palmer H, Ryder RE, Taylor KG. Uncommon presentation of asymmetrical retinopathy in diabetes type 1. *Acta Ophthalmol Scand*. 2004;82:321–323.
694. Slusher MM. Retinal sparing in diabetic retinopathy. *South Med J*. 1975;68:655–657.
695. Brown GC, Magargal LE, Simeone FA, et al. Arterial obstruction and ocular neovascularization. *Ophthalmology*. 1982;89:139–146.
696. Browning DJ, Flynn HW, Jr, Blankenship GW. Asymmetric retinopathy in patients with diabetes mellitus. *Am J Ophthalmol*. 1988;105:584–589.
697. UK Prospective Diabetes Study Group. Tight blood pressure control and risk of macrovascular and microvascular complications in type 2 diabetes: UKPDS 38. UK Prospective Diabetes Study Group. *BMJ*. 1998;317:703–713.
698. Stratton IM, Kohner EM, Aldington SJ, et al. UKPDS 50: risk factors for incidence and progression of retinopathy in Type II diabetes over 6 years from diagnosis. *Diabetologia*. 2001;44:156–163.
699. McCrary JA, III. Venous stasis retinopathy of stenotic or occlusive carotid origin. *J Clin Neuroophthalmol*. 1989;9:195–199.
700. Munch IC, Larsen M. [The ocular ischemic syndrome]. *Ugeskr Laeger*. 2005;167:3269–3273.
701. Clouse WD, Hagino RT, Chiou A, et al. Extracranial cerebrovascular revascularization for chronic ocular ischemia. *Ann Vasc Surg*. 2002;16:1–5.
702. Paivansalo M, Pelkonen O, Rajala U, et al. Diabetic retinopathy: sonographically measured hemodynamic alterations in ocular, carotid, and vertebral arteries. *Acta Radiol*. 2004;45:404–410.
703. Ino-ue M, Azumi A, Yamamoto M. Ophthalmic artery blood flow velocity changes in diabetic patients as a manifestation of macroangiopathy. *Acta Ophthalmol Scand*. 2000;78:173–176.
704. Rennie CA, Flanagan DW. Resolution of proliferative venous stasis retinopathy after carotid endarterectomy. *Br J Ophthalmol*. 2002;86:117–118.
705. Bierly JR, Dunn JP. Macular edema after carotid endarterectomy in ocular ischemic syndrome. *Am J Ophthalmol*. 1992;113:105–107.
706. de Gooyer TE, Stevenson KA, Humphries P, et al. Retinopathy is reduced during experimental diabetes in a mouse model of outer retinal degeneration. *Invest Ophthalmol Vis Sci*. 2006;47:5561–5568.
707. Lai TY, Kwok AK, Lam DS, Bhende P. Progression of diabetic retinopathy after endophthalmitis. *Ophthalmology*. 2000;107:619–621.
708. Probst K, Fijnheer R, Schellekens P, Rothova A. Intraocular and plasma levels of cellular fibronectin in patients with uveitis and diabetes mellitus. *Br J Ophthalmol*. 2004;88:667–672.

709. Udono T, Takahashi K, Abe T, et al. Elevated immunoreactive-adrenomedullin levels in the aqueous humor of patients with uveitis and vitreoretinal disorders. *Peptides*. 2002;23:1865–1868.
710. Kimmel AS, Magargal LE, Goldberg RE. Unilateral proliferative sickle retinopathy: a model for photocoagulation in the proliferative retinopathies. *Ann Ophthalmol*. 1989;21:211–212, 216.
711. Scialdone A, Menchini U, Pietroni C, Brancato R. Unilateral proliferative diabetic retinopathy and uveitis in the fellow eye: report of a case. *Ann Ophthalmol*. 1991;23:259–261.
712. Dunn JP, Yamashita A, Kempen JH, Jabs DA. Retinal vascular occlusion in patients infected with human immunodeficiency virus. *Retina*. 2005;25:759–766.
713. Au A, O'Day J. Review of severe vaso-occlusive retinopathy in systemic lupus erythematosus and the antiphospholipid syndrome: associations, visual outcomes, complications and treatment. *Clin Experiment Ophthalmol*. 2004;32:87–100.
714. Saatci OA, Kocak N, Durak I, Ergin MH. Unilateral retinal vasculitis, branch retinal artery occlusion and subsequent retinal neovascularization in Crohn's disease. *Int Ophthalmol*. 2001;24:89–92.
715. Adan A, Goday A, Ferrer J, Cabot J. Diabetic retinopathy associated with acquired immunodeficiency syndrome. *Am J Ophthalmol*. 1990;109:744–745.
716. Jackson H, Bentley CR, Hingorani M, et al. Sickle retinopathy in patients with sickle trait. *Eye*. 1995;9(Pt 5): 589–593.
717. Page MM, MacKay JM, Paterson G. Sickle cell trait and diabetic retinopathy. *Br J Ophthalmol*. 1979;63: 837–838.
718. Koduri PR, Patel AR, Bernstein HA. Concurrent sickle cell hemoglobin C disease and diabetes mellitus: no added risk of proliferative retinopathy? *J Natl Med Assoc*. 1994;86:682–685.
719. Incorvaia C, Parmeggiani F, Mingrone G, et al. Prevalence of retinopathy in diabetic thalassaemic patients. *J Pediatr Endocrinol Metab*. 1998;11(Suppl 3):879–883.
720. Takagi H, Watanabe D, Suzuma K, et al. Novel role of erythropoietin in proliferative diabetic retinopathy. *Diabetes Res Clin Pract*. 2007;77(Suppl 1):S62–S64.
721. Diskin CJ. Erythropoietin and retinopathy: the beginning of an understanding. *Br J Ophthalmol*. 2008;92:574.
722. Diskin CJ, Stokes TJ, Dansby LM, et al. A hypothesis: can erythropoietin administration affect the severity of retinopathy in diabetic patients with renal failure? *Am J Med Sci*. 2007;334:260–264.
723. Watanabe D, Suzuma K, Matsui S, et al. Erythropoietin as a retinal angiogenic factor in proliferative diabetic retinopathy. *N Engl J Med*. 2005;353:782–792.
724. Friedman EA, Brown CD, Berman DH. Erythropoietin in diabetic macular edema and renal insufficiency. *Am J Kidney Dis*. 1995;26:202–208.
725. Friedman EA, L'Esperance FA, Brown CD, Berman DH. Treating azotemia-induced anemia with erythropoietin improves diabetic eye disease. *Kidney Int Suppl*. 2003;S57–S63.
726. Liinamaa MJ, Savolainen MJ. High vitreous concentration of vascular endothelial growth factor in diabetic patients with proliferative retinopathy using statins. *Ann Med*. 2008;40:209–214.
727. Roy MS, Roy A, Affouf M. Depression is a risk factor for poor glycemic control and retinopathy in African-Americans with type 1 diabetes. *Psychosom Med*. 2007; 69:537–542.
728. Do DV, Nguyen QD, Bressler NM, et al. Hemoglobin A1c awareness among patients receiving eye care at a tertiary ophthalmic center. *Am J Ophthalmol*. 2006;141: 951–953.
729. Ferris FL, III, Chew EY, Hoogwerf BJ. Serum lipids and diabetic retinopathy. Early Treatment Diabetic Retinopathy Study Research Group. *Diabetes Care*. 1996;19:1291–1293.
730. Speicher MA, Danis RP, Criswell M, Pratt L. Pharmacologic therapy for diabetic retinopathy. *Expert Opin Emerg Drugs*. 2003;8:239–250.
731. Effect of ruboxistaurin in patients with diabetic macular edema: thirty-month results of the randomized PKC-DMES clinical trial. *Arch Ophthalmol*. 2007;125:318–324.
732. Aiello LP. The potential role of PKC beta in diabetic retinopathy and macular edema. *Surv Ophthalmol*. 2002;47(Suppl 2):S263–S269.
733. Okamoto T, Yamagishi S, Inagaki Y, et al. Incadronate disodium inhibits advanced glycation end products-induced angiogenesis in vitro. *Biochem Biophys Res Commun*. 2002;297:419–424.
734. Barile GR, Pachydaki SI, Tari SR, et al. The RAGE axis in early diabetic retinopathy. *Invest Ophthalmol Vis Sci*. 2005;46:2916–2924.
735. Pachydaki SI, Tari SR, Lee SE, et al. Upregulation of RAGE and its ligands in proliferative retinal disease. *Exp Eye Res*. 2006;82:807–815.
736. Sjolie AK, Chaturvedi N. The retinal renin-angiotensin system: implications for therapy in diabetic retinopathy. *J Hum Hypertens*. 2002;16(Suppl 3):S42–S46.
737. Yamagishi S, Matsui T, Nakamura K, et al. Olmesartan blocks inflammatory reactions in endothelial cells evoked by advanced glycation end products by suppressing generation of reactive oxygen species. *Ophthalmic Res*. 2008;40:10–15.
738. Yamagishi S, Matsui T, Nakamura K, et al. Olmesartan blocks advanced glycation end products (AGEs)-induced angiogenesis in vitro by suppressing receptor for AGEs (RAGE) expression. *Microvasc Res*. 2008;75: 130–134.
739. Deinum J, Chaturvedi N. The Renin-Angiotensin system and vascular disease in diabetes. *Semin Vasc Med*. 2002;2:149–156.
740. Sjolie AK, Klein R, Porta M, et al. Effect of candesartan on progression and regression of retinopathy in type 2 diabetes (DIRECT-Protect 2): a randomised placebo-controlled trial. *Lancet*. 2008;372:1385–1393.
741. Chaturvedi N, Porta M, Klein R, et al. Effect of candesartan on prevention (DIRECT-Prevent 1) and progression (DIRECT-Protect 1) of retinopathy in type 1 diabetes: randomised, placebo-controlled trials. *Lancet*. 2008;372:1394–1402.
742. Boehm BO. Use of long-acting somatostatin analogue treatment in diabetic retinopathy. *Dev Ophthalmol*. 2007;39:111–121.

743. Palii SS, Caballero S Jr, Shapiro G, Grant MB. Medical treatment of diabetic retinopathy with somatostatin analogues. *Expert Opin Investig Drugs*. 2007;16:73–82.
744. Shen LQ, Child A, Weber GM, et al. Rosiglitazone and delayed onset of proliferative diabetic retinopathy. *Arch Ophthalmol*. 2008;126:793–799.
745. Ozkiris A, Erkilic K, Koc A, Mistik S. Effect of atorvastatin on ocular blood flow velocities in patients with diabetic retinopathy. *Br J Ophthalmol*. 2007;91:69–73.
746. Sennlaub F, Valamanesh F, Vazquez-Tello A, et al. Cyclooxygenase-2 in human and experimental ischemic proliferative retinopathy. *Circulation*. 2003;108: 198–204.
747. McFarland TJ, Zhang Y, Appukuttan B, Stout JT. Gene therapy for proliferative ocular diseases. *Expert Opin Biol Ther*. 2004;4:1053–1058.
748. Lee SJ, Choi MG. Association of manganese superoxide dismutase gene polymorphism (V16A) with diabetic macular edema in Korean type 2 diabetic patients. *Metabolism*. 2006;55:1681–1688.
749. Lee M, Choi D, Choi MJ, et al. Hypoxia-inducible gene expression system using the erythropoietin enhancer and 3'-untranslated region for the VEGF gene therapy. *J Control Release*. 2006;115:113–119.
750. Igarashi T, Miyake K, Kato K, et al. Lentivirus-mediated expression of angiostatin efficiently inhibits neovascularization in a murine proliferative retinopathy model. *Gene Ther*. 2003;10:219–226.
751. Desmettre TJ, Mordon SR, Buzawa DM, Mainster MA. Micropulse and continuous wave diode retinal photocoagulation: visible and subvisible lesion parameters. *Br J Ophthalmol*. 2006;90:709–712.
752. Moorman CM, Hamilton AM. Clinical applications of the MicroPulse diode laser. *Eye*. 1999;13(Pt 2):145–150.
753. Priglinger SG, Haritoglou C, Palanker DV, et al. Pulsed electron avalanche knife (PEAK-fc) for dissection of retinal tissue. *Arch Ophthalmol*. 2005;123:1412–1418.
754. Priglinger SG, Haritoglou C, Mueller A, et al. Pulsed electron avalanche knife in vitreoretinal surgery. *Retina*. 2005;25:889–896.
755. Zoega GM, Gunnarsdottir T, Bjornsdottir S, et al. Screening compliance and visual outcome in diabetes. *Acta Ophthalmol Scand*. 2005;83:687–690.
756. Stefansson E. Prevention of diabetic blindness. *Br J Ophthalmol*. 2006;90:2–3.
757. Giannoukakis N, Phillips B, Trucco M. Toward a cure for type 1 diabetes mellitus: diabetes-suppressive dendritic cells and beyond. *Pediatr Diabetes*. 2008;9:4–13.
758. Chew EY, Ambrosius WT, Howard LT, et al. Rationale, design, and methods of the Action to Control Cardiovascular Risk in Diabetes Eye Study (ACCORD-EYE). *Am J Cardiol*. 2007;99:103i–111i.
759. Henricsson M, Nystrom L, Blohme G, et al. The incidence of retinopathy 10 years after diagnosis in young adult people with diabetes: results from the nationwide population-based Diabetes Incidence Study in Sweden (DISS). *Diabetes Care*. 2003;26:349–354.
760. Rand LI, Prud'homme GJ, Ederer F, Canner PL. Factors influencing the development of visual loss in advanced diabetic retinopathy. Diabetic Retinopathy Study (DRS) Report No. 10. *Invest Ophthalmol Vis Sci*. 1985;26:983–991.
761. Kaufman SC, Ferris FL, III, Swartz M. Intraocular pressure following panretinal photocoagulation for diabetic retinopathy. Diabetic Retinopathy Report No. 11. *Arch Ophthalmol*. 1987;105:807–809.
762. Ferris FL, III, Podgor MJ, Davis MD. Macular edema in Diabetic Retinopathy Study patients. Diabetic Retinopathy Study Report Number 12. *Ophthalmology*. 1987;94:754–760.
763. Kaufman SC, Ferris FL, III, Seigel DG, et al. Factors associated with visual outcome after photocoagulation for diabetic retinopathy. Diabetic Retinopathy Study Report #13. *Invest Ophthalmol Vis Sci*. 1989;30:23–28.
764. Early Treatment Diabetic Retinopathy Study Research Group. Effects of aspirin treatment on diabetic retinopathy. ETDRS report number 8. Early Treatment Diabetic Retinopathy Study Research Group. *Ophthalmology*. 1991;98:757–765.
765. Chew EY, Klein ML, Murphy RP, et al. Effects of aspirin on vitreous/preretinal hemorrhage in patients with diabetes mellitus. Early Treatment Diabetic Retinopathy Study report no. 20. *Arch Ophthalmol*. 1995; 113:52–55.
766. Braun CI, Benson WE, Remaley NA, et al. Accommodative amplitudes in the Early Treatment Diabetic Retinopathy Study. *Retina*. 1995;15:275–281.
767. Rice TA, Michels RG, Rice EF. Vitrectomy for diabetic traction retinal detachment involving the macula. *Am J Ophthalmol*. 1983;95:22–33.

Chapter 10
Cataract Surgery and Diabetic Retinopathy

David J. Browning

10.1 Scope of the Problem of Diabetic Retinopathy Concomitant with Surgical Cataract

Diabetes mellitus is increasing around the world with 171 million affected persons in 2000 and projected prevalences of 221 and 366 million affected patients by 2010 and 2030, respectively.[1,2] In the United States, an estimated 7.8% of the population has diabetes.[3] Diabetic patients have an increased risk of developing cataract and develop cataract at an earlier age than patients without diabetes.[1,4–8] In developed nations, 11–25% of all cataract surgery is performed in patients with diabetes and 1.2–5.0% of these patients will have concomitant diabetic retinopathy.[7,9–13] Thus, cataract surgery in patients with diabetes and with diabetic retinopathy is common, yet the interactions of cataract surgery and the diabetic eye are incompletely understood and a subject of controversy.

10.2 Visual Outcomes After Cataract Surgery in Patients with Diabetic Retinopathy

The rate of visual outcome ≥20/40 in patients without diabetes who undergo cataract surgery is ≥ 85%, and similar rates apply to patients with diabetes but no retinopathy.[14–19] Visual acuity outcomes of cataract surgery are worse in patients with diabetic retinopathy than in patients without diabetic retinopathy. In patients with nonproliferative diabetic retinopathy (NPDR), rates of visual acuity ≥20/40 have been reported from 52 to 70% and are worse the more severe the retinopathy, because increasing severity of retinopathy is associated with increasing prevalence of diabetic macular edema (DME).[16,19–25] In patients with treated proliferative diabetic retinopathy (PDR), rates of postoperative visual acuity ≥ 20/40 have been reported from 26 to 53%.[19,23,26] Visual acuity outcomes after cataract surgery are worse in patients with preoperative DME because of postoperative exacerbation of the edema and are worse in older patients because of higher rates of development of postoperative macular edema (Table 10.1).[16,20,24,25,27]

10.3 Postoperative Course and Special Considerations After Cataract Surgery in Patients with Diabetic Retinopathy

Uneventful cataract surgery in patients with diabetes has been inconsistently associated with higher rates of posterior capsular opacification and lower postoperative endothelial cell counts than in patients without diabetes.[28–32] Patients with diabetes have more anterior chamber inflammation after cataract surgery and a greater tendency to develop iris synechia and capsulorhexis contraction

D.J. Browning (✉)
Charlotte Eye Ear Nose & Throat Associates, Charlotte, NC 28210, USA
e-mail: dbrowning@ceenta.com

D.J. Browning (ed.), *Diabetic Retinopathy*, DOI 10.1007/978-0-387-85900-2_10,

Table 10.1 Rate of visual acuity ≥ 20/40 by retinopathy severity

Retinopathy status	% ≥20/40
No diabetic retinopathy	87%
Nonproliferative, no DME	80%
Quiescent PDR, no DME	57%
Nonproliferative, +DME	41%
Quiescent PDR, +DME	11%
Active proliferative	0%

DME = diabetic macular edema. PDR = proliferative diabetic retinopathy.
Reproduced with permission from Dowler.[27] Table summarizing visual outcomes of cataract surgery in patients with diabetes by retinopathy severity and presence or absence of preoperative macular edema.

than patients without diabetes.[16,32–34] These differences seem more pronounced with extracapsular and intracapsular cataract extractions and have not been as apparent with phacoemulsification and small incisions, the contemporary preferred technique.[30,35–37] More postoperative inflammation is noted in eyes with more advanced retinopathy, especially in eyes with active proliferative retinopathy. This may be related to the increasing breakdown of the blood–aqueous barrier that parallels increasing retinopathy severity.[25,38] The creation of a larger anterior capsulorhexis and the use of a more intense postoperative anti-inflammatory drop regimen than in nondiabetics have been recommended to aid in visualizing the peripheral fundus and to prevent synechiae, respectively.[39,40] Intraocular lenses with larger optics and no positioning holes are recommended to allow easier panretinal laser treatment, based on less peripheral capsular opacification and a greater optical area for viewing the fundus, should it be needed.[36,39–41] Anterior chamber lenses are not advised because of the increase in anterior chamber inflammation associated with haptic chafing. Silicone intraocular lenses should be avoided because they develop more inflammatory cellular precipitates than acrylic and polymethylmethacrylate lenses, suffer worse condensation on the posterior lens surface in the presence of an open posterior capsule during air–fluid exchange in vitrectomy surgery, and adhere to silicone oil after YAG capsulotomy, should the use of oil be needed later.[42,43] Larger YAG laser capsulotomies are recommended to facilitate possible later panretinal laser treatment.[16]

Patients with diabetic retinopathy can develop iris neovascularization (NVI) after cataract surgery.[16,44–48] The risk of this complication is increased if the posterior capsule is opened, but it occasionally develops with uncomplicated surgery and an intact capsule.[20,43,45,49] It was much more common in the era of intracapsular surgery, with a reported incidence of 7.8–8.9% in series with no selection for degree of preoperative retinopathy severity.[44,49] In the era before endolaser photocoagulation, eyes undergoing lensectomy in addition to vitrectomy for proliferative diabetic retinopathy had a threefold increased risk of developing postoperative NVI.[50] Careful inspection for any retinal neovascularization before cataract surgery or YAG capsulotomy is important, and panretinal laser photocoagulation should be applied before either procedure if new vessels are discovered.[36,43]

Rarely, cataract surgery must be performed in an eye with active NVI, because no view to the fundus is possible. Preoperative intravitreal injection of anti-vascular endothelial growth factor (VEGF) drugs such as bevacizumab causes rapid involution of the new vessels, reduces intraoperative bleeding, and allows intraoperative photocoagulation to be applied to enable more sustained regression of the new vessels.[51,52] At the end of surgery, a repeat injection of bevacizumab may be advisable because the effect of scatter photocoagulation is not immediate.

Some patients with advanced diabetic retinopathy require pars plana vitrectomy. Vitrectomy surgery can accelerate progression of cataract and lead to a subsequent need for cataract surgery.[53,54] The visual prognosis in such cases is guarded because of the limitations imposed by the underlying retinopathy, but 90% of eyes can expect improved visual acuity after cataract surgery and 45–50% can expect an outcome ≥ 20/40.[26,54,55] In addition, the technical aspects of the surgery can be different, including significant intraoperative fluctuations in anterior chamber depth, unexpected zonular dehiscence, and higher rates of a dropped nucleus.[36,54,55] In some patients, combined cataract surgery and vitrectomy may be needed because of concomitant cataract and active proliferative retinopathy with vitreous hemorrhage. As in the case of NVI, preoperative use of anti-VEGF drugs can reduce the risk of intraoperative bleeding, but anecdotal evidence suggests that any pre-existing retinal traction may be worsened with these agents.[56,57]

10.4 The Influence of Cataract Surgery on Diabetic Retinopathy

It has been long suspected that intracapsular and extracapsular cataract surgeries can exacerbate diabetic retinopathy, but relevant evidence has been inconsistent.[9,21,23,24,34,48,58–67] The more recent literature, applicable to phacoemulsification, supports the view that, on average, uncomplicated surgery does not cause clinically important retinopathy progression when the preoperative retinopathy is less advanced than severe nonproliferative.[1,9,10,30,37,58,60,62,64,68–73] There are, however, exceptional case reports in which exacerbation of retinopathy has occurred with contemporary, uncomplicated phacoemulsification technique.[74] Preoperative presence of diabetic retinopathy, duration of diabetes, worse glycemic control, surgery by residents, and use of insulin have been reported as risk factors for progression of retinopathy after cataract surgery.[23,30,34,73] There is little evidence regarding the effect of uncomplicated phacoemulsification surgery on retinopathy progression in eyes with untreated severe NPDR or PDR because of clear evidence of retinopathy progression from the era of intracapsular or extracapsular surgery and therefore intentional avoidance of this situation.[20,44,48,75] In a series of eyes undergoing intracapsular cataract extraction in the presence of active PDR, 20% developed vitreous hemorrhage within 6 weeks of surgery.[44] This has been extrapolated to the phacoemulsification era, and such eyes are typically treated with panretinal photocoagulation (PRP) first to reduce the levels of intraocular angiogenic growth factors before cataract surgery.[20] There is evidence, however, that uncomplicated phacoemulsification cataract surgery can be associated with the induction or exacerbation of DME.[62,63,68–70,76–78] Little evidence exists associating uncomplicated phacoemulsification cataract surgery and exacerbation of macular ischemia in patients with diabetic retinopathy, although reports existed of this association after extracapsular surgery.[20,64,66,79] Before the phacoemulsification era, anterior segment neovascularization was reported to follow cataract surgery in 6–8% of cases with most of the evidence implicating primary capsulotomy as increasing the incidence of this complication.[20,44,49] The rate has been less since the widespread adoption of phacoemulsification.

The association between cataract surgery and development or exacerbation of macular edema in diabetics is complicated to unravel because there are two types of macular edema in these situations – pseudophakic cystoid macular edema (PCME) and DME. In patients without diabetic retinopathy undergoing uncomplicated cataract surgery, the rate of clinically recognized macular thickening due to perioperative inflammation, PCME, has been reported to be 1–5%.[34,80–82] PCME usually spontaneously resolves within 6 months.[83,84] Uneventful cataract surgery in nondiabetics who do not develop PCME is generally associated with a mild, clinically unimportant, and transitory increase in macular thickness less than 10 μm.[80,81,84–87] Patients with diabetes have higher rates of PCME ranging from 13 to 24% in different series, and more severe retinopathy at baseline has been associated with higher postoperative rates of PCME.[34,59,73,81,82,88–90] Rates of fluorangiographic but not clinical PCME are also higher in eyes of diabetics undergoing cataract surgery than in eyes of nondiabetics and higher than rates of clinical PCME. In eyes of patients with diabetes but no retinopathy, rates of fluoroangiographic PCME at 1 month and 1 year were 69% and 24% for diabetics without retinopathy compared to 63% and 0% for nondiabetic eyes, respectively.[90] Patients with pre-existing diabetic retinopathy who develop PCME are more recalcitrant to treatment than those who do not have pre-existing diabetic retinopathy.[91]

DME considered as distinct from PCME can be induced or exacerbated by cataract surgery, with reported rates that vary according to many variables.[21,27,59,63,64,71,77] Diabetes causes a breakdown of the blood–ocular barrier before overt retinopathy is seen.[31,37,92] Vascular permeability increases with increasing retinopathy severity. Increased intraocular concentrations of inflammatory cytokines associated with cataract surgery added to the diathesis of increased permeability in diabetes translate into an increased incidence of postcataract surgery macular thickening.[64–66,70,77,93] Patel and colleagues prospectively assessed aqueous humor concentrations of growth factors after uncomplicated cataract surgery in seven eyes of six patients with diabetic retinopathy. Pro-angiogenic growth factors (VEGF, hepatocyte growth factor (HGF), and interleukin 1β (IL-1β)) and anti-angiogenic growth factors (pigment epithelial-derived growth factor (PEDF)) were assayed. VEGF, IL-1β, and PEDF rose at 1 day after surgery and declined by 1 month. HGF increased progressively over the first month after surgery. One patient developed DME. Although the number of eyes studied was small, the evidence suggests a possible mechanism for the development or exacerbation of DME after cataract surgery. Others have reported elevated intraocular levels of leukotrienes and endothelin after cataract surgery, which could enhance breakdown of the blood–retina barrier.[66] Surgically induced inflammation is less with small incision phacoemulsification than large incision extracapsular or intracapsular technique, which may explain the clinical impression that exacerbations of DME by cataract surgery are less common in the phacoemulsification era.[94] Rapid control of diabetes shortly before performing cataract surgery has been associated with an increased risk of new DME or exacerbation of pre-existing DME in the 12 months following uncomplicated cataract surgery and should be avoided.[78]

It can be difficult to define postsurgical increases in macular thickness as purely PCME or as purely DME.[20,66,95] Presence of disk hyperfluorescence on fluorescein angiography has in the past been said to be helpful in distinguishing DME from PCME, but the observation in prospective studies that the optic disk becomes more hyperfluorescent after cataract surgery in diabetic eyes that do not develop clinical macular edema undermines the usefulness of this suggested pearl.[70,96] Dowler and colleagues did not find that disk hyperfluorescence allowed discrimination of PCME from DME.[68] Presence of associated hemorrhage and lipid, a multifocal rather than a foveocentric pattern of edema, and petalloid late macular staining may help to distinguish DME from PCME, but again are subjective signs of questionable reliability (Fig. 10.1).[9,36,64,96] Thus, the relative contributions of DME versus PCME in postsurgical macular thickening can be difficult to assess in mixed clinical pictures.[9,96] In the past, when it was thought that the treatments differed for the two conditions, discriminating the components had greater importance. With the discovery that anti-inflammatory drugs can improve DME and that anti-VEGF drugs can improve PCME, the importance of the distinction has diminished.[82,97–101]

Eyes of diabetics with a range of retinopathy severities and no clinical DME preoperatively develop postoperative macular thickening that is greater than that of nondiabetics undergoing uncomplicated cataract surgery. Table 10.2 shows the results of four prospective studies involving a total of 160 eyes with average grades of retinopathy severity ranging from no-DR to mild NPDR before surgery. At 1–3 months after surgery, the macular thickness increase ranged from 10 to 69 μm and more severe retinopathy was associated with a larger increase in macular thickness.[70,77,93,102] Thus, even in diabetic eyes without clinical macular edema after cataract surgery, subclinical edema predictably develops. None of these studies makes an attempt to distinguish the macular thickening associated with the cataract surgery as PCME or DME.

Prospectively acquired data on the effect of cataract surgery on DME are available from the Early Treatment Diabetic Retinopathy Study (ETDRS) in which 81% of 270 eyes of 205 patients had laser photocoagulation for DME or PDR before cataract surgery.[58] In this series, there was no adverse effect of cataract surgery on the prevalence of DME. The proportions of eyes with photographically documented clinically significant diabetic macular edema (CSME) at the nearest annual visit were 29% before cataract surgery and 31% after cataract surgery.[58] The authors attributed this lack of effect of cataract surgery on rates of CSME to the high rate of preoperative macular laser treatment.[58] This publication has been the basis for the widely accepted principle that in a patient with concomitant surgical

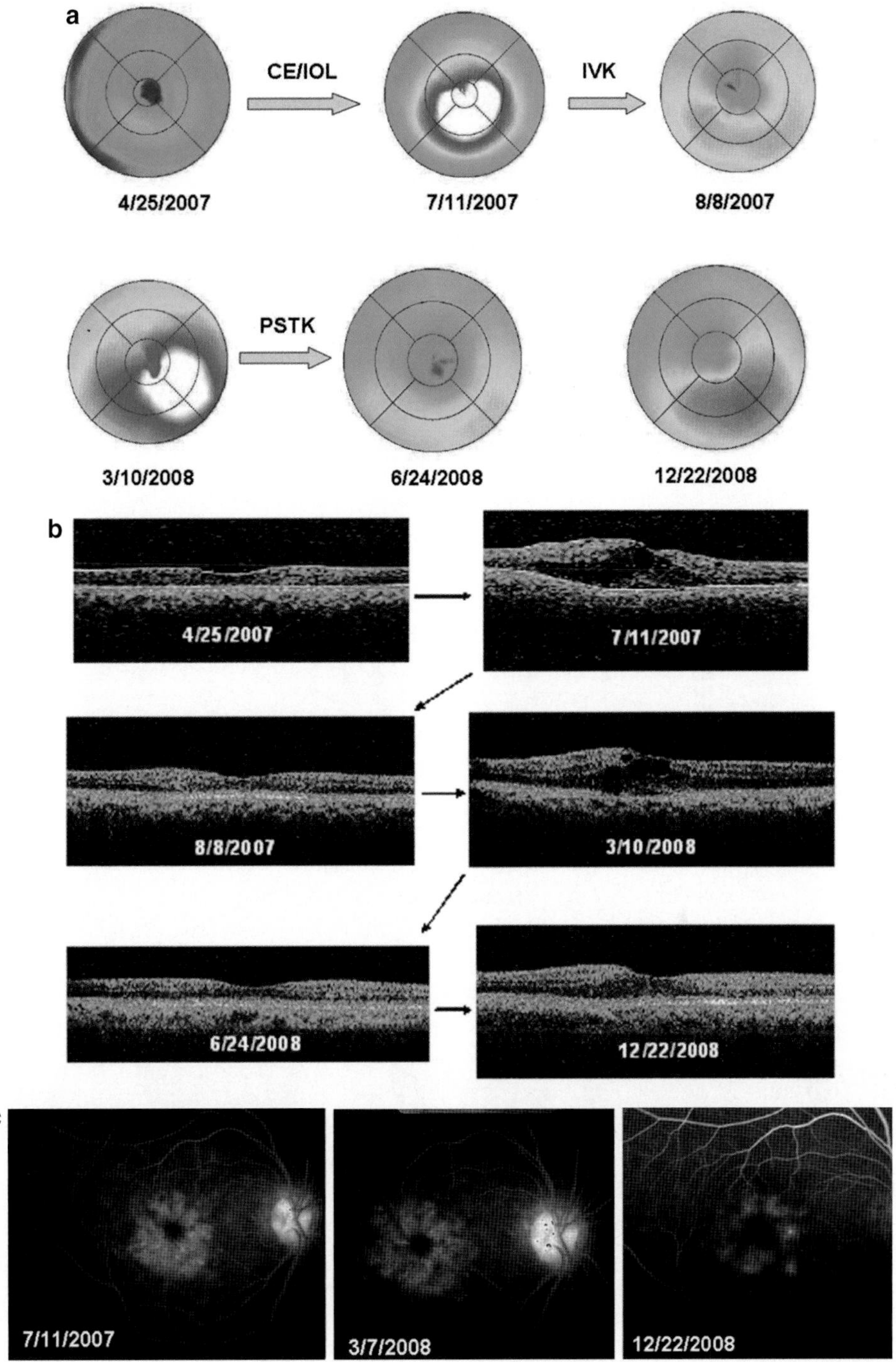

Fig. 10.1 A 67-year-old man with mild NPDR and no macular edema had 20/50 best corrected visual acuity of the right eye and a visually significant cataract. A preoperative OCT on April 25, 2007, showed no macular edema (Panels **a** and **b**). Uncomplicated phacoemulsification cataract extraction with posterior chamber intraocular lens implant on May 30, 2007, was followed by macular edema that was considered to be purely postoperative PCME. The disk was hyperfluorescent and the pattern of late macular hyperfluorescence was petalloid (Panel **c**). It did not respond to topical prednisolone acetate and ketorolac therapy, but did respond to intravitreal triamcinolone injection, 4 mg. It reoccurred and responded to posterior subtenon's triamcinolone injection, 40 mg. The macular edema reoccurred 6 months later, and consideration was given to the possibility that this was at least in part DME and not PCME. Focal laser photocoagulation was given to the leaky microaneurysms on September 9, 2009

cataract and CSME, the DME should be treated with focal/grid laser until it resolves or until maximal treatment has been applied before cataract surgery is performed. If this management pathway has been followed, on average one can expect that the cataract surgery will not adversely affect the prevalence of macular edema. An example of this common situation is illustrated in Fig. 10.2 in which an eye has been treated with maximal laser, continues to have DME, and yet does not have the feared exacerbation of edema by cataract surgery. There are, however, particular patients in which worsening will occur and adjunctive pharmacologic treatments may have a role in these cases.

One prospective study has suggested a difference in course for DME existing before cataract surgery and that developing de novo after surgery.[68] The edema occurring de novo after surgery has been hypothesized to be PCME, which is known to spontaneously remit in a high percentage of cases.[83] De novo CSME developed in the first year after cataract surgery in 13 of 27 (48%) eyes.[68] In 9 of these 13 eyes (69%), this CSME resolved spontaneously within the first postoperative year.[68] None of five eyes with preoperative CSME showed spontaneous resolution.[68] Some have suggested that macular edema in eyes with diabetic retinopathy after cataract surgery be treated as PCME for 3–6 months, and then treated as DME if it persists beyond 6 months.[9,41,103]

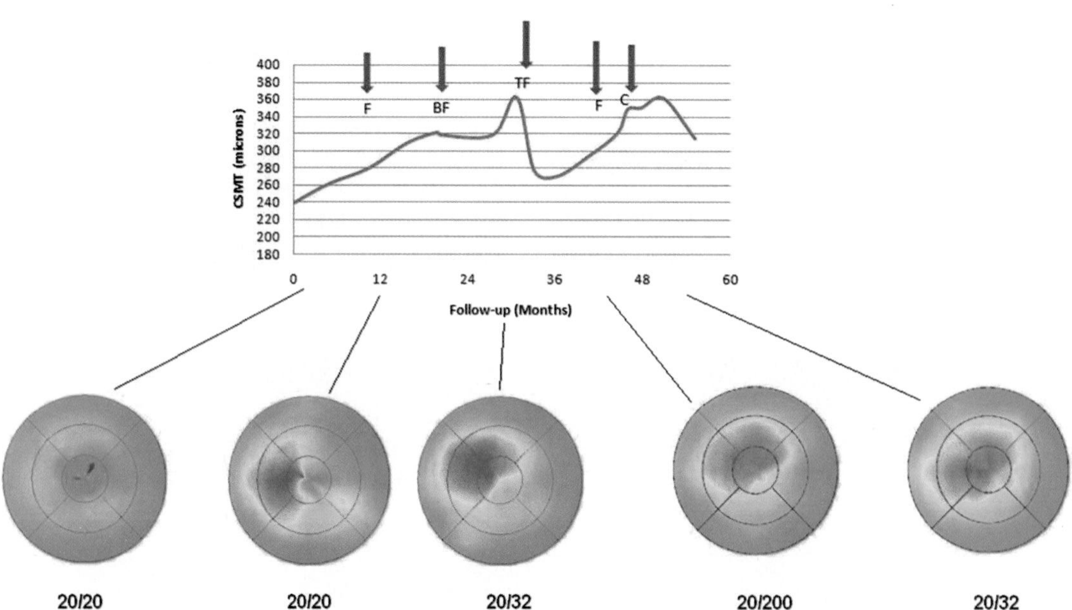

Fig. 10.2 In this figure, the *Y*-axis represents central subfield mean thickness in microns (CSMT). The *X*-axis represents time of follow-up (months), and illustrative OCT studies over the 4-year span illustrated are shown below at the times corresponding to the graphed CSMTs. Associated best corrected visual acuities are shown beneath the false color maps. This 66-year-old woman developed DME in 2004 and despite multiple focal laser treatments, some with adjunctive intravitreal bevacizumab (Avastin) and triamcinolone, continued to have refractory DME. Cataract developed, accelerated by the triamcinolone, and she underwent uneventful phacoemulsification with posterior chamber intraocular lens implantation 4 years later. Because her DME had been refractory to previous intravitreal triamcinolone injection, no repeat injection was given immediately preceding her surgery, and no worsening of the DME was noted after cataract surgery. Refractory, persistent DME remains, but the patient is content with her improved visual acuity following surgery and prefers no further intravitreal injection therapy although the option was presented. Vitrectomy surgery was also presented as a possible option should the DME worsen and vision decline, but was not recommended in this eye with visual acuity of 20/32. F = focal laser photocoagulation; BF = intravitreal bevacizumab injection followed by focal laser treatment 1 week later; TF = intravitreal triamcinolone injection followed by focal laser treatment 1 week later; C = cataract surgery

In an Eye with Diabetic Retinopathy but No Preoperative Macular Edema, Should One Wait 6 Months Before Considering PostCataract Surgery Macular Thickening to Be De Novo DME and Employing Focal/Grid Laser?

Because management recommendations to wait for 6 months before proceeding to laser treatment were made in a time when treatments for PCME and DME were considered to be different, their underlying rationales may be outdated.[37,41] An alternate management plan to consider might be to treat all edema in eyes with diabetic retinopathy after cataract surgery as some combination of PCME and DME. There seems little reason to omit focal/grid laser treatment within the first 6 months after surgery if there are clearly treatable lesions such as microaneurysms centered in areas of macular thickening. Omitting laser has a stronger rationale the less severe the degree of diabetic retinopathy and may safeguard against the opposite pitfall of unnecessary focal/grid laser in eyes destined to spontaneously resolve their macular edema if given adequate time.[9] Prospective clinical trials are needed to place management guidelines on firmer evidential footing. Consider the case illustrated in Fig. 10.3. This 68-year old man with type 2 diabetes for 20 years developed a cataract reducing best corrected visual acuity in the right eye to 20/40 and significantly interfering with his reading ability and driving at night. Preoperatively, a macular examination by a retina specialist revealed no DME, and there was mild NPDR with a few microaneurysms clustered temporal to the macula. The first day after surgery his visual acuity was 20/20. Two months later he noted blurring. Visual acuity had dropped to 20/30, and de novo DME was present (Figs. 10.3A–D). According to Dowler and colleagues, this patient might be treated as PCME for 6 months before considering focal/grid laser. Instead, the patient was treated with focal photocoagulation and subsequent combined peribulbar triamcinolone injection plus focal photocoagulation. Visual acuity 9 months later had returned to 20/20 (Fig. 10.3E).

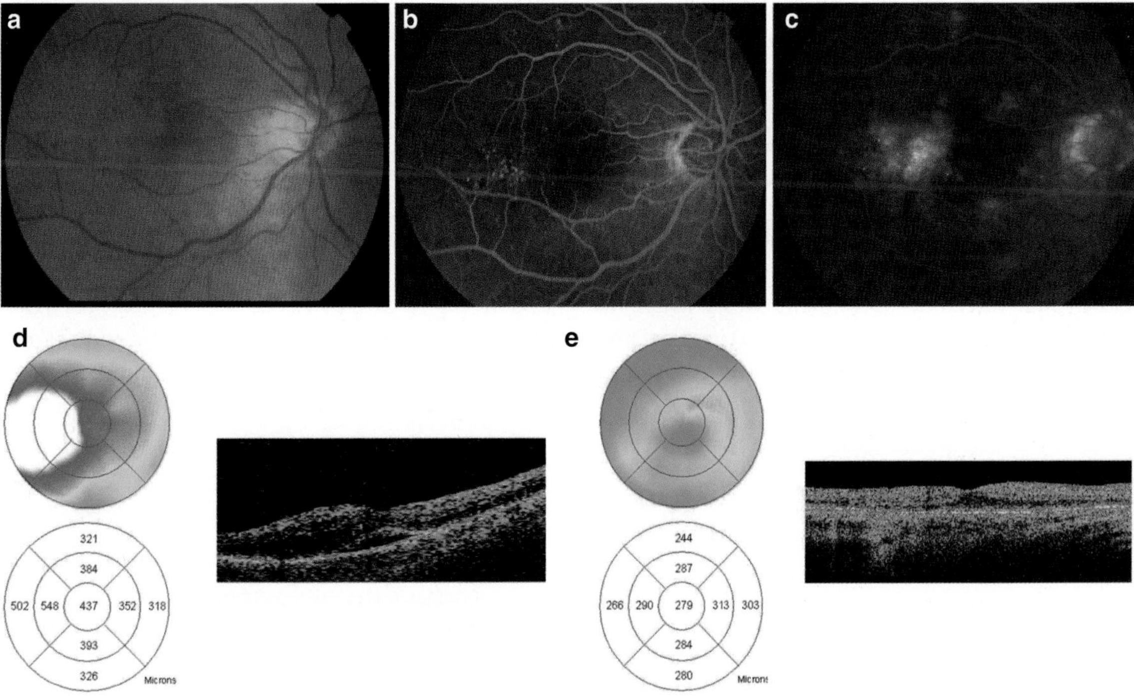

Fig. 10.3 Example of a patient in whom de novo macular thickening following cataract surgery was unlikely to be PCME and in which a favorable outcome followed treatment of leaking microaneurysms under the alternate assumption that the situation represented DME instead

Table 10.2 Preoperative and postoperative macular thickness in eyes of diabetics undergoing uncomplicated cataract surgery

Study	Mean DR severity	*N* (eyes)	Mean preop macular thickness ± SD (μm)	Mean 1–2 months postop macular thickness ± SD (μm)
Kim[77]	1.3	46	205 ± 39	274 ± 91
Kim[93]	1.0	50	275*	322*
Escaravage[70]	1.0	30	221 ± 50	260 ± 68
Hayashi[102]	0	34	170 ± 29**	180 ± 36

DR = diabetic retinopathy; Preop = preoperative; Postop = postoperative; * = the SD was not stated.** = the value was the foveal thickness rather than the central subfield mean thickness. Retinopathy severity is defined as follows: 0 = no retinopathy; 1 = mild to moderate NPRD; 2 = severe NPRD. Fractional gradings between these integer values arise from calculating the mean severity for the sample of eyes in the respective studies.

From these studies, one might hazard the following synthesis of the relationship of cataract surgery and DME. Eyes of diabetic patients have a predisposition to breakdown of the blood–retina barrier. Pre- and postoperative treatment with nonsteroidal anti-inflammatory drops and postoperative treatment with steroid drops are rational, but unproven to reduce rates of postoperative macular edema and improve visual outcomes. Eyes with treated and resolved DME are unlikely to undergo re-exacerbation with uncomplicated phacoemulsification cataract extraction and posterior chamber intraocular lens implantation.[58] Macular thickening arising de novo after uncomplicated cataract surgery often spontaneously resolves and therefore need not be immediately treated if minimal retinopathy is present, although treatment as PCME is rational.[68] DME present at the time of contemplated cataract surgery is unlikely to spontaneously resolve, may get worse after surgery, and therefore should be treated before the cataract surgery[68,93] PCME occurs more commonly in eyes with more advanced degrees of retinopathy and therefore anti-inflammatory treatment approaches such as peribulbar or intravitreal triamcinolone have a rationale in such eyes, even if focal/grid laser is the foundation of treatment for DME.[17]

10.5 The Role of Ancillary Testing in Managing Cataract Surgery in Eyes with Diabetic Retinopathy

The clinical assessment of mild DME in eyes with clear media is problematic, and retina specialists increasingly rely on optical coherence tomography (OCT) to detect mild DME.[104,105] In the presence of a cataract, the clinical examination becomes even less reliable in the detection of mild macular thickening, but the OCT remains reliable until the signal strength drops (the threshold level depends on the OCT machine, but for the Stratus OCT, this might be below a signal strength of 4). Others have advocated using OCT rather than clinical criteria in decisions regarding perioperative management of DME.[106] In the presence of cataract and diabetic retinopathy, it is the author's opinion that OCT should be routinely obtained preoperatively to prevent the occurrence of a postoperative surprise of DME that was present but unsuspected in the preoperative state. The use of fluorescein angiography has been advocated as a way to distinguish PCME from DME.[9] Because the evidence is weak that the findings of disk hyperfluorescence or petalloid macular staining discriminate PCME from DME with reproducible specificity, this recommendation seems costly and imprudent.[68,70]

In eyes with dense cataracts preventing a view of the fundus, a useful ancillary study is iris fluorescein angiography.[107] Any presence of NVI should alert the surgeon to the certain presence of severe NPDR or PDR.[107] Consideration can be given to perioperative intravitreal bevacizumab injection and prompt PRP in such a case. Absence of NVI, however, is still compatible with the presence of advanced diabetic retinopathy, and a careful fundus evaluation in the early postoperative period is necessary.

10.6 Candidate Risk and Protective Factors for Diabetic Macular Edema Induction or Exacerbation Following Cataract Surgery and Suggested Management Actions

Review of retrospective series leads to a list of factors which have been associated with greater risk of macular edema induction or worsening in diabetic patients after cataract surgery. These include female sex[76] (and counterevidence[59]), obesity,[76] control of diabetes with oral agents[76] (and counterevidence[59]), control of diabetes with insulin,[59] age ≥ 64,[20] longer duration of diabetes,[59] more severe retinopathy,[25] poor control of diabetes,[73] any macular edema before cataract surgery,[20] complicated cataract surgery,[72] and rapid control of poorly controlled blood glucose before surgery.[78] Several factors have been cited as possibly protective against postoperative DME, including previous vitrectomy,[54] posterior chamber intraocular lens implantation placement in the capsular bag rather than the sulcus,[108] and previous macular photocoagulation.[58,109] Prospective studies are needed to more definitively address which of these factors have the greatest predictive importance.

Based on these factors, specific suggestions for preventing DME following cataract surgery have been published. These include intensive preoperative topical steroids or nonsteroidal anti-inflammatory drugs,[24,48,80,95,110] delaying cataract surgery in patients with diabetes until a more advanced visual handicap relative to nondiabetic patients,[64,76] the opposite approach of operating on patients with diabetes and cataract earlier rather than later to capitalize on the evidence of lack of harm when diabetic retinopathy is absent or minimal,[1,9,37,68] avoidance of anterior chamber intraocular lenses,[72] recusal of surgeons who have relatively high rates of posterior capsule rupture,[72] avoidance of cataract surgery in patients with diabetic retinopathy by beginning-level residents,[23] and scrupulous examination for DME in the preoperative examination and treatment with laser photocoagulation before proceeding to surgery.[58,76] These all seem to be reasonable suggestions, subject to rigorous testing in better designed prospective studies, but the conflicting recommendations regarding when to operate cannot be wise. In the absence of a study addressing the issue, the author suggests that the threshold for cataract surgery be the same as for eyes of patients without diabetes – when the cataract is judged sufficiently advanced to interfere with the patient's visual quality of life.

Suggestions for mitigating the possible effects of cataract surgery on retinopathy progression and DME include weekly or biweekly retinopathy checks for 3 months following cataract surgery,[64] fluorescein angiography at 1, 3, and 6 months postcataract surgery in patients with diabetic retinopathy,[64] aggressive laser photocoagulation for any deterioration in retinopathy following cataract surgery, and an intravitreal injection of bevacizumab at the time of cataract surgery.[64,75] Some of these suggested measures, such as biweekly checks and frequent fluorescein angiography, arose in a time of extracapsular and intracapsular surgeries, and seem excessive now, when phacoemulsification is the technique universally used. Modifications of these ideas may be worth considering for cases at particularly high risk rather than in routine uncomplicated cataract surgery in patients with diabetes. The widespread availability of OCT and its sensitivity for macular thickening make it the most important modality in analyzing diabetic eyes after cataract surgery.

10.7 The Problem of Adherence to Preferred Practice Guidelines

In addition to the problem of accurately assessing the extent of cataract surgery induced or exacerbated DME and PCME, there is the practical problem of how frequently clinicians depart from delivering evidence-based care. There is consensus that cataract surgery should not be performed in patients with untreated DME if it can be avoided, because visual acuity outcomes are worse.[41,73] Nevertheless, many ophthalmologists do not follow this recommendation (Fig. 10.4). McCarty et al. found that 10–16% of surveyed Australian ophthalmologists would remove the cataract of a patient with combined cataract and DME first and then address the DME.[111] Indeed, it has been stated that problem of DME induced or exacerbated by cataract surgery is more accurately characterized as a problem of insufficient diagnostic accuracy by cataract surgeons in recognizing presence of DME or ignorance or disagreement with clinical practice guidelines.[1,9,64]

10.8 Management of the Diabetic Eye Without Macular Edema About to Undergo Cataract Surgery

In contemporary ophthalmic practice, there is no agreement that any measures beyond usual perioperative cataract care should be used in eyes with diabetic retinopathy and no preoperative

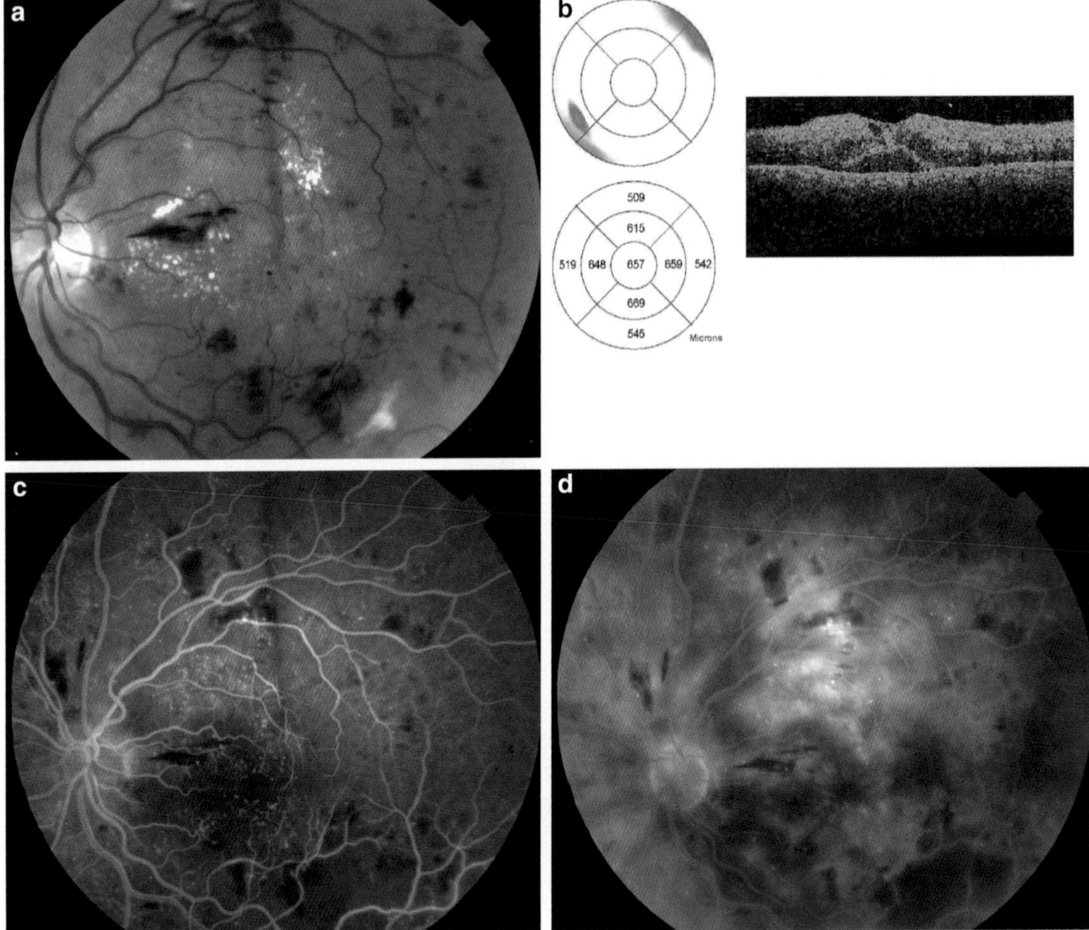

Fig. 10.4 Exemplary case demonstrating lack of awareness of guidelines regarding management of DME and cataract. A 65-year-old man with type 2 diabetes for 12 years and hypertension for 10 years saw his ophthalmologist with complaints of gradual blurring of the left eye for a year. The best corrected visual acuities were 20/30 and 20/200 of the right and left eyes, respectively. The ophthalmologist noted a cataract on the left but had a clear view of the macula and noted that diabetic macular edema was present. Left eye cataract surgery was done 2 days later without complication, but the visual acuity was unchanged at the first postoperative examination. The fundus examination at this visit was identical to that of the preoperative examination. The patient was referred to the author to manage the diabetic retinopathy. Marked macular edema with lipid exudates and severe diabetic retinopathy were present of the left eye on clinical examination (**a**). Marked macular thickening was shown on OCT (**b**). Fluorescein angiography showed marked fluorescein leakage (**c** and **d**). The patient was treated with intravitreal triamcinolone injection and focal/grid photocoagulation

macular edema. Nevertheless, the evidence that subclinical macular thickening occurs after cataract surgery more often and more severely in such eyes than in the eyes of nondiabetics has led to studies of alternative approaches to perioperative management. Kim and colleagues have shown that a single posterior subtenon injection of triamcinolone is associated with a statistically significant decrease in OCT-measured macular thickening and best corrected visual acuity at 1 month but not 6 months.[77]

10.9 Treatment of Diabetic Macular Edema Detected Before Cataract Surgery When the Macular View Is Clear

The most effective treatment for DME in general is focal/grid laser photocoagulation.[98,112] In refractory cases, adjunctive modalities such as peribulbar triamcinolone injection, intravitreal triamcinolone injection, intravitreal injection of anti-VEGF drugs, and sometimes vitrectomy surgery can be employed.[113–115] The best order of intervention is an active area of research and remains unclear.[116] Sometimes the cataract obscures the view for delivery of laser photocoagulation. In such cases, pharmacologic therapy can be used to reduce macular edema preoperatively, and prompt focal/grid laser treatment can be provided in the early postoperative period. If a taut hyaloid is present and is considered to be etiologic, a combined cataract operation with pars plana vitrectomy may be a reasonable option.

10.10 Management When Cataract Sufficient to Obscure the Macular View and DME Coexist or When Refractory DME and Cataract Coexist

There is no debate regarding the management of eyes with concomitant cataract and DME when an excellent view to the macula is present. In these eyes, it should be treated and the edema should have resolved before proceeding with the cataract surgery.[96] However, there are cases in which DME is present but the cataract precludes an adequate view to the macula to allow treatment of the DME or in which DME refractory to maximal focal/grid laser treatment exists. In these cases, there are several management options; the option associated with the best visual outcome is unknown. If submaximal focal/grid photocoagulation has been applied, the possible options include preoperative injection of peribulbar or intravitreal triamcinolone or bevacizumab followed by focal/grid laser photocoagulation in the early postoperative period, cataract surgery with intraoperative peribulbar or intravitreal triamcinolone injection followed by focal/grid photocoagulation in the early perioperative period, or cataract surgery without preoperative pharmacologic treatment with focal/grid photocoagulation.[68,75,96] If maximal focal/grid laser has already been applied and refractory DME exists, the options include serial preoperative and postoperative injections of peribulbar or intravitreal triamcinolone, serial preoperative and postoperative injections of intravitreal anti-VEGF drugs, or combined cataract and vitrectomy surgery, the latter of which may include an array of possible steps including internal limiting membrane peeling, panretinal laser photocoagulation, and intravitreal injection with triamcinolone or anti-VEGF drugs. An example of the clinical management of refractory DME and cataract was shown in Fig. 10.2.

When DME exists and a taut posterior vitreous hyaloid is also determined to be present, consideration may be given to a combined procedure involving both phacoemulsification cataract surgery and vitrectomy with separation of the tautly adherent posterior hyaloid. The indications for this procedure are controversial even when the complicating factor of a visually significant cataract is not present. The reader is referred to Chapter 7 for perspective on this controversy. Here, we will emphasize the variables associated with combining vitrectomy and cataract surgery. Combined phacoemulsification cataract extraction and pars plana vitrectomy is a widely practiced technique.[117–119] All variations of the technique employ removal of posterior hyaloid. Variations include removal of the internal limiting membrane, either aided by staining with indocyanine green or marked by triamcinolone, with or without panretinal laser treatment and with or without adjunctive intravitreal triamcinolone or anti-VEGF drugs. The disadvantages of combined surgery include increased operative time, possible need for two surgeons, and potential for increased fibrin response in the postoperative period.[118] Prospective studies are needed to determine the management choices associated with the best outcomes.

10.11 Patients with Simultaneous Indications for Panretinal Photocoagulation and Cataract Surgery

Traditionally, it has been taught that eyes with severe NPDR and PDR concomitant with cataract be treated with PRP first, and that cataract surgery be deferred until angiogenically active retinopathy has been rendered quiescent.[13,20] The greatest fear in these earlier studies was NVI and neovascular glaucoma.[13,20] Before anti-VEGF drugs were available, preoperative scatter laser with the laser indirect ophthalmoscope was recommended to avoid the inability to apply laser due to the heavy fibrinous iritis that sometimes occurs in such eyes after cataract surgery.[13] Currently, an intravitreal injection of bevacizumab can be given shortly before anticipated cataract surgery and PRP laser applied shortly after surgery as an office procedure.

More recently, worry has shifted from NVI to induced DME. Suto and colleagues reported that patients with simultaneous severe NPDR or early PDR and visually significant cataracts had a statistically significant higher rate of attaining ≥ 20/40 vision and lower rate of DME progression postoperatively if the order of interventions was cataract surgery first followed by PRP 3 months postoperatively compared to the alternative order of PRP first followed by cataract surgery 1–3 months later.[10] Rates of application of focal/grid laser for DME were lower in the surgery first group. Eyes in the study were mixed with regard to presence or absence of DME, and if DME was present, focal laser was used before PRP was performed in the PRP group and shortly after cataract surgery in the cataract surgery first group. Breakdown of the blood–aqueous barrier was higher in the PRP first group based on aqueous flare intensity measurement.[10] As this study did not use OCT, it is possible that CSME existed simultaneously with the cataract in a significant proportion of eyes, and that the PRP exacerbated this DME more than cataract surgery did.

10.12 Management of Cataract in Patients with Diabetic Retinopathy Undergoing Vitrectomy

Some patients undergoing vitrectomy surgery for various indications have concomitant cataract that interferes with the ability to achieve the goals of the vitrectomy surgery.[120,121] In such cases, possible management options include standard phacoemulsification cataract extraction with intraocular lens implantation followed by a second vitrectomy procedure at a later time or combined operations in which both the cataract surgery and the vitrectomy are completed with a single anesthesia. There are many variations on the theme of combined surgery. For example, the cataract extraction may be done first without insertion of the intraocular lens, followed by the vitrectomy, and lastly insertion of the implant. Alternatively, a complete cataract procedure with implant insertion may be done first followed by the vitrectomy.[39,120] One or two surgeons may be involved, usually based on cultural differences. In the United States, retinologists rarely perform cataract surgery and sequential or two-surgeon single combined procedures are more common.[120] Outside the United States, it is common for retinologists to perform cataract surgery and retina surgery, and single-surgeon combined procedures are more common. Visual acuity results depend on the underlying severity of the retinal disease. Rates of visual acuity ≥ 20/40 have been reported from 7 to 29%.[120,121] In the era before endophotocoagulation, vitrectomy surgery for complications of PDR was associated with postoperative NVI in 20–30% of cases, and simultaneous cataract extraction (lensectomy) increased the rate two to three times compared to vitrectomy without simultaneous cataract extraction.[50] Application of complete panretinal endophotocoagulation at the time of vitrectomy and use of intraocular anti-VEGF drugs as surgical adjuncts have reduced this effect of concomitant cataract extraction dramatically.[122] There is evidence from one case series that in the contemporary era of vitreoretinal surgery with endophotocoagulation capability reoperation rates are decreased when the crystalline lens has been removed before or during the vitrectomy procedure. The hypothesis advanced for this result is that more complete epiretinal proliferation resection and endophotocoagulation are possible in an eye without the crystalline lens.[122]

10.13 Influence of Vitrectomy Surgery on Cataract Formation

The traditional teaching has been that vitrectomy surgery for any indication increases the rate of development of cataract. In a recent series of cases undergoing vitrectomy for complications of diabetic retinopathy, 49.1% of 72 phakic eyes developed significant cataract within 6 months of vitrectomy and 23.7% of phakic eyes underwent cataract extraction with intraocular lens implantation over a mean follow-up of 9.6 months, which would tend to support traditional teaching.[122] Hutton and colleagues analyzed a retrospective series of 289 phakic eyes that had been subjected to diabetic vitrectomy. Moderate to severe cataract developed in 37% of eyes at an average of 1.1 years after surgery.[54] On the other hand, Smiddy and Feuer reported a 15% incidence of cataract extraction 2 years after diabetic vitrectomy compared to 53–66% rates for comparative cohorts of eyes undergoing vitrectomy for macular pucker and macular hole, respectively, and the rates in diabetic eyes remained significantly lower after statistically adjusting for the effect of age.[123] The issue remains controversial and unresolved.

10.14 Summary Flow Chart of Management Principles and Estimated Outcomes for Diabetic Eyes Facing Cataract Surgery

A summary of management principles and average outcomes when cataract surgery is contemplated in a patient with diabetes is illustrated in the flow charts in Figs. 10.5 and 10.6.

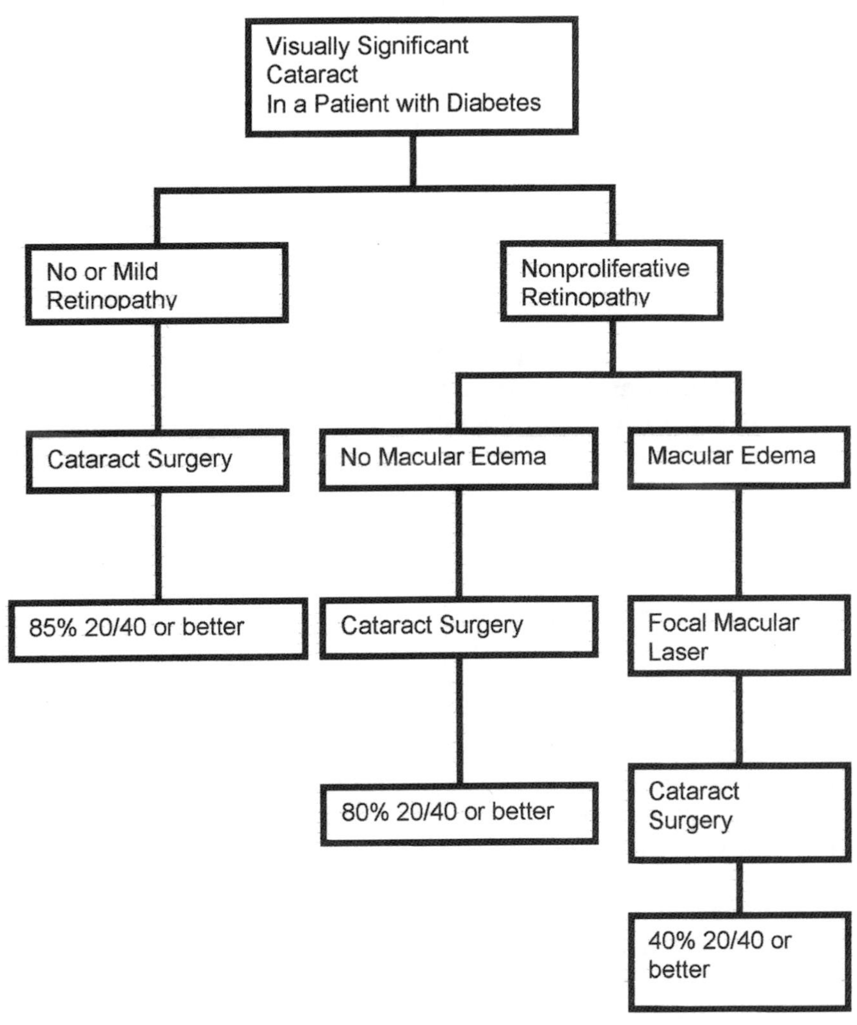

Fig. 10.5 Flow chart with suggested management of an eye with cataract in a patient with diabetes and less than proliferative retinopathy. Average outcomes by retinopathy classification group are indicated. Reproduced with permission from Fineman and Benson[36]

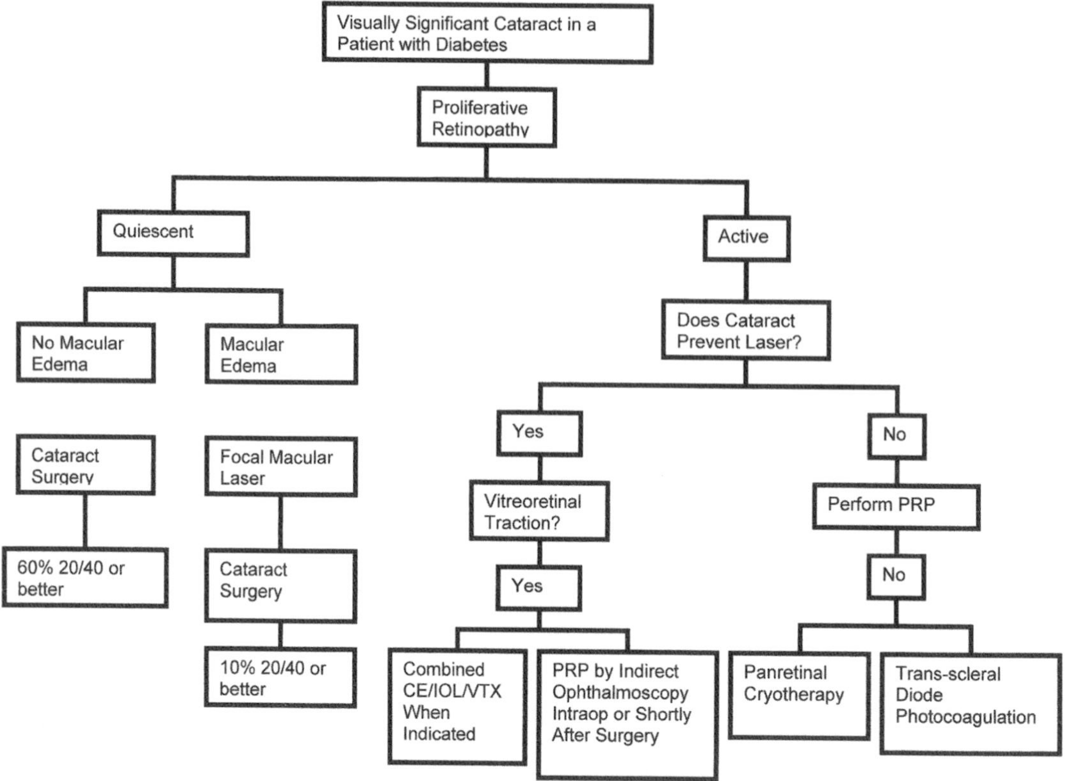

Fig. 10.6 Flow chart with suggested management of an eye with cataract in a patient with diabetes and proliferative retinopathy that is active or regressed. Average outcomes by retinopathy classification group are indicated. Reproduced with permission from Fineman and Benson[36]. CE = cataract extraction, IOL = intraocular lens, implantation, VTX = vitrectomy, Intraop = intraoperative.

10.15 Postoperative Endophthalmitis in Patients with Diabetic Retinopathy

There is some controversy regarding whether patients with diabetes undergoing cataract surgery develop endophthalmitis at a higher rate than nondiabetics.[36,124,125] The severity of diabetic retinopathy and diabetic macular edema are exacerbated by endophthalmitis, however, and it is generally agreed that visual results after endophthalmitis in diabetic eyes are worse than in nondiabetic eyes.[61,126] The rates of achieving ≥ 20/40 visual acuity after endophthalmitis are 39% and 55% for diabetic and nondiabetic eyes, respectively, and similar worse outcomes for diabetic eyes were found at every level of visual acuity.[126] Diabetic eyes suffering endophthalmitis have higher rates of culture positivity, have higher rates of growth of coagulase negative staphylococci, and respond less well to therapy, requiring more frequent additional injections and other procedures to manage the endophthalmitis.[126] There is a suggestion that visual acuity outcomes are improved in eyes of diabetics suffering endophthalmitis and having visual acuity better than light perception if vitrectomy with intravitreal antibiotic injection is used rather than a vitreous tap with antibiotic injection, a result not found in nondiabetic eyes.[126] Not enough eyes were studied to allow a more definitive statement to be made. [126]

10.16 Summary of Key Points

- Eyes of patients with diabetes have a pre-existing tendency toward vascular endothelial hyperpermeability. The effects of normal postsurgical inflammation are therefore superimposed on a diathesis for macular edema. Moreover, eyes of patients with diabetes have higher levels of postsurgical inflammation even after technically perfect surgery. The net effect is a higher rate of postoperative clinical and subclinical macular edema in diabetic eyes.

- It is difficult to distinguish a PCME component from a DME component of macular thickening after cataract surgery in eyes of diabetics. Disk hyperfluorescence and a petalloid pattern of fluorescein leakage are not specific for PCME.
- The practical consequence of the above considerations is that all eyes of diabetic patients about to undergo cataract surgery need to have a painstaking examination of the macula both clinically and by OCT. If any macular thickening is detected, every effort should be made to eliminate it before cataract surgery. This may involve focal/grid laser and use of peribulbar and intraocular steroids or intraocular anti-VEGF drugs.
- Careful examination of the macula after cataract surgery is also important, and treatment should be applied promptly for macular thickening that might have been precluded by a suboptimal view through the cataract.
- Complicated cataract surgery is a particularly negative influence relative to both DME and PCME; thus, cataract surgery in patients with diabetes is best performed by surgeons with low complication rates and specifically not by beginning residents.
- If cataract surgery in a patient with diabetes is complicated, the early involvement of a retina specialist is worthwhile to facilitate detection of retinopathy progression and induction or worsening of DME.
- Preoperative discussions of prognosis before cataract surgery are more complex in patients with diabetic retinopathy and expectations of patients need to be appropriately modulated based on the pertinent risk factors.
- Active PDR at the time of cataract surgery is particularly dangerous, as it can be associated with heavy fibrinous iritis and pupillary membrane formation after surgery. Early postoperative scatter laser should be considered in such cases when preoperative treatment is not possible, and preoperative intravitreal injection of anti-VEGF drugs is prudent.

10.17 Future Directions

Further investigations are needed to resolve several questions.

1. How often do cataract surgeons misassess the presence or absence of DME in their patients being considered for cataract surgery? Should preoperative assessment for DME by a retina specialist become a standard in patients with diabetic retinopathy?
2. What is the rate of development of DME in patients without DME who undergo cataract surgery?
3. What is the rate of development of worsened DME in patients with mild DME who undergo cataract surgery?
4. Do pharmacologic or combined pharmacologic and laser treatments reduce the rate of DME worsening in patients with refractory DME undergoing cataract surgery?
5. In patients with DME and a poor macular view, what management plan produces the best visual acuity outcomes?
6. In patients with DME associated with a taut posterior hyaloid, which management plan produces the best visual acuity outcomes?
7. Does vitrectomy surgery in a diabetic patient accelerate cataract formation as it does in a nondiabetic patient?

References

1. Dowler J, Hykin PG. Cataract surgery in diabetics. *Curr Opin Ophthalmol*. 2001;12:175–178.
2. Williams R, Airey M, Baxter H, et al. Epidemiology of diabetic retinopathy and macular edema: a systematic review. *Eye*. 2004;18(963):983.
3. US Diabetes Prevalence. http://www.cdc.gov/diabetes/pubs/pdf/ndfs_2005.pdf9-20-2008. Accessed 9-20-2008.
4. Kleinbek R, Moss SE. Prevalence of cataracts in a population-based study of patients with diabetes mellitus. *Ophthalmology*. 1985;92:1191–1196.
5. Nielsen NV, Vinding T. The prevalence of cataract in insulin-dependent and non-insulin-dependent diabetes mellitus. *Acta Ophthalmol Scand*. 1984;62:595–602.
6. Ederer F, Hiller R, Taylor HR. Senile lens changes and diabetes in two population studies. *Am J Ophthalmol*. 1981;91:381–395.
7. Harding JJ, Egerton M, van Heyningen R, Harding RS. Diabetes, glaucoma, sex and cataract: analysis of

combined data from two case control studies. *Br J Ophthalmol.* 1993;77:2–6.
8. Klein BE, Klein R, Wang Q, Moss SSE. Older-onset diabetes and lens opacities: the Beaver Dam Eye Study. *Ophthalmic Epidemiol.* 1995;2:49–55.
9. Squirrell D, Bhola R, Bush J, et al. A prospective, case controlled study of the natural history of diabetic retinopathy and maculopathy after uncomplicated phacoemulsification cataract surgery in patients with type 2 diabetes. *Br J Ophthalmol.* 2002;86:565–571.
10. Suto C, Hori S, Kato S. Management of type 2 diabetics requiring panretinal photocoagulation and cataract surgery. *J Cataract Refract Surg.* 2008;34:1001–1006.
11. The Eye Diseases Prevalence Research Group. The prevalence of diabetic retinopathy among adults in the United States. *Arch Ophthalmol.* 2004;122:552–563.
12. Royal College of Ophthalmologists. Cataract Surgery Guidelines. 2004. http://www.rcophth.ac.uk/docs/publications/CataractSurgeryGuidelinesMarch2005Updated.pdf. Accessed 9-20-2008.
13. Flanagan DW. Progression of diabetic retinopathy following cataract surgery: can it be prevented? *Br J Ophthalmol.* 1996;80:777–779.
14. Schein OD, Steinberg EP, Javitt JC, et al. Variation in cataract surgery practice and clinical outcomes. *Ophthalmology.* 1994;101:1142–1152.
15. Straatsma BR, Pettit TH, Wheeler N, Miyamasu W. Diabetes and intraocular lens implantation. *Ophthalmology.* 1983;90:336–343.
16. Cunliffe IA, Flanagan DW, George NDL, et al. Extracapsular cataract surgery with lens implantation in diabetics with and without proliferative retinopathy. *Br J Ophthalmol.* 1991;75:9–12.
17. Zaczek A, Olivestedt G, Zetterstrom C. Visual outcome after phacoemulsification and IOL implantation in diabetic patients. *Br J Ophthalmol.* 1999;83:1036–1041.
18. Shah DP, Krishnan AA, Albanis CV, et al. Visual acuity outcomes following vitreous loss in glaucoma and diabetic patients. *Eye.* 2002;16:271–274.
19. Wagner T, Knaflic D, Rauber M, Mester U. Influence of cataract surgery of the diabetic eye: a prospective study. *German J Ophthalmol.* 1996;5:79–83.
20. Benson WE, Brown GC, Tasman W, et al. Extracapsular cataract extraction with placement of a posterior chamber lens in patients with diabetic retinopathy. *Ophthalmology.* 1993;100:730–738.
21. Sebestyen JG, Wafai MZ. Experience with intraocular lens implants in patients with diabetes. *Am J Ophthalmol.* 1983;96:94–96.
22. Klein R, Klein BEK, Moss SE, et al. The Wisconsin epidemiologic study of diabetic retinopathy IV. Diabetic macular edema. *Ophthalmology.* 1984;91:1464–1474.
23. Mittra RA, Borrillo JL, Dev S, et al. Retinopathy progression and visual outcomes after phacoemulsification in patients with diabetes mellitus. *Arch Ophthalmol.* 2000;118:912–917.
24. Chiu DW, Meusemann RA, Kaufman DV, et al. Visual outcome and progression of retinopathy after cataract surgery in diabetic patients. *Austral NZ J Ophthalmol.* 26:129–133.
25. Hykin PG, Gregson RMC, Stevens JD, Hamilton PAM. Extracapsular cataract extraction in proliferative diabetic retinopathy. *Ophthalmology.* 1993;100:394–399.
26. Ruiz RS, Saatci OA. Posterior chamber intraocular lens implantation in eyes with inactive and active proliferative diabetic retinopathy. *Am J Ophthalmol.* 1991;111:158–162.
27. Dowler JGF, Hykin PG, Lightman SL, Hamilton AM. Visual acuity following extracapsular cataract extraction in diabetes: a meta-analysis. *Eye.* 1995;9:313–317.
28. Ebihara Y, Kato S, Oshika T, et al. Posterior capsule opacification after cataract surgery in patients with diabetes mellitus. *J Cataract Refract Surg.* 2006;32:1184–1187.
29. Lee JS, Lee JE, Choi HY, et al. Corneal endothelial cell change after phacoemulsification relative to the severity of diabetic retinopathy. *J Cataract Ref Surg.* 2005;31:742–749.
30. Romero-Aroca P, Fernandez-Ballart J, Almena-Garcia M, et al. Nonproliferative diabetic retinopathy and macular edema progression after phacoemulsification: prospective study. *J Cataract Refract Surg.* 2006;32:1438–1444.
31. Ionides A, Dowler JG, Hykin PG, et al. Posterior capsular opacification following diabetic extracapsular cataract extraction. *Eye.* 1994;8:535–537.
32. Zaczek A, Zetterstrom C. Aqueous flare intensity after phacoemulsification in patients with diabetes mellitus. *Cataract Refract Surg.* 1998;24:1099–1106.
33. Tennant MTS, Connolly BP. Cataract surgery in patients with retinal disease. *Curr Opin Ophthalmol.* 2002;13:19–23.
34. Kodama T, Hayasaka S, Setogawa T. Plasma glucose levels, postoperative complications, and progression of retinopathy in diabetic patients undergoing intraocular lens implantation. *Graefe's Arch Clin Exp Ophthalmol.* 1993;231:439–443.
35. Krupsky S, Zalish M, Oliver M, Pollack A. Anterior segment complications in diabetic patients following extracapsular cataract extraction and posterior chamber intraocular lens implantation. *Ophthalmic Surg.* 1991;22:526–530.
36. Fineman MS, Benson WE. Cataract surgery in patients with diabetes mellitus. *Comp Ophthalmol Update.* 2000;1:259–269.
37. Dowler JGF, Hykin PG, Hamilton AMP. Phacoemulsification versus extracapsular cataract extraction in patients with diabetes. *Ophthalmology.* 2000;107:457–462.
38. Moriarty AP, Spalton DJ, Moriarty BJ, et al. Studies of the blood-aqueous barrier in diabetes mellitus. *Am J Ophthalmol.* 1994;117:766–771.
39. Menchini U, Azzolini C, Camesasca FI, Brancato R. Combined vitrectomy, cataract extraction, and posterior chamber intraocular lens implantation in diabetic patients. *Ophthalmic Surg.* 1991;22:69–73.
40. Jaffe GJ, Burton TC, Kuhn E, et al. Reply to Progression of nonproliferative diabetic retinopathy and visual outcome after extracapsular cataract extraction and intraocular lens implantation. *Am J Ophthalmol.* 1993;115:401–402.

41. Benson WE. Cataract surgery and diabetic retinopathy. *Curr Opin Ophthalmol*. 1992;3:396–400.
42. Apple DJ, Federman JL, Krolicki TJ, et al. Irreversible silicone oil adhesion to silicone lenses. A clinicopathologic analysis. *Ophthalmology*. 1996;103:1555–1561.
43. Pavese T, Insler MS. Effects of extracapsular cataract extraction with posterior chamber lens implantation on the development of neovascular glaucoma in diabetics. *J Cataract Ref Surg*. 1987;13:197–201.
44. Aiello LM, Wand M, Liang G. Neovascular glaucoma and vitreous hemorrhage following cataract surgery in patients with diabetes mellitus. *Ophthalmology*. 1983;90: 814–820.
45. Prasad P, Setna PH, Dunne JA. Accelerated ocular neovascularisation in diabetics following posterior chamber lens implantation. *Br J Ophthalmol*. 1990; 74:313–314.
46. Parodi MB, Iacono P. Photodynamic therapy with verteporfin for anterior segment neovascularizations in neovascular glaucoma. *Am J Ophthalmol*. 2004;138:157–158.
47. Kubota T, Tawara A, Hata T, et al. Neovascular tissue in the intertrabecular spaces in eyes with neovascular glaucoma. *Br J Ophthalmology*. 1996;80:750–754.
48. Coyle JT. Progression of nonproliferative diabetic retinopathy and visual outcome after extracapsular cataract extraction and intraocular lens implantation. *Am J Ophthalmol*. 1993;115:824–825.
49. Poliner L, Christianson D, Escoffery R, et al. Neovascular glaucoma after intracapsular and extracapsular cataract extraction in diabetic patients. *Am J Ophthalmol*. 1985;100:637–643.
50. Rice TA, Michels RG, Maguire MG, Rice EF. The effect of lensectomy on the incidence of iris neovascularization and neovascular glaucoma after vitrectomy for diabetic retinopathy. *Am J Ophthalmol*. 1983;95:1–11.
51. Oshima Y, Sakaguchi H, Gomi F, Tano Y. Regression of iris neovascularization after intravitreal injection of bevacizumab in patients with proliferative diabetic retinopathy. *Am J Ophthalmol*. 2006;142:155–158.
52. Eren E, Kucukerdonmez C, YIlmaz G, Akova YA. Regression of neovascular posterior capsule vessels by intravitreal bevacizumab. *J Cataract Ref Surg*. 2007;33:1113–1115.
53. Blankenship G, Machemer R. Long-term diabetic vitrectomy results: report of 10 year follow-up. *Ophthalmology*. 1985;92:503–506.
54. Hutton WL, Pesicka GA, Fuller DW. Cataract extraction in the diabetic eye after vitrectomy. *Am J Ophthalmol*. 1987;104:1–4.
55. Grusha YO, Masket S, Miller KM. Phacoemulsification and lens implantation after pars plana vitrectomy. *Ophthalmology*. 1998;105:287–294.
56. Spaide RF, Fisher YL. Intravitreal Bevacizumab (Avastin) Treatment of proliferative diabetic retinopathy complicated by vitreous hemorrhage. *Retina*. 2006;26: 275–278.
57. Mason JO III, Nixon PA, White MF. Intravitreal injection of bevacizumab (avastin) as adjunctive treatment of proliferative diabetic retinopathy. *Am J Ophthalmol*. 2006;142:685–688.
58. Chew EY, Benson WE, Remaley NA, et al. Results after lens extraction in patients with diabetic retinopathy-Early treatment diabetic retinopathy study report number 25. *Arch Ophthalmol*. 1999;117:1600–1606.
59. Pollack A, Leiba H, Oliver M. Cystoid macular oedema following cataract extraction in patients with diabetes. *Br J Ophthalmol*. 1992;76:221–224.
60. Chung J, Kim MY, Kim HS, et al. Effect of cataract surgery on the progression of diabetic retinopathy. *J Cataract Refract Surg*. 2002;25:626–630.
61. Dev S, Pulido JS, Tessler HH, et al. Progression of diabetic retinopathy after endophthalmitis. *Ophthalmology*. 1999;106:774–781.
62. Chatterjee S, Savant VV, Stavrou P. Diabetic retinopathy progression and visual outcome after phacoemulsification in South-Asian and Afro-Caribbean patients with diabetes. *Eye*. 2004;18:575–579.
63. Flesner P, Sander B, Henning V, et al. Cataract surgery on diabetic patients. A prospective evaluation of risk factors and complications. *Acta Ophthalmol Scand*. 2002;80:19–24.
64. Pollack A, Dotan S, Oliver M. Course of diabetic retinopathy following cataract surgery. *Br J Ophthalmol*. 1991;75:2–8.
65. Schatz H, Atienza D, McDonald HR, Johnson RN. Severe diabetic retinopathy after cataract surgery. *Am J Ophthalmol*. 1994;117:314–321.
66. Pollack A, Dotan S, Oliver M. Progression of diabetic retinopathy after cataract extraction. *Br J Ophthalmol*. 1991;75:547–551.
67. Hauser D, Katz H, Pokroy R, et al. Occurrence and progression of diabetic retinopathy after phacoemulsification cataract surgery. *J Cataract Refract Surg*. 2004; 30:428–432.
68. Dowler JGF, Sehmi KS, Hykin PG, Hamilton AMP. The natural history of macular edema after cataract surgery in diabetes. *Ophthalmology*. 1999;106:663–668.
69. Kurtschan A, Heinz P, Wiegand W. Extrakapsulare kataraktoperation mittels kernexpression mit hinterkammerlinsenimplantation bei patienten mit diabetes mellitus – eine retrospektive studie an 145 patienten. *Klin Monatsnl Augenheilkd*. 2002;219:117–124.
70. Escaravage GK, Cohen KL, Patel SB, et al. Quantification of macular and optic disc hyperfluorescence after phacoemulsification in diabetes mellitus. *J Cataract Refract Surg*. 2006;32:803–811.
71. Patz A. Photocoagulation of retinal, vascular, and macular diseases through intraocular lenses. *Ophthalmology*. 1981;88:398–406.
72. Levin ML, Kincaid MC, Eifler CW, et al. Effect of cataract surgery and intraocular lenses on diabetic retinopathy. *J Cataract Refract Surg*. 1998; 14:642–649.
73. Henricsson M, Heijl A, Janzon L. Diabetic retinopathy before and after cataract surgery. *Br J Ophthalmol*. 1996; 80:789–793.
74. Bressler NM, Bressler SB. Exacerbation of diabetic macular edema after cataract surgery. The Wilmer Retina Update. 1996;2:69–85.
75. Cheema RA, Al-Mubarak MM, Amin YM, Cheema MA. Role of combined cataract surgery and intravitreal bevacizumab injection in preventing progression of diabetic retinopathy. A prospective randomized study. *J Cataract Refract Surg*. 2009;35:18–25.

76. Jaffe GJ, Burton TC, Kuhn E, et al. Progression of nonproliferative diabetic retinopathy and visual outcome after extracapsular cataract extraction and intraocular lens implantation. *Am J Ophthalmol.* 1992;114: 448–456.
77. Kim SY, Yang J, Lee YC, Park YH. Effect of a single intraoperative sub-Tenon injection of triamcinolone acetonide on the progression of diabetic retinopathy and visual outcomes after cataract surgery. *J Cataract Refract Surg.* 2008;34:823–826.
78. Suto C, Hori S, Kato S, et al. Effect of perioperative glycemic control in progression of diabetic retinopathy and maculopathy. *Arch Ophthalmol.* 2008;124: 38–45.
79. Jaffe GJ, Burton TC. Progression of nonproliferative diabetic retinopathy following cataract extraction. *Arch Ophthalmol.* 1988;106:745–749.
80. Henderson BA, Kim JY, Ament CS, et al. Clinical pseudophakic cystoid macular edema. Risk factors for development and duration after treatment. *J Cataract Refract Surg.* 2007;33:1550–1558.
81. Degenring RF, Vey S, Kamppeter B, et al. Effect of uncomplicated phacoemulsification on the central retina in diabetic and non-diabetic subjects. *Graefes Arch Clin Exp Ophthalmol.* 2007;245:18–23.
82. Johnson MW. Etiology and treatment of macular edema. *Am J Ophthalmol.* 2009;147:11–21.
83. Gass JDM, Norton EWD. Cystoid macular edema and papilledema following cataract extraction: a fluorescein funduscopic and angiographic study. *Arch Ophthalmol.* 1966;76:396–400.
84. Stark WJ J, Maumenee AE, Fagadau W, et al. Cystoid macular edema in pseudophakia. *Surv Ophthalmol.* 1984;28:442–451.
85. Lee YC, Chung FL, Chen CC. Intraocular pressure and foveal thickness after phacoemulsification. *Am J Ophthalmol.* 2007;144:203–208.
86. von Jagow B, Ohrloff C, Kohnen T. Macular thickness after uneventful cataract surgery determined by optical coherence tomography. *Graefe's Arch Clin Exp Ophthalmol.* 2007;245:1765–1771.
87. Lobo CL, Faria PM, Soares MA, et al. Macular alterations after small-incision cataract surgery. *J Cataract Refract Surg.* 2004;30:752–760.
88. Alpar JJ. Diabetes: cataract extraction and intraocular lens. *J Cataract Refract Surg.* 1987;13:43–46.
89. Menchini U, Cappelli S, Virgili G. Cataract surgery and diabetic retinopathy. *Semin Ophthalmol.* 2003;18: 103–108.
90. Menchini U, Bandello F, Brancato R, et al. Cystoid macular oedema after extracapsular cataract extraction and intraocular lens implantation in diabetic patients without retinopathy. *Br J Ophthalmol.* 1993; 77:208–211.
91. Nelson ML, Martidis A. Managing cystoid macular edema after cataract surgery. Curr Opin Ophthalmol. 2003;14:39–43.
92. Lobo CL, Bernardes RC, Cunha-Vaz JG. Alterations of the blood-retinal barrier and retinal thickness in preclinical retinopathy in subjects with type 2 diabetes. *Arch Ophthalmol.* 2000;118:1364–1369.
93. Kim SJ, Equi R, Bressler NM. Analysis of macular edema after cataract surgery in patients with diabetes using optical coherence tomography. *Ophthalmology.* 2007;114:881–889.
94. Laurell CG, Zetterstrom C, Lundgren B, et al. Inflammatory response in the rabbit after phacoemulsification and intraocular lens implantation using a 5.2 or 11.0 mm incision. *J Cataract Ref Surg.* 1997;23:126–131.
95. Shimura M, Nakazawa T, Yasuda K, Nishida K. Diclofenac prevents an early event of macular thickening after cataract surgery in patients with diabetes. *J Ocul Pharmacol Ther.* 2007;23:284–291.
96. Browning DJ. Diabetic macular edema: a critical review of the early treatment diabetic retinopathy study (ETDRS) series and subsequent studies. *Comp Ophthalmol Update.* 2000;1:69–83.
97. Gillies MC, Sutter FK, Simpson JM, et al. Intravitreal triamcinolone for refractory diabetic macular edema: two-year results of a double-masked, placebo-controlled, randomized clinical trial. *Ophthalmology.* 2006;113: 1533–1538.
98. Diabetic Retinopathy Clinical Research Network. A randomized trial comparing intravitreal triamcinolone acetonide and focal/grid photocoagulation for diabetic macular edema. *Ophthalmology.* 2008;115:1447–1459.
99. Arevalo JF, Garcia-Amaris RA, Roca JA, et al. Primary intravitreal bevacizumab for the management of pseudophakic cystoid macular edema: pilot study of the Pan-American Collaborative Retina Study Group. *J Cataract Refract Surg.* 2007;33:2098–2105.
100. Mason JO III, Albert MA Jr, Vail R. Intravitreal bevacizumab (Avastin) for refractory pseudophakic cystoid macular edema. *Retina.* 2006;26:356–358.
101. Cervera E, Diaz-Llopis M, Udaondo P, Garcia-Delpech S. Intravitreal pegaptanib sodium for refractory pseudophakic macular edema. *Eye.* 2008;22:1180–1182.
102. Hayashi K, Igarashi C, Hirata A, Hayashi H. Changes in diabetic macular oedema after phacoemulsification surgery [epub ahead of print] [Record Supplied By Publisher]. *Eye.* 2007;23:389–396.
103. Gupta A, Gupta V. Diabetic maculopathy and cataract surgery. *Ophthalmol Clin North Am.* 2001;14:625–637.
104. Browning DJ, McOwen MD, Bowen RM Jr, O'Marah TL. Comparison of the clinical diagnosis of diabetic macular edema with diagnosis by optical coherence tomography. *Ophthalmology.* 2004;111:712–715.
105. Brown JC, Solomon SD, Bressler SB, et al. Detection of diabetic foveal edema; contact lens biomicroscopy compared with optical coherence tomography. *Arch Ophthalmol.* 2004;122:330–335.
106. Lam DS, Chan CK, Mohamed S, et al. Phacoemulsification with intravitreal triamcinolone in patients with cataract and coexisting diabetic macular oedema: a 6-month prospective pilot study. *Eye.* 2005;19:885–890.
107. Bandello F, Brancato R, Lattanzio R, et al. Relation between iridopathy and retinopathy in diabetes. *Br J Ophthalmology.* 1994;78:542–545.
108. Mackool RJ. Progression of nonproliferative diabetic retinopathy and visual outcome after extracapsular cataract extraction and intraocular lens implantation. *Am J Ophthalmol.* 1993;115:400–401.

109. Browning DJ, Zhang Z, Benfield JM. The effect of patient characteristics on response to focal laser treatment for diabetic macular edema. *Ophthalmology*. 1997;104:466–472.
110. Hariprasad SM, Callanan D, Gainey S, et al. Cystoid and diabetic macular edema treated with nepafenac 0.1%. *J Ocul Pharmacol Ther*. 2007;23:585–590.
111. McCarty CA, Wright S, McKay R, et al. Changes in management of diabetic retinopathy by Australian ophthalmologists as a result of the NHMRC clinical guidelines. *Clinical and Exp Ophthalmol*. 2001;29:230–234.
112. Early Treatment Diabetic Retinopathy Study Research Group. Photocoagulation for Diabetic Macular Edema. *Arch Ophthalmol*. 1985;103:1796–1806.
113. Tunc M, Onder HI, Kaya M. Posterior sub-tenon's capsule triamcinolone injection combined with focal laser photocoagulation for diabetic macular edema. *Ophthalmology*. 2005;112:1086–1091.
114. Martidis A, Duker JS, Greenberg PB, et al. Intravitreal triamcinolone for refractory diabetic macular edema. *Ophthalmology*. 2002;109:920–927.
115. Lewis H. The role of vitrectomy in the treatment of diabetic macular edema. *Am J Ophthalmol*. 2001; 131:123–125.
116. Browning DJ, Fraser CM, Powers ME. Comparison of the magnitude and time course of macular thinning induced by different interventions for diabetic macular edema: implications for sequence of application. *Ophthalmology*. 2006;113:1713–1719.
117. Mamalis N, Teske MP, Kreisler KR, et al. Phacoemulsification combined with pars plana vitrectomy. *Ophthalmic Surg*. 1991;22:194–198.
118. Lahey JM, Francis RR, Kearney JJ. Combining phacoemulsification with pars plana vitrectomy in patients with proliferative diabetic retinopathy; a series of 223 cases. *Ophthalmology*. 2003;110:1335–1339.
119. Koenig SB, Mieler WF, Han DP, Abrams GW. Combined phacoemulsification, pars plana vitrectomy, and posterior chamber intraocular lens insertion. *Arch Ophthalmol*. 1992;110:1101–1104.
120. Benson W, Brown G, Tasman W, McNamara J. Extracapsular cataract extraction, posterior chamber lens insertion, and pars plana vitrectomy in one operation. *Ophthalmology*. 1990;97:918–921.
121. Blankenship GW, Flynn HW Jr, Kokame GT. Posterior chamber intraocular lens insertion during pars plana lensectomy and vitrectomy for complications of proliferative diabetic retinopathy. *Am J Ophthalmol*. 1989; 108:1–5.
122. Schiff WM, Barile GR, Hwang JC, et al. Diabetic vitrectomy: influence of lens status upon anatomic and visual outcomes. *Ophthalmology*. 2007;114:544–550.
123. Smiddy WE, Feuer W. Incidence of cataract extraction after diabetic vitrectomy. *Retina*. 2004;24: 574–581.
124. Montan PG, Koranyi G, Setterquist HE, et al. Endophthalmitis after cataract surgery: risk factors relating to technique and events of the operation and patient history-A retrospective case-control study. *Ophthalmology*. 1998;105:2171–2177.
125. Doft B, Wisniewski SR, Kelsey SF, et al. Diabetes and postoperative endophthalmitis in the endophthalmitis vitrectomy study. *Arch Ophthalmol*. 2001;119: 650–656.
126. Doft BH, Wisniewski SR, Kelsey SF, et al. Diabetes and postoperative endophthalmitis in the endophthalmitis vitrectomy study. *Arch Ophthalmol*. 2001;119:650–656.

Chapter 11
The Relationship of Diabetic Retinopathy and Glaucoma

David J. Browning and Michael H. Rotberg

11.1 Interaction of Diabetes and Glaucoma

Diabetes, diabetic retinopathy, and their various treatments can each influence a patient's risk of developing not only neovascular glaucoma, but open angle, narrow angle, and secondary glaucoma as well. After reviewing the connections between these types of glaucoma and diabetes, the pathogenesis and management of neovascular glaucoma will be discussed in detail.

Quigley et al. estimated that there are more than 60 million people with glaucoma worldwide.[1] While 171 million people had diabetes in 2004, by 2030 this number is expected to more than double.[2] How many of these diabetics also have glaucoma, and whether having diabetes increases the risk of developing glaucoma, remains unresolved. Bonovas performed a meta-analysis of studies that attempted to determine whether diabetes is a risk factor for open angle glaucoma and found that patients with diabetes were at increased risk of developing glaucoma.[3] Other studies have determined that the presence of type 2 diabetes and the duration of disease were each independently associated with a higher risk of having open angle glaucoma.[4] And in another recent study higher hemoglobin A1c levels were correlated with higher intraocular pressures.[5]

The mechanism by which diabetes may increase the risk of glaucoma remains speculative. Nakamura postulated that diabetes may not only increase the incidence of elevated intraocular pressure and the risk of vascular compromise but also impair neuronal and glial metabolism and promote apoptosis.[6] Corneal elasticity may also be abnormal in diabetics, causing falsely elevated intraocular pressure measurements.[7]

But while many studies have found an association between diabetes and open angle glaucoma[5,8–21] others do not confirm this finding.[22–29] Pache and Flammer[30] reviewed the literature and concluded that evidence does not yet exist to be able to claim conclusively that diabetes is a risk factor for the development of open angle glaucoma. In fact, the Ocular Hypertension Treatment Study[31] actually found diabetes to be protective and to reduce the likelihood of having glaucoma. Quigley has hypothesized that locally elevated VEGF concentrations in diabetic retinas may provide a neuroprotective environment for retinal ganglion cells, possibly explaining the paradoxical results. But since this is still the only study to have found diabetes to be advantageous in this way, the authors postulated that they may have been misled by having enrolled an unrepresentative group of diabetic patients, since only those without diabetic retinopathy were included.

Diabetes may also be directly implicated in the pathogenesis of some cases of narrow angle glaucoma. Rapid correction of hyperglycemia has been associated with the onset of acute angle closure glaucoma.[32–34] In Singapore, diabetes was found to be associated with the risk of developing narrow angle glaucoma, which is the variety most commonly found in this predominantly Asian population.[35] In this population of Singapore residents of Chinese ancestry, diabetics had shallower anterior

D.J. Browning (✉)
Charlotte Eye Ear Nose & Throat Associates, Charlotte, NC 28210, USA
e-mail: dbrowning@ceenta.com

D.J. Browning (ed.), *Diabetic Retinopathy*, DOI 10.1007/978-0-387-85900-2_11,

chambers and thicker lenses than an age- and gender-matched group of nondiabetics, even though axial length, refractive error, and vitreous chamber depth did not differ.[36] Wiemer et al.[37,38] also found increased lens thickness in a northern European population, but only in patients with type 1 diabetes, and the amount of thickening was also correlated with the duration of disease.

In addition, certain treatments of diabetic retinopathy and its complications may predispose to narrowing of the anterior chamber angles in ways unrelated to the specifics of the underlying disease. Panretinal photocoagulation and scleral buckling can both lead to transient choroidal thickening and forward rotation of the ciliary body with secondary narrowing of the anterior chamber angle. Silicone oil and intraocular gas can also push the iris forward and obstruct aqueous outflow.

Most well known, however, is the ability of steroids, by any route, to provoke elevated intraocular pressure. In general, diabetics are at higher risk than nondiabetics to develop a steroid response.[39] Intravitreal injection of triamcinolone, which places a long-term depot of the drug into the eye, has recently become a frequent cause of elevated intraocular pressure. The incidence of intraocular pressure rise after intravitreal triamcinolone (IVT) injection ranges from 30 to 68%,[40–44] with the elevation beginning between 7 and 60 days after injection. The risk is higher in younger patients, in males, and in those with a fluocinolone implant.[45–47] Most of these pressure spikes are clinically insignificant and self-limited, but in some cases glaucoma medications need to be started, and in others glaucoma filtration surgery or other interventions may be indicated.

When glaucoma medicine fails to control the intraocular pressure spike following IVT both argon laser trabeculoplasty[48,49] and selective laser trabeculoplasty can be effective.[50,51] Another novel approach is the anterior subtenons injection of anecortave acetate. Robin reported that four eyes of three patients with elevated IOP due to IVT responded to a single injection of anecortave acetate, with IOP falling within a month by an average of 48%, the effect lasting 6 months.[52] Further investigations of this approach to nonsteroid-related open angle glaucoma are also ongoing.[53,54]

Not only does diabetes influence the development of glaucoma, but intraocular pressure has a relationship to the development of diabetic retinopathy. Eyes with proliferative retinopathy on average have lower intraocular pressures than eyes with nonproliferative retinopathy.[55] High intraocular pressures can be protective with respect to the development of diabetic retinopathy, and many years ago the purposeful induction of a steroid response was seriously discussed as a possible treatment approach for diabetic retinopathy.[56] Conversely, low intraocular pressures are associated with worse diabetic macular edema as a logical consequence of Starling's law (see Chapter 7).[57] For unknown reason, diabetic patients who are steroid responders have slower rates of progression of diabetic retinopathy despite absence of differences in baseline intraocular pressures. That is, factors associated with the steroid response other than increased intraocular pressure may confer this relative resistance to diabetic retinopathy progression.[58]

11.2 Iris and Angle Neovascularization Pathoanatomy and Pathophysiology

The most clinically significant and vision-threatening link between diabetes and glaucoma is the propensity of diabetes to lead to neovascular glaucoma. The remainder of this chapter will review the anatomy, pathogenesis, and management of this challenging disorder.

The normal iris and angle structures are shown in Fig. 11.1. The iris has zones denoted as the pupillary margin, the collarette, the ciliary zone, and the iris root. The iris vascular endothelium is nonfenestrated with tight junctions, which comprise part of the blood–aqueous barrier. Fluorescein does not typically leak across the endothelium of iris vessels, but often does in the elderly, in pseudoexfoliation, and in inflamed eyes.[59,60]

The innermost angle structure is the trabecular meshwork, which bridges between the peripheral cornea (Schwalbe's line) and the scleral spur. Aqueous percolates through the meshwork as it leaves the anterior chamber, and then reaches Schlemm's canal, a circumferential channel that rests against

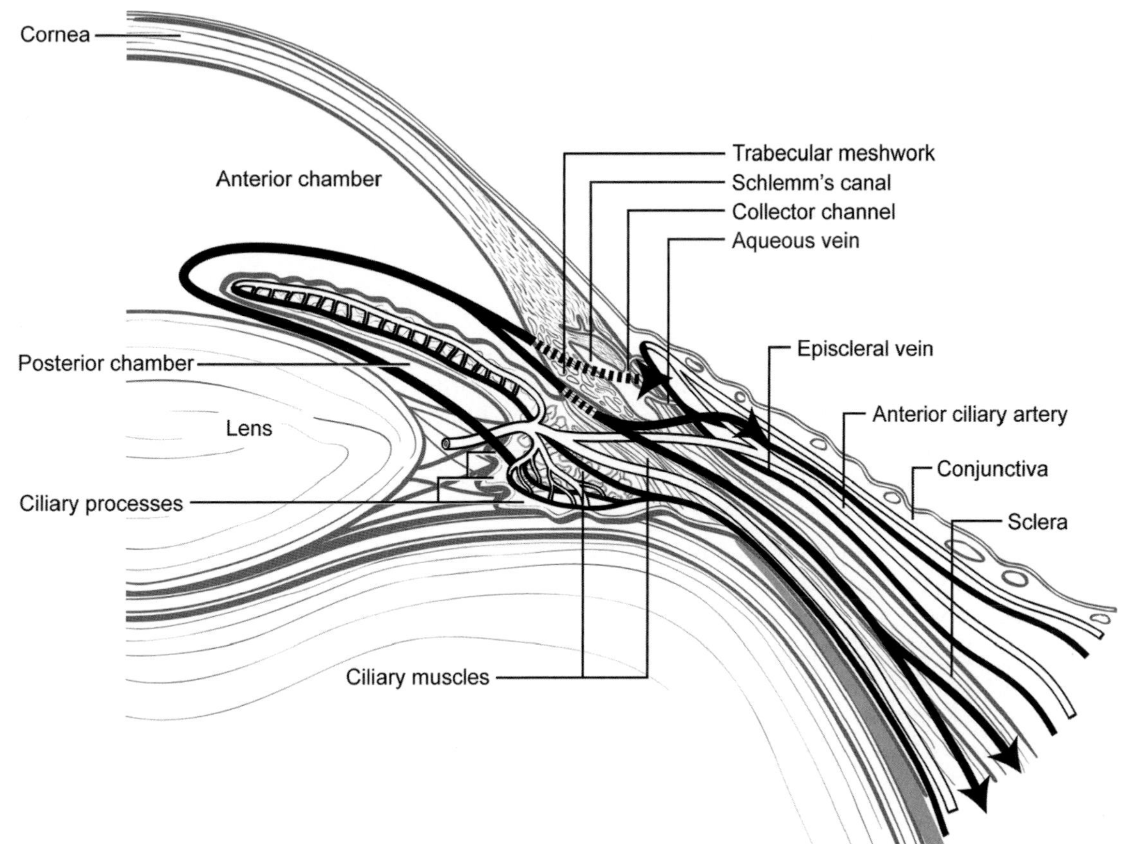

Fig. 11.1 Anatomy of the iris and anterior chamber angle showing the vascular supply and the structures through which aqueous humor passes in its route through the eye

the sclera. Aqueous leaves this canal through collector channels that carry it back into the bloodstream via aqueous veins, with a smaller amount leaving by a transconjunctival route. Aqueous also leaves the eye by a nontrabecular outflow pathway, primarily through the iris and the portion of the ciliary body that faces the anterior chamber.

Neovascularization occurring anterior to the retina in diabetic retinopathy arises secondary to retinal ischemia, which preferentially involves the midperipheral and peripheral retina in diabetic retinopathy.[61–63] Several varieties of the condition exist including entry site neovascularization after pars plana vitrectomy, anterior hyaloidal fibrovascular proliferation, cyclitic membrane formation, iris neovascularization (NVI), and anterior chamber angle neovascularization (NVA).[64] Retinal ischemia induces production of vascular endothelial growth factor (VEGF) in the retina and ciliary body, which diffuses into the vitreous gel and ultimately into the aqueous humor.[65] Other growth factors may also be involved.[66] Bathing the anterior and posterior surfaces of the iris and the anterior chamber angle, VEGF induces neovascularization in all these tissues with secondary scarring, synechiae formation, hemorrhage, obstruction of aqueous outflow, elevated intraocular pressure, and eventually ciliary body detachment and hypotony with phthisis bulbi.[67–69] Antibodies to VEGF can block this cascade of events in animal models and in clinical reports.[70–72]

The single most important factor in anterior segment neovascularization in association with diabetic retinopathy is the concentration of vascular endothelial growth factor (VEGF) in the aqueous humor.[73] Vitreous levels of VEGF are significantly correlated with the severity of diabetic retinopathy, and it is thought that the aqueous humor VEGF originates from the retina and the ciliary body, diffuses into the vitreous, and thence into the aqueous humor.[63–67]

Eyes with NVI are frequently observed to have dilated retinal vessels traversing zones of nonperfused retina ending in broom-like expanses of new vessels feeding a ridge of neovascularization just posterior to the ora serrata.[63] These findings have been described best by intraoperative fluorescein angiography employing an ophthalmic endoscope, and the descriptions and photographs resemble findings in retinopathy of prematurity.[63]

Neovascularization of the iris is associated with a myofibroblastic membrane on the iris surface that effaces iris surface crypts and contraction furrows and produces the tractional forces leading to ectropion uvea and angle synechia.[74] The new vessels lie beneath this myofibroblastic membrane (Figs. 11.2 and 11.3).[67] Although the new vessels predominantly grow on the anterior iris surface, cases have been reported in which they grow on the posterior surface and on the surface of the ciliary body.[75,76] They also can grow over the pupil and adhere to the lens (seclusio pupillae).[74] Untreated cases of NVI often progress to hyphema.[74]

The pathophysiology of anterior segment neovascularization explains how treatment has beneficial effects. The photoreceptor–retinal pigment epithelial complex consumes two-thirds of the oxygen used by the retina. Laser photocoagulation selectively destroys the retinal pigment epithelium and photoreceptor layers, thus decreasing oxygen consumption of the outer retina and allowing more choroidal oxygen to diffuse to the remaining, viable inner retina.[77] This downregulates the production of VEGF and leads to regression of anterior segment neovascularization.[78]

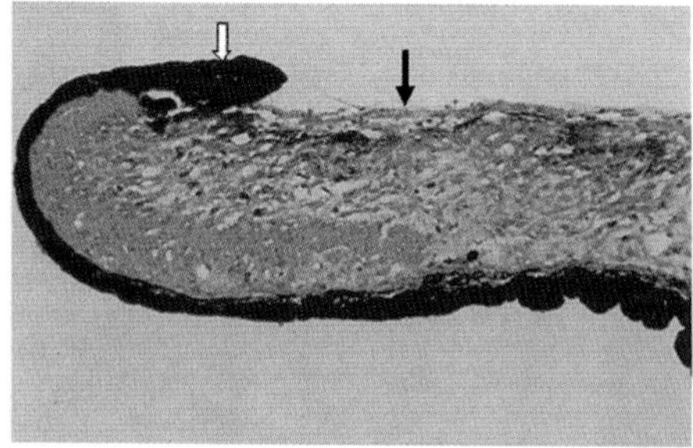

Fig. 11.2 A myofibroblastic membrane (*black arrow*) is present on the iris surface with subjacent iris new vessels. Ectropion uvea is indicated by the *open arrow*. Reprinted with permission from Roth and Brown[172]

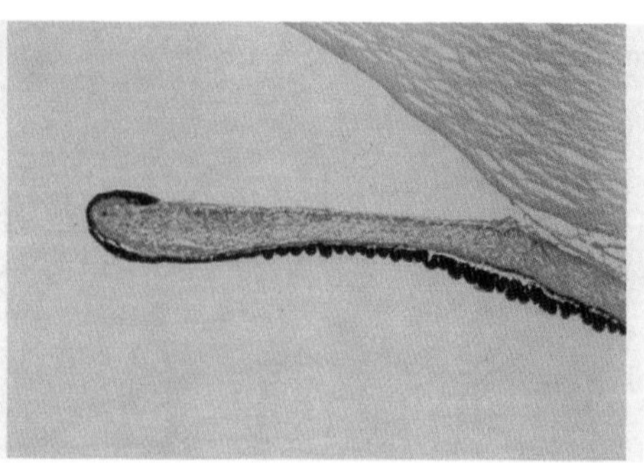

Fig. 11.3 Anterior synechia secondary to neovascularization of the iris causing effacement of the anterior chamber angle. Reprinted with permission from Roth and Brown[172]

11.3 Epidemiology

Presence of NVI and NVA in a diabetic patient is a sign of advanced diabetic retinopathy, and often is also a sign that diabetes treatment has not been adequate. Using the slit lamp examination for diagnosis, Ohrt[79] found no case of NVI without diabetic retinopathy, and 64% of cases of PDR had NVI. Using fluorescein gonioangiography, Ohnishi et al.[80] found NVA in 24% of eyes with NPDR and 73% of eyes with PDR. Consecutive series of eyes undergoing vitrectomy surgery for complications of diabetic retinopathy report preoperative NVI in 4–27% of eyes.[81,82] In a clinical series of eyes examined with iris fluorangiography and having varying degrees of retinopathy, the prevalence of NVI when severe NPDR and PDR were present was 44 and 66%, respectively.[83] No patients with less advanced retinopathy than severe NPDR had NVI.[83] In an unselected series of patients with untreated diabetic retinopathy from the 1950s, NVI was present in 6.8% of patients.[79] A similar series from 1980 was a lower prevalence of 3.8%.[84] This percentage is probably still higher than the true value as it derived from a tertiary referral clinic and was not population based.[84] In the DRS, 2.3% of eyes with PDR had NVI by clinical examination.[85] A higher percentage of cases of NVI are bilateral in association with diabetic retinopathy than other causes of NVI, reflecting the generally symmetric nature of diabetic retinopathy.[79] Bilateral involvement of NVI in association with diabetic retinopathy has been reported in 5–76%.[74] NVI occasionally spontaneously resolves clinically, although histological evidence of the vessels may be detected.[74,86,87]

11.4 Clinical Detection

Iris neovascularization usually follows the development of proliferative diabetic retinopathy, but cases have been described in which NVI was seen in the absence of PDR.[83,88,89] In these cases, however, severe nonproliferative retinopathy was present or intracapsular cataract extraction had been performed.[83,89] Studies have reported widespread areas of peripheral retinal capillary nonperfusion in eyes with PDR and in eyes with NVI.[62,63] There is a controversy regarding the sequence of anterior segment neovascularization.

Why the Difference in Sequence of Ocular Neovascularization in Different Diseases?

We have noted that in diabetic retinopathy, retinal neovascularization typically precedes iris and angle neovascularization and that typically pupillary margin neovascularization precedes angle neovascularization.[90] Why, then, in ischemic central retinal vein occlusion, is retinal neovascularization rare, but anterior segment neovascularization common, and why is it much more common in central retinal vein occlusion to find NVA before pupillary margin NVI?[91] And why, in retinoblastoma, is NVI present in 44–80% of cases, yet retinal neovascularization absent?[92,93] Henkind[93] hypothesized that the iris vessels are more sensitive to a diffusible factor, not known at the time, but now known to be VEGF. This seems too simple an explanation, as there is no evidence in the experimental models that iris vessels have greater sensitivity than retinal vessels to neovascularization to intravitreal injections of VEGF, and the gradient of VEGF is decreasing from vitreous to aqueous. Although VEGF is upregulated in necrotic retinoblastoma cells and in outer nuclear layer cells in adjacent areas of detached retina, it is possible that other molecules than VEGF contribute to NVI in cases of retinoblastoma.[92] Intraocular fluid samples have not been available to sample in this condition. In central retinal vein occlusion, the ischemic retina may have insufficient viability to respond to VEGF with neovascularization, in contrast to the iris vessels.

Most authors report that in diabetic patients pupillary margin iris neovascularization consistently precedes angle neovascularization, pathological evidence exists to support this sequence, and some classification schemes are based on this presumption.[59,75,79,83,87,90,74,94,80,95] In five clinical series comprising 245 eyes, no case of NVA was seen without concomitant NVI.[59,83,86,96,80] Based on Hanley's rule of three, we can be 95% confident that the probability of NVA without NVI is at most 3/245 (1.2%).[96,97] However, rare cases have been reported in which angle new vessels were seen in the absence of pupillary margin new vessels.[63,98] The authors consider the general clinical rule to be true, conceding that rare counterexamples may exist, and we have illustrated our understanding of the clinical sequence of anterior segment neovascularization in association with diabetic retinopathy based on this understanding (Fig. 11.4).

Unlike the situation with diabetic retinopathy, NVA is often found before pupillary margin NVI in central retinal vein occlusion, occurring in 12% of cases developing anterior segment neovascularization.[91] If it can occur in diabetic retinopathy, the frequency of its occurrence is much less, and there seems to be little reason to do undilated

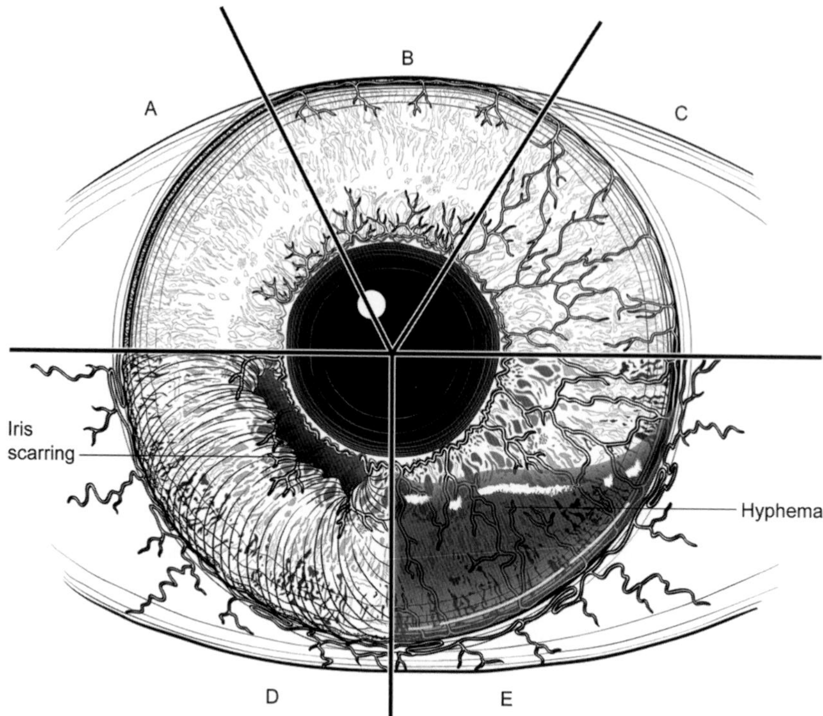

Fig. 11.4 Diagram illustrating the natural history of uninhibited anterior segment neovascularization associated with diabetic retinopathy. *A* – new vessels begin at the pupillary margin. *B* – next new vessels can appear in the angle. *C* – next the iris stroma is involved with new vessels and angle synechiae develop. *D* – pupillary margin posterior synechia to the lens capsule develop and iris bombe may occur. *E* – hyphema may occur when iris neovascularization bleeds. Adapted from and reproduced with permission from Roth and Brown[172]

gonioscopy in search of NVA in diabetic eyes with no pupillary margin NVI.[99] NVI in association with diabetic retinopathy behaves differently from NVI in association with central retinal vein occlusion. In the latter, the course of NVI is compressed and neovascular glaucoma can occur rapidly, whereas on an average the course is slower in the case of diabetic retinopathy.[88,100] This general observation may reflect the generally lower levels of intraocular VEGF seen in diabetic retinopathy compared with ischemic central retinal vein occlusion.

Actual Practice Patterns for Undilated Slit Lamp Examination in Patients with Diabetic Retinopathy

Preferred practice patterns are published by the American Academy of Ophthalmology "to identify characteristics and components of quality eye care."[101] It is of interest, therefore, to know if the intent of these patterns is being met in actual practice. An undilated slit lamp examination is considered part of the preferred practice, in part to detect NVI in patients with diabetic retinopathy. Regarding undilated slit lamp examination to check for NVI in diabetic patients, one of the authors (DJB) performed a survey in North Carolina to estimate congruence between preferred and actual practice patterns. Of 369 ophthalmologists polled, 335 (91%) responded. Forty-one percent of ophthalmologists report omitting undilated slit lamp examination in at least 25% of patients. Of the 138 ophthalmologists in this group, when asked if they modify their practice if they know the patient has had diabetes for at least 10 years, 44 (32%) responded that they do not. A potential problem exists in omitting undilated examination of the iris in patients with long duration of diabetes. It is likely that detection of NVI is impaired by dilation. An example is shown in Figs. 11.5 and 11.6.

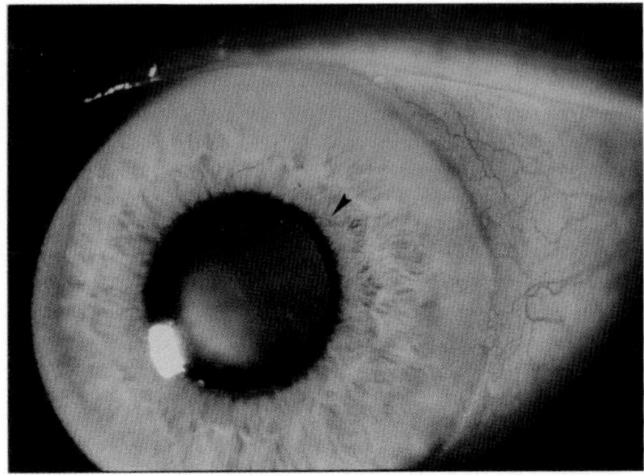

Fig. 11.5 In the undilated state, NVI is shown (*arrowhead*)

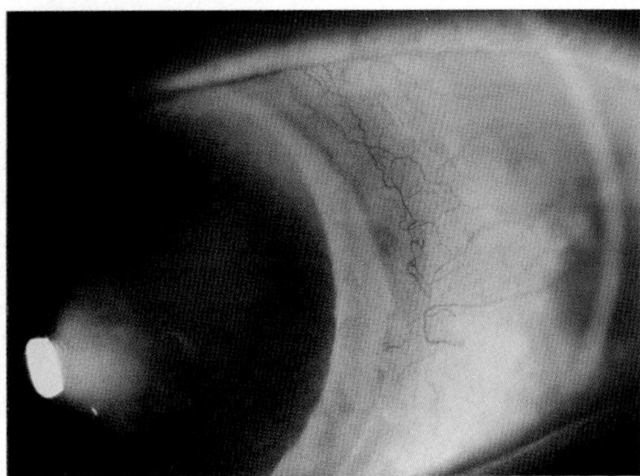

Fig. 11.6 In the dilated state, the NVI cannot be detected

Clinical detection of NVI is clouded by the difficulty of distinguishing dilated normal iris vessels from NVI. Eyes with inflammation can have dilated iris vessels that may masquerade as NVI. Iris neovascularization must also be distinguished from iris vascular tufts, which are located along the pupillary margin and do not occur on the surface of the iris stroma or in the angle.[90,102]

Iris color influences the ease of detection of NVI.[79] Clinical detection at the slit lamp is easier in a light-colored iris.[74] Subtle NVI may be difficult to discern in a dark-colored iris. Red-free light may make detection of the red NVI easier.[103] In difficult cases, iris fluorescein angiography and gonioangiography can make detection of NVI and NVA easier.[62,80] Iris fluorescein angiography is more sensitive than slit lamp biomicroscopy in the detection of NVI and NVA, but is also less specific.[80,104,105] Dilated iris vessels in eyes with iritis, normal iris vessels in older patients, and eyes of diabetics with retinopathy but no NVI can leak fluorescein on angiography just as does NVI, thus iris fluorescein angiography is not always a reliable method for distinguishing the two conditions.[59,106–108] Iris fluorangiography is an often forgotten method of assessing the presence of diabetic retinopathy in eyes with dense cataracts before proceeding to surgery. Presence of NVI implies that severe NPDR or worse is present and allows for preoperative planning such as use of intravitreal bevacizumab or early postoperative PRP.[83] Indocyanine green iris angiography has also been investigated in patients with diabetic retinopathy and is not as useful as iris fluorescein angiograms.[109]

Figures 11.7, 11.8, and 11.9 show standards useful in interpreting iris fluorescein angiograms.

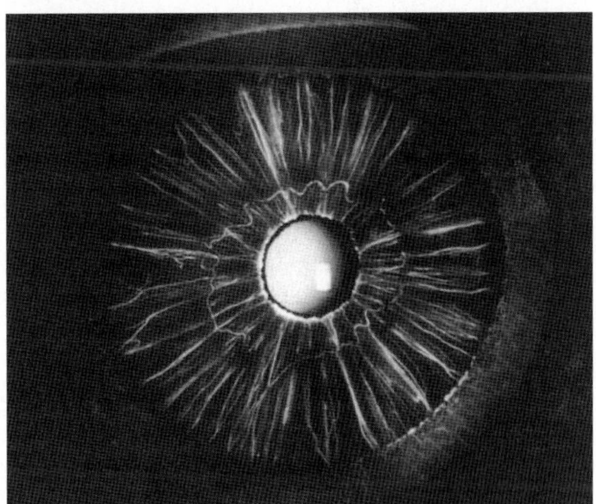

Fig. 11.7 Example of a normal iris fluorescein angiogram. No dye leakage is present, although in patients over the age of 50 years, a small amount of pupillary margin leakage of fluorescein can be considered normal. Reprinted with permission from Bandello et al.[83]

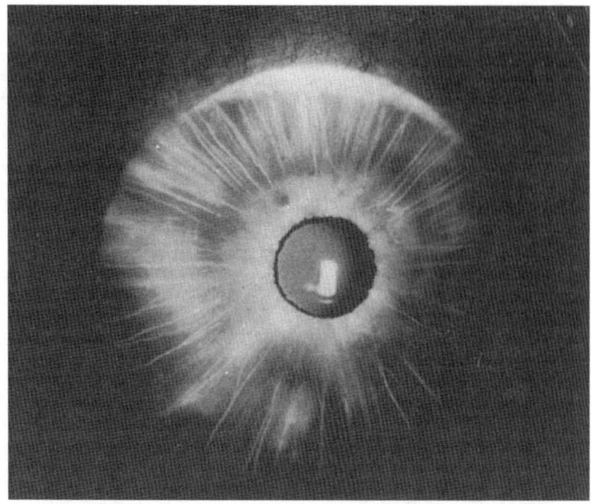

Fig. 11.8 Example of nonproliferative diabetic iridopathy. Dye leakage is prominent in the late phase but neovascularization is absent. Reprinted with permission from Bandello et al.[83]

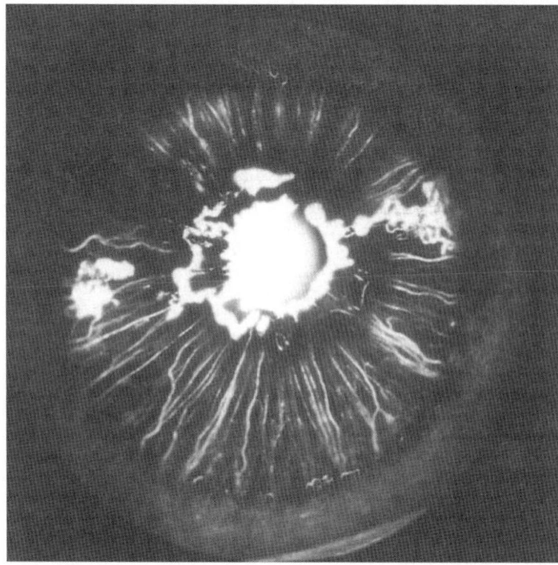

Fig. 11.9 Example of iris neovascularization present around the entire pupillary margin and at several places on the iris stroma. Reprinted with permission from Bandello et al.[83]

11.5 Classification

Several classification schemes for NVI and NVA have been proposed and none is accepted by the majority of clinicians.[62,83,88,110] There are also different classification schemes for the clinical and histopathological stages of NVA (Fig. 11.10).[82,111,112] The purpose of these schemes is to attempt to provide a prognosis for visual outcome and to allow correlations to be made with stages of diabetic retinopathy.[88,80] They differ not only in conception, but in the method used for detecting NVI and NVA. Although standardized classifications have attraction in common conditions such as diabetic retinopathy, the relative uncommonness of NVI makes the ability to recall details of any system difficult for the clinician, and we favor a method of straightforward description of pupillary margin and angle involvement by neovascularization as being most practical (Tables 11.1 and 11.2).

11.6 Risk Factors for Iris Neovascularization

Several risk factors for NVI relate to characteristics of diabetic retinopathy severity and fluorescein angiography. Hamanaka and colleagues performed nearly simultaneous goniofluorescein angiography and panoramic fundus fluorescein angiography in a series of eyes with proliferative diabetic retinopathy.[62] They graded eyes as having any capillary nonperfusion in the temporal raphe and radial peripapillary capillary network regions and graded whether midperipheral retinal capillary nonperfusion exceeded 50% or not. Figure 11.11 illustrates these regions. Presence of disk neovascularization (NVD) was also noted. They then correlated the presence of NVA with the findings on fundus fluorescein angiography and the status of NVD. The strongest risk factor for the presence of NVA was midperipheral capillary nonperfusion greater than 50% by area with a relative risk of 16.7 compared to eyes without this characteristic (Table 11.3). The relative risk is much higher for this factor because of the rarity of finding an eye with NVA when capillary nonperfusion of the midperiphery falls below 50%. Only 1 out of 28 such eyes had NVA.

Risk factors for development of NVI in eyes with diabetic retinopathy include previous vitrectomy and previous cataract extraction, both of which remove a diffusion barrier for VEGF access to the aqueous humor.[89,115] Attempts to predict postoperative NVI after vitrectomy by using preoperative iris fluorescein angiography have not been successful. Aphakia has been reported to be a risk factor for NVI in eyes with diabetic retinopathy in

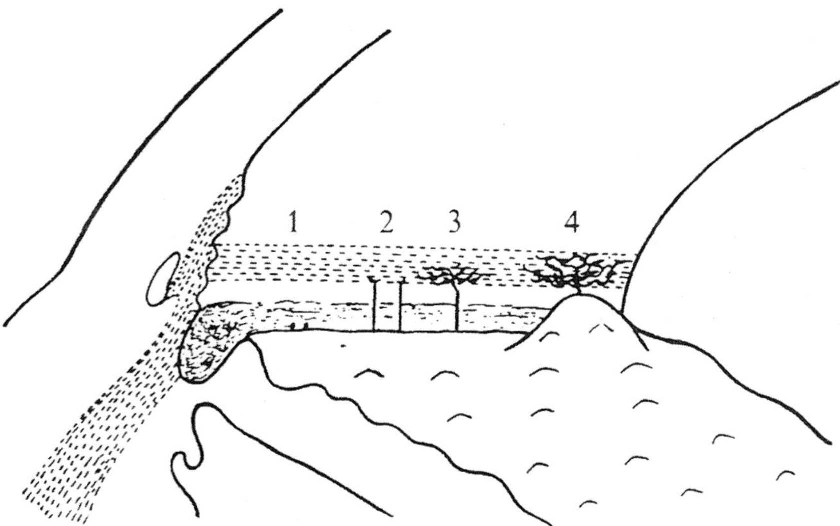

Fig. 11.10 Classification of NVA from Ohnishi et al. using fluorescein gonioangiography for detection. In grade 1, dot proliferations are seen at the iris root. In grade 2, a linear vessel arising from these dot proliferations rises at a perpendicular to the iris root to connect to the trabecular meshwork. In grade 3, an arborization of the vessel over the surface of the trabecular meshwork is seen. In grade 4, contracture of the neofibromyovascularization occurs with synechia. Reprinted with permission from Ohnishi et al.[80]

the past, but is rarely encountered in recent years because almost all eyes receive intraocular lens implants.[89,115] Posterior pseudophakia is probably not a risk factor for NVI, although anterior pseudophakia may be.[116] Silicone oil present in the vitreous cavity can reduce the risk of NVI in such cases, but not eliminate it.[117] Rhegmatogenous or peripheral tractional retinal detachment in an eye with diabetic retinopathy increases the risk of NVI, and repair of such detachments can lead to NVI regression.[68,118] Neodymium-YAG capsulotomy after extracapsular cataract extraction is a potential risk factor for anterior segment neovascularization.[119]

In eyes with diabetic retinopathy undergoing vitrectomy, the risk factors for postoperative development of rubeosis are intraoperative lensectomy, increased preoperative retinopathy severity, and absence of preoperative PRP associated with relative risks of 3.3 (95% CI 2.0, 5.4), 2.1 (95% CI 1.3, 3.4), and 1.7 (95% CI 1.1, 2.6), respectively.[68] If an eye undergoing vitrectomy has preoperative NVI, the odds are increased that it will have postoperative NVI.[95] In these cases, presence of a postoperative retinal detachment negatively affects regression of NVI.[95]

Table 11.1 Iris neovascularization grading systems

		Grades			
Reference	Detection method	0	1	2	3
Teich[88], Weiss[113]	Slit lamp biomicroscopy	Pupillary margin NVI <2 quadrants	Pupillary margin NVI >2 quadrants	Ciliary zone NVI or ectropion uvea of 1–3 quadrants	Ciliary zone NVI or ectropion uvea of 4 quadrants
Bandello[83]	Iris FA	No fluorescein leakage	Dilated iris capillaries that leak fluorescein	Pupillary margin or stromal new vessels that leak fluorescein	New vessels in the angle with elevated IOP
Tauber et al.[110]	Slit lamp biomicroscopy and gonioscopy	1 quadrant involved; pupillary margin, iris stroma, and angle involvement graded	2 quadrants involved; pupillary margin, iris stroma, and angle involvement graded	3 quadrants involved; pupillary margin, iris stroma, and angle involvement graded	4 quadrants involved; pupillary margin, iris stroma, and angle involvement graded

Not all the grading systems use the same numbering. Some start at zero and some start at 1. For comparison purposes, they have all been converted into a scale starting at zero. Ciliary zone – the outer zone of the iris separated from the pupillary zone by the collarette.

Table 11.2 Angle neovascularization grading systems

		Grades			
Reference	Detection method	0	1	2	3
Teich [88] Weiss[113]	Slit lamp biomicroscopy	NV twigs cross the scleral spur ≤ 2 quadrants	NV twigs cross the scleral spur > 2 quadrants	PAS of 1–3 quadrants	PAS of 4 quadrants
Little et al.[114]	Slit lamp gonioscopy	Few or no PAS without glaucoma	Few or many PAS with glaucoma	360° closed angle	
Ohnishi et al.[80]	Fluorescein		gonioangiography	Hyperfluorescent dots in the angle	
	Hyperfluorescent line in the angle perpendicular to the iris root	Hyperfluorescent network spreads over the trabecular meshwork	Peripheral anterior synechia present		

Not all the grading systems use the same numbering. Some start at zero and some start at 1. For comparison purposes, they have all been converted into a scale starting at zero.

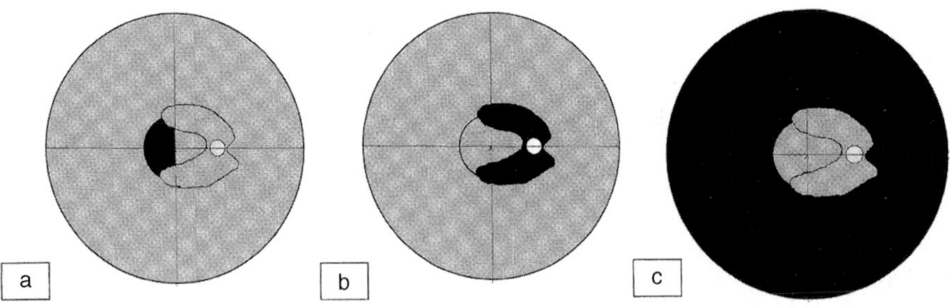

Fig. 11.11 Three regions of the fundus are depicted. The *black areas* represent the temporal raphe region (**a**), the radial peripapillary capillary network regions (**b**), and the midperipheral retina (**c**). Eyes were graded as to whether retinal capillary nonperfusion exceeded 50% or not. Reprinted with permission from Hamanaka et al.[62]

Table 11.3 Risk Factors for Angle Neovascularization

Fundus risk factor	Rate of occurrence of angle neovascularization (%)	Relative risk
Temporal raphe nonperfusion present	50	1.5
RPC area nonperfusion present	48	1.6
Midperipheral capillary nonperfusion >50%	60	16.7
Neovascularization of the disk	50	1.8

Data from Hamanaka et al.[62] The relative risk means risk when this factor is present compared to the case when it is not present.

Not only does lensectomy during vitrectomy increase the odds of postoperative development of NVI, if an eye has preoperative NVI and undergoes vitrectomy, the odds of postoperative regression of NVI decrease from 55 to 28% if an intraoperative lensectomy is performed.[95]

11.7 Entry Site Neovascularization After Pars Plana Vitrectomy

Entry site neovascularization after pars plana vitrectomy for proliferative diabetic retinopathy has been reported to occur in 18% of sclerotomies. Three configurations of proliferations have been described – spheroidal, tent shaped, and trapezoidal. The trapezoidal configuration is associated with the highest incidence of clinically important postvitrectomy vitreous hemorrhage requiring vitreous cavity washout. Rates for requiring vitreous cavity washout of postvitrectomy hemorrhage have ranged from 7.5 to 23.7% over ≥6 months of follow-up.[64,96] These rates are probably influenced by the case mixes of the eyes in the series. Unlike the situation with iris neovascularization, a possible confounding variable is the presence of vitreous incarceration in the entry site acting as a scaffold for proliferation. Surgeons generally make special efforts to prevent this occurrence by using maneuvers such as scleral depression to better view and access the vitreous base during surgery, and sometimes simultaneous cataract surgery to allow better access to this location. Other steps used to minimize the occurrence of entry site neovascularization include near-confluent laser photocoagulation to the anterior retina or peripheral retinal cryotherapy.[64,120,121] Iris neovascularization is sometimes associated with cases of entry site neovascularization.[122,120]

11.8 Anterior Hyaloidal Fibrovascular Proliferation

Anterior hyaloidal fibrovascular proliferation is the most common severe postoperative complication following vitrectomy for diabetic retinopathy occurring in approximately 13% of eyes within the first 12 months after vitrectomy. Neovascularization originating from the anterior retina grows into the anterior hyaloid and extends along the posterior lens surface causing early recurrent vitreous hemorrhage, cataract formation, peripheral retinal traction detachment, ciliary body detachment with hypotony, and often progressing to phthisis bulbi.[97,98] The typical patient developing this complication is a young male with poorly controlled diabetes mellitus, severe retinal ischemia, and frequently traction retinal detachment. Placement of a scleral buckle may increase the frequency of this complication.[97] Early recognition with lensectomy, repeat vitrectomy with aggressive dissection of anterior fibrovascular membranes, placement of confluent panretinal laser photocoagulation up to the ora serrata, and sometimes instillation of silicone oil may salvage such eyes.[97]

11.9 Treatments for Iris Neovascularization

The foundation for treatment of iris neovascularization is panretinal photocoagulation, which destroys ischemic retina and leads to reduced intraocular production of VEGF.[59,63,84,117,123] Although often effective, and differentially effective in NVI associated with diabetic retinopathy as opposed to central vein occlusion, PRP is not universally effective, and its effect is not immediate.[84,124,125] The effect of PRP is dose dependent.[125,126] Full PRP is more effective than partial PRP in causing regression of NVI.[125,126] Occasionally there is insufficient time for the effect of PRP to develop before irreversible damage such as angle synechia and optic atrophy from elevated pressure supervenes.[127] In these cases, a regression of neovascularization within 24 h can be effected by intravitreal or intracameral injection of bevacizumab or another anti-VEGF agent (Figs. 11.12a and b).[128–132] Bevacizumab is also helpful in cases in which PRP fails to cause regression of NVI.[128,129]This regression of NVI can boost the success rates of filtering surgeries, but the effects vanish as the drug leaves the eye, usually within 6 weeks.[128,133] Bevacizumab is best viewed as a bridge to allow more complete and sustainable reduction in intraocular VEGF concentrations through PRP or cryotherapy. Bevacizumab alters wound healing, reduces postoperative bleeding, and may augment the effectiveness of filtering surgery through these mechanisms.[128,133] Photodynamic therapy of NVI with intravenous verteporfin has also been used as a treatment to cause regression of NVI and prevent angle closure while the effect of PRP takes effect.[127] In some cases with vitreous hemorrhage precluding a view for office PRP, regression of NVI can be effected by vitrectomy with endolaser photocoagulation, or in eyes with poor visual potential, transscleral cryotherapy, or transscleral diode laser photocoagulation.[124,134–136]

The outcome of treatment of NVI and NVA is related to the severity of the anterior segment signs present before treatment. In general, the more

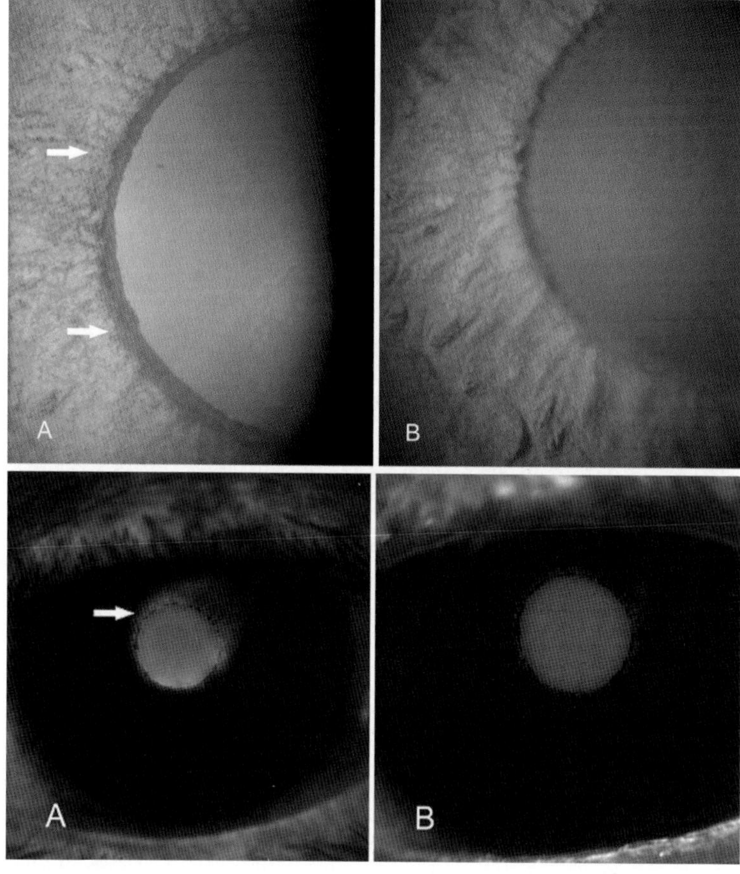

Fig. 11.12 Effect of Intravitreal Bevacizumab on Iris Neovascularization. (A) Neovascularization of the iris is shown at the white arrows in the iris photograph and iris fluorescein angiogram. (B) After intravitreal bevacizumab injection the neovascularization has regressed. Reprinted with permission from Grover[130]

extensive the PAS, the less likely that intraocular pressure control can be achieved with retinal ablation and medical therapy. For eyes with no PAS, 94% show regression of NVI with PRP and 12% have persistent elevation of IOP. For eyes with <270 degrees of angle closure, 25% have persistent IOP elevation after peripheral retinal ablation. Of eyes with >270 degrees of PAS, persistent IOP elevation was present in 67% of eyes.[88]

A subset of eyes with NVI progress to neovascular glaucoma. These eyes frequently require filtering surgery or tube shunt surgery to control the intraocular pressure. Adequate preoperative PRP and induced regression of anterior segment neovascularization are considered important to increase the chance of success of these procedures.[137] Presence of active intraocular neovascularization and presumptively elevated VEGF levels are thought to produce an exaggerated wound-healing response that mitigates the effectiveness of glaucoma surgery.[138]

In experimental models of NVI, systemic α-interferon injections and intravenous injections of squalamine, an antiangiogenic aminosterol, led to regression of NVI and prevention of NVI, respectively.[139,140] The side effects of interferon therapy in humans for other indications have been significant, and this experimental result has not translated into a practical treatment in human disease. Intravenous squalamine therapy has been tested in a phase 1 clinical trial for neovascular age-related macular degeneration, but has not been used in NVI.

11.10 Modifiers of Behavior of Iris Neovascularization

Removal of the lens in eyes with diabetic retinopathy undergoing vitrectomy surgery has traditionally been considered to raise the risk of subsequent development of NVI, but more recent reports in the era of endolaser photocoagulation suggest that this traditional teaching is no longer true.[119] In modern series, rates of postoperative development of NVI following vitrectomy surgery have been <5% whether the eyes are phakic or pseudophakic.[119] The postoperative NVI in these cases typically regresses with office PRP.[119]

Iris neovascularization secondary to diabetic retinopathy progresses less rapidly and responds better to PRP than that following retinal venous occlusions.[88] Because patients with diabetic retinopathy can have concomitant retinal venous occlusive disease, awareness of this relationship is important, and follow-up interval and heaviness of treatment adjusted as needed in the presence of two conditions.

Carotid artery occlusive disease can exacerbate a tendency for an eye with diabetic retinopathy to develop NVI and, paradoxically, may ameliorate the tendency in some cases.

11.11 Management of Neovascular Glaucoma

It was only a few decades ago that a textbook could say of neovascular glaucoma "the only practical treatment, if a retrobulbar injection of alcohol or cyclodiathermy fails to relieve the pain, is enucleation."[133] Fortunately, the prognosis for patients with NVG is much less grim today. The management of neovascular glaucoma has evolved dramatically since then, especially over the past few years as the emerging role of anti-VEGF medications has come into better focus.

In evaluating a patient with neovascular glaucoma it is first critical to determine the cause of the new vessels, since definitive treatment of the underlying disorder, whether it is diabetes, ocular ischemia, uveitis, radiation, or some other condition, makes management of the glaucoma more successful and preservation of vision more likely.[134] A dilated fundus exam is mandatory, and other studies including fluorescein angiography, noninvasive carotid ultrasound, or B-scan may provide additional useful information about the etiology.

Once the causative condition has been identified and addressed, the appropriate approach to a patient with neovascular glaucoma depends upon the stage at which the disease presents. The essential diagnostic test in staging NVG is gonioscopy. In Stage 1 NVG, there is rubeosis or angle neovascularization but the angle remains open and the IOP is still normal. Stage 2 NVG has iris or angle NV with elevated IOP. Stage 3 NVG is characterized in addition by peripheral anterior synechiae, and some degree of irreversible angle closure.[137] However, even before there are clinically visible peripheral anterior synechiae neovascular tissue can insinuate itself into intertrabecular spaces and disturb aqueous outflow.[115] All three stages of NVG may be associated with anterior chamber flare, conjunctival injection, hyphema, or photophobia, but ectropion uveae, corneal edema, decreased vision, headache, and eye pain more frequently appear in the advanced stages.

In Stage 1 NVG, the priority is to induce the new vessels to regress before they cause angle closure. Until recently, this meant applying urgent panretinal photocoagulation, which can, within 3–6 weeks, lead to resolution of rubeosis.[123] If the view of the retina is inadequate, other options include transscleral retina cryoablation or, more often, pars plana vitrectomy with endophotocoagulation, and possibly cataract extraction.

Now, however, the availability of medications to counteract the effect of VEGF has altered the therapeutic algorithm. An intravitreal or intracameral injection of an anti-VEGF medication such as bevacizumab can cause very rapid and long-lasting resolution of new vessels even before PRP can take effect. A growing literature, still mostly case reports and small series, attests to the utility of these medications in arresting the neovascular process and in causing rapid regression of the new vessels. The first case report appeared as recently as 2006. Avery reported regression of retinal and iris neovascularization when intravitreal bevacizumab was given after PRP. No side effects were noted.[71] Since then, many other reports have confirmed this impression.[72,136–143] Typical are the findings reported by Wakabayashi et al., whose large series of 41 eyes showed that intravitreal bevacizumab often leads to complete regression of neovascularization within a week.[144] Although many eyes had recurrent rubeosis within 6 months, beginning on average after 2 months, repeat injections were usually effective. In eyes with elevated IOP but open angles, the typical result of a single injection was not only regression of rubeosis but also normalization of IOP within a week as well. Eyes with synechial angle closure due to NVG had resolution of rubeosis but no improvement in IOP. Martinez-Carpio surveyed the burgeoning literature in this area.[145] In the 26 articles he compiled, none of which were randomized studies, the use of intravitreal bevacizumab injections for NVG was associated with no systemic complications and less than 1% ocular complications.

This medication may also be given as an intracameral injection with similarly dramatic reductions in new vessels, IOP, and aqueous VEGF levels.[130–132] When cultured human corneal endothelial cells were exposed to a normal therapeutic concentrations of bevacizumab, no toxic effects were identified.[146,147]

It is uncertain whether such injections by either route are better given before, after, or on the same day as PRP, since publications report rapid regression of NV regardless of the sequence.[71,140,141] In some eyes PRP may be easier to perform after new vessels have regressed, IOP has normalized, the cornea has cleared, and hyphema has resolved. But in general, when retinal ischemia is the cause of iris neovascularization, the sooner the underlying disorder can be treated the better, and PRP should be applied as soon as possible to begin to build a long-term solution upon the acute improvement that anti-VEGF medication can provide.

In Stage 2 NVG, which presents with rubeosis, elevated IOP, and open angles, the IOP needs to be controlled medically until the new vessels regress. Once the neovascular process has been arrested and reversed the IOP may return to normal, allowing glaucoma medications to be tapered and discontinued. As in Stage 1 NVG, the first priority is to treat the underlying cause of the rubeosis, to do aggressive PRP, and to consider injection of an anti-VEGF medication either into the vitreous or into the anterior chamber. At the same time medications to lower the IOP and to control inflammation can be started to prevent optic nerve damage and to encourage corneal edema to clear, so the eye can be more fully examined.

Aqueous suppressants, such as beta-blockers, carbonic anhydrase inhibitors, and alpha-2 agonists, are all often effective. Prostaglandin analogues may also be helpful, but can aggravate inflammation in these eyes. Miotics (cholinergic drops) should not be used. The pain that NVG patients experience is just as often due to inflammation as to high IOP and may persist even after the IOP is controlled. It is also important to begin topical corticosteroid drops and cycloplegics to reduce inflammation, relieve pain, and stabilize the blood–aqueous barrier.

Patients presenting with synechial angle closure (Stage 3 NVG) will almost always have persistent elevated IOP even after their new vessels regress, and most soon require some sort of glaucoma surgery to lower IOP and preserve vision. In fact, whichever Stage NVG the patient has at presentation, if IOP cannot be controlled medically glaucoma surgery is indicated, but deciding upon the appropriate procedure depends upon the eye's vision potential. Incisional surgery, such as trabeculectomy or a glaucoma drainage implant, is best reserved for eyes in which vision can be preserved. Nonpenetrating glaucoma procedures, such as viscocanalostomy or canaloplasty, are unlikely to be helpful in these cases, especially if the angle is closed. If vision is expected to remain very poor because of extensive retinal ischemia or advanced optic nerve damage, the risks of incisional surgery may not be acceptable, and a cyclodestructive procedure should be considered. Blind painful eyes may be treated with retrobulbar injections or by evisceration or enucleation.[148] Each of these approaches will be discussed.

Trabeculectomy surgery has historically had a very poor success rate in neovascular glaucoma. Full PRP improves the prognosis for trabeculectomy, but the vessels may take several weeks to regress.[149] Surgery in such eyes is complicated by excessive risk of inflammation and hemorrhage. Even with the help of 5-FU or mitomycin-C, the chance of long-term filtration is minimal in an eye with active rubeosis, since aqueous containing high levels of VEGF will leave the eye through the sclerostomy and promote neovascularization that can cause the bleb to scar. For this reason, many glaucoma surgeons have preferred to perform trabeculectomy with mitomycin for immediate IOP control soon after PRP, while at the same time placing a glaucoma implant, expecting that the trabeculectomy would be scarring closed and beginning to fail by the time the temporary ligature around the implant tube opened after 1–2 months.

Recent reports of the adjunctive use of anti-VEGF medications suggest that they may improve the outlook for filtration surgery in eyes with NVG. Bevacizumab has been injected into the vitreous,[121,127,150,128,133] into the anterior chamber,[151] and subconjunctivally[152] to good effect. These medications also have an inhibitory effect on fibroblasts[153,154] and have been used post-operatively to rescue failing filtering blebs, taking advantage of this effect of the drugs.[155,156] While very promising, the appropriate role for anti-VEGF medications to augment trabeculectomy is being clarified.

Prior to the use of anti-VEGF drugs, most patients needing filtering surgery for NVG had glaucoma implant procedures, using the Ahmed, Baerveldt, Molteno, or Krupin valves (Fig. 11.13). Even so, long-term success rates were poor, with reported 5-year control of IOP in only 25–30% of patients with NVG.[157,158] Progression of underlying ischemia can lead to vision loss even when IOP is well treated.[159] Glaucoma implants can be placed either after or at the same time as pars plana vitrectomy and endophotocoagulation, with or without intravitreal bevacizumab. The tube can be placed into the anterior chamber, or if the angle is closed into the sulcus, or through the pars plana.[160–162] Placement of a glaucoma implant may be technically difficult in an eye that has an encircling band. In these eyes, a drainage tube without a plate can be threaded from the anterior chamber into the capsule that encases the scleral buckle (anterior chamber tube shunt to encircling band).[163–165]

As in trabeculectomy, there is an increased chance of success if the neovascular stimulus can be diminished before venting aqueous from the eye through a tube. Bevacizumab has been reported to be helpful in improving the outcome of glaucoma implant surgery as well. Two investigators have reported good results performing glaucoma implant surgery after intravitreal injection of anti-VEGF medication.[166,167] Eid reported a series of 20 eyes in which he gave intravitreal bevacizumab, followed 1–2 weeks later by Ahmed glaucoma implant surgery. Successful IOP control was achieved in 85% of those who were treated with PRP and bevacizumab prior to glaucoma implant, compared to a 70% success rate in those who were given PRP alone. Again, more work remains to be done before the role of bevacizumab in glaucoma implant surgery for NVG.

In spite of the improving results being reported with trabeculectomy and glaucoma implant for NVG, in eyes that have a poor visual prognosis the risk of incisional surgery may not be justified. In such eyes, cyclophotocoagulation may be the most appropriate procedure. The diode laser, applied to the surface of the eye, can reduce IOP in patients with NVG as effectively as can trabeculectomy (Fig. 11.14).[168,169]

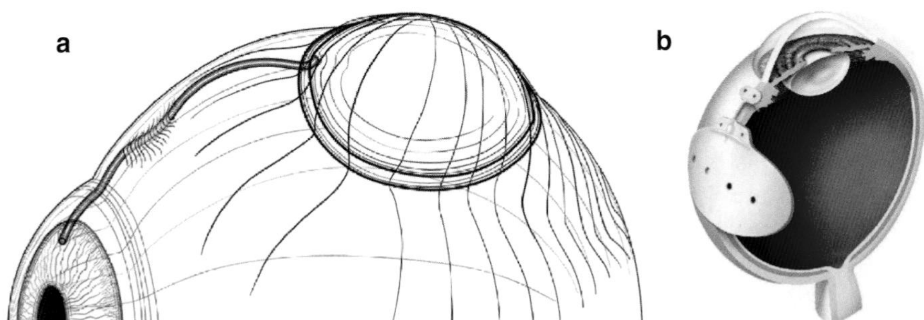

Fig. 11.13 (**a**) Diagram of an Ahmed glaucoma implant with the drainage tube placed in the anterior chamber, covered by a patch graft of sclera, and ending in a reservoir sutured to the sclera allowing posterior filtration. (**b**) Diagram of a Baerveldt glaucoma implant with the drainage tube placed through the pars plana into the vitreous cavity following vitrectomy and ending in a reservoir sutured to the sclera

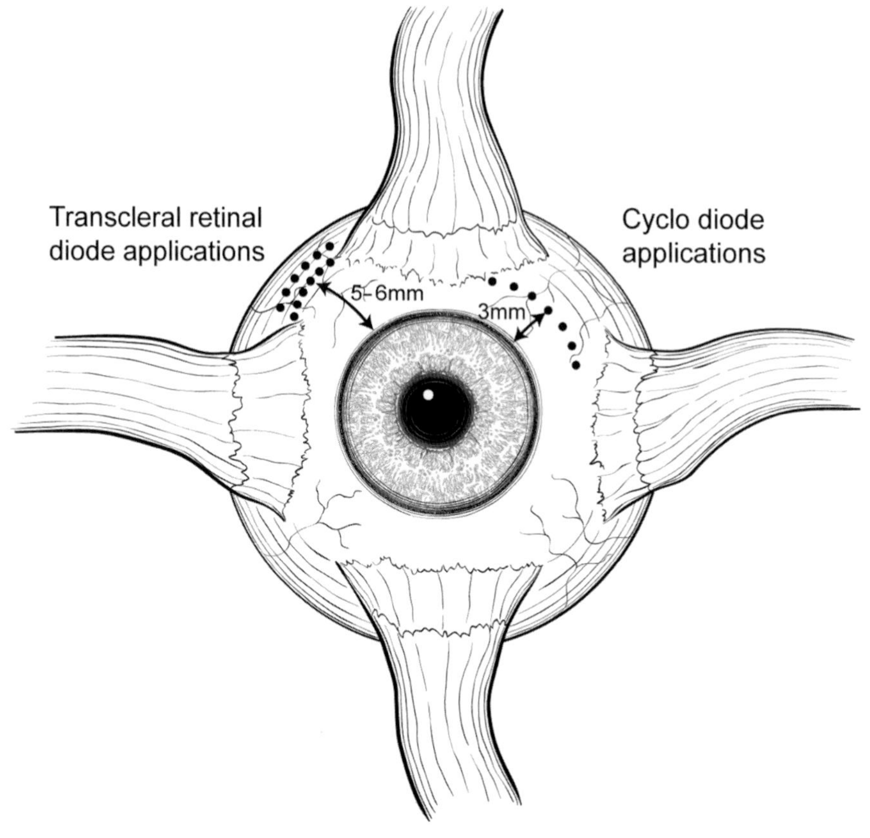

Fig. 11.14 Diagram illustrating location and spacing of transscleral photocoagulation spots for retinal and ciliary body treatment in cases with iris neovascularization with or without neovascular glaucoma

How to Perform Transscleral Cyclophotocoagulation

A retrobulbar anesthetic injection using either Lidocaine 2% or Lidocaine combined with Bupivacaine 0.75% is given and allowed to take effect. The diode laser is portable and durable and allows treatments to be done in the office or hospital. A fiber with a special handpiece is used; the handpiece features a footplate specifically designed for this procedure. When this footplate is placed along the limbus the fiberoptic tip sits on the surface of the eye directly over the ciliary body, the energy focused more than a millimeter from the tip, concentrating laser energy in the target tissue. A lid speculum is placed. With the laser set to deliver pulses lasting 2 s, with power settings of between 1,500 and 2,000 mW, a total of 20–30 applications of the laser are given to the full circumference of the limbus, sparing only the horizontal meridians to avoid damaging the long posterior ciliary arteries. Subconjunctival decadron as well as topical prednisolone and atropine are placed on the eye. All glaucoma medications are continued. Postoperative pain is usually not severe. Intraocular pressure typically falls for 6–8 weeks, and a single treatment gives adequate pressure reduction in about two of three patients. The treatment may be repeated if the IOP remains too high a few months after the initial treatment.[170]

Another way to ablate the ciliary body is the older technique of cyclocryotherapy, which tends to provoke more inflammation and pain than does the diode laser. Also, diode laser energy may be delivered directly to the ciliary processes using the ocular endoscope. While endocyclophotocoagulation (ECP) has the advantage of being able to place laser treatment precisely where it is needed without damaging adjacent structures, and may cause even less inflammation than transscleral treatment, the cost of the equipment and the fact that this is an intraocular procedure have limited its acceptance.[171]

When dealing with a blind and painful eye caused by NVG, the goal of IOP reduction is simply to improve patient comfort. There are reports that cyclophotocoagulation may lead to sympathetic ophthalmia, and therefore some physicians feel it should not be used in blind eyes.[170] Topical steroids and cycloplegics can provide long-term pain control in some patients. Retrobulbar alcohol or chlorpromazine injection[171] is another way to control pain and avoid enucleation or evisceration, although in some badly damaged eyes this is the definitive approach.

11.12 Summary of Key Points

- Whether diabetes predisposes to primary open angle glaucoma is an unresolved issue, a surprising change from a long-held notion linking the two diseases.
- Intravitreal triamcinolone injection, commonly used for complications of diabetic retinopathy, is associated with secondary intraocular pressure elevation in a large fraction of cases and must be monitored. Most cases that develop can be successfully treated with topical therapy.
- Neovascularization of the iris (NVI) arises in response to retinal hypoxia. Vascular endothelial growth factor (VEGF) produced in the retina diffuses into the vitreous and thence to the aqueous, which bathes the iris and angle. They in turn respond with growth of new vessels.
- NVI is usually associated with proliferative diabetic retinopathy. Neovascularization of the angle (NVA) rarely develops without preceding NVI.
- NVI will be often missed if the eye is examined after pupillary dilation. If no pupillary margin NVI is present before dilation, it is unnecessary to perform routine gonioscopy to search for NVA.
- In a diabetic eye with a dense cataract, iris angiography to look for NVI can allow the clinician to infer the severity of the diabetic retinopathy.
- No single classification system for NVI or NVA has been widely adopted.
- Injection of anti-VEGF drugs into the eye can cause rapid, temporary regression of NVI and NVA. Panretinal ablation by laser or cryotherapy is required to cause sustained regression.
- If angle structures have been damaged by NVA, various glaucoma treatments can be used to control the intraocular pressure, starting with topical therapy, progressing to surgical therapy, and in eyes with little visual potential sometimes involving ciliary body destruction.

11.13 Future Directions

The question of diabetes as a risk factor for primary open angle glaucoma will be resolved by large population-based studies that adequately control for confounding variables. The use of anecortave acetate as a therapy for steroid-induced glaucoma is a promising development in need of further study. Longer duration anti-VEGF drugs and sustained delivery devices may be developed that overcome the short-term effect of intraocular injections of bevacizumab and ranibizumab. Surgical therapy for neovascular glaucoma will continue to be refined.

References

1. Quigley HA, Broman AT. The number of people with glaucoma worldwide in 2010 and 2020. *Br J Ophthalmol*. 2006;90:262–267.
2. Wild S, Green A, Sicree R, King H. Global prevalence of diabetes: estimates for the year 2000 and projections for 2030. *Diabetes Care*. 2004;27:1047–1053.
3. Bonovas S, Peponis V, Filioussi K. Diabetes mellitus as a risk factor for primary open-angle glaucoma: a meta-analysis. *Diabetes Med*. 2004;21:609–614.
4. Chopra V, Varma R, Francis BA et al. Type 2 diabetes mellitus and the risk of open-angle glaucoma. The Los Angeles Latino Eye Study. *Ophthalmology*. 2008;115: 227–232.

5. Memarzadeh F, Ying-Lai M, Azen SP, Varma R, on behalf of the Los Angeles Latino Eye Study Group. Associations with intraocular pressure in Latinos: the Los Angeles Latino Eye Study. *Am J Ophthalmol.* 2008;146:69–76.
6. Nakamura M, Kanamori A, Negi A. Diabetes mellitus as a risk factor for glaucomatous optic neuropathy. *Ophthalmologica.* 2005;219:1–10.
7. Krueger RR, Ramos-Esteban JC. How might corneal elasticity help us understand diabetes and intraocular pressure? *J Refract Surg.* 2007;23:85–88.
8. The Advanced Glaucoma Intervention Study (AGIS):12. Baseline risk factors for sustained loss of visual field and visual acuity in patients with advanced glaucoma. *Am J Ophthalmol.* 2002;134:499–512.
9. Armstrong JR, Daily RK, Dobson HL, Girard LJ. The incidence of glaucoma in diabetes mellitus. A comparison with the incidence of glaucoma in the general population. *Am J Ophthalmol.* 1960;50:55–63.
10. Becker B. Diabetes mellitus and primary open-angle glaucoma. The XXVII Edward Jackson Memorial Lecture. *Am J Ophthalmol.* 1971;1:1–16.
11. De Voogd S, Ikram MK, Wolfs RC, et al. Is diabetes mellitus a risk factor for open-angle glaucoma? The Rotterdam Study. *Ophthalmology.* 2006;113:1827–1831.
12. Klein BE, Klein R, Jensen SC. Open-angle glaucoma and older-onset diabetes. The Beaver Dam Eye Study. *Ophthalmology.* 1994;101:1173–1177.
13. Klein BE, Klein R, Moss SE. Intraocular pressure in diabetic persons. *Ophthalmology.* 1984;91:1356–1360.
14. Klein BE, Klein R, Moss SE. Incidence of self reported glaucoma in people with diabetes mellitus. *Br J Ophthalmol.* 1997;81:743–747.
15. Mitchell P, Smith W, Chey T, et al. Open-angle glaucoma and diabetes: the Blue Mountains Eye Study. Australia. *Ophthalmology.* 1997;104:712–718.
16. Nielsen NV. The prevalence of glaucoma and ocular hypertension in type 1 and 2 diabetes mellitus. An epidemiological study of diabetes mellitus on the island of Falster, Denmark. *Acta Ophthalmol.* 1983;61:662–672.
17. Leske MC. The epidemiology of open-angle glaucoma: a review. *Am J Epidemiol.* 1983;118:166–191.
18. Wu SY, Leske MC. Associations with intraocular pressure in the Barbados Eye Study. *Arch Ophthalmol.* 1997;115:1572–1576.
19. Bonomi L, Marchini G, Marraffa M, Bernardi P, Morbio R, Varotto A. Vascular risk factors for primary open-angle glaucoma: the Egna–Neumarkt Study. *Ophthalmology.* 2000;107:1287–1293.
20. Hennis A, Wu SY, Nemesure B, Leske MC. Hypertension, diabetes, and longitudinal changes in intraocular pressure. *Ophthalmology.* 2003;110:908–914.
21. Dielemans I, de Jong PT, Stolk R, Vingerling JR, Grobbee DE, Hofman A. Primary open-angle glaucoma, intraocular pressure, and diabetes mellitus in the general elderly population: the Rotterdam Study. *Ophthalmology.* 1996;103:1271–1275.
22. Bankes JL. Ocular tension and diabetes mellitus. *Br J Ophthalmol.* 1967;51:557–561.
23. Grødum K, Heijl A, Bengtsson B. Optic disc hemorrhages and generalized vascular disease. *J Glaucoma.* 2002;11:226–230.
24. Kahn HA, Leibowitz HM, Ganley JP, et al. The Framingham Eye Study. II. Association of ophthalmic pathology with single variables previously measured in the Framingham Heart Study. *Am J Epidemiol.* 1977;106:33–41.
25. Leibowitz HM, Krueger DE, Maunder LR, et al. The Framingham Eye Study monograph: an ophthalmological and epidemiological study of cataract, glaucoma, diabetic retinopathy, macular degeneration, and visual acuity in a general population of 2631 adults, 1973–1975. *Surv Ophthalmol.* 1980;24:335–610.
26. Leske MC, Connell AM, Wu SY, et al. Risk factors for open angle glaucoma. The Barbados Eye Study. *Arch Ophthalmol.* 1995;113:918–924.
27. Tielsch JM, Katz J, Quigley HA, et al. Diabetes, intraocular pressure, and primary open-angle glaucoma in the Baltimore Eye Survey. *Ophthalmology.* 1995;102: 48–53.
28. Wilson MR, Hertzmark E, Walker AM, et al. A case–control study of risk factors in open angle glaucoma. *Arch Ophthalmol.* 1987;105:1066–1071.
29. Ellis JD, Morris AD, MacEwen CJ. Should diabetic patients be screened for glaucoma? DARTS/MEMO Collaboration. *Br J Ophthalmol.* 1999;83:369–372.
30. Pache M and Flammer J. A sick eye in a sick body? Systemic findings in patients with primary open-angle glaucoma. *Surv Ophthalmol.* 2006;51:179–212.
31. Gordon MO, Beiser JA, Brandt JD, Heuer DK, Higginbotham EJ, Johnson CA, Keltner JL, Miller JP, Parrish RK, Wilson MR, Kass MA, for the Ocular Hypertension Treatment Study Group. The ocular hypertension treatment study: baseline factors that predict the onset of primary open-angle glaucoma. *Arch Ophthalmol.* 2002;120:714–720.
32. Blake DR, Nathan DM. Acute angle closure glaucoma following rapid correction of hyperglycemia. *Diabetes Care.* 2003;26:3197–3198.
33. Sorokanich S, Wand M, Nix HR. Angle closure glaucoma and acute hyperglycemia. *Arch Ophthalmol.* 1986;104:1434.
34. Smith JP. Angle closure glaucoma and acute hyperglycemia (Letter). *Arch Ophthalmol.* 1987;105:454–455.
35. Clark CV. Diabetes mellitus in primary glaucomas. *Ann Acad Med Singapore.* 1989;18:190–194.
36. Saw SM, Wong TY, Ting S, Foong AW, Foster PJ. The relationship between anterior chamber depth and the presence of diabetes in the Tanjong Pagar Survey. *Am J Ophthalmol.* 2007;144:325–326.
37. Wiemer NGM, Dubbelman M, Kostense PJ, Ringens PF, Polak BCP. The influence of diabetes mellitus type 1 and 2 on the thickness, shape, and equivalent refractive index of the human crystalline lens. *Ophthalmology.* 2008;115:1679–1686.
38. Wiemer NGM, Dubbelman M, Hermans EA, Ringens PF, Polak BCP. Changes in the internal structure of the human crystalline lens with diabetes mellitus type 1 and type 2. *Ophthalmology.* 2008;115:2017–2023.
39. Jones R, Rhee DJ. Corticosteroid-induced ocular hypertension and glaucoma: a brief review and update of the literature. *Curr Opin Ophthalmol.* 2006;17: 163–167.

40. Jermak CM, Dellacroce JT, Heffez J, Peyman GA. Triamcinolone acetonide in ocular therapeutics. *Surv Ophthalmol*. 2007;52:503–522.
41. Kramar M, Vu L, Whitson JT, He YG. The effect of intravitreal triamcinolone on intraocular pressure. *Curr Med Res Opin*. 2007;23:1253–1258.
42. Batioglu F, Ozmert E, Parmak N, Celik S. Two year results of intravitreal triamcinolone acetonide injection for the treatment of diabetic macular edema. *Int Ophthalmol*. 2007;27:299–306.
43. Vasconcelos-Santos DV, Nehemy PG, Schachat AP, Nehemy MB. Secondary ocular hypertension after intravitreal injection of 4 mg of triamcinolone acetonide: incidence and risk factors. *Retina*. 2008;28:573–580.
44. Gillies MC, Sutter FK, Simpson JM, Larsson J, Ali H, Zhu M. Intravitreal triamcinolone for refractory diabetic macular edema: two year results of a double masked, placebo controlled, randomized clinical trial. *Ophthalmology*. 2006;113:1533–1538.
45. Lau LI, Chen KC, Lee FL, Chen SJ, Ko YC, Liu CJL, Hsu WM. Intraocular pressure elevation after intravitreal triamcinolone acetonide injection in a Chinese population. *Am J Ophthalmol*. 2008;146:573–578.
46. Cunningham MA, Edelman JF, Kaushal S. Intravitreal steroids for macular edema: the past, the present, and the future. *Surv Ophthalmol*. 2008;53:139–149.
47. Callanan DG, Jaffe GJ, Martin DF, Pearson PA, Comstock TL. Treatment of posterior uveitis with a fluocinolone acetonide implant. *Arch Ophthalmol*. 2008;126: 1191–1201.
48. Ricci F, Missiroli F, Parravano M. Argon laser trabeculoplasty in triamcinolone acetonide induced ocular hypertension refractory to maximal medical treatment. *Eur J Ophthalmol*. 2006;16:756–757.
49. Viola F, Morescalchi F, Staurenghi G. Argon laser trabeculoplasty for intractable glaucoma following intravitreal triamcinolone. *Arch Ophthalmol*. 2006;124: 133–134.
50. Rubin B, Taglienti A, Rothman RF, Marcus CH, Serle JB. The effect of selective laser trabeculoplasty on intraocular pressure in patients with intravitreal steroid-induced elevated intraocular pressure. *J Glaucoma*. 2008;17:287–292.
51. Realini T. Selective laser trabeculoplasty: a review. *J Glaucoma*. 2008;17:497–502.
52. Robin AL, Sjaarda R, Suan EP. A novel long-lasting therapy for glaucoma caused by intravitreal triamcinolone acetonide: anterior juxtascleral depot of anecortave acetate. Presented at Annual Meeting of the American Glaucoma Society, Charleston, SC, March 2006.
53. Robin AL, et al. Anterior juxtascleral delivery of anecortave acetate in eyes with primary open angle glaucoma: a pilot investigation. *Am J Ophthalmol*. 2009;147:45–50.
54. Katz GJ, et al. A study of anecortave acetate (7.5 and 15 mg) vs vehicle in patients with open angle glaucoma. Presented at American Academy of Ophthalmology meeting, November 2008.
55. Eid TM, Radwan A, el-Manawy W, el-Hawary I. Outcome of intravitreal bevacizumab (Avastin) followed by aqueous shunting tube surgery for management of intractable neovascular glaucoma. Poster at American Academy of Ophthalmology November 2008.
56. Kuang TM, Liu CJ, Chou CK, Hsu WM. Clinical experience in the management of neovascular glaucoma. *J Chin Med Assoc*. 2004;67:131–135.
57. Nabili S, Kirkness CM. Trans-scleral diode laser cyclophoto-coagulation in the treatment of diabetic neovascular glaucoma. *Eye*. 2004;18:352–256.
58. Sothornwit N. Intravitreal bevacizumab for Ahmed glaucoma valve implantation in neovascular glaucoma: a case report. *J Med Assoc Thai*. 2008;91(Suppl 1): S162–S165.
59. Wand M, Dueker DK, Aiello LM, Grant WM. Effects of panretinal photocoagulation on rubeosis iridis, angle neovascularization, and neovascular glaucoma. *Am J Ophthalmol*. 1978;86:332–339.
60. Ringvold A, Davanger M. Iris neovascularization in eyes with pseudoexfoliation syndrome. *Br J Ophthalmol*. 1981;65:138–141.
61. Shimizu K, Kobayashi K, Muraoka K. Midperipheral fundus involvement in diabetic retinopathy. *Ophthalmology*. 1981;88:601–612.
62. Hamanaka T, Akabane N, Yajima T, et al. Retinal ischemia and angle neovascularization in proliferative diabetic retinopathy. *Am J Ophthalmol*. 2001;132: 648–658.
63. Terasaki H, Miyake Y, Mori M, et al. Fluorescein angiography of extreme peripheral retina and rubeosis iridis in proliferative diabetic retinopathy. *Retina*. 1999;19:302–308.
64. Steel DHW, Habib MS, Park S, et al. Entry site neovascularization and vitreous cavity hemorrhage after diabetic vitrectomy the predictive value of inner sclerostomy site ultrasonography. *Ophthalmology*. 2008;115: 525–532.
65. Tolentino MJ, McLeod DS, Taomoto M, et al. Pathologic features of vascular endothelial growth factor-induced retinopathy in the nonhuman primate. *Am J Ophthalmol*. 2002;133:373–385.
66. Meyer-Schwickerath R, Pfeiffer A, Blum WF, et al. Vitreous levels of the insulin-like growth factors I and III, and the insulin-like growth factor binding proteins 2 and 3, increase in neovascular eye disease. Studies in nondiabetic and diabetic patients. *J Clin Invest*. 1993;92: 2620–2625.
67. John T, Sassani JW, Eagle RC. The myofibroblastic component of rubeosis iridis. *Ophthalmology*. 1983;90: 721–728.
68. Rice TA, Michels RG, Maguire MG, Rice EF. The effect of lensectomy on the incidence of iris neovascularization and neovascular glaucoma after vitrectomy for diabetic retinopathy. *Am J Ophthalmol*. 1983;95:1–11.
69. Tolentino MJ, Miller JW, Gragoudis ES, et al. Vascular endothelial growth factor is sufficient to produce iris neovascularization and neovascular glaucoma in a nonhuman primate. *Arch Ophthalmol*. 1996;114: 964–970.
70. Adamis AP, Shima DT, Tolentino MJ, et al. Inhibition of vascular endothelial growth factor prevents retinal ischemia-associated iris neovascularization in a nonhuman primate. *Arch Ophthalmol*. 1996;114:66–71.

71. Avery RL. Regression of retinal and iris neovascularization after intravitreal bevacizumab (avastin) treatment. *Retina, J Retin Vitreous Dis*. 2006;26:352–356.
72. Davidorf FH, Mouser JG, Derick RJ. Rapid improvement of rubeosis iridis from a single bevacizumab (Avastin) injection. *Retina*. 2006;26:354–356.
73. Tripathi RC, Li J, Tripathi BJ, et al. Increased level of vascular endothelial growth factor in aqueous humor of patients with neovascular glaucoma. *Ophthalmology*. 1998;105:232–237.
74. Gartner S, Henkind P. Neovascularization of the iris (rubeosis iridis). *Surv Ophthalmol*. 1978;22:291–312.
75. Anderson DM, Morin JD, Hunter WS. Rubeosis iridis. *Can J Ophthalmol*. 1971;6:183–188.
76. Schulze RR. Rubeosis iridis. *Am J Ophthalmol*. 1967;63:487–495.
77. Weiter J, Zuckerman R. The influence of the photoreceptor–RPE complex on the inner retina. *Ophthalmology*. 1980;87:1133–1139.
78. Aiello LP, Arrigg PG, Keyt BA, et al. Vascular endothelial growth factor in ocular fluid of patients with diabetic retinopathy and other retinal disorders. *New Eng J Med*. 1994;331:1480–1487.
79. Ohrt V. Rubeosis iridis diabetica. *Acta Ophthalmol*. 1958;36:556–558.
80. Ohnishi Y, Ishibashi T, Sagawa T. Fluorescein gonioangiography in diabetic neovascularization. *Graefe's Arch Clin Exp Ophthalmol*. 1994;232:199–204.
81. Helbig H, Kellner U, Bornfeld N, Foerster MH. Rubeosis iridis after vitrectomy for diabetic retinopathy. *Graefe's Arch Clin Exp Ophthalmol*. 1998;236:730–733.
82. Michels R. Vitrectomy for complications of diabetic retinopathy. *Arch Ophthalmol*. 1978;96:237–246.
83. Bandello F, Brancato R, Lattanzio R, et al. Relation between iridopathy and retinopathy in diabetes. *Br J Ophthalmol*. 1994;78:542–545.
84. Tasman W, Magargal LE, Augsburger JJ. Effects of argon laser photocoagulation on rubeosis iridis and angle neovascularization. *Ophthalmology*. 1980;87:400–402.
85. Diabetic Retinopathy Study Research Group. Diabetic retinopathy study, report number 6: design, methods, and baseline results. *Invest Ophthalmol Vis Sci*. 1981;21:149–209.
86. Ohrt V. The frequency of rubeosis iridis in diabetic patients. *Ophthalmologica*. 1971;49:301–307.
87. Murphy RP, Egbert PR. Regression of iris neovascularization following panretinal photocoagulation. *Arch Ophthalmol*. 1979;97:700–702.
88. Teich SA, Walsh JB. A grading system for iris neovascularization-prognostic implications for treatment. *Ophthalmology*. 1981;88:1102–1106.
89. Aiello LM, Wand M, Liang G. Neovascular glaucoma and vitreous hemorrhage following cataract surgery in patients with diabetes mellitus. *Ophthalmology*. 1983;90:814–820.
90. Browning DJ. Risk of missing angle neovascularization by omitting screening gonioscopy in patients with diabetes mellitus. *Am J Ophthalmol*. 1991;112:212.
91. Browning DJ, Scott AQ, Peterson CB, et al. The risk of missing angle neovascularization by omitting screening gonioscopy in acute central retinal vein occlusion. *Ophthalmology*. 1998;105:776–784.
92. Pe'er J, Neufeld M, Baras M, et al. Rubeosis in retinoblastoma – histologic findings and the possible role of vascular endothelial growth factor in its induction. *Ophthalmology*. 1997;104:1251–1258.
93. Henkind P. Ocular neovascularization. The Krill Memorial Lecture. *Am J Ophthalmol*. 1978;85:287–301.
94. Ehrenberg M, McCuen BW, Schindler RH, Machemer R. Rubeosis iridis: preoperative iris fluorescein angiography and periocular steroids. *Ophthalmology*. 1984;91:321–325.
95. Scuderi JJ, Blumenkranz MS, Blankenship G. Regression of diabetic rubeosis iridis following successful surgical reattachment of the retina by vitrectomy. *Retina*. 1982;2:193–196.
96. Tolentino FI, Cajita VN, Gancayco T, Skates S. Vitreous hemorrhage after closed vitrectomy for proliferative diabetic retinopathy. *Ophthalmology*. 1989;96:1495–1500.
97. Lewis H, Abrams GW, Williams GA. Anterior hyaloidal fibrovascular proliferation after diabetic vitrectomy. *Am J Ophthalmol*. 1987;104:607–613.
98. Lewis H, Abrams GW, Foos RY. Clinicopathologic findings in anterior hyaloidal fibrovascular proliferation after diabetic vitrectomy. *Am J Ophthalmol*. 1987;104:614–618.
99. Hanley JA, Lippman-Hand A. If nothing goes wrong, is everything alright? *JAMA*. 1983;259:1743–1745.
100. Eypasch E, Lefering R, Kum CK. Probability of adverse events that have not yet occurred: a statistical reminder. *BMJ*. 1995;311:619–620.
101. Blinder KJ, Friedman SM, Mames RN. Diabetic iris neovascularization. *Am J Ophthalmol*. 1998;120:393–395.
102. Brancato R, Bandello F, Lattanzio R. Iris fluorescein angiography in clinical practice. *Surv Ophthalmol*. 1997;42:41–70.
103. Mandelbaum S, Chew EY, Christman LM, et al. Comprehensive adult medical eye evaluation. 2008. American Academy of Ophthalmology.
104. Coleman SL, Green WR, Patz A. Vascular tufts of the pupillary margin of the iris. *Am J Ophthalmol*. 1977;83:881–883.
105. Dahlmann AH, Benson MT. Spontaneous hyphema secondary to iris vascular tufts. *Arch Ophthalmol*. 2001;119:1728.
106. Davies N. Letter. *Eye*. 2001;15:688–691.
107. Bandello F, Brancato R, Lattanzio R, et al. Biomicroscopy versus fluorescein angiography of the iris in the detection of diabetic iridopathy. *Graefes Arch Clin Exp Ophthalmol*. 1993;231:444–448.
108. Sanborn GE, Symes DJ, Magaragal LE. Fundus-iris fluorescein angiography: evaluation of its use in the diagnosis of rubeosis iridis. *Ann Ophthalmol*. 1986;18:52–58.
109. Jensen VA, Lundbaek K. Fluorescence angiography of the iris in recent and long-term diabetics. *Acta Ophthalmol*. 1968;46:584–585.

110. Kottow MH. Iris neovascular tufts. *Arch Ophthalmol.* 1980;98:2084.
111. Vannas A. Fluorescein angiography of the vessels of the iris. *Acta Ophthalmol.* 1969;105:1–75.
112. Parodi MB, Bondel E, Russo D, Ravalico G. Iris indocyanine green video angiography in diabetic iridopathy. *Br J Ophthalmol.* 1996;80:416–419.
113. Tauber J, Lahav M, Erzurum SA. New clinical classification for iris neovascularization. *Ophthalmology.* 1987;94:542–544.
114. Nomura T, Furukawa H, Kurinoto S. Development and classification of neovascular glaucoma in diabetic eye disease: histopathological study. *Acta Ophthalmol Soc Jpn.* 1976;86:166–175.
115. Kubota T, Tawara A, Hata T, et al. Neovascular tissue in the intertrabecular spaces in eyes with neovascular glaucoma. *Br J Ophthalmol.* 1996;80:750–754.
116. Weiss DI, Gold D. Neofibrovascularization of iris and anterior chamber angle: a clinical classification. *Ann Ophthalmol.* 1978;10:488–491.
117. Little HL, Rosenthal AR, Dellaporta A, Jacobson DR. The effect of panretinal photocoagulation on rubeosis iridis and neovascular glaucoma. *Am J Ophthalmol.* 1976;81:804–809.
118. Beasley H. Rubeosis iridis in aphakic diabetics. *JAMA.* 1970;213:128.
119. Schiff WM, Barile GR, Hwang JC et al. Diabetic vitrectomy: influence of lens status upon anatomic and visual outcomes. *Ophthalmology.* 2007;114:544–550.
120. Yang CM, Yeh PT, Yang CH. Intravitreal long-acting gas in the prevention of early postoperative vitreous hemorrhage in diabetic vitrectomy. *Ophthalmology.* 2007;114:710–715.
121. Yeh PT, Yang CM, Yang CH, Huang JS. Cryotherapy of the anterior retina and sclerotomy sites in diabetic vitrectomy to prevent recurrent vitreous hemorrhage. *Ophthalmology.* 2005;112:2095–2102.
122. Azzolini C, Brancato R, Camesasca FI, August 1993 (Vol.100 I8PP). Influence of silicone oil on iris microangiopathy in diabetic vitrectomized eyes. *Ophthalmology.* 1993;100:1152–1158.
123. Laatikainen L. Preliminary report on effect of retinal panphotocoagulation on rubeosis iridis and neovascular glaucoma. *Br J Ophthalmol.* 1977;61:278–284.
124. Vernon SA, Cheng H. Panretinal cryotherapy in neovascular disease. *Br J Ophthalmol.* 1988;72:401–405.
125. Pauleikhoff D, Gerke E. Photocoagulation in diabetic rubeosis iridis and neovascular glaucoma. *Klin Monatsbl Augenheil.* 1987;190:11–16.
126. Striga M, Ivanisevic M. Comparison between efficacy of full- and mild-scatter (panretinal) photocoagulation on the course of diabetic rubeosis iridis. *Ophthalmologica.* 1993;207:144–147.
127. Parodi MB, Iacono P. Photodynamic therapy with verteporfin for anterior segment neovascularizations in neovascular glaucoma. *Am J Ophthalmol.* 2004;138: 157–158.
128. Spiteri Cornish K, Ramamurthi S, Saidkasimova S, Ramaesh K. Intravitreal bevacizumab and augmented trabeculectomy for neovascular glaucoma in young diabetic patients. *Eye.* 2008;23:979–981.
129. Avery RL, Pearlman J, Pieramici DJ et al. Intravitreal bevacizumab (Avastin) in the treatment of proliferative diabetic retinopathy. *Ophthalmology.* 2006;113:1695–1705.
130. Grover S, Gupta SK, Sharma RK, Brar VS, Chalam KV. Intracameral bevacizumab effectively reduces aqueous VEGF levels in neovascular glaucoma. *Br J Ophthalmol.* 2009;93:1273–1274.
131. Chalam KV, Gupta SK, Grover S, Brar VS, Agarwal S. Intracameral Avastin dramatically resolves iris neovascularization and reverses neovascular glaucoma. *Eur J Ophthalmol.* 2008;18:255–262.
132. Grisanti S, Biester S, Peters S, Tatar O, Ziemssen F, Bartz-Schmidt KU, Tuebingen Bevacizumab Study Group. Intracameral bevacizumab for iris rubeosis. *Am J Ophthalmol.* 2006;142:158–160.
133. Miki A, Oshima Y, Otori Y, et al. Efficacy of intravitreal bevacizumab as adjunctive treatment with pars plana vitrectomy, endolaser photocoagulation, and trabeculectomy for neovascular glaucoma. *Br J Ophthalmol.* 2008;92:1431–1433.
134. May DR, Bergstrom TJ, Parmet AJ, Schwartz JG. Treatment of neovascular glaucoma with transscleral panretinal cryotherapy. *Ophthalmology.* 1980;87: 1106–1111.
135. Flaxel CJ, Larkin GB, Broadway DB, et al. Peripheral transscleral retinal diode laser for rubeosis iridis. *Retina.* 1997;17:421–429.
136. Hilton GF. Panretinal cryotherapy for diabetic rubeosis. *Arch Ophthalmol.* 1979;97:776.
137. Allen RC, Bellows AR, Hutchinson BT, Murphy SD. Filtration surgery in the treatment of neovascular glaucoma. *Ophthalmology.* 1982;89:1181–1187.
138. Skuta GL, Parrish RK II. Wound healing in glaucoma filtering surgery. *Surv Ophthalmol.* 1987;32:149–170.
139. Miller JW, StinsonWG, Folkman J. Regression of experimental iris neovascularization with systemic alpha-interferon. *Ophthalmology.* 2008;100:9–14.
140. Genaidy M, Kazi A, Peyman G, et al. Effect of squalamine on iris neovascularization in monkeys. *Retina.* 2002;22:772–778.
141. Sir Duke-Elder S., Jay B. eds. Haemorrhagic glaucoma. In: *System of Ophthalmology.* Vol. 9. London: Henry Kimpton;1969:667.
142. Sivak-Callcott JS, O'Day DM, Gass JDM, Tsai JC. Evidence based recommendations for the diagnosis and treatment of neovascular glaucoma. *Ophthalmology.* 2001;108:1767–1778.
143. Ehlers JP, Shah CP, Fenton GL, Hoskins EN, Shelsta HN. *The Wills Eye Manual: office and Emergency Room Diagnosis and Treatment of Eye Disease.* 5th ed. Philadelphia: Lippincott Williams & Wilkins; 2008:214–217.
144. Silva Paula J, Jorge R, Alves Costa R, Rodrigues Mde L, Scott IU. Short-term results of intravitreal bevacizumab (Avastin) on anterior segment neovascularization in neovascular glaucoma. *Acta Ophthalmol Scand.* 2006;84:556–557.
145. Oshima Y, Sakgauchi H, Gomi F, Tano Y. Regression of iris neovascularization after intravitreal injection of bevacizumab in patients with proliferative diabetic retinopathy. *Am J Ophthalmol.* 2006;142:155–158.

146. Beutel J, Peters S, Luke M, Aisenbrey S, Szurman P, Spitzer MS, Yoeruek E, The Bevacizumab Study Group, Grisanti S. Bevacizumab as adjuvant for neovascular glaucoma. *Acta Ophthalmol.* Sept 20, 2008 (E-pub).
147. Jiang Y, Liang X, Li X, Tao Y, Wang K. Analysis of the clinical efficacy of intravitreal bevacizumab in the treatment of iris neovascularization caused by proliferative diabetic retinopathy. *Acta Ophthalmol.* 2008 Sep 18 (E-pub)
148. Ehlers JP, Spirn MJ, Lam A, Sivalingam A, Samuel MA, Tasman W. Combination intravitreal bevacizumab/panretinal photocoagulation versus panretinal photocoagulation alone in the treatment of neovascular glaucoma. *Retina.* 2008;28:696–702.
149. Gheith ME, Siam GA, de Barros DS, Garg SJ, Moster MR. Role of intravitreal bevacizumab in neovascular glaucoma. *J Ocul Pharmacol Ther.* 2007;23:487–491.
150. Iliev ME, Domig D, Wolf-Schnurrbursch U, Wolf S, Sarra G-M. Intravitreal bevacizumab (Avastin) in the treatment of neovascular glaucoma. *Am J Ophthalmol.* 2006;142:1054–1056.
151. Chilov MN, Grigg JR, Playfair TJ. Bevacizumab (Avastin) for the treatment of neovascular glaucoma. *Clin Exp Ophthalmol.* 2007;35:494–496.
152. Wakabayashi T, Oshima Y, Sakaguchi H, Ikuno Y, Miki A, Gomi F, Otori Y, Kamei M, Kusada S, Tano Y. Intravitreal bevacizumab to treat iris neovascularization and neovascular glaucoma secondary to ischemic retinal diseases in 41 consecutive cases. *Ophthalmology.* 2008;115:1571–1580.
153. Martinez-Carpio PA, Bonafonte-Marquez E, Heredia-Garcia CD, Bonafonte-Rovo S. Efficacy and safety of intravitreal injection of bevacizumab in the treatment of neovascular glaucoma: systemic review. *Arch Soc Esp Oftalmol.* 2008;83:579–588.
154. Yoeruek E, Spitzer MS, Tatar O, Aisenbrey S, Bartz-Schmidt KU, Szurman P. Safety profile of bevacizumab on cultured human corneal cells. *Cornea.* 2007;26: 977–982.
155. Sharma, RK, Chalam, KV, et al. Evaluation of cytotoxic effects of bevacizumab on human corneal endothelial cells. *Cornea.* 2009;28:328–333.
156. Netland PA. The Management of Neovascular Glaucoma in 2008. Presentation at the annual meeting of the American Academy of Ophthalmology, Atlanta, GA. November 10, 2008.
157. Al Obeidan SA, Osman EA, Al-Amro SA, Kangave D, Abu El-Asrar AM. Full preoperative panretinal photocoagulation improves the outcome of trabeculectomy with mitomycin C for neovascular glaucoma. *Eur J Ophthalmol.* 2008;18:758–764.
158. Kitnarong N, Chindasub P, Metheetrairut A. Surgical outcome of intravitreal bevacizumab and filtration surgery in neovascular glaucoma. *Adv Ther.* 2008;25: 438–443.
159. Pappas GD, Panagiotoglou T, Kounali VD, Koukoulasis MG, Fanouriakis CD. Intracameral bevacizumab and augmented trabeculectomy with mitomycin C for the treatment of neovascular glaucoma. Poster at American Academy of Ophthalmology November 2008.
160. Grewal DS, Jain R, Kumar H, Grewal SPS. Evaluation of subconjunctival bevacizumab as an adjunct to trabeculectomy. *Ophthalmology.* 2008;115:2141–2145.
161. Welsandt GR, Mietz H, Becker M, et al. Effect of bevacizumab on 3T3 fibroblasts in vitro: possible role in wound healing modulation. *Invest Ophthalmol Vis Sci* 48:E-abstract 836, 2007.
162. Icchpujani P, Ramasubramanian A, Kaushik S, Pandav SS. Bevacizumab in glaucoma: a review; *Can J Ophthalmol.* 2007;42:812–815.
163. Kapetansky F, et al. Subconjunctival injection(s) of bevacizumab for failing filtering blebs. Poster at American Academy of Ophthalmology November 2008.
164. Wang J, Harasymowycz PJ. Subconjunctival bevacizumab injection for glaucoma filtering surgery: a case series. Poster at American Academy of Ophthalmology November 2008.
165. Yalvac IS, Eksioglu U, Satana B, Duman S. Long term results of Ahmed glaucoma valve and Molteno implant in neovascular glaucoma. *Eye.* 2007;21:65–70.
166. Lloyd MA, Sedlak T, Heuer DK, et al. Clinical experience with the single-plate Molteno implant in complicated glaucomas. *Ophthalmology.* 1992;99:679–687.
167. Every SG, Molteno AC, Bevin TH, Herbison P. Long term results of Molteno implant insertion in cases of neovascular glaucoma. *Arch Ophthalmol.* 2006;124: 355–360.
168. Luttrul JK, Avery RL. Pars plana implant and vitrectomy for treatment of neovascular glaucoma. *Retina.* 1995;15:379–387.
169. Faghihi H, Hajizadeh F, Hahammadi SF, Kadkhoda A, Peyman GA, Riazi-Esfahani M. Pars plana Ahmed valve implant and vitrectomy in the management of neovascular glaucoma. *Opthalmic Surg Lasers Imaging.* 2007;38:292–300.
170. Smith MF, Doyle JW, Fanous MM. Modified aqueous drainage implants in the treatment of complicated glaucomas in eyes with pre-existing episcleral bands. *Ophthalmology.* 1998;105:2237–2242.
171. Schocket SS. The 'taco' tube shunt. In: Chen TC ed. *Surgical Techniques in Ophthalmology: Glaucoma Surgery.* Philadelphia: Saunders Elsevier; 2008:143–152.
172. Roth SM, Brown GC. The diagnosis and management of rubeosis iridis. *Clin Signs Ophthalmol.* 1989;10:1–15.

Chapter 12
The Cornea in Diabetes Mellitus

S. Akbar Hasan

12.1 Introduction

Although the cornea may appear disease free in the diabetic, marked biochemical and ultrastructural abnormalities are present altering form and function. Awareness of these manifestations of corneal disease in diabetes can lead to steps that prevent more overt complications.

Corneal manifestations of diabetes mellitus have been studied less extensively than diabetic retinopathy. Early clinical observations of the diabetic cornea included endothelial changes such as Descemet's folds and pigment deposition on the endothelium.[1] In addition, diabetics were noted to have impaired corneal sensitivity resulting in a neurotrophic keratitis with corneal ulceration.[2,3] Over the last few decades, a more detailed knowledge of the pathophysiological changes to the cornea has been gained.

12.2 Pathophysiology

Early studies examined the polyol pathway and its effects in diabetic corneal disease.[4–6] In the polyol pathway, aldose reductase is the rate-limiting enzyme in which glucose is converted into sorbitol. Elevated glucose levels spur an increase in aldose reductase activity resulting in sorbitol accumulation. These products have been identified in corneal epithelial and endothelial cells in animal models of diabetes.[7–9] Furthermore, studies have revealed faster re-epithelialization rates after abrasion as well as improved epithelial morphological changes in animals treated with aldose reductase inhibitors, confirming the enzyme's role in diabetic corneal disease.[10,11] Evidence suggests that the inhibition of aldose reductase reduces dysmorphological changes in the corneal endothelium as well.[12,13] Nonetheless, the mechanism linking the accumulation of by-products of the polyol pathway to ultrastructural corneal changes has not been elucidated.

Other studies have identified the role of matrix metalloproteinases (MMP) in corneal disease.[14] These zinc enzymes are responsible for the degradation of the extracellular matrix components and play an essential role in corneal wound healing.[15] Increased expression of MMPs has been demonstrated in hyperglycemia.[16] Enhanced production and activity of MMPs likely damages basement membrane, including type IV collagen and limits epithelial cell migration resulting in poor epithelial healing.

Advanced glycation end products (AGEs) may also have a role in diabetic corneal disease, just as they have been linked to diabetic retinopathy and cataract.[17–19] Chronic hyperglycemia results in the formation of AGEs on proteins, through a process of nonenzymatic glycation. N-(carboxymethyl) lysine (CML) has been identified as a dominant AGE antigen in tissue proteins.[20] CML immunoreactivity is increased in the epithelial basement membrane of diabetic corneas, resulting from the nonenzymatic glycation of laminin, the major basement membrane component.[21] The accumulation of AGEs on the epithelial basement membrane may therefore be involved in diabetic corneal epitheliopathy.

S.A. Hasan (✉)
Department of Ophthalmology, Mayo Clinic, Jacksonville, FL 32082, USA
e-mail: hasan.saiyid@mayo.edu

D.J. Browning (ed.), *Diabetic Retinopathy*, DOI 10.1007/978-0-387-85900-2_12,

12.3 Anatomy and Morphological Changes

Anatomically overlaying the cornea and safeguarding its health and stability, the tear film is comprised of three layers: aqueous, mucin, and lipid. The cornea consists of three cellular layers, separated by two basement membranes. The corneal epithelium is composed of a layer of stratified squamous cells and has an underlying basement membrane. The stroma consists of an extracellular matrix of collagen and glycoaminoglycans, keratocytes, and nerve cells. Its anterior portion is known as Bowman's layer and consists of collagen fibers and proteoglycans. Descemet's membrane is the basement membrane of the corneal endothelium and consists primarily of type IV collagen. Lastly, the corneal endothelium is comprised of a single layer of cells in a uniform mosaic pattern.[22] Diabetes alters the tear film as well as producing ultrastructural changes throughout the cornea.

Diabetics may suffer from tear film abnormalities resulting in ocular discomfort, burning, and foreign body sensation. All components of the tear film in diabetes are altered resulting in abnormal tear film breakup time (BUT), fluorescein staining, Schirmer I testing and Rose Bengal or Lissamine Green staining.[22,25] The severity of the tear film dysfunction correlates with the severity of the diabetic retinopathy, with proliferative diabetic changes associated with a more diminished tear film function. In addition, conjunctival impression cytology demonstrates a higher grade of conjunctival squamous metaplasia as well as a lower goblet cell density in the diabetic patient.[23] These changes have been related to the status of metabolic control and stage of diabetic retinopathy. The tear lipid layer is also less uniform in the diabetic. Increasing derangement of the tear lipid layer has been correlated with the degree of diabetic keratoepitheliopathy.[24] Abnormalities in aqueous, mucin, and lipid tear film layers contribute significantly to the poor ocular surface seen in diabetics.

Corneal epithelial changes in the diabetic include degeneration of basal epithelial cells resulting in a decrease in cell density.[26,27] In addition, abnormal glucose metabolism in the corneal epithelium and its basement membrane results in thickening of the epithelial basement membrane as well as deterioration of basal cell adhesions.[11] This loss of cellular adhesion likely limits cellular migration and can be partially explained by a reduction in the area of the basal cell membrane occupied by hemidesmosomes.[28,29] In addition, in the diabetic cornea, nonenzymatic glycation of components in the epithelial basement membrane involved in adhesion complexes, such as nidogen-1/entactin, laminin-1, laminin-10, and of an epithelial integrin [alpha]$_3$[beta]$_1$, has been demonstrated. This accumulation of AGEs in the corneal epithelial basement membrane may represent a molecular mechanism leading to abnormalities in epithelial cell adhesion.[30–32]

In the diabetic corneal stroma, keratocytes display degeneration of intracellular organelles and cytoplasmic vacuoles of various sizes with deposition of an amorphous material. Furthermore, collagen fibers demonstrate variable thickness.[33] These ultrastructural changes are also likely a result of increased corneal AGEs, which leads to protein cross-linking and causes the destruction of cellular structures.[34] Iclal et al. recently demonstrated the use of aminoguanidine (AG), an AGE inhibitor, prevented corneal stromal changes, confirming the importance of AGEs in inducing stromal changes. Within the stroma, abnormalities in the corneal nerves are also evident. Studies have demonstrated basal lamina thickening of Schwann cells and axonal degeneration. Morphological damage of the corneal subbasal nerve plexus in diabetic patients has been confirmed with confocal microscopy.[35,36] These ultrastructural changes may be involved in corneal neuropathy.

Assessment of the posterior cornea in diabetes may reveal faint vertical lines at the level of Descemet's membrane, a change initially described by Waite and Beetham.[1,36] The etiology of Waite–Beetham lines, whether metabolic or mechanical, has yet to be elucidated. Corneal endothelial studies in the diabetic demonstrate a decrease in endothelial cell density and a greater coefficient of variation of cell area with greater polymegathism and pleomorphism.[12,13,37–40] In animal studies, the diabetic endothelium has demonstrated significant reduction in Na^+/K^+ ATPase activity, the key transport enzyme of the endothelial cell pump.[41] In addition, studies of central corneal thickness in the diabetic, although somewhat inconsistent, seem to suggest a small increase in thickness as measured by pachymetry.[39,40,42–48] However, no association between corneal thickness and retinopathy or diabetic control has been reported. These findings indicate that the corneal endothelium is probably more vulnerable to stress and trauma in the diabetic.

12.4 Clinical Manifestations

The effects of diabetes on the tear film and cornea produce many clinical manifestations. Numerous studies have demonstrated aqueous tear deficiency in diabetes (Fig. 12.1).[49–60] The primary cause of the aqueous tear deficiency may be due to the diminished sensitivity caused by neuropathy. This leads to a slowing of the corneal reflex with a consecutive decrease in blinking frequency and tear secretion.[61–63] In addition, a worsening of keratoconjunctivitis sicca correlates with the severity of diabetic retinopathy.[64] Alterations in the tear lipid and mucin layer as measured by tear break up time and impression cytology contribute to a poor quality tear film and abnormal ocular surface manifested as fluctuation in vision and ocular discomfort. Slit-lamp examination of the cornea, with the assistance of vital staining, provides an accurate assessment of the status of the tear film and degree of superficial punctate keratopathy.

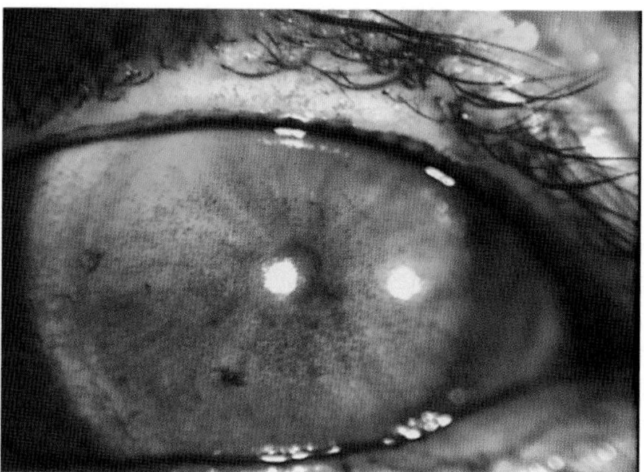

Fig. 12.1 Marked staining with Lissamine Green confirming severe aqueous tear deficiency in a poorly controlled diabetic patients

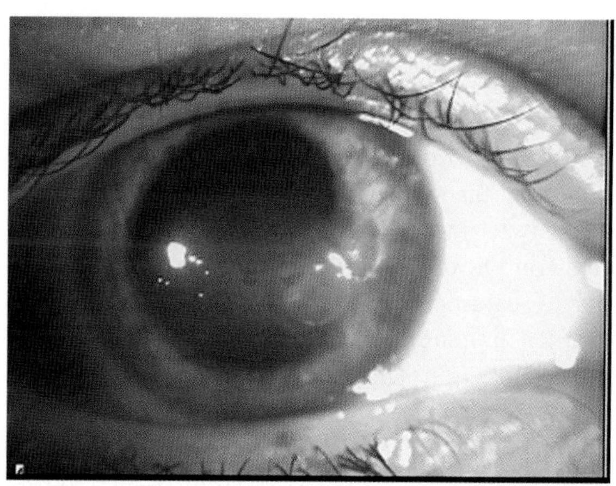

Fig. 12.2 Loose epithelium resulting in a recurrent corneal erosion in a long-standing diabetic patient

Diabetics are also prone to have epithelial healing problems exhibiting a loose and fragile epithelium (Fig. 12.2). Schultz et al. noted that about half of all diabetic patients will experience problems and present with diabetic epitheliopathy.[64] Hyperglycemia-induced epithelial basement membrane abnormalities result in poor epithelial adhesion. This can lead to corneal abrasions, recurrent erosions, and persistent epithelial defects.[65] The extent of epithelial fragility correlates with the degree of retinopathy. Patients with proliferative diabetic retinopathy demonstrated 84% greater fragility than diabetics without retinopathy and patients with nonproliferative retinopathy exhibited 41% greater corneal epithelial fragility.[66]

Diabetic corneal neuropathy, a manifestation of diabetic polyneuropathy, also plays a significant role in limiting epithelial wound healing. Diabetes-induced alterations in corneal nerves decreases corneal sensitivity, resulting in corneal hypothesia.[3,61–63,67,68] Corneal hypothesia disrupts epithelium architecture and function, further delaying epithelialization in the stressed cornea.[61,69,70] In severe cases, diabetics may suffer from atraumatic, sterile neurotrophic corneal ulcers.

Endothelial changes in the diabetic can alter function. Abnormal corneal endothelial morphology, polymegathism, and pleomorphism, coupled with an increase in corneal thickness in the diabetic, are indications of corneal endothelial dysfunction. Alterations in endothelial pump function may place the cornea at greater risk for decompensation following stress-related injury and surgical trauma.

12.5 Ocular Surgery

Ocular surgery places the diabetic cornea at risk. Recognition of the clinical manifestations of diabetes on the cornea is essential in developing a strategy to minimize intraoperative and postoperative complications. Anterior segment surgery, primarily cataract surgery with phacoemulsification and lens implantation, is associated with endothelial cell loss.[71–73] This mechanically induced cell loss is greater in the diabetic cornea.[74,75] As such, greater effort and care should be utilized to minimize surgical trauma, by avoiding phaco power near the cornea and using viscoelastics generously to cushion the endothelium. Attention to wound construction and manipulation is also important in an attempt to minimize epithelial injury as well.

Posterior segment surgery, pars plana vitrectomy, in the diabetic places much greater stress on an already compromised corneal epithelium. The need for vitrectomy often suggests the presence of significant diabetic retinopathy, which is associated with a marked increase in epithelial fragility as well as an increase in corneal hypothesia.[61,66] Vitrectomy also requires increased operative time, which further traumatizes the epithelium. These factors increase the rate and severity of intraoperative epithelial defect formation. In complex cases, pars plana vitrectomy in diabetics may require intraoperative corneal epithelial debridement to aid in visualization of the posterior pole, often resulting in a poorly healing abrasion and persistent epithelial defect.[76,77] Whether inadvertent or intentional, an epithelial defect in this setting may result in delayed visual recovery, predispose patients to infection, and result in a persistent epithelial defect with associated stromal scarring and thinning. In early studies, diabetes accounted for 80–100% of all postvitrectomy keratopathy and diabetic postvitrectomy keratopathy was identified in up to 65% of patients.[76–80] More recent studies, however, reported 6–15% of diabetic eyes had postoperative corneal complications suggesting that improved preoperative surgical preparation and intraoperative technique to minimize corneal trauma likely accounts for the decrease.[46,81–83]

Improvements in viewing lens systems, surgical technique, and recognition of avoiding corneal epithelial trauma have reduced the rate of postvitrectomy keratopathy. Handheld infusion lenses have been demonstrated to induce greater corneal epithelial injury than sew-on lenses. Noncontact lens systems do not physically touch the cornea and have the lowest rate of epithelial injury.[84] In difficult cases, intraepithelial corneal edema may obscure visualization of the retina and require intraoperative debridement. Greater awareness in protecting and preserving an intact corneal epithelium will decrease the need for debridement and can lead to better postvitrectomy outcomes. Garcia-Valenzuela et al.[85] report suggestions to minimize epithelial debridement rates. The use of GenTeal gel instead of Goniosol as a lubricant decreased the rate of epithelial debridement from 54 to 14%. This decrease is likely related to the preservatives found in Goniosol, especially benzalkonium chloride, which are toxic to the corneal epithelium.

The corneal endothelium can also be compromised during pars plana vitrectomy in the diabetic. Endothelial cell loss may lead to corneal decompensation limiting visual acuity and possibly requiring the need for endothelial transplantation. The causes of postoperative endothelial cell dysfunction are multifactorial and include intraocular irrigating solutions, lens status, capsular integrity, and the use of adjunctive intraocular gas.[46,82,86–90] These factors, coupled with the effects of diabetes on endothelium cell function, place the diabetic at greater risk of long-term corneal compromise with decompensation and the development of bullous keratopathy.

Severe diabetic retinopathy can result in complex tractional detachments requiring the use of silicone oil. The effects of silicone oil on the cornea can result in band keratopathy, epithelial irregularities, corneal neovascularization, and persistent stromal edema with endothelial cell damage.[91,92] The risk of endothelial dysfunction may be reduced by avoiding silicone oil overfill and subsequent damage with the corneal endothelium. In addition, to prevent contact of oil with the cornea, supine positioning of the patient with aphakia should be avoided. Furthermore, an inferior iridectomy is important to permit the flow of aqueous, avoiding pupillary block. In the Silicone Study Report 7, preoperative and postoperative risk factors for the development of corneal complications associated with silicone oil use included aphakia or pseudophakia, iris neovascularization, corneal touch with silicone oil, absence of fluid–gas exchange, additional surgery, and anterior chamber inflammation.[92]

Laser photocoagulation is commonly used to treat proliferative diabetic retinopathy and has been associated with corneal decompensation in some diabetics. Argon laser photocoagulation can result in decreased corneal sensitivity.[61,93] This decreased sensitivity coupled with fundus contact lens-induced hypoxia can traumatize an already compromised cornea resulting in worsening of keratopathy. Lastly, corneal burns have been reported stemming from intraoperative laser indirect ophthalmoscope treatment.[94]

The emergence of refractive surgery as a widely accepted and popular procedure has raised questions regarding its use in the diabetic patient. Diabetes is a relative contraindication to refractive surgery. Studies have demonstrated its safety and efficacy in the well-controlled diabetic patient.[95,96] Nevertheless, patients with diabetes who undergo LASIK are at a significantly higher risk of developing postoperative epithelial complications and are more likely to require additional laser treatment to achieve emmetropia.[96,97] In this setting, a surface ablation, photorefractive keratectomy (PRK) may be a safer alternative. The diabetic patient should be carefully counseled and well informed regarding the disease-specific risks of refractive surgery.

12.6 Treatment of Corneal Disease in Diabetes Mellitus

Protecting and preserving the ocular surface limits the impact of diabetic keratopathy in altering vision and comfort. As diabetes affects all components of the tear film, the role of artificial tears and lubricants is valuable.[50–57] Use of preservative-free lubricants is particularly important in the postoperative period as the cornea is a greater risk of epithelial breakdown.[76–80] Recalcitrant keratopathy may require the use of anti-inflammatory as well. There is increasing evidence that decreased tear secretion and epithelial injury promote inflammation on the ocular surface, resulting in an increase in cytokines and proteases in the tear fluid.[98] Moreover, T-cell infiltration of the conjunctiva has been observed. The use of cyclosporine A, corticosteroids, and doxycycline in keratopathy has been demonstrated to be efficacious in curbing inflammation and improving signs and symptoms of ocular surface disease.[99–101] Additional therapy for severe keratopathy such as erosions and persistent epithelial defects with neurotrophic keratopathy includes bandage contact lens, amniotic membrane grafts, and tarsorrhaphy.[102–104] A stepwise approach to managing keratopathy with timely referral to a cornea specialist can avoid corneal stromal scarring and possible thinning with subsequent compromise of vision. Early recognition and prompt treatment of diabetic corneal disease is vital.

12.7 Conclusion

Diabetes has a significant impact on the cornea. Recognizing the pathophysiological and morphological changes in the diabetic cornea provides greater insight into the clinical manifestations and implications of ocular surgery. An altered tear film and greater epithelial fragility in conjunction with decreased corneal sensitivity leave the diabetic cornea more prone to trauma and injury that may result in complications such as infectious keratitis, neurotrophic ulcers, and stromal scarring. Endothelial cell dysfunction may place the cornea at risk for decompensation following stress. This unique constellation of properties of the diabetic cornea warrants careful understanding as diabetic retinopathy is one of the primary indications for pars plana vitrectomy and surgery can further traumatize a compromised cornea. Identifying the signs and symptoms of diabetic keratopathy is essential in establishing the appropriate treatment plan, thereby preventing further complications and minimizing visual loss.

12.8 Summary of Key Points

- The diabetic cornea may appear normal, but it is not. The abnormalities correlate with the severity of diabetic retinopathy.
- Accumulation of advanced glycation end products in the corneal epithelial basement membrane may be the basis of poor healing of diabetic corneal epithelial defects.

- Corneal neuropathy leads to reduced blink frequency, reduced tear secretion, and hypoesthesia.
- In pars plana vitrectomy for advanced diabetic retinopathy, the use of noncontact lens systems reduces the incidence of intraoperative and postoperative problems with corneal epitheliopathy.
- If silicone oil is used in surgery for advanced diabetic retinopathy, special care is warranted to avoid contact between the corneal endothelium and the silicone oil.
- A low threshold for consultation with a corneal specialist is warranted for retinal specialists managing patients with advanced diabetic retinopathy having concomitant diabetic keratopathy.
- Diabetes is a relative contraindication for refractive surgery. In the situation of a well-controlled diabetic being considered for a refractive procedure, photorefractive keratectomy may be the preferred option.

12.9 Future Directions

Improved understanding of the molecular abnormalities underlying diabetes mellitus should improve our ability to treat diabetic keratopathy in concert with other end-organ abnormalities. In particular, improved treatment of tear insufficiency and corneal neuropathy will be valuable in themselves, but also as aids in the management of advanced diabetic retinopathy in which corneal and retinal challenges often intersect.

References

1. Henkind P, Wise GN. Descemet's wrinkles in diabetes. *Am J Ophthamol.* 1961;52:371.
2. Armaly MF, Baloglou PJ. Diabetes mellitus and the eye: I. Changes in the anterior segment. *Arch Opthalmol.* 1967;77:485–492.
3. Schwartz DE. Corneal sensitivity in diabetics. *Arch Ophthalmol.* 1974;91:174–178.
4. Marano CW. Matschinsky FM. Biochemical manifestations of diabetes mellitus in microscopic layers of the cornea and retina. *Diabetes Metabol Rev.* 1989;5:1–15.
5. Narayanan S. Aldose reductase and its inhibition in the control of diabetic complications. *Ann Clin Lab Sci.* 1993;23:148–158.
6. Jacot JL, Hosotani H, Glover JP, Lois N, Robison WG Jr. Diabetic-like corneal sensitivity loss in galactose-fed rats ameliorated with aldose reductase inhibitors. *J Ocul Pharmacol Ther.* 1998;14:169–180.
7. Kern TS, Engerman RL. Distribution of aldose reductase in ocular tissues. *Exp Eye Res.* 1981;33:175–181.
8. Friend J, Kiorpes TC, Thoft RA. Diabetes mellitus and the rabbit corneal epithelium. *Invest Ophthalmol Vis Sci.* 1987;21:317–321.
9. Ludvigson MJ, Sorenson RL. Immunohistochemical localization on aldolase reductase. II. Rat eye and kidney. *Diabetes.* 1980;29:450–459.
10. Cobo LM, Hatchell DL. Treatment of severe diabetic keratopathy with a topical aldose reductase inhibitor: clinical response and electron microscopy (ARVO Abstract). *Invest Ophthalmol Vis Sci.* 1980;26(suppl):176.
11. Fukushi S, Merola LO, Tanaka M. Reepithelialization of denuded corneas in diabetic rats. *Exp Eye Res.* 1980; 31:611–621.
12. Matsuda M, et al. The effects of aldose reductase inhibitor on the corneal endothelial morphology in diabetic rats. *Curr Eye Res.* 1987;6:391–397.
13. Meyer LA, Ubels JL, Edelhauser HF. Corneal endothelial morphology in the rat. Effects of aging, diabetes, and topical aldose reductase inhibitor treatment. *Invest Ophthalmol Vis Sci.* 1988;29:940–948.
14. Ramamurthi S, Rahman MQ, Dutton GN, Ramaesh K. Pathogenesis, clinical features and management of recurrent corneal erosions. *Eye.* 2006;20:635–644.
15. Woessner JF, Jr. Matrix metalloproteinases and their inhibitors in connective tissue remodeling. *Faseb J.* 1991;5:2145–2154.
16. Takahashi H, Akiba K, Noguchi T, Ohmura T, Takahashi R, Ezure Y, Ohara K, Zieske JD. Matrix metalloproteinase activity is enhanced during corneal wound repair in high glucose condition. *Curr Eye Res.* 2000;21:608–615.
17. Murata T, Nagai R, Ishibashi T, Inomata H, Ikeda K, Horiuchi S. The relationship between accumulation of advanced glycation end products and expression of vascular endothelial growth factor in human diabetic retinas. *Diabetologia.* 1997;40:764–769.
18. Dunn JA, Patrick JS, Thorpe SR, Baynes JW. Oxidation of glycated proteins: age-dependent accumulation of Ne-(carboxymethyl) lysine in lens proteins. *Biochemistry.* 1989;28:9464–9468.
19. Araki N, Ueno N, Chakrabarti B, Morino Y, Horiuchi S. Immunochemical evidence for the presence of advanced glycation end products and its positive correlation with aging. *J Biol Chem.* 1992;267:10211–10214.
20. Horiuchi S, Araki N, Morino Y. Immunochemical approach to characterize advanced glycation end products of the Maillard reaction: evidence for the presence of a common structure. *J Biol Chem.* 1991;266:7329–7332.
21. Yuichi K, Tomohiko U, Tetsuro O, et al. Advanced glycation end products in diabetic corneas. *Invest Ophthalmol Vis Sci.* 2000;41:362–368.
22. Nishida, T. Cornea. *Cornea.* 2nd ed. Vol. 1. Chapter 1. Philadelphia: Elsevier Mosby; 2005.
23. Yu L. Chen X. Qin G. Xie H. Lv P. Tear film function in type 2 diabetic patients with retinopathy. *Ophthalmologica.* 2008;222:284–291.

24. Yoon KC, Im SK, Seo MS. Changes of tear film and ocular surface in diabetes mellitus. Korean J Ophthalmol. 2004;18:168–174.
25. Inoue K, Kato S, Ohara C, Numaga J, Amano S, Oshika T. Ocular and systemic factors relevant to diabetic keratoepitheliopathy. *Cornea*. 2001;20:798–801.
26. Quadrado MJ, Popper M, Morgado AM, Murta JN, Van Best JA. Diabetes and corneal cell densities in humans by in vivo confocal microscopy. Cornea. 2006;25:761–768.
27. Hosotani H, Ohashi Y, Yamada M, et al. Reversal of abnormal corneal epithelial cell morphological characteristics and reduced corneal sensitivity in diabetic patients by aldose reductase inhibitor, CT-112. *Am J Ophthalmol*. 1995;119:288–294.
28. Azar DT, Spurr-Michaud SJ, Tisdale AS, et al. Altered epithelial-basement membrane interactions in diabetic corneas. *Arch Ophthalmol*. 1992;110:537–540.
29. Tabatabay CA, Bumbacher M, Baumgartner B, et al. Reduced number of hemidesmosomes in the corneal epithelium of diabetics with proliferative vitreoretinopathy. *Graefes Arch Clin Exp Ophthalmol*. 1988;226:389–392.
30. Ljubimov AV, Huang ZS, Huang GH, et al. Human corneal epithelial basement membrane and integrin alterations in diabetes and diabetic retinopathy. *J Histochem Cytochem*. 1998;46:1033–1041.
31. Kabosova A, Kramerov AA, Aoki AM, et al. Human diabetic corneas preserve wound healing, basement membrane, integrin and MMP-10 differences from normal corneas in organ culture. *Exp Eye Res*. 2003;77:211–217.
32. Saghizadeh M, Brown DJ, Castellon R, et al. Overexpression of matrix metalloproteinase-10 and matrix metalloproteinase-3 in human diabetic corneas: a possible mechanism of basement membrane and integrin alterations. *Am J Pathol*. 2001;158:723–734.
33. Ishii Y, Lahav M, Mukai Y. Corneal changes in diabetic patients and streptozotocin diabetic rats: an ultrastructural correlation. *Invest Ophthmol Vis Sci*. 1981;20(suppl):154.
34. Bierhaus A, Hofmann MA, Ziegler R, Nawroth PP. AGEs and their interaction with AGE-receptors in vascular disease and diabetes mellitus. I. The AGE concept. *Cardiovasc Res*. 1998;37:586–600.
35. Midena E, Brugin E, Ghirlando A, Sommavilla M, Avogaro A. Corneal diabetic neuropathy: a confocal microscopy study. *J Refract Surg*. 2006;22(9 Suppl):S1047–S1052.
36. Waite JH, Beetham WP. The visual mechanism in diabetes mellitus (a comparative study of 2002 diabetics, and 457 non-diabetics for control). *N Engl J Med*. 1935;212:367–443.
37. Chang PY, Carrel H, Huang JS, et al. Decreased density of corneal basal epithelium and subbasal corneal nerve bundle changes in patients with diabetic retinopathy. *Am J Ophthalmol*. 2006;142(3):488–490.
38. Inoue K, Kato S, Inoue Y, Amano S, Oshika T. The corneal endothelium and thickness in type II diabetes mellitus. *Jpn J Ophthalmol*. 2002;46:65–69.
39. Keoleian JM, et al. Structural and functional studies of the corneal endothelium and diabetes mellitus. *Am J Ophthalmol*. 1992;113:64–70.
40. Schultz RO, Matsuda M, et al. Corneal endothelial changes in type I, type II diabetes mellitus. *Am J Ophthalmol*. 1984;98:401–410.
41. Schultz RO, Peters MA, Sobocinski K, et al. Diabetic corneal neuropathy. *Trans Am Opthalmol Soc*. 1983;81: 107–124.
42. Pardos JG, Krachmer JH. Comparison of endothelial cell density in diabetics and a control population. *Am J Ophthalmol*. 1980;90:172–174.
43. Lass JH, et al. A morphological and fluorophotometric analysis of the corneal endothelium in type I diabetes mellitus and cystic fibrosis. *Am J Ophthalmol*. 1985;100: 783–788.
44. Busted N, Olsen T, Schmitz O. Clinical observations on the corneal thickness and the corneal endothelium in diabetes mellitus. *Br J Ophthalmol*. 1981;65:687–690.
45. Matsuda M, et al. Relationship of corneal endothelial morphology to diabetic retinopathy, duration of diabetes, and glycemic control. *Jpn J Opthalmol*. 1990;34: 53–56.
46. Buettner H, Bourne WM. Effect of trans pars plana surgery on the corneal endothelium. *Dev Ophthalmol*. 1981;2:28–34.
47. Itoi M, et al. Specular microscopic studies of the corneal endothelia of Japanese diabetics. *Cornea*. 1989;8:2–6.
48. Olsen T, Busted N. Corneal thickness in eyes with diabetic and nondiabetic neovascularisation. *Br J Ophthalmol*. 1981;65:691–693.
49. Hoshino M, Hoshino T. Schirmer test in diabetic patients. *Jpn J Clin Ophthalmol*. 1989;43:1917–1920.
50. Binder A, Maddison PJ, Skinner P, Kurtz A, Isenberger DA. Sjogren's syndrome: association with type-1 diabetes mellitus. *Br J Rheumatol*. 1989;28:516–520.
51. Barrera R, Cinta-Mane-M, Rodriguez-JF, Jimenez A. Keratoconjunctivitis sicca and diabetes mellitus in a dog. *J Am Vet Med Assoc*. 1992;200:1967–1968.
52. Sreebny LM, Yu A, Green A, Valdini A. Xerostomia in diabetes mellitus. *Diabetes Care*.199215:900–904.
53. Stolwijk TR, Kuizenga A, van-Haeringen NJ, Kijlstra A, Oosterhuis JA, van Best JA. Analysis of tear fluid proteins in insulin dependent diabetes mellitus. *Acta Ophthalmol Copenh*. 1994;72:357–362.
54. Ramos RC, Suarez AM, Russell AS. Low tear production in patients with diabetes mellitus. *Clin Exp Rheum*. 1994;12:375–380.
55. Stolwijk TR, van Best JA, Lemkes HH, de-Keizer RJ, Oosterhuis JA. Determination of basal tear turnover in insulin dependent diabetes mellitus patients by fluorophotometry. *Int Ophthalmol*. 1991;15:377–382.
56. Sullivan DA, Edwards JA, Wickham LA, et al. Identification and endocrine control of sex steroid binding sites in the lacrimal gland. *Curr Eye Res*. 1996;15:279–291.
57. Takeuchi K, Hori Y, Hayakawa T, et al. A case of an old woman with Sjogren's syndrome associated with insulin dependent diabetes mellitus. *Ryumachi*. 1996;36:769–774.
58. Ekgardt VF, Tarasova LN, Teplova SN, Alekhina TV. Systemic and local immunity in patients with diabetic retinopathy. *Vestn Oftalmol*. 1998;114:46–48.
59. Robinson CP, Yamachika S, Bounous DI, et al. A novel NOD-derived murine model of primary Sjogren's syndrome. *Arthritis Rheum*. 1998;41:150–156.

60. Grus FH, Augustin AJ, Evangelou NG, Toth-Sagi K. Analysis of tear protein pattern as a diagnostic tool for the detection of dry eyes. *Eur J Ophthalmol.* 1998;18:90–97.
61. Rogell JD. Corneal hypesthesia and retinopathy in diabetes mellitus. *Ophthalmology.* 1980;87:229–233.
62. Nielsen NV. Corneal sensitivity and vibratory perception in diabetes mellitus, *Acta Ophthalmol.* 1978;56:406–411.
63. Riss B, Binder S. Corneal sensitivity after photocoagulation for diabetic retinopathy. *Graefes Arch Klin Exp Ophthalmol.* 1981;217:143–147.
64. Schultz R, Van Horn D, Peters M, et al. Diabetic keratopathy. *Trans Am Ophthalmol Soc.* 1982;79:180–199.
65. Nepp J, et al. Is there a correlation between the severity of diabetic retinopathy and keratoconjunctivitis sicca? *Cornea.* 2000;19(14):487–491.
66. Saini JS, Khandalavia B. Corneal epithelial fragility in diabetes mellitus. *Can J Ophthalmol.* 1995;30(3):142–146.
67. Schultz RO, Peters MA, Sobocinski K, et al. Diabetic keratopathy as a manifestation of peripheral neuropathy. *Am J Ophthalmol.* 1983;96:368–371.
68. Ishida N, Rao GN, Del Cerro M, Aquaella JV. Corneal nerve alterations in diabetes mellitus. *Arch Ophthalmol.* 1984;102(9):1380–1384.
69. Beuerman RW, Schimmelpfennig B, Burstein N. Anatomy of the denervated corneal epithelium. *Invest Ophthalmol Vis Sci.* 1979;18(suppl):126.
70. Paton L. The trigeminal and its ocular lesions. *Br J Ophthalmol.* 1926;10:305–342.
71. Diaz-Valle D, Benitez del Castillo Sanchez JM, Castillo A, Sayagues O, Moriche M. Endothelial damage with cataract surgery techniques. *J Cataract Refract Surg.* 1998;24:951–955.
72. Walkow T, Anders N, Klebe S. Endothelial cell loss after phacoemulsification: relation to preoperative and intraoperative parameters. *J Cataract Refract Surg.* 2000;26(5): 727–732.
73. Dick HB, Kohnen T, Jacobi FK, Jacobi KW. Long-term endothelial cell loss following phacoemulsification through a temporal clear corneal incision. *J Cataract Refract Surg.* 1996;22:63–71.
74. Morikubo S, Takamura Y, Kubo E, Tsuzuki S, Akagi Y. Corneal changes after small-incision cataract surgery in patients with diabetes mellitus. *Arch Ophthalmol.* 2004; 122(7):966–969.
75. Lee JS, Lee JE, Choi HY, et al. Corneal endothelial cell change after phacoemulsification relative to the severity of diabetic retinopathy. *J Cataract Ref Surg.* 2005;31:742–749.
76. Faulborn J, Conway BP, Machemer, R. Surgical complications of pars plana vitreous surgery. *Ophthalmology.* 1978;185:116–125.
77. Perry HD, Foulks GN, Thoft RA, Tolentino FI. Corneal complications following closed vitrectomy through the pars plana. *Arch Ophthalmol.* 1978;96:1401–1403.
78. Mandelcorn MS, Blankenship J, Machemer R. Pars plana vitrectomy for the management of severe diabetic retinopathy. *Am J Opthalmol.* 1976;81:561–570.
79. Foulks GN, et al. Factors related to corneal epithelial complications after closed vitrectomy in diabetics. *Arch Ophthalmol.* 1979;97:1076–1078.
80. Brightbill FS. Myers FL. Bresnick GH. Postvitrectomy keratopathy. *Am J Ophthalmol.* 1978;85:651–655.
81. Chung H, Tolentino FI, Cajita VN, Acosta J, Refojo MF. Reevaluation of corneal complications after closed vitrectomy. *Arch Ophthalmol.* 1988;106(7):916–919.
82. Friberg TR, Doran DL, Lazenby FL. The effect of vitreous and retinal surgery on corneal endothelial cell density. *Ophthalmology.* 1984;91:1166–1169.
83. Schachat AP, Oyakawa RT, Michels RG, Rice TA. Complications of vitreous surgery for diabetic retinopathy. II. Postoperative complications. *Ophthalmology.* 1983;90:522–530.
84. Virata SR, Kylstra JA, Singh HT. Corneal epithelial defects following vitrectomy surgery using hand-held, sew-on, and noncontact viewing lenses. *Retina.* 1999;19(4):287–290.
85. Garcia-Valenzuela E, et al. Reduced need for corneal epithelial debridement during vitreo-retinal surgery using two different viscous surface lubricants. *Am J Ophthalmol.* 2003;136(6):1062–1066.
86. McDermott M, et al. Effects of intraocular irrigants on the preserved human corneal endothelium. *Cornea.* 1991;10(5):402–407.
87. Benson WE, Diamond JG, Tasman W. Intraocular irrigating solutions for pars plana vitrectomy: a prospective, randomized, double-blind study. *Arch Ophthalmol.* 1981;99(6):1013–1015.
88. Diddie KR, Schanzlin DJ. Specular microscopy in pars plana vitrectomy. *Arch Ophthalmol.* 1983;101(3):408–409.
89. Mittl RN, et al. Endothelial cell counts following pars plana vitrectomy in pseudophakic and aphakic eyes. *Ophthalmic Surg.* 1989;20(1):13–16.
90. Mitamura Y, Yamamoto S, Yamazaki S. Corneal endothelial cell loss in eyes undergoing lensectomy with and without anterior lens capsule removal combined with pars plana vitrectomy and gas tamponade. *Retina.* 2000;20(1):59–62.
91. Sternberg Jr P, et al. The effect of silicone oil on the cornea. *Arch Ophthalmol.* 1985;103(1):90–94.
92. Abrams GW, et al. The incidence of corneal abnormalities in the silicone study: silicone study report 7. *Arch Ophthalmol.* 1995;113(6):764–769.
93. Makitie J, Koskenvuo M, Vannas A, et al. Corneal endothelium after photocoagulation in diabetic patients. *Acta Ophthalmol.* 1985;63:355–360.
94. Irvine WD, Smiddy WE, Nicholson DH. Corneal and iris burns with the laser indirect ophthalmoscope. *Am J Ophthalmol.* 1990;110(3):311–313.
95. Cobo-Soriano R, Beltran J, Baviera J. LASIK outcomes in patients with underlying systemic contraindications: a preliminary study. *Ophthalmology.* 2006; 113(7):1124.e1.
96. Halkiadakis I, Belfair N, Gimbel HV. Laser in situ keratomileusis in patients with diabetes. *J Cataract Refract Surg.* 2005;31(10):1895–1898.
97. Fraunfelder FW, Rich LF. Laser-assisted in situ keratomileusis complications in diabetes mellitus. *Cornea.* 2002;21(3):246–248.
98. Pflugfelder SC. Antiinflammatory therapy for dry eye. *Am J Ophthalmol.* 2004;137(2):337–342.
99. Laibovitz RA, Solch S, Andrianao J. Pilot trial of cyclosporin 1% ophthalmic ointment in the treatment of keratoconjunctivitis sicca. *Cornea.* 1993;12:315–323.

100. Frucht-Pery J, Sagi E, Hemo I, Ever-Hadani P. Efficacy of doxycycline and tetracycline in ocular rosacea. *Am J Ophthalmol*. 1993;116:88–92.
101. Marsh P, Pflugfelder SC. Topical non-preserved methylprednisolone therapy of keratoconjunctivitis sicca in Sjogren's syndrome. *Ophthalmology*. 1999;106: 811–816.
102. Prabhasawat P, Tesavibul N, Komolsuradej W. Single and multilayer amniotic membrane transplantation for persistent corneal epithelial defect with and without stromal thinning and perforation. *Br J Ophthalmol*. 2001;85(12):1455–1463.
103. Khokhar S, Natung T, Sony P, Sharma N, Agarwal N, Vajpayee RB. Amniotic membrane transplantation in refractory neurotrophic corneal ulcers: a randomized, controlled clinical trial. *Cornea*. 2005;24(6): 654–660.
104. Cosar CB, Cohen EJ, Rapuano CJ, Maus M, Penne RP, Flanagan JC, Laibson PR. Tarsorrhaphy: clinical experience from a cornea practice. *Cornea*. 2001;20(8):787–791.

Chapter 13
Optic Nerve Disease in Diabetes Mellitus

David J. Browning

13.1 Relevant Normal Optic Nerve Anatomy and Physiology

The vascular supply of the optic nerve depends on the stratum of the optic nerve head under consideration. The optic nerve head is divided into four strata – superficial nerve fiber layer, prelaminar layer, laminar layer, and retrolaminar layer. Fine retinal arterioles arising in the peripapillary retina and derived from the central retinal artery supply the superficial nerve fiber layer of the optic nerve; there is no posterior ciliary contribution.[1]The prelaminar and laminar optic nerve derive their blood supply primarily from the paraoptic short posterior ciliary arteries and the circumferential vessels of the circle of Zinn-Haller (Fig. 13.1).[2–5] The circle of Zinn-Haller, where it exists, is an intermediary between the posterior ciliary arteries and the anterior optic nerve small vessels.[1,6] There may be smaller and inconsistent contributions from peripapillary choroidal arteries.[1,2,6,7] Although the circle of Zinn-Haller is present in the peripapillary sclera in most eyes studied by plastic cast studies in cadaver eyes, there is some controversy about whether the circle is functional and whether it serves as an intermediary between the short posterior ciliary arteries and the optic disk blood supply.[1,8] In vivo, the perfusion of the circle of Zinn-Haller can only be seen in highly myopic eyes with peripapillary crescents by using ICG angiography.[9] In such eyes, the circle of Zinn-Haller has been found to be incomplete, but one cannot generalize to the case of normal eyes. The mesh of capillaries in the anterior optic nerve has spacing of 30–50 μm to 50–85 μm and connects with the capillary mesh of the laminar portion of the optic disk and the overlying superficial nerve fiber layer.[1,2,10] The capillaries themselves have a luminal diameter of 7–10 μm.[2] Electron microscopy shows tight junctions between capillary endothelial cells of the optic nerve, thus a blood–optic nerve barrier exists in analogy to the blood–retina barrier.[11,12] The retrolaminar optic nerve head is supplied both by the short posterior ciliary arteries via branches to the circle of Zinn-Haller and thence to pial arteries and by branches of the central retinal artery.[13]

The intravascular pressure of the short posterior ciliary artery branches to the anterior optic nerve has been deduced to be somewhat lower than the intravascular pressure of branches of the central retinal artery based on fluorescein angiograms of primates performed with elevated, controlled intraocular pressure in an experimental model suggesting vulnerability of the optic nerve head should perfusion pressure fall.[3]

The optic nerve shares the property of autoregulation with the retina.[12,14–16] Systemic controls on optic nerve blood flow are absent or minor, but local factors mediated by nitric oxide, endothelin, prostaglandins, and the renin–angiotensin system are important.[17] The ocular perfusion pressure (OPP) is defined as follows:

OPP = mean rterial blood pressure – intraocular pressure
= [diastolic blood pressure + 1/3 (systolic blood pressure – diastolic blood pressure)] – intraocular pressure [14,18]

D.J. Browning (✉)
Charlotte Eye Ear Nose & Throat Associates, Charlotte, NC 28210, USA
e-mail: dbrowning@ceenta.com

D.J. Browning (ed.), *Diabetic Retinopathy*, DOI 10.1007/978-0-387-85900-2_13,

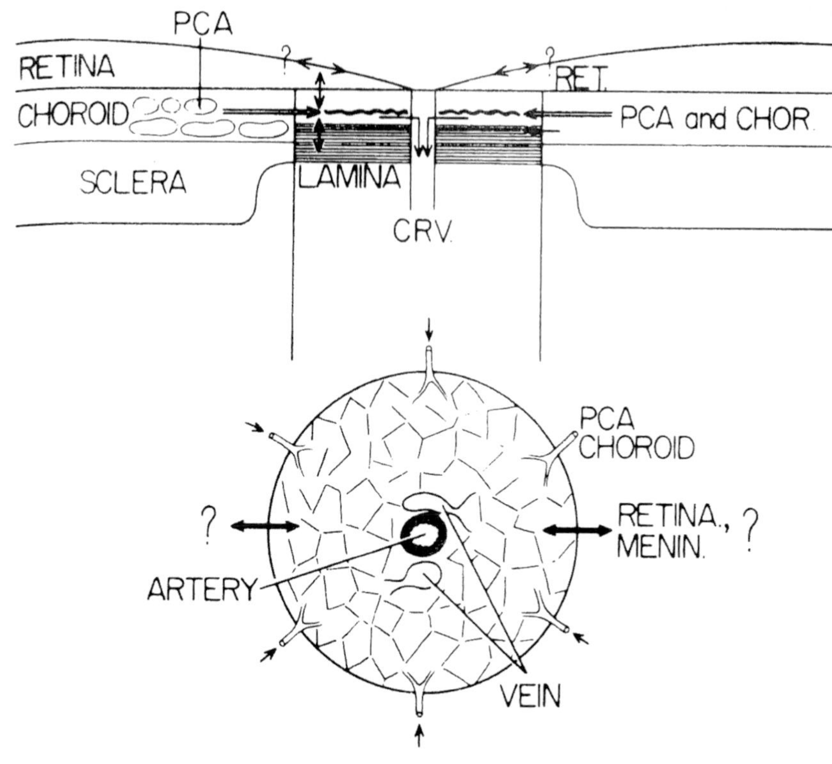

Fig. 13.1 Schematic of the vascular supply of the anterior optic nerve. Contributions from the paraoptic short posterior ciliary arteries (PCA) and the choroid are important, whereas contributions from peripapillary retinal arterioles (RETINA) and perineural meningeal arterioles (MENING) are inconsistent or questionable (signified by ?). CRV = central retinal vein. Reprinted with permission from Henkind[2]

In most, but not all, humans, the optic nerve vascular response to an increase in perfusion pressure of up to 45 mm Hg is vasoconstriction such that optic nerve head blood flow tends to remain constant. Likewise, with a fall in perfusion pressure by raising intraocular pressure, the optic disk arterioles tend to dilate and protect optic disk oxygen tension.[12] Some persons seem to have a reduced optic nerve autoregulatory capacity and may be more susceptible to ischemia of the optic nerve. Although both arterial blood pressure and intraocular pressure affect the ocular perfusion pressure, it is not known if changes induced by the two factors produce equivalent responses.[14]

13.2 The Effect of Diabetes on the Optic Nerve

The retinal nerve fiber layer thickness is reduced in diabetes mellitus compared to control eyes with increasing atrophy as retinopathy severity increases. Thus diabetes can be a source of overestimation of glaucomatous optic neuropathy when scanning laser polarimetry is used to monitor progression of glaucomatous optic atrophy.[19]

The neuroretinal rim area of the optic nerve has been studied longitudinally in a subset of photographs taken as part of the Wisconsin Study of Diabetic Retinopathy.[20] In younger onset and older onset diabetics, the neuroretinal rim area increased over a 4-year period. In addition, the neuroretinal rim area was larger in eyes with more severe retinopathy at baseline. It is possible that diabetes is associated with subclinical optic disk swelling in general.

Although rare, optociliary shunt vessels can arise de novo in diabetic retinopathy, perhaps signifying a relative venous obstruction at the lamina cribrosa. The more common causes of optociliary shunt vessels are spheno-orbital meningiomas, central retinal vein occlusions, primary open angle glaucoma, papilledema, optic nerve glioma, optic disk drusen, arachnoid cyst of the optic nerve, phakomatoses, and rarely congenital abnormality.[21]

13.3 Nonarteritic Anterior Ischemic Optic Neuropathy and Diabetes

Nonarteritic anterior ischemic optic neuropathy (NAION) is generally considered to occur as a response to hypoperfusion of the branches of the posterior ciliary arteries that supply the optic disk.[22–25] An alternative hypothesis – that the primary disorder is relative central venous occlusion – has been advanced but not embraced.[26] The annual incidence of NAION is 2.3–10.3 per 100,000 persons.[24,25] Although more common in the elderly with the median age of affected patients being 62 years, it can strike the young (range 12–92 years).[27] Visual loss is most frequently noted upon awakening from sleep suggesting that nocturnal hypotension may have a role in the condition.[28] Hypoxia induces axoplasmic flow stasis, neural swelling, and dilated capillaries on the surface of the disk with peripapillary splinter hemorrhages more prominent in patients with diabetes than in those without (Fig. 13.2).[29,30] Because the space through which the optic nerve passes is typically restricted as reflected in a small optic disk cup, the axonal swelling is thought to compress the capillaries further, in turn exacerbating ischemia and producing a vicious spiral ending in tissue infarction.[30–32] Diabetes mellitus is a risk factor for NAION, and others include hypertension, nocturnal or post-surgical hypotension, older age, smoking, sleep apnea, and anemia.[23,33–42] Cataract surgery may be a minor risk factor.[43] The role of thrombophilic factors has been inconsistent. Although thrombophilic risk factors have been absent in most studies, one study reported elevated levels of lipoprotein (a), von Willebrand antigen, factor V Leiden, cholesterol, and fibrinogen in patients with NAION.[44–46]

Central scotomata are present in 55.3% and 36.2% of eyes with the I-2e and V-4e targets, respectively.[47] Inferonasal sector loss is the most common sectoral defect (22.4%).[47] An inferior altitudinal field defect is seen in 8.0% of eyes.[47] Many other visual field defects can be seen and in 6.4% of eyes no field defect is present.[47] The sector of optic disk edema and the location of the visual field defects correlate early in the condition.[30] As the edema resolves, however, the correlation vanishes.[25] At a later stage, the correlation of sectoral optic pallor and the observed visual field defects is also poor.[30] A relative afferent pupillary defect is usually present.[33]

Before visual dysfunction occurs, there may be asymptomatic optic disk edema, which has been termed incipient nonarteritic anterior ischemic optic neuropathy (Fig. 13.2).[22,48,49] Twenty five to 31% of cases of incipient NAION resolve with the rest progressing to NAION and some visual loss involving acuity or field or both.[22,50]

Previous fellow eye involvement at baseline is seen in 21.1% of patients and new fellow eye involvement occurs in 14.7% of patients over 5 years of follow-up with half the cases occurring in the first year after first eye involvement.[23] Presence of diabetes mellitus increases the incidence of fellow eye involvement.[23] Recurrences in the same eye are uncommon.[51,52]

NAION in patients with diabetes has some differences compared to the condition in nondiabetics. Diabetic patients with NAION have a higher prevalence of hypertension, ischemic heart disease, transient ischemic attacks, and second eye involvement than patients who have NAION without diabetes.[23,53] Time to resolution of disk edema is longer in patients with diabetes than in patients without diabetes.[30,53] Median time to second eye involvement is shorter in patients with diabetes than in patients without diabetes.[53] In some respects, diabetic and nondiabetic patients are similar. The fluorescein angiographic findings are the same. The optic disk shows fluorescein leakage of swollen sectors in both groups of patients.[30,53] Both groups of patients have small cup-to-disk ratios. At 6 months after diagnosis, the visual acuity and visual field outcomes are similar in diabetic and nondiabetic groups.[53]

Subsequent optic disk pallor after the acute hyperemia of NAION occurs approximately 6–12 weeks later.[30,33] Atrophic cupping of the optic nerve after NAION is not seen, in contrast to arteritic ION, where subsequent optic cupping can be part of the clinical picture.[33]

Although controversial, some have linked the use of phosphodiesterase-5 inhibitors for the treatment of erectile dysfunction and the development of

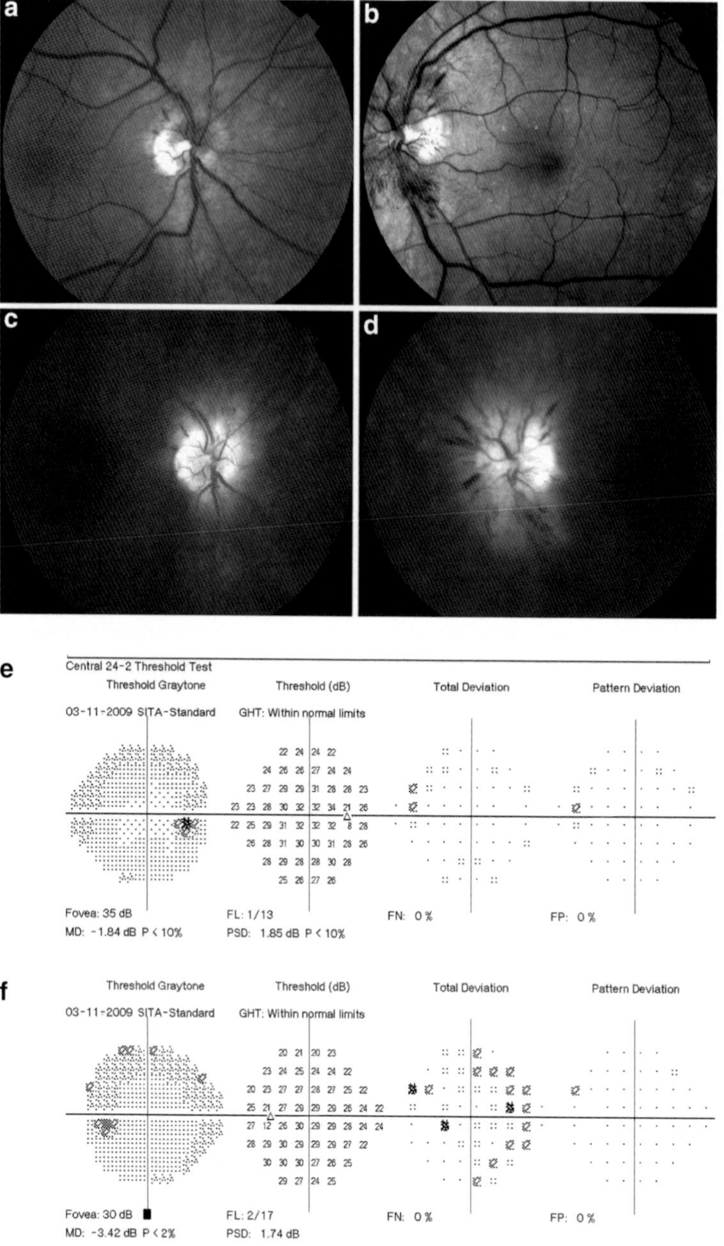

Fig. 13.2 Example of incipient nonarteritic ischemic optic neuropathy. The patient was a 65-year-old man with type 2, insulin-requiring diabetes mellitus, hypertension, and sleep apnea. He had had uneventful cataract surgery in the right eye 8 months earlier and in the left eye 3 months earlier. He complained of acute onset of painless, blurred vision of the left eye for 3 weeks and had no complaints with regard to the right eye. Best corrected visual acuity was 20/20 in each eye. Both eyes had optic disk edema, more prominent on the left than the right (**a** and **b**); on the right only the superior pole of the nerve was involved. Fluorescein angiography showed late disk hyperfluorescence bilaterally, more prominent on the left than the right (**c** and **d**). The visual field was normal on the right (mean defect –1.94 db) and showed some patchy superior scotomata on the left (mean defect –3.42 db) (**e** and **f**)

NAION.[54–57] These drugs increase the level of cyclic guanosine monophosphate in vascular smooth muscle cells which leads to vasodilation of arterioles and subsequent arterial hypotension. Because arterial hypotension, especially during sleep, is thought to be associated with NAION, it is conceivable that these drugs could add to the risk of NAION.[18,58] Hayreh states that diabetic patients should be counseled against their use for this reason. Similar concerns have been raised about nocturnal use of beta-blocker eyedrops for glaucoma.[59]

Posterior ischemic optic neuropathy is much less common than anterior ischemic optic neuropathy, comprising perhaps 2% of the cases of ischemic optic neuropathy.[33] Affected patients tend to fall into three groups: perioperative cases, temporal arteritis-associated cases, and cases associated with nonarteritic systemic vascular disease.[60] Because the condition is much rarer than anterior ischemic optic neuropathy, little data are available regarding the role of diabetes.[60] The optic nerve appearance is normal at the time of the acute event. Optic disk pallor is seen approximately 6 weeks after the event.[33] Central nervous system imaging is advisable to exclude a compressive lesion.

There is no proven effective therapy for NAION.[61] Optic nerve sheath decompression is of no benefit and may be harmful.[62] Other therapies tried have included levodopa, hyperbaric oxygen, aspirin, and prednisone.[30,63–66]

13.4 Diabetic Papillopathy

Diabetic papillopathy is a clinical description of unilateral or bilateral optic disk edema with or without decreased visual function that improves with time in diabetics.[67,68] Although no population-based studies exist to provide reliable prevalence data, an estimate of 0.4% of diabetics seen by ophthalmologists has been published.[69] In the 42% of cases with bilateral involvement, the two eyes may be affected by simultaneously or sequentially involvement.[69–71] As with NAION, the disk in diabetic papillopathy often has a small cup and dilated radial peripapillary capillaries (Fig. 13.3).[29,68,70] Although early reports suggested that the condition usually occurs in patients under age 30 who have had longstanding type 1 diabetes mellitus, more recent reports suggest that older patients and patients with type 2 diabetes may actually comprise the majority of cases.[67,70,72,73] A history of poor metabolic control is elicited in 50% of patients, but the condition can occur in patients with good glycemic control and in pregnancy.[67,68,73–75] The optic disk edema does not correlate with the degree of diabetic retinopathy. It usually resolves within 3–6 months, although it can persist for 1 year or more, and is not followed by dramatic optic atrophy, although mild pallor may be seen.[67,68,71,76]

Although diabetic retinopathy can be mild in affected eyes, accelerated retinopathy progression to the point of proliferative disease occurs in 17%, thus close follow-up is warranted.[69,73,77] Macular edema and significant capillary nonperfusion are frequently present in affected eyes.[70] Care must be taken to distinguish the macular edema associated with diabetic papillopathy from concomitant diabetic macular edema. In the former, the edema resolves spontaneously and no treatment is necessary.[78] In the latter, focal/grid laser is of proven benefit.[79] Visual field examinations reveal blind spot enlargement alone or no abnormality in approximately equal proportions; occasionally arcuate or central scotomata are seen.[68–70,73] Although visual acuity is usually unaffected after resolution of edema, a decrease may be seen in approximately 8% of patients.[73] Relative afferent pupillary defects are absent or rare and spontaneous venous pulsations may be seen.[68] Cerebrospinal fluid pressure is normal in such cases, as is computed tomography of the brain.[67–69] Recurrence of diabetic papillopathy is rare or unreported once the initial episode has resolved.[68] Because the appearance of the optic disk is indistinguishable from the papilledema arising from increased intracranial pressure or hypertension, these latter conditions need to be excluded before making the diagnosis of diabetic papillopathy.[68,71,75,77]

Some authors consider diabetic papillopathy to be incipient NAION in a patient with diabetes mellitus and not a distinct entity, although others disagree.[30,67,68,70,71,80] Incipient NAION in patients with diabetes can be accompanied by telangiectatic disk vessels easily confused with disk neovascularization.[53] A distinction needs to be made, because panretinal photocoagulation is needed for the one but not the other.[30,53] The distinction can be made

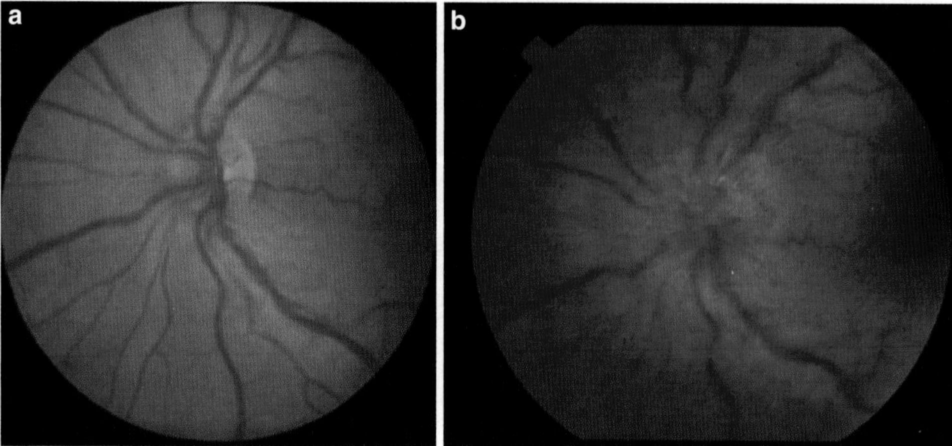

Fig. 13.3 (**a**) Normal optic nerve head appearance of the left eye of a 30-year-old woman with type 1 diabetes of 27 years duration and poor glycemic control before the development of diabetic papillopathy (see Fig. 13.3b). Mild nonproliferative diabetic retinopathy was present and the visual acuity was 20/20. The optic nerve head cup is small. (**b**) Appearance of the left optic nerve head of the patient shown in Fig. 13.3a when diabetic papillopathy developed. The visual acuity was 20/30. Prominent dilation of capillaries on the superficial optic nerve head is seen. The patient had a normal opening pressure on lumbar puncture

by assessing the degree of midperipheral capillary nonperfusion of the retina that is commonly present with disk neovascularization, and not characteristically present, although possibly present, in diabetic papillopathy. Another distinguishing characteristic is the location of the vessels. Disk neovascularization is found in the preretinal space, whereas the dilated capillaries of diabetic papillopathy are present within the plane of the retina.[70] The leakage of dye from the vessels on fluorescein angiography is not a useful test for distinguishing the two, as it occurs in both.[80] The late frames of the fluorescein angiogram can be helpful, however. The retinal arteries and veins of the disk are dark against the hyperfluorescent disk substance in the case of diabetic papillopathy. In contrast, in the case of disk neovascularization the fluorescein in front of the disk obscures the underlying arteries and veins of the disk.[74]

Although lumbar punctures in case reports have uniformly shown normal opening pressures, some have speculated that a mildly elevated cerebrospinal fluid pressure may contribute to the condition. Few patients have been studied with serial lumbar punctures to investigate this possibility.[76] There is no known treatment for diabetic papillopathy, although excellent glycemic and blood pressure control are recommended, as for all patients with diabetes.[69,71,75,81]

13.5 Disk Edema Associated with Vitreous Traction

Vitreopapillary traction associated in a patient with diabetic retinopathy can rarely be the cause of optic disk edema. With spontaneous posterior vitreous detachment, the edema resolves.[82]

13.6 Superior Segmental Optic Hypoplasia (Topless Optic Disk Syndrome)

Superior segmental optic hypoplasia is a congenital, stable optic disk anomaly often but not always occurring in the offspring of mothers with type 1 diabetes mellitus.[83–85,86] Although affected patients have been predominantly female in some case series, the gender imbalance did not reach statistical significance in a population-based study.[83,87] Bilateral disk involvement occurs in 22–67% of cases.[86,87] Familial clustering has been reported suggesting a genetic component to the disorder.[88,89] Short gestation time, low birth weight, and poor maternal diabetic control seem to be risk factors.[83] Patients typically have good visual acuity, but inferior visual field defects are present and the optic nerves and sometimes chiasm are small on MRI scanning.[86,87]

Fundus findings include a superior disk entrance of the central retinal artery, superior disk pallor, and a superior scleral halo (Fig. 13.4).[83,84,90] Optical coherence tomography shows retinal nerve fiber layer thinning superiorly.[84] The appearance of the optic disk can be subtly abnormal and can be confused with the disk in normal tension glaucoma, although in the latter disorder the neural rim thinning is usually located inferiorly. The reported prevalence has been from 0.08 to 0.3%, approximately one-tenth the prevalence of normal tension glaucoma.[84,87]

13.7 Wolfram Syndrome

Wolfram syndrome is an autosomal recessive, progressive neurodegenerative syndrome consisting of insulin-dependent diabetes mellitus, diabetes insipidus, sensorineural hearing loss, ataxia, peripheral neuropathy, urinary tract atrophy, psychiatric illness, and progressive optic nerve atrophy (Fig. 13.5).[91,98] It is also called DIDMOAD (diabetes insipidus, diabetes mellitus, optic atrophy, and deafness).[92] Diabetes mellitus and optic atrophy are the major features, present in 98–99% of cases, whereas diabetes insipidus and deafness are minor features, occurring in 32–35% and 12% of cases, respectively.[93] Its manifestations occur in stages

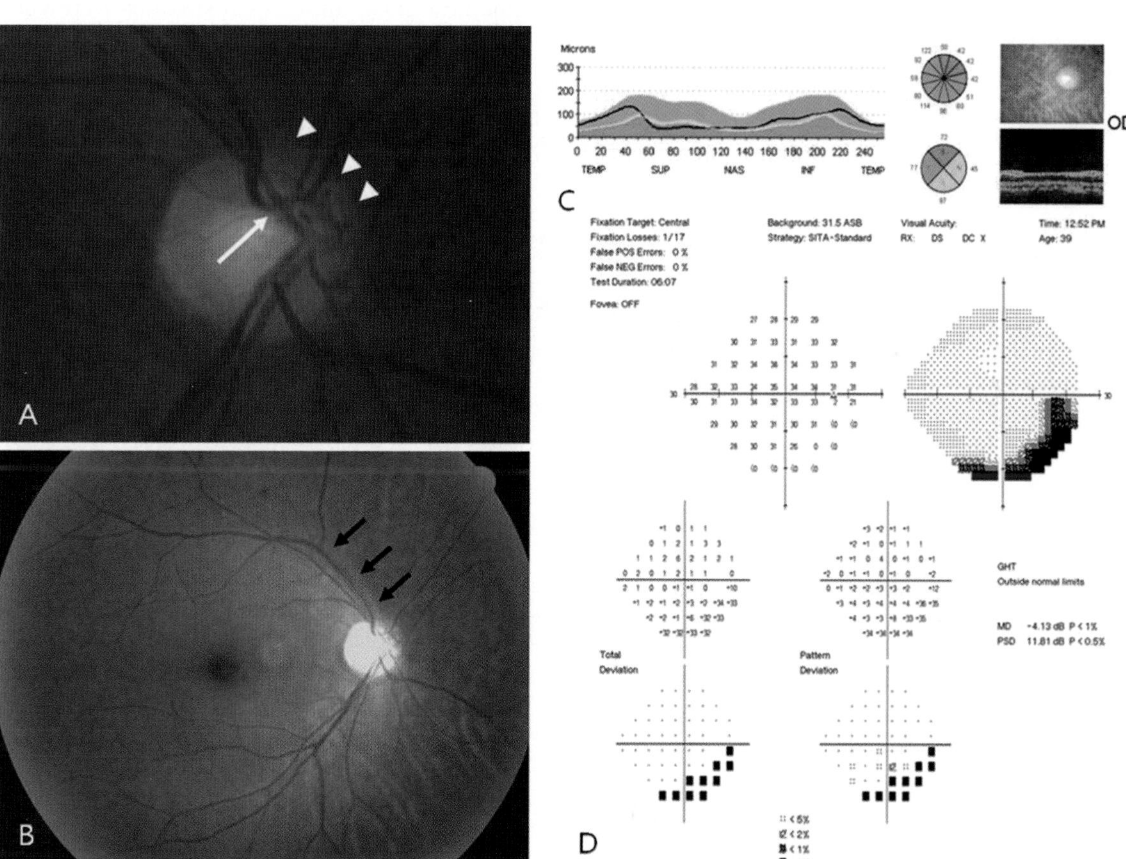

Fig. 13.4 Characteristic features of superior segmental optic hypoplasia are illustrated. (**a**) The central retinal artery enters the optic disk superiorly (*arrow*). There is a superior peripapillary scleral halo (*arrowheads*). (**b**) Red free fundus photograph shows thinning of the superior nerve fiber layer (*arrows*). (**c**) The optical coherence tomography shows retinal nerve fiber layer thinning in the superonasal quadrant. (**d**) Humphrey 24-2 visual field testing shows an inferior arcuate scotoma. Reprinted with permission from Han.[84]

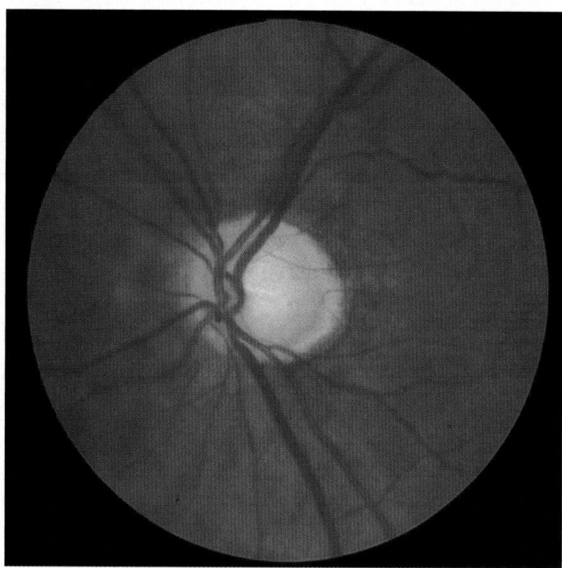

Fig. 13.5 Optic disk atrophy in an 8-year-old boy with Wolfram syndrome. Reprinted with permission from Wake[98]

with diabetes mellitus and optic atrophy by age 10; diabetes insipidus and deafness by age 20; renal tract abnormalities by age 30; cerebellar ataxia, myoclonus, and psychiatric illness by age 40; and death from central respiratory failure usually by age 50.[92] Estimates of incidence range from 1:100,000 to 1:770,000 in South America and the United Kingdom, respectively.[94] MRI studies of the brains of affected persons can show cerebellar and pontine atrophy, shrinkage of the optic nerves and chiasm, and foci of high signal on PD- and T2-weighted images in the substantia nigra.[93,95] Neuropathology shows atrophy of the olfactory tracts, optic nerves and chiasm, loss of neurons in the lateral geniculate body, atrophy of the superior colliculus, cochlear nerve fiber loss, olivopontocerebellar atrophy, and demyelination of pyramidal tracts.[91]

The responsible gene, *WFS1* on the short arm of chromosome 4, has no known function as yet, but more than 50 mutations have already been described in affected individuals.[92,94,96] Multiple deletions of mitochondrial DNA have also been associated with the condition.[97] There is no known treatment for the disease. Management consists of treating the complications of the genetic defect as they arise over a lifetime.[94]

13.8 Summary of Key Points

- The vascular supply of the anterior optic nerve is primarily derived from the short posterior ciliary arteries. The vessels show autoregulation by locally released molecules such as nitric oxide, endothelin, prostaglandins, and members of the renin–angiotensin pathway.
- Blood pressure and intraocular pressure influence anterior optic nerve perfusion pressure. Diurnal variation in blood pressure is an important variable to consider in the use of vasoactive medications.
- Optic disk cup size is a risk factor for nonarteritic anterior ischemic optic neuropathy (NAION). The mechanism seems to be ischemia → axoplasmic flow stasis and axonal swelling→ crowding of axons as they exit the eye→compression of optic disk capillaries→worse ischemia (a vicious cycle).
- The peripapillary nerve fiber layer thickness is increasingly reduced in diabetes as retinopathy severity worsens.
- Evidence exists for subclinical optic disk neuroretinal rim edema in diabetic eyes.
- Diabetes is a risk factor for NAION and is associated with more florid disk capillary dilation and peripapillary splinter hemorrhage, a longer course until edema resolution, and a shorter time until fellow eye involvement with NAION than in nondiabetic eyes with NAION. Other treatable risk factors include sleep apnea and nocturnal use of anti-hypertensive medications. Male patients at risk for NAION should probably avoid the use of phosphodiesterase-5 inhibitors to treat erectile dysfunction.
- Diabetic papillopathy, a syndrome of unilateral or bilateral disk edema with or without visual dysfunction that spontaneous resolves, is controversially related to NAION.
- Superior segmental optic hypoplasia is a rare congenital disk anomaly associated in many cases with maternal type 1 diabetes mellitus. It can masquerade as normal tension glaucoma, but unlike the latter, is nonprogressive.
- Wolfram syndrome is a rare neurodegenerative disorder caused by a mutation in the *WFS1 gene*

found on chromosome 4 causing optic atrophy, diabetes mellitus, and other neurological and endocrinologic signs.

13.9 Future Directions

The absence of effective therapy for NAION and of prophylactic treatment of proven efficacy for the fellow eye is potentially superable. Geographically widespread networks such as the Diabetic Retinopathy Clinical Research Network may provide the infrastructure to address potential therapies requiring large sample sizes for proper evaluation. Potentially promising therapies will probably arise from a better understanding of the physiology of the vascular supply to the anterior optic nerve. In particular, the hypothesis that central venous insufficiency in the setting of a small optic disk cup may be the causative insult is worthy of further exploration.[26] Anti-vascular endothelial growth factor drugs given intravitreally may be a way to test this hypothesis, because it has been shown that they decrease venous congestion and disk edema in central retinal vein occlusion.[99] These drugs may be able to abort the vicious cycle of disk edema, increased compression of capillaries, worsened ischemia, and further edema in a confined space.

It has been proposed that laser panretinal photocoagulation might cause optic atrophy and decompress the crowded scleral canal of patients who have had an episode of NAION in one eye.[29] This hypothesis could be tested in a randomized clinical trial.

References

1. Onda E, Cioffi GA, Bacon DR, Van Busckirk EM. Microvasculature of the human optic nerve. *Am J Ophthalmol.* 1995;120:92–102.
2. Henkind P, Levitzky M. Angioarchitecture of the optic nerve I. The papilla. *Am J Ophthalmol.* 1969;68: 979–986.
3. Ernest JT, Potts AM. Pathophysiology of the distal portion of the optic nerve II. Vascular relationships. *Am J Ophthalmol.* 1968;66:380–387.
4. Gitter KA, Blumenthal M, Best M, Galin MA. Origin of the peripapillary vascular network. *Am J Ophthalmol.* 1970;69:249–251.
5. Hayreh SS. Posterior ciliary artery circulation in health and disease. The Weisenfeld Lecture. *Invest Ophthalmol Vis Sci.* 2004;45(3):749–757.
6. Anderson DR. Vascular supply to the optic nerve of primates. *Am J Ophthalmol.* 1970;70:341–351.
7. Lieberman MF, Maumenee AE, Green WR. Histologic studies of the vasculature of the anterior optic nerve. *Am J Ophthalmol.* 1976;82:405–423.
8. Ruskell G. Blood flow in the Zinn-Haller circle. *Br J Ophthalmol.* 1998;82:1351.
9. Ohno-Matsui K, Futagami S, Yamashita S, Tokoro T. Zinn-Haller arterial ring observed by ICG angiography in high myopia. *Br J Ophthalmol.* 1998;82: 1357–1362.
10. Levitsky M, Henkind P. Architecture of the optic nerve II. Lamina cribrosa. *Am J Ophthalmol.* 1969;68: 986–996.
11. Anderson DR. Ultrastructure of human and monkey lamina cribrosa and optic nerve head. *Arch Ophthalmol.* 1969;82:800–814.
12. Levin LA. Optic nerve. In: Kaufman PL, Alm A, eds. *Adler's Physiology of the Eye. Clinical Application.* St. Louis, Mo: Mosby; 2003:603–638.
13. Harris A, Kagemann L, Cioffi GA. Assessment of human ocular hemodynamics. *Surv Ophthalmol.* 1998;42: 509–533.
14. Harris A, Cuilla TA, Chung HK, Martin B. Regulation of retinal and optic nerve blood flow. *Arch Ophthalmol.* 1998;116:1491–1495.
15. Anderson DR. Introductory comments on blood flow autoregulation in the optic nerve head and vascular risk factors in glaucoma. *Surv Ophthalmol.* 1999;43: S5–S9.
16. Hayreh SS. Blood flow in the optic nerve head and factors that may influence it. *Prog Retin Eye Res.* 2001;20:596–624.
17. Rockwood EJ, Fantes F, Davis EB, Anderson DR. The response of retinal vasculature to angiotensin. *Invest Ophthalmol Vis Sci.* 1987;28:676–682.
18. Hayreh SS, Zimmerman MB, Podhajsky P, Alward WLM. Nocturnal arterial hypotension and its role in optic nerve head and ocular ischemic disorders. *Am J Ophthalmol.* 1994;117:603–624.
19. Takahashi H, Goto T, Shoji T, et al. Diabetes associated retinal nerve fiber damage evaluated with scanning laser polarimetry. *Am J Ophthalmol.* 2006;142:88–94.
20. Klein B, Moss S, Klein R, Magli Y, Hoyer C. Neuroretinal rim area in diabetes mellitus. *Invest Ophthalmol Vis Sci.* 1990;31:805–809.
21. Cullen J. Pituitary ablation for advancing diabetic retinopathy. E.E.N.T Digest. 1968;47–54.
22. Hayreh SS, Zimmerman MB. Incipient nonarteritic anterior ischemic optic neuropathy. *Ophthalmology.* 2007;114: 1763–1772.
23. Newman NJ, Scherer R, Langenberg P, et al. The fellow eye in NAION: Report from the ischemic optic neuropathy decompression trial follow-up study. *Am J Ophthalmol.* 2002;134:317–328.

24. Hattenhauer MG, Leavitt JA, Hodge DO, Grill R, Gray DT. Incidence of nonarteritic anterior ischemic optic neuropathy. *Am J Ophthalmol*. 1997;123: 103–107.
25. Arnold AC, Hepler RS. Fluorescein angiography in acute nonarteritic anterior ischemic optic neuropathy. *Am J Ophthalmol*. 1994;117:222–230.
26. Levin LA, Danesh-Meyer HV. Hypothesis. A venous etiology for nonarteritic anterior ischemic optic neuropathy. *Arch Ophthalmol*. 2008;126:1582–1584.
27. Beri M, Klugman MR, Kohler JA, Hayreh SS. Anterior ischemic optic neuropathy VII. Incidence of bilaterality and various influencing factors. *Ophthalmology*. 1987;94:1020–1028.
28. Hayreh SS, Podhajsky PA, Zimmerman B. Nonarteritic anterior ischemic optic neuropathy: time of onset of visual loss. *Am J Ophthalmol*. 1997;124:641–647.
29. Burde RM. Optic disk risk factors for nonarteritic anterior ischemic optic neuropathy. *Am J Ophthalmol*. 1993;116:759–764.
30. Hayreh SS, Zimmerman MB. Optic disk edema in nonarteritic anterior ischemic optic neuropathy. *Graefe's Arch Clin Exp Ophthalmol*. 2007; 245:1107–1121.
31. Feit RH, Tomsak RL, Ellenberger C Jr. Structural factors in the pathogenesis of ischemic optic neuropathy. *Am J Ophthalmol*. 1984;98:105–108.
32. Beck RW, Savino PJ, Repka MX, Schatz NJ, Sergott RC. Optic disk structure in anterior ischemic optic neuropathy. *Ophthalmology*. 1984;91:1334–1337.
33. Cullen JF, Por YM. Ischemic optic neuropathy: the Singapore scene. *Singapore Med J*. 2007;48:281–286.
34. Sadaba LM, Garcia-Layana A, Maldonado MJ, Berian JM. Bilateral ischemic optic neuropathy after transurethral prostatic resection: a case report. *BMC Ophthalmology*. 2006;6:32–36.
35. Hayreh SS. Anterior ischemic optic neuropathy VIII. Clinical features and pathogenesis of post-hemorrhagic amaurosis. *Ophthalmology*. 1987;94:1488–1502.
36. Palombi K, Renard E, Levy P, et al. Non-arteritic anterior ischaemic optic neuropathy is nearly systematically associated with obstructive sleep apnoea. *Br J Ophthalmol*. 2006;90:879–882.
37. Repka MX, Savino PJ, Schatz NJ, Sergott RC. Clinical profile and long-term implications of anterior ischemic optic neuropathy. *Am J Ophthalmol*. 1983; 96:478–483.
38. Behbehani R, Matthews MK, Sergot RC, Savino PJ. Nonarteritic anterior ischemic optic neuropathy in patients with sleep apnea while being treated with continuous positive airway pressure. *Am J Ophthalmol*. 2005;139:518–521.
39. Hayreh SS, Joos KM, Podhajsky PA, Long CR. Systemic diseases associated with nonarteritic anterior ischemic optic neuropathy. *Am J Ophthalmol*. 1994; 118:766–780.
40. Mansour AM, Awwad ST, Najjar DM, et al. Anterior ischemic optic neuropathy after coronary artery bypass graft: the role of anemia in diabetics. *Eye*. 2006;20: 706–711.
41. Jacobson DM, Vierkant RA, Belongias EA. Nonarteritic canterior ischemic optic neuropathy. A case-control study of potential risk factors. *Arch Ophthalmol*. 1997;115:1403–1407.
42. Mojon DS, Hedges TR III, Ehrenberg B, et al. Association between sleep apnea syndrome and nonarteritic anterior ischemic optic neuropathy. *Arch Ophthalmol*. 2002;120:601–605.
43. McCulley TJ, Lam BL, Feuer WJ. Incidence of nonarteritic anterior ischemic optic neuropathy associated with cataract extraction. *Ophthalmology*. 2001;108: 1275–1278.
44. Salomon O, Huna-Baron R, Kurtz S, et al. Analysis of prothrombotic and vascular risk factors in patients with nonarteritic anterior ischemic optic neuropathy. *Ophthalmology*. 1999;106:739–742.
45. Feldon SE. Anterior ischemic optic neuropathy: trouble waiting to happen. *Ophthalmology*. 1999;106: 651–652.
46. Nagy V, Steiber Z, Takacs L, et al. Thrombophilic screening for nonarteritic anterior ischemic optic neuropathy. *Graefe's Arch Clin Exp Ophthalmol*. 2006;244: 3–8.
47. Hayreh SS, Zimmerman B. Visual field abnormalities in nonarteritic anterior ischemic optic neuropathy. Their pattern and prevalence at initial examination. *Arch Ophthalmol*. 2005;123:1554–1562.
48. Burde RM, Slamovits T. Asymptomatic optic disc edema. *J Neuro-ophthalmology*. 1997;17:29–32.
49. Hayreh SS. Anterior ischemic optic neuropathy V. Optic disk edema an early sign. *Arch Ophthalmol*. 1981;99:1030–1040.
50. Almog Y, Goldstein M. Visual outcome in eyes with asymptomatic optic disk edema. *J Neuro-ophthalmol*. 2003;23:204–207.
51. Borchert M, Lessell S. Progressive and recurrent nonarteritic anterior ischemic optic neuropathy. *Arch Ophthalmol*. 1988;106:443–449.
52. Beck RW, Savino PJ, Schatz NJ, et al. Anterior ischemic optic neuropathy: recurrent episodes in the same eye. *Br J Ophthalmol*. 1983;67:705–709.
53. Hayreh SS, Zimmerman MB. Nonarteritic anterior ischemic optic neuropathy: clinical characteristics in diabetic patients versus nondiabetic patients. *Ophthalmology*. 2008;115:1818–1825.
54. Hayreh SS. Non-arteritic anterior ischaemic optic neuropathy and phosphodiesterase-5 inhibitors. *Br J Ophthalmol*. 2008;92:1577–1580.
55. Escaravage GK, Wright JD Jr, Givre SJ. Tadalafil associated with anterior ischemic optic neuropathy. *Arch Ophthalmol*. 2005;123:399–400.
56. Pomeranz HD, Smith KH, Hart WM Jr, Egan RA. Sildenafil-associated nonarteritic anterior ischemic optic neuropathy. *Ophthalmology*. 2002;109: 584–587.
57. Bollinger K, Lee MS. Recurrent visual field defect and ischemic optic neuropathy associated with tadalafil rechallenge. *Arch Ophthalmol*. 2005;123: 400–401.
58. Landau K, Winterkorn JMS, Mailloux LU, Vetter W, Napolitano B. 24-hour blood pressure monitoring in patients with anterior ischemic optic neuropathy. *Arch Ophthalmol*. 1996;114:570–575.

59. Hayreh SS, Podhajsky P, Zimmerman MB. Beta-blocker eyedrops and nocturnal arterial hypotension. *Am J Ophthalmol*. 1999;128:301–309.
60. Sadda SR, Nee M, Miller NR, Biousse V, Newman NJ, Kouzis A. Clinical spectrum of posterior ischemic optic neuropathy. *Am J Ophthalmol*. 2001;132: 743–750.
61. Arnold A. Anterior ischemic optic neuropathy. *Sem Ophthalmol*. 1995;10:221–233.
62. The Ischemic-Optic Neuropathy Decompression Trial Research Group. Optic nerve decompression surgery for nonarteritic anterior ischemic optic neuropathy (NAION) is not effective and may be harmful. *JAMA*. 1995;273:625–632.
63. Johnson LN, Gould TJ, Krohel GB. Effect of levodopa and carbidopa on recovery of visual function in patients with nonarteritic anterior ischemic optic neuropathy of longer than six months' duration. *Am J Ophthalmol*. 1996;121:77–83.
64. Arnold AC, Hepler RS, Lieber M, Alexander JM. Hyperbaric oxygen therapy for nonarteritic anterior ischemic optic neuropathy. *Am J Ophthalmol*. 1996;122:535–541.
65. Beck RW, Hayreh SS, Podhajsky PA, Tan ES, Moke PS. Aspirin therapy in nonarteritic anterior ischemic optic neuropathy. *Am J Ophthalmol*. 1997;123: 212–217.
66. Botelho PJ, Johnson LN, Arnold AC. The effect of aspirin on the visual outcome of nonarteritic anterior ischemic optic neuropathy. *Am J Ophthalmol*. 1996;121:450–451.
67. Lubow M, Makley TA. Pseudopapilledema of juvenile diabetes mellitus. *Arch Ophthalmol*. 1971;85:417–422.
68. Pavan P, Aiello L, Wafai M, Briones J, Sebestyen J, Bradbury M. Optic disc edema in juvenile-onset diabetes. *Arch Ophthalmol*. 1980;98:2193–2195.
69. Barr CC, Glaser JS, Blankenship G. Acute disc swelling in juvenile diabetes: a clinical profile and natural history of 12 cases. *Arch Ophthalmol*. 1980;98: 2185–2192.
70. Regillo C, Brown G, Savino P, et al. Diabetic papillopathy: patient characteristics and fundus findings. *Arch Ophthalmol*. 1995;113:889–895.
71. Valphiades MS. The disk edema dilemma. *Surv Ophthalmol*. 2002;47:183–188.
72. Hayreh SS, Zahoruk RM. Anterior ischemic optic neuropathy VI. In juvenile diabetics. *Ophthalmologica*. 1981;182:13–28.
73. Bayraktar Z, Alacali N, Bayraktar S. Diabetic papillopathy in type 2 diabetic patients. *Retina*. 2002;22:752–758.
74. de Ungria JM, Del Priore LV, Hart W. Abnormal disk vessels after diabetic papillopathy. *Arch Ophthalmol*. 1995;113:245–246.
75. Ward SC, Woods DR, Gilstrap LC III, Hauth JC. Pregnancy and acute optic disc edema of juvenile-onset diabetes. *Obstet Gynecol*. 1984;64:816–818.
76. Katz B. Disc swelling in an adult diabetic patient. *Surv Ophthalmol*. 1990;35:158–163.
77. Ho AC, Maguire AM, Yanuzzi LA, et al. Rapidly progressive optic disk neovascularization after diabetic papillopathy. *Am J Ophthalmol*. 1995;120:673–675.
78. Friedrich Y, Feiner M, Gawi H, Friedman Z. Diabetic papillopathy with macular star mimicking clinically significant diabetic macular edema. *Retina*. 2001;21: 80–82.
79. Early Treatment Diabetic Retinopathy Study Research Group. Photocoagulation for diabetic macular edema. *Arch Ophthalmol*. 1985;103:1796–1806.
80. Appen RE, Chandra SR, Klein R, Myers FL. Diabetic papillopathy. *Am J Ophthalmol*. 1980;90:203–209.
81. Schatz H, McDonald HR, Johnson RN. Diagnostic and therapeutic challenges. *Retina*. 1998;18:67–69.
82. Saito Y, Ueki N, Hamanaka N, et al. Transient optic disk edema by vitreous traction in a quiescent eye with proliferative diabetic retinopathy mimicking diabetic papillopathy. *Retina*. 2005;25:83–84.
83. Landau K, Bajka JD, Kirchschlager BM. Topless optic disks in children of mothers with type I diabetes mellitus. *Am J Ophthalmol*. 1998;125:605–611.
84. Han SB, Park KH, Kim DM, Kim TW. Prevalence of superior segmental optic nerve hypoplasia in Korea. *Jpn J Ophthalmol*. 2009;53:225–228.
85. Hayashi K, Tomidokoro A, Aihara M, et al. Long-term follow-up of superior segmental optic hypoplasia. *Jpn J Ophthalmol*. 2008;52:412–414.
86. Foroozan R. Superior segmental optic nerve hypoplasia and diabetes mellitus. *J Diabetes Complications*. 2005;19:165–167.
87. Yamamoto T, Sato M, Iwase A. Superior segmental optic hypoplasia found in tajimi eye health care project participants. *Jpn J Ophthalmol*. 2004;48:578–583.
88. Unoki K, Ohba N, Hoyt WF. Optical coherence tomography of superior segmental optic hypoplasia. *Br J Ophthalmol*. 2002;86:910–914.
89. Brodsky MC, Schroeder GT, Ford R. Superior segmental optic hypoplasia in identical twins. *J Clin Neuro-ophthalmol*. 1993;13:152–154.
90. Sowka J, Vollmer L, Reynolds S. Superior segmental optic nerve hypoplasia: the topless disc syndrome 70. *Optometry*. 2008;79:576–580.
91. Genis D, Davalos A, Molins A, Ferrer I. Wolfram syndrome: a neuropathological study. *Acta Neuropathol*. 1997;93:426–429.
92. Van den Ouweland JMW, Cryns K, Pennings RJE, et al. Molecular characterization of WFS1 in patients with Wolfram Syndrome. *J Mol Diagn*. 2003;5:88–95.
93. Galluzzi P, Filosomi G, Vallone IM, Bardelli AM, Venturi C. MRI of wolfram syndrome (DIDMOAD). *Neuroradiology*. 1999;41:729–731.
94. Hong J, Zhang YW, Zhang HJ, et al. The novel compound heterozygous mutations, V434del and W666X, in WFS1 gene causing Wolfram syndrome in a Chinese family. *Endocrine*. 2009;35:151–157.
95. Barrett TG, Bundey SE, Fiedler AR, Good PA. Optic atrophy in Wolfram (DIDMOAD) Syndrome. *Eye*. 1997;11:882–888.
96. Ajlouni K, Jarrah N, El-Khateeb M, et al. Wolfram Syndrome: identification of a phenotypic and genotypic variant from Jordan. *Am J Med Genet*. 2002;115:61–65.
97. Barrientos A, Volpini V, Casademont J, et al. A nuclear defect in the 4p16 region predisposes to multiple

mitochondrial DNA deletions in families with Wolfram syndrome. *J Clin Invest*. 1996;97:1570–1576.
98. Wake DJ, Jadhav V, Whittome LR, Campbell IW. Wolfram syndrome: DIDMOAD. *Br J Diabetes Vasc Dis*. 2005;5:236–237.
99. Iturralde D, Spaide RF, Meyerle CB, et al. Intravitreal bevacizumab (Avastin) treatment for macular edema in central retinal vein occlusion: a short term study. *Retina*. 2006;26:279–284.

Chapter 14
Screening for Diabetic Retinopathy

David J. Browning

14.1 Introduction

Screening is worthwhile when certain criteria are met: a disease has public health importance; an effective treatment exists; an interval exists within which treatment can effect benefit; and the disease is neither too rare nor too common.[1] Screening for diabetes mellitus in those over 40 years of age and screening for diabetic retinopathy (DR) in those with known diabetes mellitus fulfill these criteria.[2,3] Beyond improving health-related outcomes, treatment of diabetes and DR is cost effective.[4,5,6] Thus, the value of screening for DR is widely recognized. There is, however, controversy regarding the best screening method and screening intervals.[7]

In the United States, the gold standard for screening to detect DR is a dilated fundus examination with stereoscopic biomicroscopy and indirect ophthalmoscopy annually from diagnosis of diabetes in type 2 diabetes and annually beginning 5 years after diagnosis in type 1 diabetes.[8–10] The failure of this ideal as a practical standard is exemplified by the statistic that 30–50% of patients with diabetes are not screened annually, and that 10–36% of known diabetics have never had a dilated eye examination, depending on the country.[7,11–17] In the United States, approximately half of those never having had a dilated eye examination have eye disease.[18] Across the world, failure in screening is related to economic status; worse poverty is associated with worse screening outcomes.[16,14] For example, among Chinese populations, rates of undiagnosed diabetes due to failure to screen are lower in Hong Kong and Taiwan than mainland China[19]. In the United States too, poverty is associated with lower rates of eye examinations for DR.[16,14,20] Among the poor, minorities, migrants, and others with limited access to health-care annual screening rates for DR are as low as 10%.[14,21]

A correlation exists between failure of screening for diabetes and DR and a preventable proportion of societal blindness. In Bristol, UK, 5.5% of blind registrations were due to DR, and of these, 50% had never had an eye examination and 22% were not known to be diabetic.[22] Screening for DR implies a more basic need to screen for diabetes. If diabetes has not been diagnosed, there is no possibility of screening for DR. Screening for DR should be focused on known diabetics, as the rate of referable retinopathy in newly diagnosed diabetics from screening is negligible.[23]

The goal of screening all diabetic patients has not been met in most societies across the world with the exception of Iceland.[3,11,24,25] The reasons besides poverty vary, but include inadequate numbers and regional maldistribution of ophthalmologists and optometrists, poor ability of non-eye care health professionals to recognize referable DR, lack of education and awareness of the importance of screening eye examinations in diabetes, advanced patient age, requirement to dilate the pupils, and burden of undiagnosed diabetes.[3,24,26,27] As a result, interest in screening methods is worldwide and the literature is large. The topic is complex because the optimal techniques in screening for diabetic macular edema (DME), nonproliferative diabetic retinopathy

D.J. Browning (✉)
Charlotte Eye Ear Nose & Throat Associates, Charlotte, NC 28210, USA
e-mail: dbrowning@ceenta.com

D.J. Browning (ed.), *Diabetic Retinopathy*, DOI 10.1007/978-0-387-85900-2_14,

(NPDR), and proliferative diabetic retinopathy (PDR) are not the same. The retinal lesions are often more peripheral in PDR and detection of DME is compromised by nonstereoscopic methods.[9,26,28–30] Nor are the techniques necessarily the same for types 1 and 2 diabetes. Some studies use more complicated protocols for type 1 diabetics because of their greater probability of having PDR requiring more peripheral retinal examination.[27] Comparing the results of studies is difficult because of different definitions of referable retinopathy, ungradable photographic images, gold standards, and protocols for screening.[3,9] Moreover, cameras have improved limiting comparability across studies over time.[26] Film versus digital media, red-free versus color images for grading, and grading on screens versus prints further cloud comparability of studies.[31] Despite these complexities, in this chapter we will try to identify the broad themes, while making no claim to exhaustive coverage of the topic.

The effectiveness of a screening program depends on four variables – the prevalence of the disease, the percentage of the target population actually screened (the compliance), the performance statistics of the screening method (the sensitivity and specificity), and the cost.[32] Estimates of the prevalence of sight-threatening eye disease among diabetics range from 6.0 to 14.1%.[9,32] Compliance with opportunistic screening by general practitioners and diabetologists in daily practice versus systematic photographic screening in pilot trials in the United Kingdom has been reported to be 38–85% and 80–93%, respectively.[10,32] Compliance with ophthalmic screening in the United States is 50–65%.[17] Factors that limit compliance include housebound patients, percentage of patients in rural areas, social deprivation score based on unemployment, distribution of doctors, crowding, car ownership, socioeconomic status, and rapid population turnover in mobile urban societies.[32,33] Published benchmark targets for compliance are 90–95%.[10] Sensitivity and specificity for screening by primary care physicians have been estimated to be 38–63% and 92–97%, respectively.[32,34,35] For photographic screening methods, these estimates are generally >80% and >90%, respectively (Table 14.2). As a reference benchmark, an acceptable screening technique needs to have a sensitivity for the detection of DR of $\geq$ 80%.[9,36] Cost estimates vary over time and on many assumptions such as method of screening and valuation for degrees of visual impairment.[7] We will compare the performance of the various methods of screening on these variables below.

14.2 Who Does Not Need to Be Screened

Type 1 diabetics of age less than 9–12 years do not need to be screened, because the risk of DME and PDR is near zero.[37–40] Type 1 diabetics who have been diagnosed less than 3–5 years previously also do not need to be screened for similar reasons.[8,39]

14.3 Screening for Diabetic Retinopathy by Adjunctive or Stand-Alone Visual Acuity Testing

Given the challenge of primary care providers learning ophthalmoscopic skills, there has been an interest in determining if detection of DR by simply screening for subnormal corrected visual acuity is feasible.[17] Evidence suggests that this is not the case.[35,36,41,42] The sensitivity of visual acuity testing for retinopathy as severe or more severe than moderate NPDR was 43.8% because many patients with more severe DR continue to have good visual acuity.[35] Its sensitivity for the detection of DME was 7.5–38.5%. The specificity of visual acuity screening is also low because other causes of reduced vision, such as cataract, corneal pathology, or macular degeneration, are common.[35–36,41–43] Nevertheless, because DME is 4–5 times as common as PDR, its detection is difficult for all methods, and a check of visual acuity is simple and inexpensive to perform, adding a vision check to the other methods of screening is a good strategy for reducing false negatives and prioritizing referral.[9,22,35]

14.4 Screening with Undilated Direct Ophthalmoscopy by Non-eye Care Professionals

Direct ophthalmoscopy performed by nonophthalmologist physicians has sensitivity and specificity for detecting PDR of 30–67% and 97%, respectively.[35,44,45] Experience affects the screening statistics; physicians in fellowship training performed worse than attendings with >8 years experience.[35] For DME detection by nonophthalmologists, the sensitivity and specificity were 0% and 100%, respectively.[35] For DR retinopathy detection without further subclassification, the sensitivity and specificity were 52 and 91% for a general practitioner and 67 and 97% for an endocrinologist.[46] The sensitivity and specificity of a physician's assistant for detection of DR compared to seven-field stereo fundus photography were 14 and 99%, respectively.[47] The sensitivity and specificity of experienced technicians to detect PDR compared to seven-field stereo fundus photography were 50 and 90%, respectively.[29]

The practicality of non-eye care professionals screening for DR has been in turn defended and deprecated.[17,35] The best case scenario has been studied using the photographic files of the Early Treatment Diabetic Retinopathy Study (ETDRS).[17] Bresnick and colleagues assumed that such professionals could be trained to correctly identify retinal lesions of DR in the area covered by ETDRS photographic fields 1–3 (roughly the posterior pole and peripapillary retina). If this were the case, in the older onset diabetic population, the best case sensitivity and specificity for detecting PDR were 87 and 80%, respectively.[17] The fundus characteristic associated with this level of performance was the presence of hemorrhages and microaneurysms temporal to the macula as severe as or more severe than ETDRS standard photograph 3 (see chapter 5). For clinically significant macular edema (CSME), the sensitivity and specificity were 94 and 54%, respectively.[17] The characteristic associated with this performance was presence of any hard exudates within 1 disk diameter of the center of the macula. Assuming it were practical and that nonophthalmologists could detect vision-threatening retinopathy (PDR and DME) reliably, the number of referrals for ophthalmologic examination would drop an estimated 47% for younger onset patients and 62% for older onset patients.[17] The bulk of the evidence suggests that actual performance by nonophthalmic physicians will continue to fall far short of this best case scenario.[48]

14.5 Screening with Dilated Ophthalmoscopy by Ophthalmic Technicians or Optometrists

With special training and unrestricted ability to consult among themselves, an optometrist and an ophthalmic technician were able to perform on par with an ophthalmologist in detecting DR by direct ophthalmoscopy and indirect ophthalmoscopy as needed.[49] DR severity was collapsed into three categories: none, NPDR, and PDR. The agreement between all three examiner types and graded seven-field stereo fundus photographs was 85.7% and the chance-corrected agreement (kappa) was 0.749. There was no important difference between the performance of the ophthalmologist, the optometrist, or the technician.[49] Studies using various gold standards (e.g., ophthalmologist or retina specialist diagnosis) and levels of retinopathy detection (e.g., referable or sight threatening) have reported sensitivity and specificity for optometric detection of DR of 52–94% and 90–100%, respectively.[10,46,50,51] The sensitivity of British ophthalmic opticians for detecting any DR was 73%.[45]

14.6 Screening with Dilated Ophthalmoscopy by Ophthalmologists

With seven-field stereoscopic photography as a gold standard, the sensitivity and specificity for ophthalmologists detecting DR have ranged from 28 to 76% and 91 to 100%, respectively.[5,35,47,52,53] The wide range of sensitivity reflects differences in study designs and types of retinopathy assessed. Chance-corrected agreement has been poor (0.38–0.40), primarily because ophthalmoscopy is insensitive to the presence of microaneurysms and small intraretinal hemo-rrhages.[5,47,54] For DME, the sensitivity and specificity are 40 and 100%, respectively.[35] For detecting PDR, these statistics were 61–80% and 98–99%, respectively.[53,55] Whether direct plus indirect ophthalmoscopy or slit-lamp biomicroscopy with a fundus non-contact lens plus indirect ophthalmoscopy is employed seems not to matter.[47] Although a few studies disagree, most suggest that dilated ophthalmoscopy is inferior to single-field nonmydriatic photography for detecting DR, although ophthalmoscopy and the attendant co-examination have co-advantages not found with photographic screening.[5,47,55,56]

Referable Retinopathy – A Strange Situation

In clinical practice, the gold standard for the detection of DR in need of treatment is a dilated eye examination by an ophthalmologist. Screening is an issue only because too many diabetics fail to undergo this type of examination. It may seem odd, therefore, to discover that the clinical gold standard performs poorly compared to digital photography in detecting referable retinopathy, i.e., retinopathy bad enough to need to have the very technique that was inferior at detecting it in the first place. This paradox reflects the difference between any retinopathy and sight-threatening retinopathy in need of treatment. The former category includes far more patients than the latter. It is a fair question, however, to ask if eventually some other technique will supplant clinical examination as the gold standard for sight-threatening retinopathy. For example, there is accumulating evidence that OCT may become the gold standard for detecting treatable DME – that biomicroscopy leads to undertreatment of DME.[57] Until a randomized trial is done, however, comparing visual outcomes of patients detected and treated according to OCT rather than slit-lamp biomicroscopy guidelines, the clinical detection of DME remains the gold standard.

Readers of the literature on screening for DR are warned that the definition for referable retinopathy varies widely. In some studies, anything other than absence of retinopathy is a basis for referral. In others, particularly in settings where access to care is poor and poverty high, referable retinopathy has been set at severe NPDR.[21] The results of studies are difficult to compare given the wide variation in cutpoints for referring patients for ophthalmologic examination.

14.7 Screening with Dilated Ophthalmoscopy by Retina Specialists

The chance adjusted agreement for a retina specialist's detection of DR by dilated indirect and direct ophthalmoscopy versus grading by a trained photographic grader at a reading center of seven-field stereoscopic fundus photographs has been reported to be 0.49.[54] The kappa for assessing severity of retinopathy has been reported to be 0.55–0.62.[54,58] The sensitivity and specificity of a retina specialist for detecting PDR were 50 and 100%, respectively.[34] Using direct and indirect ophthalmoscopy and contact lens stereoscopic biomicroscopy through a dilated pupil, the sensitivity and specificity for detection of CSME by retina specialists compared to reading center grading of stereo fundus photographs were 82 and 79% in the ETDRS.[59]

Sensitivity, Specificity, and Chance-Corrected Agreement

The reader will have noticed that the performance statistics cited from different publications vary. Sometimes reports use sensitivity and specificity and sometimes chance-corrected agreement (kappa). The relationship between these performance measures is complex. Sensitivity is defined as the fraction of true positives expressed as a percentage. Specificity is the fraction of true negatives expressed as a percentage. It helps to consider a 2 × 2 table expressing the agreement between a gold standard method of detection and another (test) method of detection (Table 14.1).

Table 14.1 Definition of Chance-Corrected Agreement (Kappa)

		Gold standard method	
		+	–
Test	+	A	B
Method	–	C	D

With this framework,

$$\text{sensitivity} = \text{A}/(\text{A} + \text{C})$$
$$\text{specificity} = \text{D}/(\text{B} + \text{D})$$

$$\text{kappa} = [\text{observed agreement} - \text{expected agreement}]/[1 - \text{expected agreement}],$$
$$\text{where observed agreement} = (\text{A} + \text{D})/(\text{A} + \text{B} + \text{C} + \text{D})$$
$$\text{and expected agreement} = (\text{A} + \text{B})(\text{A} + \text{C})/(\text{A}+\text{B}+\text{C}+\text{D})^2 + (\text{C}+\text{D})(\text{B}+\text{D})/(\text{A}+\text{B}+\text{C}+\text{D})^2.$$

Sensitivity and specificity do not depend on prevalence of the condition in the population, but kappa does. As the prevalence decreases, kappa decreases for any given values of the sensitivity and specificity.[60]

14.8 Photographic Screening

The gold standard for photographically detecting DR is seven-field stereoscopic fundus photography covering 65–75 degrees of the fundus. This method is costly, not liked by patients because of its higher flash intensity than digital imaging and need for more photographs, and impractical for screening purposes; it is used in research protocols rather than clinical care.[3,5,28,29,36] There are many strategies for photoscreening, making comparison of different techniques difficult. Several of the strategies that have undergone pilot trials follow:

1. Mydriatic fundus photography with various numbers of fields (2, 3, 5, 6) and various degrees captured per field (30, 45, 60).[36,61,9,24,28,42,48]
2. Nonmydriatic 45 degree fundus photography with various numbers of fields (1, 2, 4).[3,21,61,62,63,64,11]
3. Staged screening comprised of stage single-field nonmydriatic photography followed by single-field mydriatic photography for ungradable images with stage 1 efforts followed by slit-lamp biomicroscopy by an ophthalmologist for ungradable images with stage 1 and 2 efforts.
4. Single-field nonmydriatic fundus photography for patients < 50 years old and single-field mydriatic fundus photography for patients ≥ 50 years old.
5. For type 2 diabetics, three-field 45 degree nonmydriatic fundus photographs with dilation as needed to obtain satisfactory image quality. For type 1 diabetics, five-field 45-degree mydriatic fundus photographs.[26]

An understanding of the trade-offs incurred by different strategies compared to seven-field imaging is helpful in choosing a preferred method of photoscreening. Underascertainment of DR by methodologies using fewer than seven fields has been estimated to range from 5 to 15%.[65] Using TIFF and JPEG compressed images, digital images are associated with 86–92% and 72–74% sensitivity, respectively, compared to using color slides.[36] Approximately 27% of cases of PDR and 8–15% of all DR lesions occur outside the area photographed with single-field 45 degree nonmydriatic photography.[39] Over time and after weighing these relative drawbacks, the trend has been toward single-image screening methods (Table 14.2). Adding more fields adds to the cost, increases the probability of poor quality images and

Table 14.2 Performance characteristics of two single-image photographic screening methods

	NPDR		PDR		Referable DR	
Technique	Sensitivity (%)	Specificity (%)	Sensitivity (%)	Specificity (%)	Sensitivity (%)	Specificity (%)
Single-field nonmydriatic 45 degree	61[56], 96.7[29]	92.9,[29] 82[56]	92.0[29]	97.6,[29] 100[56]	38,[69] 61,[47] 77,[61] 78,[5] 89,[21] 85,[70] 85,[71] 96,[56]	85,[47] 86,[5] 93,[71] 95,[61] 95,[69] 97,[21] 97,[70]
Single-field mydriatic 45 degree	97.5[29]	93.3[29]	96.6[29]	100[29]	81,[61] 84.4[72]	79.2,[72] 92[61]

The definitions of referable retinopathy, the reference standard technique, the rates of ungradable photographs, the rates of referable retinopathy, whether eyes or patients are used in calculation of referral rates, and whether the ungradable photographs are included in the referable category vary among studies, and therefore comparison of sensitivities and specificities must be guarded. Some studies had a mixture of nonmydriatic and mydriatic photographs taken. For purposes of classification, they are put into the group for which most of the photographs were taken. NPDR = nonproliferative diabetic retinopathy. PDR = proliferative diabetic retinopathy. DR = diabetic retinopathy.

leads to extra referrals for ophthalmic examination without sufficient compensatory improvement in case finding.[66]

The settings for screening have varied, but include university diabetes clinics, private practice offices, hospital endocrinology clinics, nursing homes, community health clinics, and mobile units in vans.[3,21,36,42,66–68] Methods of notifying the target population that screening will occur may be important.[27] In some models multimedia advertisement of screening is used, whereas in others there is no advertising, but only routine use of a modality in the course of diabetic, nonophthalmic care.[11] The assessment of screening techniques may need to take into account the social environment. A successful screening approach in an urban environment with tertiary care medical centers may differ from the approach adapted to a rural environment with few eye care professionals.[24] Screening for certain subgroups of the population, while a laudable goal, has proven impractical. For example, in nursing homes, the relatively high proportion of subjects who are unable to cooperate or undergo treatment even if amenable disease is discovered has rendered the cost per case too high.[42]

Different Definitions of Diabetic Retinopathy Severity in Screening Studies

Defining severity of DR is challenging, and many different sets of definitions have been established (see Chapter 5). The ETDRS definitions are difficult for any but professional graders to employ. Predictably, definitions designed for clinical use are simpler, as are those designed for screening purposes. One example of definitions of severity for screening purposes by nonophthalmologists follows (Table 14.3).

Table 14.3 Simplified classification of diabetic retinopathy

Stage	Retinal pathology
1	Mild nonproliferative (occasional microaneurysms and/or hemorrhages and/or exudates)
2	Moderate nonproliferative (intraretinal hemorrhages and/or cotton wool spots and/or venous anomalies in one to three quadrants)
3	Severe nonproliferative (intraretinal hemorrhages and/or cotton wool spots and/or venous anomalies in all quadrants)
4	Proliferative noncomplicated (new vessels on disk or retina)
5	Proliferative complicated (tractional retinal detachment, preretinal, or vitreous hemorrhage)
Maculopathy	Presence of hard exudates within 1 disk diameter of the foveola
Treated	Presence of photocoagulation scars anywhere (sectoral, panretinal, focal, grid)

Reproduced with permission from Deb-Joarder[24]

Even simpler classifications are in use. Kuo and colleagues have a four level system: no retinopathy, background retinopathy, pre-proliferative retinopathy, and proliferative or post-photocoagulation retinopathy.[3] Comparison of screening outcomes among studies using different systems is fraught with uncertainty.

Technical and practical issues arise in photographic screening. Because the photographs are taken by ancillary staff in a general clinic, training is important in recognizing unusable images and repeating photography until a usable image can be obtained. With training, such staff perform as well as ophthalmic photographers in producing gradable images.[36] Staff must be trained on the importance of physiologic mydriasis in a darkened room, and feedback on photographic quality is necessary to reduce the number of artifacts that degrade image quality. Photography of the second eye may need to be delayed for a time after the first eye photograph to allow for spontaneous redilation. It seems to be necessary to photograph both eyes and not one. A strategy of photographing only one eye results in a 9% rate of false negatives.[62] Although DR is usually a symmetric condition, it is asymmetric often enough that both eyes need to be screened.[62,73] Many have worried that nonstereoscopic photographic screening methods will miss DME, yet the presence of hard lipid exudates within 1 disk diameter of the center of the macula is >90% sensitive in detecting DME, and lipid can be sensitively detected with nonstereoscopic fundus photography.[36] Moreover, most of the cases of DME without lipid exudates are recommended for referral based on other screening criteria.[36]

Film-based photographic screening methods are now a chapter in history, not a viable method.[68] Digital methods allow for the possibility of machine-based interpretation, teleophthalmic interpretation, and more rapid turnaround in interpretation compared to film-based systems.[5] Who should interpret the digital fundus images remains controversial, but it appears that nonophthalmologists can perform well. With 40 h of training by an ophthalmologist, grading of fundus photographs by endocrinologists matched the gold standard results of consensus gradings by two experienced ophthalmologists in detecting DR.[24] Various systems have used technicians, opticians, nurse practitioners, internists, and optometrists for grading.[9,47,74]

14.9 Nonmydriatic Photography

The reported rates of ungradable images using a nonmydriatic camera range from 4 to 34%.[11,21,30,68,75] These cameras are easy to use; training to a reasonable standard of proficiency can be attained within 1 h. Level of training in ophthalmic photography does not seem to influence image quality much, a favorable attribute for consideration in screening programs.[76] Higher rates of ungradable images lead to higher rates of referral for dilated eye examinations by eye care professionals because of doubt by the photography graders regarding adequacy of the image to exclude the risk of missing referable retinopathy. This is seen by different subgroups in the care team as a positive or a negative. Where numbers of professionals are high relative to the proportion of patients to be seen, a higher rate of referral is seen as a positive. Where numbers of professionals are low relative to the number of patients to be seen, a higher rate of referral is seen as a negative and has led to adoption of mydriatic screening over nonmydriatic screening as a response.[24] In Singapore, where national photographic screening for DR by trained family practitioners using a 45 degree fundus photograph obtained with a nonmydriatic camera has been in place since the early 1990s, only 38% of the patients referred actually had DR, reflecting a much poorer specificity for the technique in practice than under idealized study conditions.[77] Similarly, in Gloucestershire, UK, the actual percentages of patients referred based on screening who, in fact, had no DR on actual clinical examination varied from 47.8 to 56.7% over the first 4 years of implementing a systematic screening program.[78] It is recognized that most screening tests perform less well in real-world settings than in settings based on a study design.[55] In a study from Colorado, USA, family physicians reading nonmydriatic 45 degree fundus photographs failed to refer 10.2% of patients deemed needing a referral to an ophthalmologist by a secondary image grader who was an ophthalmologist.[21] Nonmydriatic photography often requires placing the patient in a darkened room for a time and has been found to lengthen the screening process compared to a mydriatic screening procedure.[24] There are metrics of fundus image quality other than percentage of ungradable images, such as grades of image quality and ability to detect referable DR, and all such metrics are beneficially influenced by mydriasis and negatively influenced by nonmydriasis.[24] The perils of nonmydriatic fundus photography missing sight-threatening peripheral neovascular fronds have been documented, but despite admonitions that general practitioners become better direct ophthalmoscopists, the statistical evidence favors nonmydriatic photography over nonmydriatic ophthalmoscopy for detecting referable retinopathy.[30]

14.10 Mydriatic Photography

There are several objections raised whenever mydriatic methods of screening are considered. The first is that narrow angle glaucoma attacks may be triggered. The risk is low and has been estimated to be 1 in 7,000 examinations or lower.[47,79] The second is that patients will object and refuse screening under these conditions. When mild mydriatic agents such as tropicamide 1% are used and only a single dose is given, patient acceptance has been high.[24] The ability to drive after mydriasis is a third objection, particularly in those over 55 years of age. Somewhat counterintuitively, pharmacologic dilation has been reported to speed screening for DR compared to nonmydriatic screening.[24] The choice of the mydriatic used may be important. Patient acceptance of moderate mydriasis achieved with tropicamide 1% was reported to be good.[24] Mydriatic screening methods are particularly useful in older patients with more miotic pupils. Mydriatic photography as a backup when nonmydriatic photography gives poor images can reduce the rate of ungradable images to <1%.[21]

14.11 Risk Factors for Ungradable Photographs

In nonmydriatic photoscreening, increasing the number of fields imaged above two increases the number of cases deemed to have poor quality sets of images requiring referral.[66] The rate of ungradable photographs decreases if mydriatic photoscreening is used rather than nonmydriatic photoscreening.[24,61,75] In 12 studies using nonmydriatic photography, the median and the range of ungradable photographs were 18.3% and 4.0–42.3%, respectively.[24,75,61,5,68,11,21,47,63,71,64] By comparison, among six studies using mydriatic photography, the median and the range of ungradable photographs were 3.7% and <1–5%, respectively.[24,75,61,21,47,9] Increasing age is associated with an increasing rate of ungradable photographs whether by nonmydriatic or mydriatic photographic technique, because of both an increasing effect of cataract and a decreasing pupillary diameter alone or after pharmacologic mydriasis.[5,24,61,71,75] There is a floor for the percentage of ungradable photographs. In the Wisconsin Epidemiologic Study of Diabetic Retinopathy (WESDR), in which mydriasis and professional ophthalmic photographers were used in a population-based study, 1.5% of participants had ungradable photographs.[17]

14.12 Number of Photographic Fields

Whether a greater number of photographic fields are associated with a higher rate of detection of referable retinopathy at a reasonable price of more time, expense, and increased patient dissatisfaction with bright flashes is controversial.[28] Some studies suggest that more fields increase the rates of referable retinopathy. Others suggest that no clinically important gains are made by this provision.[61] The trend in the literature seems to be that single-field photography predominates based on adequate performance and simplicity.

14.13 Criteria for Referral

The criteria for referral for a complete, dilated eye examination by an ophthalmologist are not identical across studies. All screening methodologies recommend referral for severe nonproliferative retinopathy, proliferative retinopathy, diabetic maculopathy, presence of photocoagulation scars, and presence of nondiabetic pathology discovered coincidentally. The term diabetic maculopathy includes exudates within 1 disk diameter of the fovea, any circinate or group of exudates within the macula, and any microaneurysm or hemorrhage within 1 disk diameter of the fovea.[61] At the most liberal end of the spectrum for referral criteria, some groups mandate referral for presence of any retinopathy more severe than having microaneurysms alone.[5] Others set the bar for referral at a more severe level of retinopathy. Some guidelines place all ungradable photographs in the referral category.[5,26,63] The criteria for referral will markedly impact the cost of screening programs. For example, changing the threshold for referral from very mild DR (ETDRS level 20) to mild DR (ETDRS level 35) changed rates of referral from 36.1 to 26.1% of those undergoing photographic screening in one study.[11]

14.14 Obstacles to the Use of Teleophthalmic Screening Methods

Several obstacles hinder the acceptance of teleophthalmic screening for DR. Perhaps the greatest is the concern among ophthalmologists that patients and primary care doctors will mistakenly interpret screening photographs as a substitute for a dilated eye examination by an ophthalmologist. Although these systems are implemented with explicit acknowledgment that they serve as a net to catch those non-compliant patients who will not be seen for this recommended process, in actual practice the concern seems valid.[21] Reimbursement concerns are another obstacle slowing acceptance of these methods. In countries without nationalized health-care systems, primary care physicians are reluctant to invest in the camera, although prices are falling and retinopathy screening companies have developed proformas that identify the volumes of patients required in a given time interval at prevailing rates of reimbursement to ensure no financial loss. Worry about legal liability is another issue for photographic graders. In countries with nationalized health care, photographic screening does not encounter these obstacles and implementation of these programs has progressed further.

There is evidence that poor rates of screening for DR represent an active avoidance of patients who realize the importance of a dilated eye examination for the detection of a sight-threatening condition, yet choose not to comply.[11] There is also evidence that a proportion of these patients actively prefer a nonmydriatic, teleophthalmic method for screening as an alternative to the recommended gold standard for detection of retinopathy.[11] Thus, eye care professionals may need to accept that photographic screening is the only practical way to access a fraction of the diabetic population at risk for eye disease.[21]

14.15 Combination Methods of Screening

Single-field mydriatic fundus photography interpreted by a retina specialist added to mydriatic ophthalmoscopy increased the sensitivity of general practitioners and ophthalmic opticians for detecting any DR.[45] For general practitioners, the sensitivity increased from 55 to 71%. For ophthalmic opticians, the sensitivity increased from 73 to 88%.[45] Similarly, adding a macular stereoscopic pair of fundus photographs to mydriatic direct ophthalmoscopy improved sensitivity for detecting DR from 65 to 93%.[48]

14.16 Case Yield Rates

Rates of referable retinopathy have been consistent across many studies and locales, ranging from 4.4 to 5.1%.[68,21,78] Although screening for DR is worthwhile in many venues, as adequate detection of retinopathy is widely lacking, some venues have higher yield rates for disease needing treatment. In a study from Scotland, rural screening yielded higher rates of detected advanced retinopathy than urban screening.[68]

What Is the Optimal Screening Interval and When Should Screening Begin?

Is annual screening a good use of resources in patients with noninsulin-dependent diabetes and good HbA1c?[80] Should quality measurement organizations require annual screening of pre-pubertal type 1 diabetics even though they have had diabetes for more than 5 years? Evidence suggests that annual screening of type 2 diabetics with no retinopathy at the baseline examination may be unnecessary.[50,35,81] In such patients, the 4-year incidence rates of DME and PDR in WESDR were 1.1 and 0.4%, respectively, and omission of annual screening for 4 years is logical.[35] Translating this into a practical policy, however, is fraught with difficulty, because the accurate classification of retinopathy severity by seven-field photography is not available in the community as it was used in WESDR. Practical photographic screening protocols are able to achieve sensitivities of 89–93%, however, and screening intervals could rationally be relaxed in patients with no retinopathy in places with such methods in place.[81] For example, Younis and colleagues recommended screening intervals of every 3 years for patients without retinopathy, every year for patients with mild to moderate retinopathy, and every 4 months for patients with severe nonproliferative retinopathy in Liverpool, England, based on the performance statistics of a systematic photographic screening program established in 1991.[81] In the United States, where screening programs remain rare in 2009, the uniform annual policy, once screening begins, remains intact. Although yearly screening for type 2 diabetics and type 1 diabetics beginning 5 years after diagnosis is the screening benchmark, they are unrealistic in certain clinical settings.[21] These questions become more pressing as the economic constraints become tighter.

14.17 Compliance with Recommendation to Be Seen by an Ophthalmologist

Regardless of the success of screening for detection of referable retinopathy, if advice to be seen for examination is not heeded, the screening program has failed. Rates of compliance with a recommendation to be seen for examination have ranged from 48.0 to 90.5%.[27,64,71] In one study the rate depended on reason for referral.[27,64,71] Patients referred for PDR were more likely to comply than patients referred for NPDR, possibly because the risk of visual loss was higher with PDR and this was effectively communicated to the patient.[27] Even when screening is free to the patient (although not to some alternate payor), efforts are frequently unsuccessful. In a demonstration project among medically underserved residents of rural Colorado, the screening rate increased from <10% per year to 37% over a 3-year period when free-to-the-patient screening was introduced.[21] In a study from a prepaid Health Maintenance Organization in which there was no additional cost to the patient for the ophthalmologic examination, the compliance rate was 74%.[71] If the additional examination costs the patient, the compliance rate would be expected to be less.[71] In comparing screening rates for diabetic retinopathy across managed care versus fee-for-service settings, the managed care setting did not outperform the fee-for-service setting as might have been expected based on its cost structure for patients.[82] Factors other than simple cost of screening may explain this situation, including such problems as population transience, effectiveness of communication, and variable enthusiasm among different screening sites for the screening mission.

14.18 Intravenous Fluorescein Angiography and Oral Fluorescein Angioscopy

Adding fluorescein angiography to fundus photography does not add sufficient sensitivity for the detection of early NPDR to make it worth the expense.[83] Oral fluorescein angioscopy is too time consuming and expensive to be practical for large-scale screening purposes.[36]

14.19 Automated Fundus Image Interpretation

A drawback of all operational photographic screening methods is the requirement of a human grader, who may range from a trained technician to a fully trained retina specialist. This adds to the cost of screening. Although computerized automated interpretation is a research concept only, it promises to reduce the cost of screening in the future.[84,85] One early prototype of such a system accurately classified 14 of 22 (63.6%) images of PDR and 46 of 58 (79.3%) images of NPDR compared to a human grader taken as the gold standard.[86] Another system based on an artificial neural network reading color fundus photographs achieved sensitivity and specificity of 88.4 and 83.5%, respectively, for DR detection compared to the results of an ophthalmologist's reading of the photographs.[85]

14.20 Subgroups Needing Enhanced Screening Efforts

Certain subgroups of patients with diabetes have lower rates of usage of eye care services. In a study of Medicare claims data, males, blacks, and persons living in areas with higher poverty and fewer ophthalmologists had lower rates of having an eye examination within the past year.[16] State blindness prevention programs that target persons with diabetes, who have not had eye care previously, have reported that users of these programs differ from other diabetics by a higher probability of being female, on insulin, obese, and poor.[27]

14.21 Screening in Pregnancy

Pregnant patients with preexisting diabetes should have a dilated eye examination in the first trimester and close follow-up for the remainder of pregnancy if sight-threatening retinopathy is present. Women who develop gestational diabetes do not require such screening.[35]

14.22 Economic Considerations

The cost to society of DR is high and the cost-effectiveness of screening and treatment of DR has been firmly established.[87] Economic simulations in the United States and the United Kingdom based on epidemiologic data from WESDR, treatment benefit data from the Diabetic Retinopathy Study (DRS) and ETDRS, and costs based on country-specific data show that screening is cost effective for both types 1 and 2 diabetes, but more so for the former because of the higher incidence of advanced retinopathy and the longer survival of type 1 diabetics after screening.[35] Annual screening was most cost effective, and screening by photographic methods was more cost effective than screening by ophthalmoscopy.[35] For the type 1 diabetics in the United States, the net savings was $3,300 per person screened. For the type 2 diabetics not taking insulin, annual screening with ophthalmoscopy added years of sight at a cost of $1,500 per year of sight saved.[88]

There is controversy, however, on which screening methodology and interval are preferable on economic grounds. The cost of photographic screening depends on the initial capital outlay for the camera, van, and other equipment; the salary expense of those performing the functions of the screening process; the cost of training image graders; and the ongoing cost of goods associated with screening, such as film, fuel, and disposables.[21] Indirect costs associated with the decision to screen and the interval of screening include lost productivity that may result from degrees of visual impairment.[6] When denominated per screening event and referable event, the efficiency and volume of cases screened will affect the results. Given all these variables, the reported economic costs of screening vary widely. In the United Kingdom, the cost per screening event has been reported to be £60.30 in a nursing home environment and £10–12.75 with a mobile van model among ambulatory patients.[45,68] The cost per treatable event was £3,859 in the nursing home environment compared to £1,000 with the mobile van model.[68] For the nursing home model, these costs were judged to be unsustainable, but they were judged worthwhile in the mobile van model.[42,68] Using a different method of cost assessment, the cost per true positive by photoscreening was £209 in the Liverpool Diabetic Eye Study and the cost per laser-treated patient was £1,000.[32,68] The cost per case of blindness prevented was estimated to be £1,095.[45] In Canada, the cost per screening event was 100 Canadian dollars using a mobile camera unit set up in local pharmacies.[26] In the United States, the cost per case of retinopathy detected has been estimated at $295 for mydriatic photography and $390 for dilated eye examination by an ophthalmologist.[89]

Comparing costs of systematic photographic screening to the costs of the current model of opportunistic screening revealed that systematic photographic screening is more cost effective using cost per case detected as the outcome variable. Sensitivity analyses show that this is true for all practically achievable levels of sensitivity (sensitivity < 95%) for opportunistic screening. Systematic screening is more cost effective than opportunistic screening for all levels of compliance with systematic screening >54%. Although cost-effectiveness is better with systematic screening, the total cost is slightly higher with systematic screening, because it identifies more cases.

The single most important variable in the cost of screening is the cost of the screening examination, but the costs associated with the choice of screening interval currently are also important and have not factored into the choice of the recommended interval.[7] As available economic resources increasingly constrain choices, this may change. When QALYs were used as the primary outcome variable of a modeling study based on a US population-based study of retinopathy prevalence, the marginal cost-effectiveness of various screening frequencies varied according to HbA1c levels at baseline. For the US population overall, the marginal cost-effectiveness of annual and biennial screening was $107,510 and $49,760, respectively.[7] In a study from Taiwan which examined cost per sight year gained, the cost of screening type 2 diabetics annually was 20,962 New Taiwan dollars.[83] Using this as a base, the comparative costs of screening every 2 years, 3 years, and not screening at all were 1.19, 1.47, and 3.98 times as much, respectively.[83] Modeling studies depend on assumptions such as the value of a level of vision impairment in QALYs. The values used have ranged from 0.36 to 0.69 QALYs for blindness, for example, yet sensitivity analyses of the modeling results to these assumptions have not been consistently done. Other flaws in modeling studies include failure to stratify retinopathy progression rates by ethnicity, failure to allocate value to non-screening functions of the annual visit (e.g., detection of co-morbidity and education), and using retinopathy progression rates applicable to newly diagnosed diabetics for all diabetics, which leads to an underestimate of progression.[90] For these reasons, recommendations to depart from annual examinations have been met with resistance.[90] Still, published value judgments on screening vary from unequivocal statements that the benefits of screening outweigh the costs to statements that costs may be too high for certain currently employed annual screening strategies.[6,7,65,90,91] Actually implemented screening programs vary from annual to biennial.[78] Unlike the situation regarding cost–benefit analyses, there is unanimity that screening yields medical benefits.

Screening yields patients who must be seen for management, which implies an increased workload for eye care providers as a result of screening. On the other hand, diagnosis of DR early may reduce the work required per person diagnosed, thus potentially decreasing ophthalmic workloads. When actual impact of a screening program on ophthalmic workload has been studied, the workload for eye examinations but not laser treatment increases.[78] The increase in number of patients to be seen reflects the increase in population and the increase in type 2 diabetes prevalence in recent years together with the epidemic of obesity.[78]

A separate economic consideration in screening relates to physician efforts at implementing screening guidelines. An unknown fraction of noncompliance in screening may relate to lack of efforts by primary care physicians to educate patients to have annual eye examinations. For example, McCarty et al. found that preferred practice guidelines had been successfully disseminated to physicians but had not made a difference in management practices.[39,92] Audit benchmarks with linked financial rewards or penalties related to performance have been instituted in some health-care systems to address this problem.[93] Communication about eye examination findings from eye care professionals to primary care physicians may be lacking as well, but has been little examined.

14.23 Comparisons of the Screening Methods

The contemporary ideal in screening in the United States continues to be the dilated eye examination by a professional competent to recognize and treat or appropriately refer for treatment DR.[8,55,94] Except in Iceland, this ideal seems currently beyond reach.[26] As the burden of DR is projected to outstrip the growth in ophthalmic manpower to perform examinations, more pragmatic methods of screening must be evaluated. In the United Kingdom, screening by ophthalmologists has been deemed impractical. Instead, screening by optometrists and systematic photographic screening have been judged acceptable.[95]

Modeling studies have been done in which the sensitivity and specificity of different screening methods and various screening intervals have been tested for their effects on outcomes such as years of sight saved, eye clinic workload produced, and economic cost savings.[46,96] All the screening methods examined (screening by general practitioner, endocrinologist, optometrist, and ophthalmologist) saved sight compared to a strategy of no screening, but there was little difference between the four strategies of screening in effects on outcomes (Fig. 14.1). With screening by general practitioners on a yearly basis, 3.5 years of sight were saved on average compared to 4.1 years of sight saved with screening by ophthalmologists.[46] An independent study in type 1 diabetics likewise concluded that the cost savings generated from screening vary little over the range of sensitivities of the competing methods.[96] Thus, the evidence suggests little imperative to mandating ophthalmologic screening rather than other forms of screening for DR. A more cost-effective approach that makes fewer demands on scarce ophthalmologic manpower and produces roughly equal outcomes is to allocate lower cost screening methods with slightly lower sensitivity for universal screening with use of ophthalmologists to manage cases where DR is detected.

When all of the performance characteristics of the various screening methods are compared, the trend in recommendations for a practical method is toward digital photographic screening.[10,50,95] It appears to be more sensitive and less costly than screening by examination, reduces present inequalities in service provision, and unlike the latter, produces a permanent record.[10,95] Because it is not widely available in the United States, reliance on examination-based screening methods is necessary there for now, but acceptance of photographic screening seems to be growing.[10]

Noncompliance is the major flaw in all methods of screening.[10] Suggestions for overcoming

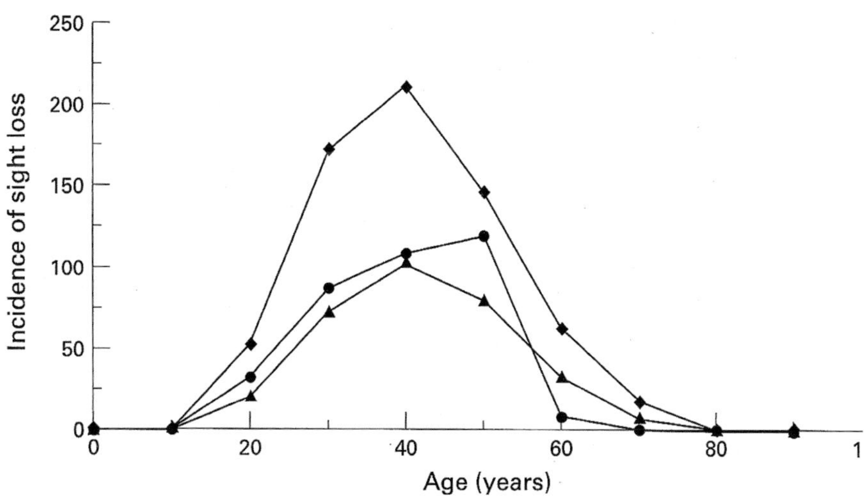

Fig. 14.1 Plot of the average number of patients out of a cohort of 1,000 patients who would develop severe vision loss from proliferative diabetic retinopathy or central visual loss from diabetic macular edema in age groups by decade by screening strategy. The *diamonds* represent outcomes with no screening, the *circles* represent screening by general practitioners every 2 years until retinopathy is detected with annual screening thereafter until referral to an ophthalmologist for treatment, and the *triangles* represent screening by ophthalmologists every 2 years until treatment is detected with annual screening thereafter. Reproduced with permission from Davies[46]

noncompliance have included developing comprehensive registries of diabetics, increasing education about the importance of screening, and increased efforts to specifically target underscreened subgroups.[10] Especially in regions underserved by eye care professionals, dilated examination by ophthalmologists is increasingly reserved for patients prescreened by digital photographic means and found to have an increased prior probability of sight-threatening retinopathy that would justify this valuable but expensive encounter.

14.24 Accountability of Screening Programs

The ultimate goal of screening programs for diabetic retinopathy is to reduce the incidence of visual loss. Provision must be made to determine if progress toward such a goal is being made.[95] This involves determination of local statistics on incidence of visual impairment and periodic audits to compare performance over time.[95] At its simplest level, these statistics may be incidence of blindness for the population and for the diabetic population. National statistics are too general to be useful given the regional variation in incidence rates of diabetes based on ethnicity, socioeconomic status, and other variables. In Great Britain, the minimum 5-year target is a 10% reduction in incidence of blindness, and an achievable target is 40%.[95]

14.25 Summary of Key Points

- Direct ophthalmoscopy through an undilated pupil by primary health-care providers is insensitive and nonspecific for detecting and classifying DR. Although with training, the performance of this method can improve to acceptable levels for screening purposes, this seems an unattainable goal as a practical matter.
- Dilated examination by ophthalmologists and optometrists competent to the task is an impractical screening goal because of poor rates of compliance by the target population of diabetics.
- Although screening methods aim for a sensitivity of at least 80% in the detection of diabetic retinopathy, modeling studies suggest that the impact both on years of sight saved and socioeconomic costs levels off for screening methods with sensitivities above 60%.
- Single-field nonmydriatic fundus photography is superior to dilated ophthalmoscopy by an ophthalmologist as a screening technique for DR. Referable cases from photographic screening then receive a focused dilated eye examination that accomplishes more than screening – education, detection of nondiabetic eye disease, and assessment for treatment.
- Mydriasis decreases the technical failure rate in photoscreening, but does not appreciably increase sensitivity or specificity for detection of DR.
- Multiple field fundus photography does not appreciably increase sensitivity or specificity in detecting DR compared to single-field fundus photography.
- Balancing all constraints, single-field nonmydriatic fundus photography appears to be the best initial screening method with single-field mydriatic fundus photography for patients with poor dilation such as the elderly.
- The ultimate goal of all methods of screening is to place the patient with DR under the care of an ophthalmologist competent to assess the disease status and implement the indicated treatment.

14.26 Future Directions

Better algorithms for automated interpretation of fundus images may reduce the cost of screening by reducing labor costs. Nonmydriatic scanning laser ophthalmoscopic imaging of the fundus may be used in lieu of dilated funduscopy in developed nations, especially by optometrists. Sensitivity and specificity for more than mild DR were 94 and 100%, respectively, compared to ophthalmologist clinical dilated examination gradings in the only study published so far, but only 51 eyes were examined.[97] Sensitivity and specificity for CSME were 89–93% and 72–89%, respectively.[97] The rate of ungradable images was 9.8%.[97] Further studies will need to be done to determine the usefulness of this screening method. The use of electronic medical records may permit improved communication between primary care physicians and eye care providers to allow detection of patients who have not been screened for diabetic retinopathy. Economic incentives in a variety of forms may improve screening rates.

References

1. Jekel JF, Elmore JG, Katz DL. *Epidemiology, Biostatistics, and Preventive Medicine*. 1st ed. Philadelphia: WB Saunders; 1996:216–217.
2. Leiter LA, Barr A, Belanger A, et al. Diabetes screening in Canada (DIASCAN) study. *Diabetes Care*. 2001;24: 1038–1043.
3. Kuo HK, Hsieh HH, Liu RT. Screening for diabetic retinopathy by one-field, non-mydriatic, 45 degrees digital photography is inadequate. *Ophthalmologica*. 2005; 219:292–296.
4. Diabetes Control and Complications Trial Research Group. Lifetime benefits and costs of intensive therapy as practiced in the diabetes control and complications trial. *JAMA*. 1996;276:1409–1415.
5. Lin DY, Blumenkranz MS, Brothers RJ, et al. The sensitivity and specificity of single field nonmydriatic monochromatic digital fundus photography with remote image interpretation for diabetic retinopathy screening: a comparison with ophthalmoscopy and standardized mydriatic color photography. *Am J Ophthalmol*. 2002; 134:204–213.
6. Tung TH, Shih HC, Chen SJ, et al. Economic evaluation of screening for diabetic retinopathy among Chinese Type 2 diabetics: a community-based study in Kinmen, Taiwan. *J Epidemiol*. 2008;18:225–233.
7. Vijan S, Hofer TP, Hayward RA. Cost-utility analysis of screening intervals for diabetic retinopathy in patients with type 2 diabetes mellitus. *JAMA*. 2000;283:889–896.
8. Chew EY, Benson WR, Boldt HC, et al. *Diabetic Retinopathy Preferred Practice Guidelines*. San Francisco: American Academy of Ophthalmology; 2003.
9. Liesenfeld B, Kohner E, Piehlmeier W, et al. A telemedicine approach to the screening of diabetic retinopathy: digital fundus photography. *Diabetes Care*. 2000;23: 345–348.
10. Harvey JN, Craney L, Nagendran S, Ng CS. Towards comprehensive population-based screening for diabetic retinopathy: operation of the North Wales diabetic retinopathy screening programme using a central patient register and various screening methods. *J Med Screen*. 2006;13:87–92.
11. Boucher MC, Nguyen QT, Angioi K. Mass community screening for diabetic retinopathy using a nonmydriatic camera with telemedicine. *Can J Ophthalmol*. 2005;40:734–742.
12. Raman R, Rani PK, Rachepalle SR, et al. Prevalence of diabetic retinopathy in India. Sankara Nethralaya diabetic retinopathy epidemiology and molecular genetics study report 2. *Ophthalmology*. 2009;116:311–318.
13. McKay R, McCarty CA, Taylor HR. Diabetic retinopathy in Victoria, Australia: the visual Impairment Project. *Br J Ophthalmol*. 2000;84:865–870.
14. Roy MS. Eye care in African Americans with type 1 Diabetes. The New Jersey 725. *Ophthalmology*. 2004;111:914–920.
15. Moss SE, Klein R, Klein BE. Factors associated with having eye examinations in persons with diabetes. *Arch Fam Med*. 1995;4:529–534.
16. Wang F, Javitt J. Eye care for elderly Americans with diabetes mellitus; failure to meet current guidelines. *Ophthalmology*. 1996;103:1744–1750.
17. Bresnick GH, Mukamel DB, Dickinson JC, Cole DR. A screening approach to the surveillance of patients with diabetes for the presence of vision-threatening retinopathy. *Ophthalmology*. 2000;107:19–24.
18. Sprafka JM, Fritsche TL, Baker R, et al. Prevalence of undiagnosed eye disease in high-risk diabetic individuals. *Arch Intern Med*. 1990;150:857–861.
19. Wong KC, Wang Z. Prevalence of type 2 diabetes mellitus of Chinese populations in mainland China, Hong Kong, and Taiwan. *Diab Res Clin Pract*. 2006;73:126–134.
20. Xie XW, Xu L, Wang YX, Jonas JB. Prevalence and associated factors of diabetic retinopathy. The Beijing Eye Study 2006. *Graefes Arch Clin Exp Ophthalmol*. 2008;246:1519–1526.
21. Farley TF, Mandava N, Prall FR, Carsky C. Accuracy of primary care clinicians in screening for diabetic retinopathy using single-image retinal photography. *Ann Fam Med*. 2008;6:428–434.
22. Clark J, Grey R, Lim K, Burns-Cox C. Loss of vision before ophthalmic referral in blind and partially sighted diabetics in Bristol. *Br J Ophthalmol*. 1994;78:741–744.
23. Bek T, Lund-Andersen H, Hansen AB, et al. The prevalence of diabetic retinopathy in patients with screen-detected type 2 diabetes in Denmark: the ADDITION study. *Acta Ophthalmologica*. 2008;E-pub ahead of print.
24. Deb-Joardar N, Germain N, Thuret G, et al. Screening for diabetic retinopathy by ophthalmologists and endocrinologists with pupillary dilation and a nonmydriatic digital camera. *Am J Ophthalmol*. 2005;140:814–821.
25. Stefansson E, Bek T, Porta M, et al. Screening and prevention of diabetic blindness. *Acta Ophthalmol Scand*. 2000;78:374–385.
26. Boucher MC, Desroches G, Garcia-Salinas R, et al. Teleophthalmology screening for diabetic retinopathy through mobile imaging units within Canada. *Can J Ophthalmol*. 2008;43:658–668.
27. Will JC, German RR, Schurman E, et al. Patient adherence to guidelines for diabetes eye care: results from the Diabetic Eye Disease Follow-up Study. *Am J Public Health*. 1994;84:1669–1671.
28. Moller F, Hansen M, Sjolie AK. Is one 60 degree fundus photograph sufficient for screening of proliferative diabetic retinopathy? *Diabetes Care*. 2002;24:2083–2085.
29. Klein R, Klein BEK, Neider MW, et al. Diabetic retinopathy as detected using ophthalmoscopy, a nonmydriatic camera and a standard fundus camera. *Ophthalmology*. 1985;92:486–491.
30. Barrie T, MacCuish AC. Assessment of non-mydriatic fundus photography in detection of diabetic retinopathy. *BMJ*. 1986;293:1304–1305.

31. von Wendt G, Summanen P, Hallnais K, et al. Detection of diabetic retinopathy: a comparison between red-free digital images and colour transparencies. *Graefes Arch Clin Exp Ophthalmol*. 2005;243:427–432.
32. James M, Turner DA, Broadbent DM, et al. Cost effectiveness analysis of screening for sight threatening diabetic eye disease. *BMJ*. 2000;320:1627–1631.
33. Leese GP, Boyle P, Feng Z, et al. Screening uptake in a well-established diabetic retinopathy screening program: the role of geographical access and deprivation. *Diabetes Care*. 2008;31:2131–2135.
34. Singer DE, Nathan DM, Fogel HA, Schachat AP. Screening for diabetic retinopathy. *Ann Intern Med*. 1992; 116:660–671.
35. Nathan DM, Fogel HA, Godine JE, et al. Role of the diabetologist in evaluating diabetic retinopathy. *Diabetes Care*. 1991;14:26–33.
36. Stellingwerf C, Hardus PLLJ, Hooymans MM. Assessing diabetic retinopathy using two-field digital photography and the influence of JPEG-compression. *Doc Ophthalmol*. 2004;108:203–209.
37. Klein R, Klein BEK, Moss SE, Cruikshanks KJ. The Wisconsin epidemiologic study of diabetic retinopathy. XIV. Ten-year incidence and progression of diabetic retinopathy. *Arch Ophthalmol*. 1994;112:1217–1228.
38. Klein R, Klein BEK, Moss SE, et al. The Wisconsin epidemiologic study of diabetic retinopathy. II. Prevalence and risk of diabetic retinopathy when age at diagnosis is less than 30 years. *Arch Ophthalmol*. 1984;102:520–526.
39. Lueder GT, Silverstein J, Section on Ophthalmology, et al. Screening for retinopathy in the pediatric patient with type 1 diabetes mellitus. *Pediatrics*. 2005;116:270–273.
40. Lueder GT, Pradhan S, White NH. Risk of retinopathy in children with type 1 diabetes mellitus before 2 years of age. *Am J Ophthalmol*. 2005;140:930–931.
41. Scanlon PH, Foy C, Chen FK. Visual acuity measurement and ocular co-morbidity in diabetic retinopathy screening. *Br J Ophthalmol*. 2008;92:775–778.
42. Anderson S, Broadbent DM, Swain JYS, et al. Ambulatory photographic screening for diabetic retinopathy in nursing homes. *Eye*. 2003;17:711–716.
43. Trautner C, Icks A, Haastert B, et al. Incidence of blindness in relation to diabetes. *Diabetes Care*. 1997;20:1147–1153.
44. Sussman E, Tsiaras W, Soper K. Diagnosis of diabetic eye disease. *JAMA*. 1982;247:3231–3234.
45. O'Hare JP, Hopper A, Madhaven C, et al. Adding retinal photography to screening for diabetic retinopathy: a prospective study in primary care. *BMJ*. 1996;312:679–682.
46. Davies R, Sullivan P, Canning C. Simulation of diabetic eye disease to compare screening policies. *Br J Ophthalmol*. 1996;80:945–950.
47. Pugh JA, Jacobson JM, Van Heuven WA, et al. Screening for diabetic retinopathy. The wide angle retinal camera. *Diabetes Care*. 1993;16:889–895.
48. Harding SP, Broadbent DM, Neoh C, et al. Sensitivity and specificity of photography and direct ophthalmoscopy in screening for sight threatening eye disease: the Liverpool Diabetic Eye Study. *BMJ*. 1995;311:1131–1135.
49. Moss SA, Klein R, Kessler SD, Richie KA. Comparison between ophthalmoscopy and fundus photography in determining severity of diabetic retinopathy. *Ophthalmology*. 1985;92:62–67.
50. Swanson M. Retinopathy screening in individuals with type 2 diabetes: who, how, how often, and at what cost – an epidemiologic review. Optometry. *J Am Optom Assoc*. 2005;76:636–646.
51. Kleinstein RN, Roseman JM, Herman WH, et al. Detection of diabetic retinopathy by optometrists. *J Am Optom Assoc*. 1987;58:879–882.
52. Schachat AP, Hyman L, Leke C, et al. Comparison of diabetic retinopathy detection by clinical examinations and photograph gradings. *Arch Ophthalmol*. 1993;111: 1064–1070.
53. Emanuele N, Klein R, Moritz T, et al. Comparison of dilated fundus examinations with seven-field stereo fundus photographs in the Veterans Affairs Diabetes Trial. *J Diabetes Complications*. 2008. doi:10.1016/j.jdiacomp. 2008.02.010
54. Kinyoun JL, Martin DC, Fujimoto WY, Leonetti DL. Ophthalmoscopy versus fundus photographs for detecting and grading diabetic retinopathy. *Invest Ophthalmol Vis Sci*. 1992;33:1888–1893.
55. Williams GA, Scott IU, Haller JA, et al. Single-field fundus photography for diabetic retinopathy screening. A report by the American Academy of Ophthalmology. *Ophthalmology*. 2004;111:1055–1062.
56. Williams R, Nussey S, Humphrey R, Thompson G. Assessment of non-mydriatic fundus photography in detection of diabetic retinopathy. *Br Med J*. 1986;293:1140–1142.
57. Browning DJ, McOwen MD, Bowen RM Jr, O'Marah TL. Comparison of the clinical diagnosis of diabetic macular edema with diagnosis by optical coherence tomography. *Ophthalmology*. 2004;111:712–715.
58. Scott IU, Bressler BN, Bressler SB, et al. Agreement between clinician and reading center gradings of diabetic retinopathy severity level at baseline in a phase 2 study of intravitreal bevacizumab for diabetic macular edema. *Retina*. 2008;28:36–40.
59. Kinyoun J, Barton FB, Fishner MR, et al. Detection of diabetic macular edema: ophthalmoscopy versus photography-early treatment diabetic retinopathy study report number 5. *Ophthalmology*. 1989;96:746–751.
60. McGinn T, Guyatt G, Cook R, Meade M. Diagnosis: measuring agreement beyond chance. In: Guyatt G, Rennie D, eds. *User's Guide to the Medical Literature*, 1st ed., Chap. 2C. Chicago: AMA Press; 2002.
61. Murgatroyd H, Ellingford A, Cox A, et al. Effect of mydriasis and different field strategies on digital image screening of diabetic eye disease. *Br J Ophthalmol*. 2004;88:920–924.
62. Chantelau E, Zwecker M, Weiss H, et al. Fundus polaroid screening for diabetic retinopathy. Is one print per patient enough? *Diabetes Care*. 1989;12:223–226.
63. Boucher MC, Gresset JA, Angioi K, Olivier S. Effectiveness and safety of screening for diabetic retinopathy with two nonmydriatic digital images compared with the seven standard stereoscopic photographic fields. *Can J Ophthalmol*. 2003;38:537–542.
64. Beynat J, Charles A, Astruc K, et al. Screening for diabetic retinopathy in a rural French population with a mobile non-mydriatic camera. *Diabetes Metab*. 2008;35:49–56.

65. The Eye Diseases Prevalence Research Group. The prevalence of diabetic retinopathy among adults in the United States. *Arch Ophthalmol*. 2004;122:552–563.
66. Perrier M, Boucher MC, Angioi K, et al. Comparison of two, three, and four 45 degrees image fields obtained with the Topcon CRW6 nonmydriatic camera for screening for diabetic retinopathy. *Can J Ophthalmol*. 2003;38: 569–574.
67. Deb-Joarder N, Germain N, Thuret G, et al. Systematic screening for diabetic retinopathy with a digital fundus camera following pupillary dilatation in a university diabetes department. *Diabet Med*. 2007;24:303–307.
68. Leese GP, Ahmed S, Newton RW, et al. Use of mobile screening unit for diabetic retinopathy in rural and urban areas. *BMJ*. 1993;306:187–189.
69. Herbert HM, Jordan K, Flanagan DW. Is screening with digital imaging using one retinal view adequate? *Eye*. 2003;17:497–500.
70. Taylor DJ, Fisher J, Jacob J, Tooke JE. The use of digital cameras in a mobile retinal screening environment. *Diabetes Care*. 1999;16:680–686.
71. Peters AL, Davidson MB, Ziel FH. Cost-effective screening for diabetic retinopathy using a nonmydriatic retinal camera in a prepaid health-care setting. *Diabetes Care*. 1993;16:1193–1195.
72. Maberly D, Cruess AF, Barile G, Slakter J. Digital photographic screening for diabetic retinopathy in the James Bay Cree. *Ophthalmic Epidemiol*. 2002;9: 169–178.
73. Leske MC, Wu SY, Hyman L, et al. Diabetic retinopathy in a black population-the Barbados eye study. *Ophthalmology*. 1999;106:1893–1899.
74. O'Hare JP, Hopper A, Madhaven C, et al. Adding retinal photography to screening for diabetic retinopathy: a prospective study in primary care. *BMJ*. 1996;312:679–682.
75. Scanlon PH, Foy C, Malhotra R, Aldington SJ. The influence of age, duration of diabetes, cataract, and pupil size on image quality in digital photographic retinal screening. *Diabetes Care*. 2005;28:2448–2453.
76. Maberly D, Morris A, Hay D, et al. A comparison of digital retinal image quality among photographers with different levels of training using a nonmydriatic fundus camera. *Ophthalmic Epidemiol*. 2004;11:191–197.
77. Lim MCC, Lee SY, Cheng BCL, et al. Diabetic retinopathy in diabetics referred to a tertiary center from a nationwide screening program. *Ann Acad Med Singapore*. 2008;37:753–759.
78. Scanlon PH, Carter S, Foy C, et al. An evaluation of the change in activity and workload arising from diabetic ophthalmology referrals following the introduction of a community based digital retinal photographic screening program. *Br J Ophthalmol*. 2005;89:971–975.
79. Pandit RJ, Taylor R. Mydriasis and glaucoma: exploding the myth. *Diabet Med*. 2000;17:693–699.
80. Brown JB, Pedula KL, Summers KH. Diabetic retinopathy. Contemporary prevalence in a well-controlled population. *Diabetes Care*. 2003;26:2637–2642.
81. Younis N, Broadbent DM, Vora JP, Harding SP. Incidence of sight-threatening retinopathy in patients with type 2 diabetes in the Liverpool Diabetic Eye Study: a cohort study. *Lancet*. 2003;361:195–200.
82. Lee PP, Meredith LS, Whitcup SM, et al. A comparison of self-reported utilization of ophthalmic care for diabetes in managed care versus fee-for-service. *Retina*. 1998;18:356–359.
83. The Diabeties Control and Complications Trial Research Group. Color photography vs fluorescein angiography in the detection of diabetic retinopathy in the diabetes control and complications trial. *Arch Ophthalmol*. 1987;105:1344–1351.
84. Abdel-Ghafar RA, Morris T. Progress towards automated detection and characterization of the optic disc in glaucoma and diabetic retinopathy. *Med Inform Internet Med*. 2007;32:19–25.
85. Gardner GG, Keating D, Williamson TH, Elliott AT. Automatic detection of diabetic retinopathy using an artificial neural network: a screening tool. *Br J Ophthalmol*. 1996;80:940–944.
86. Chaum E, Karnowski TP, Govindasamy VP, et al. Automated diagnosis of retinopathy by content-based image retrieval. *Retina*. 2008;28:1463–1477.
87. Javitt JC, Aiello LP. Cost-effectiveness of detecting and treating diabetic retinopathy. *Ann Intern Med*. 1996;124:164–169.
88. Dasbach EJ, Fryback DG, Newcomb PA, et al. Cost-effectiveness of strategies for detecting diabetic retinopathy. *Med Care*. 1991;29:20–39.
89. Lairson DR, Pugh JA, Kapadia AS, et al. Cost-effectiveness of alternative methods for diabetic retinopathy screening. *Diabetes Care*. 1992;15:1369–1377.
90. Fong DS, Gottlieh J, Ferris FL III, Klein R. Understanding the value of diabetic retinopathy screening. *Arch Ophthalmol*. 2001;119:758–760.
91. Porta M, Bandello F. Diabetic retinopathy. A clinical update. *Diabetologia*. 2002;45:1617–1634.
92. McCarty CA, Taylor KI, McKay R, et al. Diabetic retinopathy: effects of national guidelines on the referral, examination, and treatment practices of ophthalmologists and optometrists. *Clin Exp Ophthalmol*. 2001;29:52–58.
93. Diabetes Management Program. Improving multiple aspects of diabetes care. NCQA Website. 2009. 4-4-2009.
94. American College of Physicians ADAaAAoO. Screening Guidelines for Diabetic Retinopathy: clinical Guideline. *Ann Intern Med*. 1992;116:683–685.
95. Kumar N, Goyder E, McKibbin M. The incidence of visual impairment due to diabetic retinopathy in Leeds. *Eye*. 2006;20:455–459.
96. Javitt JC, Canner JK, Frank RG, et al. Detecting and treating retinopathy in patients with type 1 diabetes mellitus. *Ophthalmology*. 1990;97:483–495.
97. Neubauer AS, Kernt M, Haritoglu C, et al. Nonmydriatic screening for diabetic retinopathy by ultra-widefield scanning laser ophthalmoscopy (Optomap). *Graefes Arch Clin Exp Ophthalmol*. 2008;246:229–235.

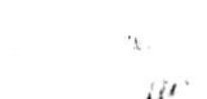

Chapter 15
Practical Concerns with Ethical Dimensions in the Management of Diabetic Retinopathy

David J. Browning

In this chapter we will cover a number of diverse, yet practical topics, rarely covered in a book on diabetic retinopathy. What ties them together is the common thread of possessing an ethical dimension. Our goal will be to identify issues that arise daily in the care of patients with diabetic retinopathy that require a response by the ophthalmologist and examine what motivates the possible alternative behaviors by ophthalmologists. Scientific studies touching these topics are few. Whereas analogous issues arise in all fields of medicine, by tying them to our emphasis here on diabetic retinopathy the author hopes to establish immediacy. The perspective will be discursive, but not directive, because in many cases, a correct answer or solution based on evidence may not be clearly discernible or may be controversial. In each case, the concept of medicine as a profession operating under a tacit social contract is crucial. This social contract states that physicians are allowed "a high degree of autonomy in their professional affairs in return for vowing to use their medical and scientific expertise solely to promote the interests of their patients and the welfare of the public."[1] In fact, the use of the word "solely" in this quotation indicates that the assertion is aspirational, not factual. Cases abound demonstrating that ophthalmologists are human and heir to self-interest. Ophthalmologists exhibit professionalism to the degree that we approach the goal and abjure self-interest and the perception of such in favor of our patients' interest and that of the public.[2]

D.J. Browning (✉)
Charlotte Eye Ear Nose & Throat Associates, Charlotte, NC 28210, USA
e-mail: dbrowning@ceenta.com

15.1 Incorporating Ancillary Testing in the Management of Patients with Diabetic Retinopathy

Optical coherence tomography and fluorescein angiography are commonly used in the management of patients with diabetic retinopathy and require time to obtain. Practical aspects of integrating these studies into a clinic setting are worthy of discussion. How commonly the tests are used will vary from practice to practice, but we can define some useful bounds for the sake of discussion. The coauthors of this text were surveyed on the matter and five responded. The data are shown in Table 15.1.

For the sake of discussion, the median values will be used. If an ophthalmologist sees 40 patients per day and works 10 h per day, then he spends on average approximately 15 min per patient. On average, in half of these patients an OCT will be obtained and 1.5 min will be spent reviewing and analyzing the images. This will involve review of the OCT, interpreting the OCT for the medical record, in some cases assisted by a scribe, and often using the OCT to educate the patient pictorially.

The review of the OCT often begins with a series of thumbnail images on a computer screen (Fig. 15.1) in offices with electronic records or may be by review of paper records in a chart. This may give a sense of progression over time by serially comparing the false color maps. A longitudinal comparison may be obtained by a spreadsheet analysis and graphical portrayal of the central subfield mean thickness or the total macular volume (Fig. 15.2).[3]

D.J. Browning (ed.), *Diabetic Retinopathy*, DOI 10.1007/978-0-387-85900-2_15,

Table 15.1 Sample data on ancillary imaging by retina specialists managing patients with diabetic retinopathy

Doctor	Number of patients seen per day	Hours in clinic per day	Time spent per patient	% with DR	% of DR patients who get an OCT	% of DR patients who get an FA	Time to analyze an OCT (min)	Time to analyze an FA (min)
1	50	10	12	23	30	*	3.0	4.0
2	47	8	10.2	20	50	25	0.5	0.5
3	40	10	15	20	17	10	5.0	5.0
4	37	10	16.2	50	80	10	1.5	3.5
5	40	10	15	25	80	5	1.0	2.0
Median	40	10	15	23	50	10	1.5	3.5

Sometimes respondents provided more than one value for a cell. For example, a Florida-based ophthalmologist saw more patients per day in the winter than the summer ("snowbird effect"). For simplicity in such cases, the midpoint of any range given was chosen for the cell entry. *= no response given.

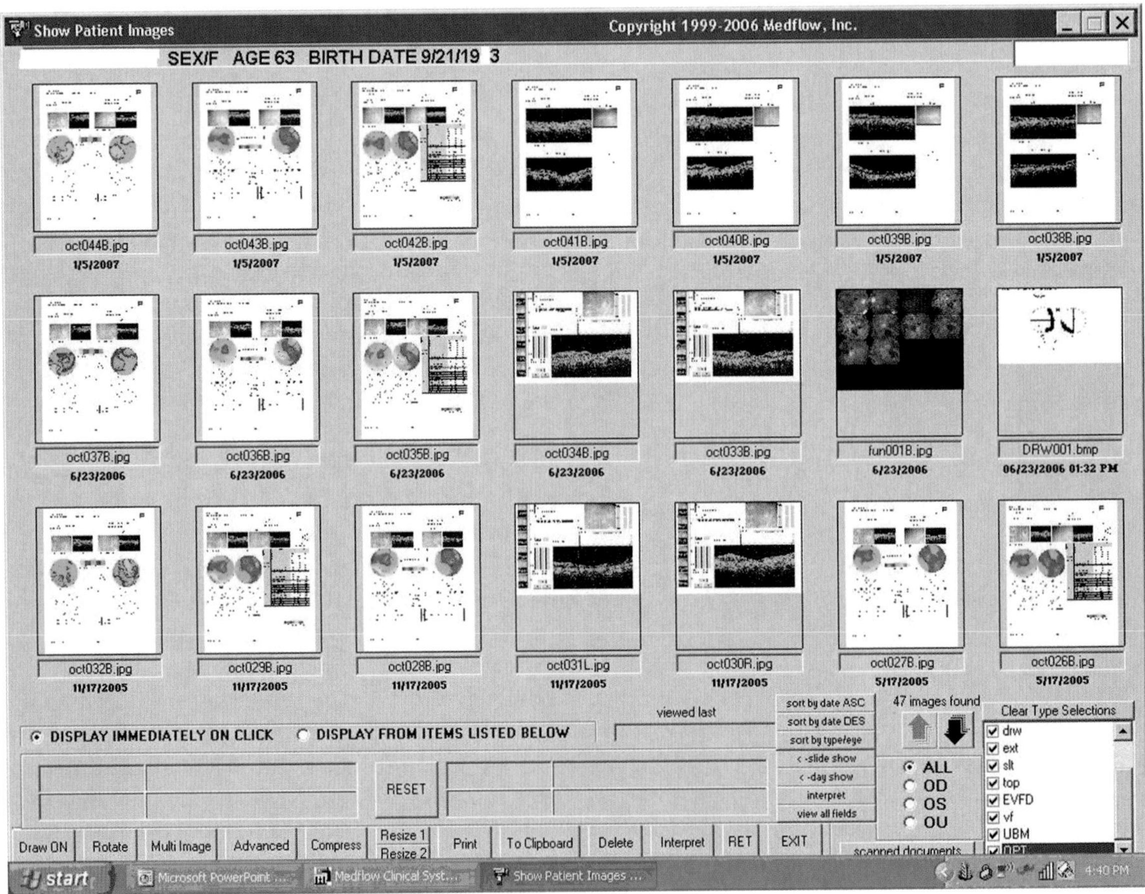

Fig. 15.1 Screenshot of a series of optical coherence tomography studies performed over time. The overall picture can be sensed quickly, and by double clicking on a particular image, the ophthalmologist can study it in detail

Finally, morphological details can be gathered by study of the individual line scans and groups of scans (e.g., macular cube, series of raster line scans). The entry of the interpretation in the record may be by free typing or by use of pick lists and drop-down menus in an electronic medical record or by ticking pre-printed options in a paper interpretation sheet or by a free handwritten note.

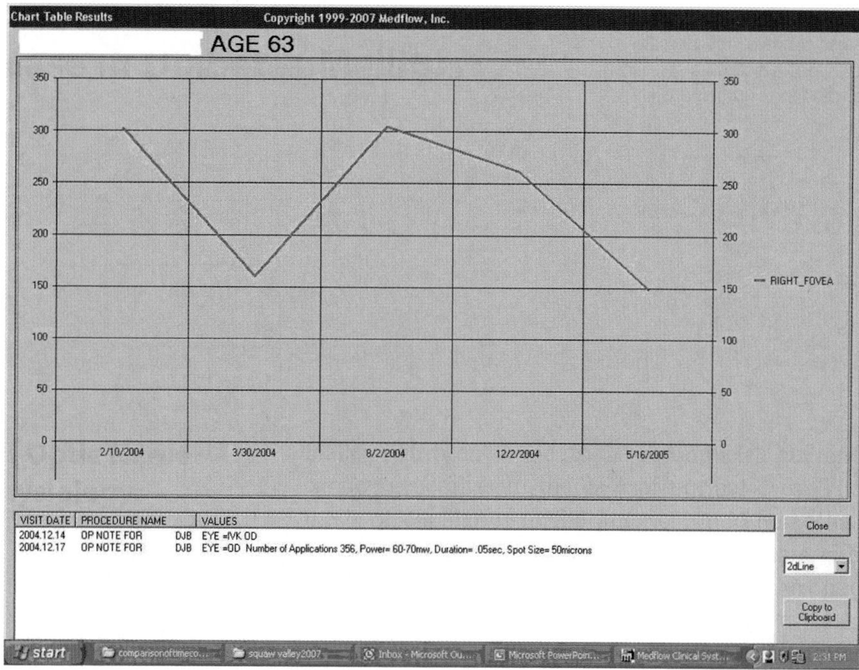

Fig. 15.2 Example of the graphical depiction of central subfield mean thickness (*Y*-axis, in microns) over time (*X*-axis, dates given). Interventions and their dates appear at the bottom of the screen. Spreadsheet software has been described for this purpose and it is included in some electronic medical records products[3]

Because the use of these studies is so common, the careful preparation of the drop-down lists can save time in the clinic.

The relationship of patient flow through the clinical encounter and imaging sequence deserves comment. Some physicians obtain OCTs on everyone, regardless of the clinical status.[4–6] Other physicians obtain OCTs selectively. There are at least two possible models for arranging patient flow. The first is shown in Fig. 15.3.

In the first model, a patient will experience anywhere from three to seven steps. In the second model (Fig. 15.4), the possibilities are three to six steps. The more time-efficient model will depend on the nature of the practice. If there are a high proportion of patients for routine examination and little pathology, then the first model is superior, because most of the patients will not require any ancillary testing. In such a practice, the second model will probably have more tests done that really were unnecessary, because it is unlikely that the technician, no matter how well trained, can make as accurate a choice as if the ophthalmologist makes all the decisions. Most of the visits in this scenario will follow the three-step pathway. The first model is inferior, however, if the ophthalmologist's practice is filled with problematic patients. In this case, few patients will travel through the three-step pathway and many more will follow the six- and seven-step paths. Under the second model, however, these problematic patients will pass through five or six steps, saving time. The disadvantage of this model is that it requires a highly trained technician who can properly execute guidelines for the ordering of ancillary tests.

There are many guidelines for the screening technician that could be used. An example is shown in Table 15.2.

In a practice in which the technician has the latitude to order an ancillary test before the patient sees the ophthalmologist, the potential exists for unnecessary testing. If the examination does not support the need for the testing, it cannot be billed, thus a certain fraction of tests will be wasted effort and will have to be written off. The compensating advantage has to do with savings in time through patient flow involving fewer steps. Fluorescein angiograms are unlikely to be treated the same way. First, they have some risk, unlike OCT. Furthermore, they are needed in approximately one-fifth the number of cases as OCT based on the survey data (Table 15.1).

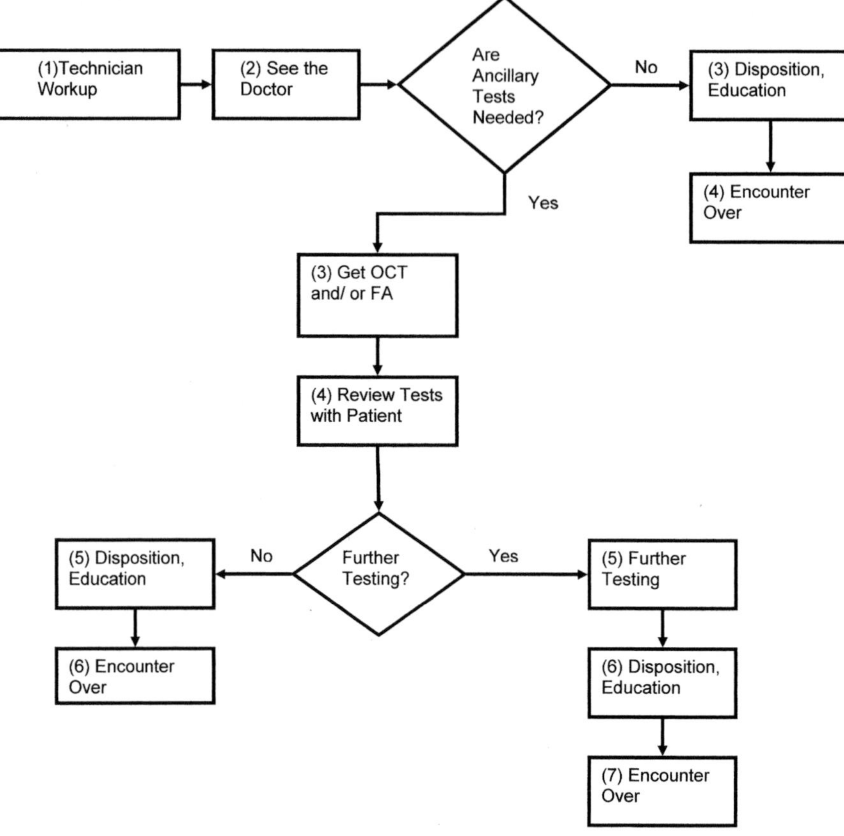

Fig. 15.3 Patient flow under a model in which decisions on ancillary imaging reside with the ophthalmologist alone

The reimbursement rules by payors of medical care for ancillary testing are interpreted by ophthalmologists with different perspectives. Some are concerned that the ophthalmologist must examine the patient first and indicate in the record an order to obtain the ancillary test. Other ophthalmologists interpret the matter such that guidelines like those listed in Table 15.2 under the supervision of the attending ophthalmologist are permissible for obtaining the OCT before the patient sees the physician.

The scientific basis for ancillary testing in management of diabetic retinopathy has been little explored. OCT and fluorescein angiography (FA) are used because ophthalmologists have these techniques, enjoy having the information they provide for documentation and education of the patient, appreciate the advantage of decision making based on objective data rather than subjective clinical examination findings, and in some healthcare systems they are a source of revenue. For FA, the randomized clinical trial proving treatment efficacy used the tests to guide treatment.[7] However, we do not know from scientific studies that our patients have better outcomes because we use FA and OCT in their management. Some evidence has been published to suggest that outcomes are similar if FA is omitted, and the effect of using OCT on outcomes has not been studied.[8,9] It may be an expensive fallacy that the paradigm chosen for the purposes of a randomized trial should be translated without modification to routine clinical practice.[10]

With respect to OCT, the cost of adding these machines to practice has indisputably added to the cost of medical care of diabetic macular edema, and yet we have no clinical trial data that justify the added expense – data showing that outcomes using OCT for management are superior to outcomes without OCT. As spectral domain OCT displaces time domain OCT at further high expense, it is again paradoxical that we have no evidence that the extra financial outlay purchases better visual outcomes for our patients.

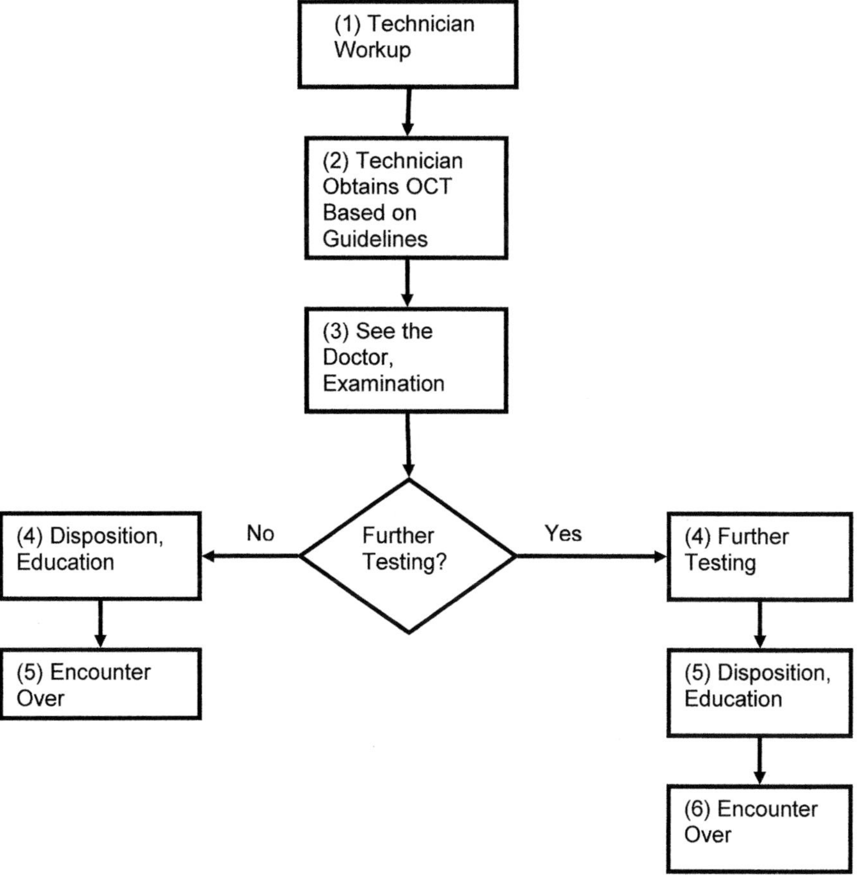

Fig. 15.4 Patient flow under a model in which decisions on ancillary imaging can be made by the technician who works up the patient based on decision rules devised by the ophthalmologist

Table 15.2 An example of indications for obtaining optical coherence tomography before the patient sees the ophthalmologist

1. Patient presents with referral note along the lines "suspect central retinal vein occlusion, branch retinal vein occlusion, macular hole, macular pucker, cystoid macular edema, macular edema, or diabetic macular edema"
2. Patient has the diagnosis of central retinal vein occlusion, branch retinal vein occlusion, or diabetic macular edema and has not had an OCT in 4 months
3. A patient with neovascular age-related macular degeneration meets the following criteria:
   a. Treatment within the past year
   b. No OCT in the past 4 weeks
4. Patient is sent for a consultation following cataract surgery performed within the previous 6 months and the vision did not return as expected
5. Patient with type 1 diabetes with duration greater than 20 years and new to the retina doctor
6. Patient with type 2 diabetes of duration greater than 10 years and new to the retina doctor
7. Patient with diabetes of any type who has vision less than 20/20 best corrected and is referred to the retina doctor to explain subnormal vision
8. For an established patient if the previous note indicates the need for OCT at the next visit

OCT = optical coherence tomography.

The situation is different for fluorescein angiography. Although the modality has seen a transition from film to digital media, the expenses associated with its use are largely unchanged over the last 30 years. The usage of FA in managing DME has diminished over time, unlike the situation with OCT (see Chapter 7). However, as with OCT, this change has not been a response to clinical trial data showing the absence of a negative effect if FA is omitted, although it may represent a response to lower level evidence.[8]

Besides the scientific aspect, the use of ancillary testing in the management of diabetic retinopathy has an economic dimension. In the modern care of patients with diabetic retinopathy and retinal diseases in general, ancillary testing provides an important source of the ophthalmologist's revenue. In the author's group practice, there are 4 retina specialists who manage all the diabetic retinopathy for patients served by the 25 ophthalmologists and 4 optometrists. The percentage of total collections provided by ancillary testing for these four retina specialists ranged from 15.7 to 21.1% in 2008. The 5.4% differential applied to the $1.5 million lower end estimated collections of a retina specialist implies a lower bound estimated $81,000 in yearly collections potentially attributable to variable use of imaging.[11] Potential financial conflicts of interest in ordering ancillary tests by physicians are well known.[12] The present example simply makes the problem specific to the management of diabetic retinopathy within a fee-for-service healthcare system.

15.2 Patients with Sight-Threatening Diabetic Retinopathy and Insufficient or No Ability to Address Medical Bills

Most ophthalmologists across the world agree on what constitutes evidence-based medicine with respect to the treatment of diabetic retinopathy (DR). For example, under ideal circumstances and without constraints of money, equipment, and logistics, most ophthalmologists would manage a case of disk neovascularization with vitreous hemorrhage similarly across the world. However, the actual circumstances in which ophthalmologists work and patients live vary widely, yet little is published on the effects that these factors have on the actual as opposed to ideal management of DR. In the United States, certain situations with socioeconomic aspects repeatedly arise and bear discussion. For these situations, there is little published literature to provide guidance, despite their daily importance in clinical practice. Two examples are discussed below, and a third will be covered in Chapter 16.

15.2.1 Case 1

A 63-year-old man with type 2 DM not on insulin, hypertension, hypercholesterolemia, a previous right-sided stroke, and amputation of the right great toe was examined on December 10, 2007, with a complaint of painless blurred vision of the right eye for 3 weeks. The visual acuity was 20/25 on the right and 20/20 on the left. Early nuclear sclerosis of both lenses was present. Both eyes had severe nonproliferative diabetic retinopathy. The right eye had clinically significant macular edema. He declined fluorescein angiography because of lack of insurance, but an OCT documented the macular thickening (Fig. 15.5A and B). Focal/grid laser photocoagulation was recommended, but the patient declined because of lack of insurance. He was offered treatment at a reduced rate (Medicaid rate) and declined. He stated that he would return for care when he became eligible for Medicare in November 2008, and he did so. By this time, his vision had dropped to 20/60 right and remained 20/20 on the left. He had worsening of clinically significant macular edema of the right eye and new CSME of the left eye. Fundus photographs, fluorescein angiography, and OCT images of both eyes are shown in Fig. 15.5C–H. Focal/grid photocoagulation was recommended in both eyes and was performed.

This case illustrates a type of clinical experience familiar to many ophthalmologists managing patients with diabetic retinopathy in the United States. The nature of the clinical problem is clear and an evidence-based course of action exists, but socioeconomic obstacles prevent proper application of known effective treatment and visual loss results. There are many possible perspectives that one might take in considering such a case. One is to deprecate the ophthalmologist. He could have provided the care as charity. This can be a solution for an occasional case, but is not a practical systemic solution. The expenses of providing care must be covered by some payor ultimately. The

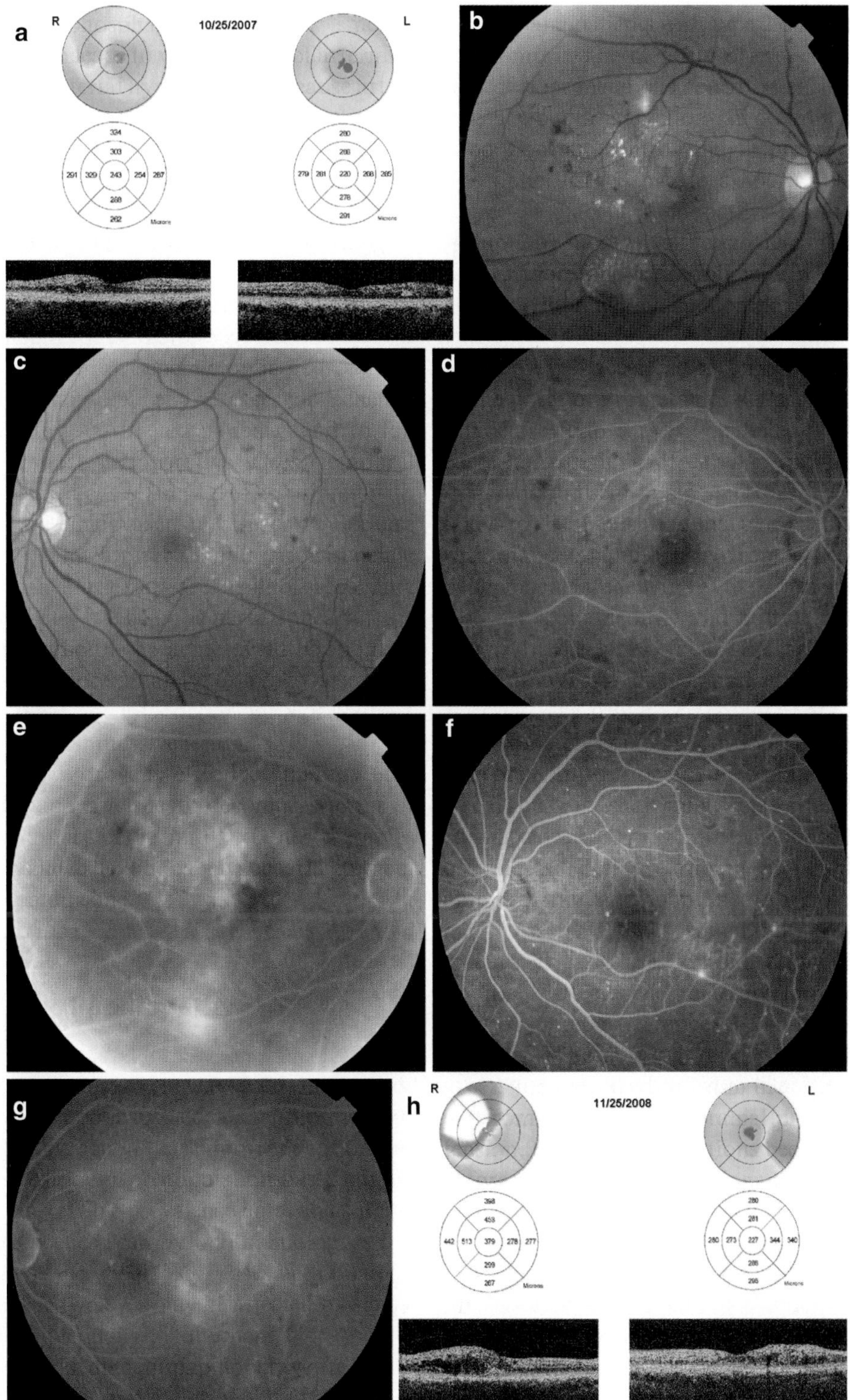

Fig. 15.5 (**a**, **b**) OCT-documented macular at the initial visit for case 1; follow-up fundus photographs, fluorescein angiography, and OCT images of both eyes are shown in **c**–**h**. Worsening of diabetic macular edema as a result of delay in treatment is documented

profligately charitable ophthalmologist will soon be out of practice for economic reasons. As stated by Cohen et al., "In countries with large numbers of such individuals, it is unreasonable to expect individual physicians to carry a burden that rightfully rests with the broader community."[1] Another perspective is to criticize the patient for putting off needed care for a year rather than accepting the offer of timely care at a reduced cost. Finally, the system of healthcare payment in the United States might be identified as the root of the problem. Such a situation would not exist in countries with nationalized health care, but those systems have their own faults, and we cannot constructively enter the debate on healthcare delivery here. The point of the case is to show how the healthcare delivery system affects the care and outcomes of patients with diabetic retinopathy as much as the patient's blood pressure and glycosylated hemoglobin.

Another relevant concern in such cases is the extent of ancillary testing to be done. Should the ophthalmologist have a standard of care and stick to it for all, or should the standard vary with the available resources? For 15 years after the Early Treatment Diabetic Retinopathy Study, DME was managed without OCT. But in 2009, when OCT is integral in the management of DME, should the ophthalmologist revert to the pre-OCT standard for economic reasons? Likewise, one can manage DME without the use of fluorescein angiography, and half or more of ophthalmologists do so.[13] Should the economic facts of a particular case influence one's practice? Our purpose here is to raise the question for discussion, not answer it. The author's practice – mentioned only for the purpose of disclosure and discussion and not put forth as a suggested norm – is to tailor the ancillary testing to the resources available. I will treat such patients without OCT or fluorescein angiography rather than defer all care because a desired standard of ancillary evidence cannot be afforded. An acknowledged pitfall of this approach in the United States is the potential for legal liability if a dissatisfied patient with a bad outcome should turn what begins as an intended act of compassion into a portrayed act of negligence. The legal system in the United States thus joins the list of considerations to be weighed in such cases.

15.2.2 Case 2

A 42-year-old woman with type 2 diabetes for 16 years and hypertension was seen with complaints of blurred vision in the left eye in association with redness, tearing, sensitivity to light, and a left-sided headache. Examination showed that she had corrected visual acuity of 20/40 right and counting fingers left. Intraocular pressures were 15 right and 45 left. She had neovascularization of the iris and a hyphema on the left. Both eyes had disk neovascularization and neovascularization of the midperipheral retina. The left eye received an intravitreal injection of bevacizumab followed by panretinal laser photocoagulation and subsequently an Ahmed tube shunt with normalization of pressure and eventual counting fingers visual acuity. The right eye received panretinal laser photocoagulation with regression of neovascularization, but contracture of a premacular membrane. Vitrectomy surgery was recommended, but the patient's coverage under the Medicaid program expired and she was unwilling to accept a recommendation to have surgery through the offices of the State Commission for Services for the Blind. As a result, lacking money, she did not return for 16 months. She did return when her visual acuity in the right eye dropped abruptly to counting fingers interfering with her ability to ambulate. A dense contracted premacular membrane with macular traction retinal detachment was found (Fig. 15.6). The patient agreed to have vitrectomy surgery. Vitrectomy, membrane peeling, laser panretinal photocoagulation, and intravitreal silicone oil instillation were done. The visual acuity returned to 20/100 on the right (Fig. 15.7).

In this case, the lack of coverage led to procrastination in applying care with compromise of the patient's final visual outcome. The primary obstacle preventing appropriate treatment was financial. In such a case, several questions arise.

1. Should the ophthalmologist have volunteered to provide the care without cost to the patient?
2. What is the responsibility of the society in which nearly 50 million persons are uninsured for the sequence of events that occurred in this case?[14]
3. Is there a solution for such cases within the current system of health care in the United States?
4. How would such a case be handled in alternate systems of health care?

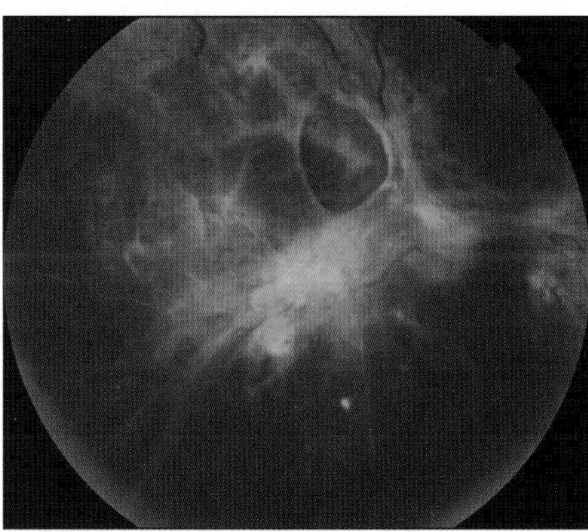

Fig. 15.6 Appearance of the right fundus of the patient in case 2. The macula is detached with a dense premacular fibrotic membrane

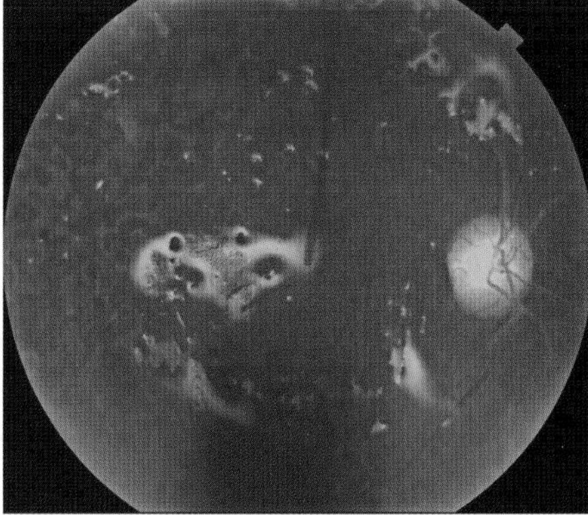

Fig. 15.7 Postoperative appearance of the right fundus of the patient in case 2. The macula is attached under silicone oil

In answer to the first question, a fair answer probably involves the proportion of charity patients in the ophthalmologist's practice. No ophthalmologist can be expected to provide charity care if the number in need renders the burden economically unviable.[1] However, as members of a profession rather than a business, ophthalmologists have a responsibility to share in providing care for the uninsured and underinsured. Where this balance is struck varies. "The tragedy of the commons" is a concept that applies to physicians as to all humans, thus it is not surprising that some physicians choose to accept little or no responsibility.[15] Questions 2 and 3 are controversial topics of debate in the United States. Historically, social beneficence in the United States has limits. The United States constitution and laws have not historically recognized a right to universal welfare or health care. In the past 50 years, other western nations have come to consider this as a newfound right, and the United States may be evolving in that direction. It is beyond the scope of this chapter to address the matter further except to emphasize that ophthalmologists caring for patients with diabetic retinopathy see examples like these daily. In answer to question 4, nationalized healthcare systems seem to be better prepared to treat such cases than is the healthcare system in the United States, but they have their own flaws such as limitations and restrictions on individualization of care, loss of attraction of the brightest students to other career choices, failure to incentivize medical innovation through low reimbursements, and rationing of care based on bureaucratic regulation and waiting. Which ensemble of flaws is worse is sharply debated.

15.3 Communications with Primary-Care Physicians

Ophthalmologists have an obligation to provide the primary-care physicians of their patients with diabetes a periodic report of the ocular status.[16] Although it is recognized that the primary physician should encourage the patient to seek annual dilated eye examination, the need for communication between primary physician and ophthalmologist has not been emphasized. Many patients do not know their glycosylated hemoglobin or their list of medications, yet knowledge of the glycosylated hemoglobin is important in developing a rational ocular prognosis for a patient and plays into decisions on re-examination intervals. Unless in-office testing of glycosylated hemoglobin becomes a reality, it would be advantageous if such information was shared. Broadening use of electronic medical records may facilitate such information sharing.

15.4 Working in a Managed Care Environment (Capitation)

The economic and ethical dimensions of ancillary testing under a fee-for-service system of medical reimbursement were acknowledged earlier. At the other extreme, managed care reimbursement systems reward physicians in such a way that underuse of diagnostic and therapeutic interventions is a possible pitfall. To simplify a complicated matter, in such systems, the physician stands to financially benefit when the care provided to patients covered by the plan is minimized.[2] In such a system, there may also be an incentive by the physician to avoid sick patients, as they will require more care with financial penalties incurred by the physician caring for the patient. Conversions between fee-for-service and capitation systems for paying physicians have been shown to produce behavioral changes in patient encounters and referral patterns in the physicians affected.[17–19]

15.5 Interactions with Medical Industry

Ophthalmologists who take care of patients with diabetic retinopathy have frequent occasions to interact with representatives of pharmaceutical and medical technology companies who spend an estimated $57.5 billion annually in the United States ($61,000/physician/year) to influence physician behavior, an amount larger than their research and development budgets.[20–22] The interactions come in several forms. Most frequent are encounters with representatives who leave samples of new and expensive topical medications, but never inexpensive generics, in return for a few minutes of the target physician's time to listen to a sales pitch in the guise of physician education.[23,24] Usually, the sales representatives have little science background and work from practiced scripts honed to produce a closing commitment from the physician to write prescriptions of the touted product.[23,25] Simultaneously, there may be gifts given, such as post-it notes, pens, computer memory sticks, a choice of textbooks, silk ties, or umbrellas. More recently, the industry has deployed increasing numbers of "medical science liaisons," who are often physicians or pharmacists and can mention off-label uses for drugs that the sales representatives cannot in their interactions with practicing physicians.[26]

Another tactic companies employ is to invite ophthalmologists to expensive restaurants to listen to an opinion leader speak on a topic relevant to a product the sponsoring company sells. The invited speaker is paid a fee, thus there is influence purchasing at the audience and speaker level in these cases.[27] Sometimes a drug company will invite physicians to an expensive hotel for a retreat, ask them their opinions about the company's drugs, call them "consultants" thereby, and pay them a fee in addition to the expenses for the retreat.[28] In another variation, the office staff of an ophthalmologist may be invited to a catered lunch or dinner at which a speaker from the company talks about a topic related to a product sold by the company. Free lunches and gifts to physicians and staff are not random, but are targeted to those with the potential to cooperate with the company's efforts and boost their sales.[29]

At a different level, pharmaceutical companies invite ophthalmologists to be investigators for company-sponsored clinical trials of investigational drugs or devices.[30] The reimbursements to the physician for encounters of patients enrolled in these studies are higher than the reimbursements for patients not in these studies.[31,32] Besides the richer reimbursements paid for subjects enrolled in studies, pharmaceutical companies will pay for the engaged ophthalmologists to travel to expensive locations to give or hear talks at meetings.[21,30,33] Patients are not informed that their participation in pharmaceutical research is associated with differentially favorable remuneration to the enrolling physician compared to remuneration associated with care outside of pharmaceutical research, although surveys indicate that many participants in clinical research would like to be informed of financial conflicts of interest.[34] In some cases a proposed research study is not validly designed, and the payment to the physician is a veiled inducement to use the drug.[35]

Financial arrangements often exist between physicians who invent or help develop medical devices and the companies that produce them. Universities may be a third party in these relationships.[34,36,37] The patents, royalties, and compensation paid by companies to these physicians can potentially bias the relationship of the physician and patient, as when a surgeon recommends a medical device to a patient in which he has a financial interest or alters research data in a study for the same reason. In the United States in 2006, the average medical industry support for medical school departmental activities was 2.1 ± SD $5.6 million.[38] Medical industries provided financial support for a wide range of activities to many medical school departmental chairmen: personal compensation for involvement in CME courses (28%); personal equity or stock options in exchange for professional services (6%); royalties, license payments, or milestone payments (11%); free or subsidized travel and expenses to meetings and conferences (16%); and research funding (21%).[38] Yet in the same survey, 25% of medical schools had no institutional conflicts of interest policy or were not working on one.[37]

Questions have been repeatedly raised about the ethical basis of these interactions.[20,39,40] They have been identified as conflicts of interest at a minimum and as bribes by some.[12,20,21,29,35,41] A conflict of interest occurs when reasonable observers of a situation could conclude that the temptation for economic gain compromises the physician's responsibility to place the patient's interest first.[41] There seems to be little doubt that the industry samples, gifts, and perks are effective from the perspective of the companies, whether the targeted physicians believe it or not.[2,21,23,29,33,41,42,42–45] The many ways that physicians attribute moral vulnerability to others but not themselves and rationalize their attitudes toward accepting free lunches, gifts, and samples-for-face-time have been studied and characterized.[43,46,47] Physicians who believe that nominal gifts are ineffective in inducing reciprocity and therefore less unethical are in error based on social science research concerning gifts.[12,29,33,47] Targeted physicians tend to change their prescribing habits and use of medical devices, and the result is higher cost for medical care.[21,33,25]

Historically, the response of the ophthalmic community has been to institute a policy of disclosure of financial conflict of interest. The assumption has been that the audience can factor this disclosure into its reception of the speaker's content and properly calibrate its granted credulity. However, there are problems with this response to the situation.[21] Counterintuitively, there is social science evidence that disclosure perversely exacerbates the effects of bias rather than ameliorating them.[12] Appraisers who disclose that they are paid based on the size of their appraisals have been found to produce inflated appraisals compared to appraisers who do not disclose.[12] This is not an argument to omit disclosure, but rather one that it is an inadequate response. Some physicians ignore disclosure rules or interpret their involvement in such a way that they think the rules do not apply. A survey of medical experts who write clinical practice guidelines found that 9 of 10 had financial ties to the pharmaceutical industry but rarely disclosed them.[48] Financial involvements and disclosures have become so widespread and the time spent on them at meetings and in publications so cursory and without detail on magnitude of financial benefit that they are ignored. Moreover, the forms of disclosure have become more opaque. For example, here is the wording of a financial disclosure of an ophthalmologist from the Johns Hopkins School of Medicine (name removed):

> The author has no financial interest in any of the material discussed. Dr [X]'s employer, the Johns Hopkins University, but not Dr [X], receives funding for research and other sponsored projects from Eyetech Pharmaceuticals, Inc, New York, NY, Genentech, Inc, South San Francisco, Calif, the National Eye Institute of the National Institutes of Health, Bethesda, Md, the US Department of Health and Human Services, Washington, DC, Novartis Pharma AG, Basel, Switzerland, QLT, Inc, Vancouver, British Columbia, and Carl Zeiss Meditec AG, Jena, Germany. The terms of these institutional consulting agreements are managed by the Johns Hopkins University in accordance with its conflict of interest policies.[49]

In the arrangement here, the money from the recipient's work flows to the employing medical school. It sounds less likely to be ethically questionable inasmuch as the potential benefit to the recipient is indirect. Yet without knowing what the cited policies of the university are, the reader cannot assess how likely the recipient is to be influenced by the money. If the university policy is a direct pass-through to the faculty member, then the potential for bias is higher than if his compensation is completely disengaged from the funding the recipient brings into the university through his involvement with the companies. The disclosure is in fact no disclosure, because it is opaque. Few if any readers will spend the effort to pierce the veil of this disclosure statement, although technically, with enough digging, they could do so. As Brennan and colleagues note, "Because declarations of conflict are usually unverified, their accuracy is uncertain."[41] Many authors argue that disclosure is a half-measure response to the apparent ethical challenge; avoidance is the more appropriate ethical response.[2,50] As an analogy, when someone embezzles money, we wish for them to stop it, not to disclose that they are embezzling. In a different profession – the judiciary – disclosure is not an option; if a judge has a conflict of interest, he must recuse himself from the case.[23]

The growing proportion of continuing medical education expenses underwritten by pharmaceutical companies that view the practice as good marketing has been noted and deprecated.[50] Relman asks, "Does anyone really believe that medical educators are properly doing their job when they allow the pharmaceutical industry not only to subsidize their educational costs but also to help prepare the curriculum, recommend and pay the speakers, indirectly pay students and residents to attend, lavish free meals and favors on attendees, and then promote the company's products at the meetings?"[50] Calls to physicians to refuse to attend industry-sponsored continuing medical education events (CME) have been published.[20] Others have suggested that accreditation for offering CME be restricted to member institutions of the Accreditation Council for Continuing Medical Education and be denied to industry-sponsored public relations firms.[51] Recommendations to eschew gifts and samples from industry representatives have been published.[41] There is insufficient evidence to conclude that any of these recommendations has gained traction.

The conflicts of interest discussed herein are not abstract. They are concrete and occur on a daily basis in ophthalmic practice. Physicians have repetitive chances to affect the ethical landscape of the profession by their choices. Historically, the American Medical Association has issued guidelines in which the ethical propriety of gifts is determined based on type and monetary value.[47] Gifts with a benefit to patients (e.g., samples) and related to a physician's work (e.g., a pen) have received a pass, despite evidence that these are intended to affect and do affect prescribing practices.[47] Based on history, pessimists contend that physicians and their professional societies are unlikely to change their behavior internally and that federal regulation with penalties for infractions lies in the future.[24,46]

In managing patients with proliferative diabetic retinopathy (PDR) and diabetic macular edema (DME), the ophthalmologist has the discretion to choose among a menu of injectable intravitreal drugs in many cases. Reviewing the actions of drug companies in this environment is relevant to the discussion. For example, Genentech makes both bevacizumab, an oncological antivascular endothelial growth factor (VEGF) drug widely co-opted for off-label use by ophthalmologists, and ranibizumab, an anti-VEGF drug specifically designed for ophthalmic use.[52,53] Both drugs show a biological effect in PDR and DME.[54] The potential profit margin for Genentech is much greater for ranibizumab with a retail price over 20 times that of bevacizumab. The company has spent and continues to spend large sums of money supporting clinical trials to demonstrate efficacy of ranibizumab for diabetic retinopathy indications, but not for bevacizumab. This financial support has been a factor in the selection of ranibizumab, and not bevacizumab, by the National Institutes of Health-funded Diabetic Retinopathy Clinical Research Network for its phase 3 clinical trials with an anti-VEGF drug component. The logic presented to the Network investigators by the Network leadership for this choice goes as follows. By accepting the Genentech subsidy of free ranibizumab other valuable research can be conducted with the dollars not spent on bevacizumab. This logic perhaps underweights the expected future argument by Genentech that should anti-VEGF therapy with ranibizumab be shown to be valuable in PDR and DME, it would be an act based on faith rather than evidence to extrapolate the results to the untested, less-expensive bevacizumab, even though the mechanism of action of the two drugs is the same. At present, well-funded pharmaceutical representatives of Genentech assiduously court retina specialists by the methods listed previously to tilt their decision making in anti-VEGF therapy for neovascular macular degeneration. They would not do so were their efforts fruitless. In the future, they will undoubtedly expand their efforts to diabetic indications should the diabetic clinical trial results turn out in their favor.

15.6 Interactions with Ambulatory Surgery Centers

A frequent component in the care of patients with diabetic retinopathy is the injection of intravitreal drugs and application of focal/grid and panretinal photocoagulation. In 2008, these procedures were added to the list of approved procedures that can be done in ambulatory surgery centers (ASC) in the United States. There are differential rates of reimbursement for these procedures when done in an ASC or in an office setting. Generally speaking, the reimbursement is higher when they are done in an ambulatory surgery center because a facility fee is generated that does not apply to the office setting. If the ophthalmologist is an investor in an ASC and directs his patient to that setting to receive the treatment, the issue of conflict of interest arises, especially if the patient is left to pay a higher out-of-pocket expense in an ASC setting compared to the office setting. As Tonelli has written, "arrangements that both increase physician remuneration and improve the care of patients are theoretically possible, and if patient care can be demonstrated to improve, would be ethically preferred. But such arrangements demand a high burden of proof demonstrating that patients, and not simply clinicians, are benefited."[2]

15.7 Comanagement of Patients

Comanagement of patients with diabetic retinopathy has not been an issue in the management of patients with diabetic retinopathy as it has been in the management of patients undergoing cataract surgery; however, related concerns have begun to arise.[55] For example, networks have been developed in which primary-care physicians take nonmydriatic fundus photographs to screen for diabetic retinopathy (see Chapter 14).[56] These are graded by ophthalmologists, and if DR is detected, the patient is sent to an ophthalmologist. If the patient has an ophthalmologist, they are directed there, but if not, relationships between the grading ophthalmologist and the screening ophthalmologist may exist that direct referrals. These relationships may be influenced by external factors, including affiliation with hospital networks that own physician practices. Referrals may be governed by concerns such as emergency room coverage.

15.8 Relationships with Investment Firms

Perhaps no month goes by without an e-mail requesting an ophthalmologist to participate in a survey or a conference call sponsored by an investment firm in which money is offered for expert opinions on the prospects of drugs and devices used to treat diabetic retinopathy. Many ophthalmologists participate in clinical research networks and know the results of clinical research before they are published in peer-reviewed journals. Inside information from unpublished clinical trials is sought and used by investment firms to make money for the firms and their clients. Is it ethical to participate in and receive fees from these activities? Recommendations have ranged from disclosure alone to non-participation in such activities.[57,58]

15.9 Summary of Key Points

- Daily clinical care of patients with diabetic retinopathy involves practical issues with an ethical dimension that are rarely covered in textbooks about diabetic retinopathy.
- These issues have the common thread of professionalism – the duty of the ophthalmologist to abjure self-interest and to act in the interest of the patient and, to a lesser and poorly defined extent, society.
- Specific examples are presented and used as a springboard for discussion.
- There are instances where the ophthalmologist's actions are immediately relevant, and instances where the issues are broader and involve the social organization of health care.

15.10 Future Directions

Studies that determine if value is added by expensive ancillary testing in the management of diabetic retinopathy may be coming in an environment of decreasing financial resources. The ophthalmological groundswell of commentary regarding ethical aspects of physician relationships with drug companies and in the conduct of research is likely to grow. The prospect of increasing federal regulation of these relationships is significant. Whether the traditional model of physician behavior based on professionalism will be displaced by a different model based on a buyer–vendor relationship is difficult to predict, but there seems to be a trend in that direction. All of these issues will have direct consequences for the care of diabetic retinopathy.

References

1. Cohen JJ, Cruess S, Davidson C. Alliance between society and medicine. The public's stake in medical professionalism. *JAMA*. 2007;298:670–673.
2. Tonelli MR. Conflict of interest in clinical practice. *Chest*. 2007;132:664–670.
3. Browning DJ, Fraser CM, Powers ME. A spreadsheet template for the analysis of optical coherence tomography in the longitudinal management of diabetic macular edema. *Ophthalmic Surg Lasers Imaging*. 2006;37:399–405.
4. Lattanzio R, Brancato R, Pierro L, et al. Macular thickness measured by optical coherence tomography (OCT) in diabetic patients. *Eur J Ophthalmol*. 2002;12:482–487.
5. Hussain A, Hussain N, Nutheti R. Comparison of mean macular thickness using optical coherence tomography and visual acuity in diabetic retinopathy. *Clin Exp Ophthalmol*. 2005;33:240–245.
6. Gaucher D, Tadayoni R, Erginay A, et al. Optical coherence tomography assessment of the vitreoretinal relationship in diabetic macular edema. *Am J Ophthalmol*. 2005;139:807–813.
7. Early Treatment Diabetic Retinopathy Study Research Group. Photocoagulation for Diabetic Macular Edema. *Arch Ophthalmol*. 1985;103:1796–1806.
8. Abu El Asrar AM, Morse PH. Laser photocoagulation control of diabetic macular edema without fluorescein angiography. *Br J Ophthalmol*. 1991;75:97–99.
9. Diabetic Retinopathy Clinical Research Network. Comparison of the modified early treatment diabetic retinopathy study and mild macular grid laser photocoagulation strategies for diabetic macular edema. *Arch Ophthalmol*. 2007;125:469–480.
10. Browning DJ. Diabetic macular edema: a critical review of the early treatment diabetic retinopathy study (ETDRS) series and subsequent studies. *Comp Ophthalmol Update*. 2000;1:69–83.
11. Pinto JB. The retina practice: economics, benchmarks, and career issues. *Retin Phys*. 6-26-2009. http://www.retinalphysician.com/article.aspx?article = 100065
12. Dana J, Loewenstein G. A social science perspective on gifts to physicians from industry. *JAMA*. 2003;290: 252–255.
13. Diabetic Retinopathy Clinical Research Network, Scott IU, Edwards AR, Beck RW, Bressler NM, Chan CK, et al. A phase II randomized clinical trial of intravitreal bevacizumab for diabetic macular edema. *Ophthalmology*. 2007;114:1860–1867.
14. The Economist. This is going to hurt. The Economist 2009 Jun 27; p.13.
15. Hardin G. The tragedy of the commons. *Science*. 1968;162:1243–1248.
16. Eye care: percentage of patients aged 18 years and older with a diagnosis of diabetic retinopathy who had a dilated macular or fundus exam performed with documented communication to the physician who manages the on-going care of the patient with diabetes regarding the findings of the macular or fundus exam at least once within 12 months. 6-20-2009. http://www.qualitymeasures.ahrq.gov/summary/summary.aspx?doc_id = 10290
17. Rothman D. The Effect of Financial Incentives on Physician Behavior and Physician Groups. Abstr Academy Health Meet. volume 21. 2004. http://gateway.nlm.nih.gov/MeetingAbstracts/ma?f = 103624520.html
18. Super N. From capitation to fee-for-service in Cincinnati: a physician group responds to a changing marketplace. *Health Aff*. 2006;25:219–225.
19. Kralewski JE, Rich EC, Feldman R, et al. The effects of medical group practice and physician payment methods on costs of care. *Health Serv Res*. 2000;35:591–613.
20. Lichter PR. Continuing medical education, physicians, and Pavlov: can we change what happens when industry rings the bell? *Arch Ophthalmol*. 2008;126:1593–1597.
21. Lichter P. Debunking myths in physician–industry conflicts of interest. *Am J Ophthalmol*. 2008;146:159–171.
22. Harris G. In article, doctors back ban on gifts from drug makers. *New York Times* 2006 Jan 25. http://www.nytimes.com/2006/01/25/national/25doctor.html
23. Millard WB. Docking the tail that wags the dog: banning drug reps from academic medical facilities. *Ann Emerg Med*. 2007;49:785–791.
24. Chren MM. Interactions between physicians and drug company representatives. *Am J Med*. 1999;107:182–183.
25. Krasner J. Mass. group links drug costs, marketing. *Boston Globe* A.D. Jan 17. http://www.boston.com/business/healthcare/articles/2008/01/17/mass_group_links_drug_costs_marketing/
26. Wang SS. Drug firms' medical staffs say what salespeople can't. *Wall Street Journal* 2009 Jun 26; B3.
27. Ferguson J. My $100,000 sideline. *Med Econ*. 2009;81:28–29.
28. Petersen M. Merck is said to limit perks in marketing to physicians. *New York Times* 2002 Jan 18. http://www.nytimes.com/2002/01/18/business/merck-is-said-to-limit-perks-in-marketing-to-physicians.html
29. Wall LL, Brown D. The high cost of free lunch. *Obstet Gynecol*. 2007;110:169–173.
30. Birch DM, Cohn G. Standing up to industry. Baltimore Sun 2001. http://www.newsday.com/topic/bal-te.research26jun26,0,6517965.story
31. Shimm DS. Human Trials. Scientists, Investors, and Patients in the Quest for a Cure. 7-31-2001.
32. Galewitz P. Cutting-edge option: doctors paid by drugmakers, but say trials not about money. Palm Beach Post 9 A.D. Feb 22.
33. Orlowski JP, Wateska L. The effects of pharmaceutical firm enticements on physician prescribing patterns. There's no such thing as a free lunch. *Chest*. 1992;102:270–273.

34. Camilleri M, Cortese DA. Managing conflicts of interest in clinical practice. *Mayo Clin Proc*. 2007;82:607–614.
35. Leary WE. Doctors given millions by drug companies. *New York Times* 1990 Dec 12; B13.
36. Lempert P, Packer S. Ethical conflicts in university-based research. *Arch Ophthalmol*. 2000;118(1):148–149.
37. Ehringhaus SH, Weissman JS, Sears JL, Goold SD, Feibelmann S, Campbell EG. Responses of medical schools to institutional conflicts of interest. *JAMA*. 2008;299:665–671.
38. Campbell EG, Weissman JS, Ehringhaus S, et al. Institutional academic–industry relationships. *JAMA*. 2007;298:1779–1786.
39. Packer S, Parke DW, II. Ethical concerns in industry support of continuing medical education: the con side. *Arch Ophthalmol*. 2004;122(5):773–776.
40. Flach AJ. Letter regarding debunking myths in physician – industry conflicts of interest. *Am J Ophthalmol*. 2009;147:562–563.
41. Brennan TA, Rothman DJ, Blumenthal DJ, et al. Health industry practices that create conflicts of interest. A policy proposal of academic medical centers. *JAMA*. 2006;295:429–433.
42. Wazana A. Physicians and the pharmaceutical industry: is a gift ever just a gift? *JAMA*. 2000; 283(3): 373–380.
43. Zipkin DA, Steinman MA. Interactions between pharmaceutical representatives and doctors in training. A thematic review. *J Gen Intern Med*. 2005;20:777–786.
44. Morelli D, Koenigsberg MR. Sample medication dispensing in a residency practice. *J Fam Pract*. 1992;34:42–48.
45. Spingarn RW, Berlin JA, Strom BL. When pharmaceutical manufacturers' employees present grand rounds, what do residents remember. *Acad Med*. 1996;71:86–88.
46. Chimonas S, Brennan TA, ROthman DJ. Physicians and drug representatives: exploring the dynamics of the relationship. *J Gen Int Med*. 2007;22:184–190.
47. Brett AS, Burr W, Moloo J. Are gifts from pharmaceutical companies ethically problematic? A survey of physicians. *Arch Intern Med*. 2003;163:2213–2218.
48. Stolberg SG. Study says clinical guides often hide ties of doctors. *New York Times* 2002 Feb 6. http://www.nytimes.com/2002/02/06/health/06DRUG.html
49. Bressler NM. Retinal Anastomosis to Choroidal Neovascularization: A Bum Rap for a Difficult Disease. *Arch Ophthalmol*. 2005;123:1741–1743.
50. Relman AS. Separating continuing medical education from pharmaceutical marketing. *JAMA*. 2001;285: 2009–2012.
51. Heaphy DP, Marrow VB. Industry funding for continuing medical education: is it ethical? *Arch Ophthalmol*. 2004;122:771–773.
52. Chun DW, Heier JS, Topping TM, Duker JS, Bankert JM. A pilot study of multiple intravitreal injections of ranibizumab in patients with center-involving clinically significant diabetic macular edema. *Ophthalmology*. 2006;113:1706–1712.
53. Arevalo JF, Fromow-Guerra J, Quiroz-Mercado H, et al. Primary intravitreal bevacizumab (Avastin) for diabetic macular edema results from the Pan-American collaborative retina study group at 6-month follow-up. *Ophthalmology*. 2007;114:743–750.
54. Ehlers JP, Spirn MJ, Lam A, Sivalingam A, Samuel MA, Tasman W. Combination intravitreal bevacizumab/panretinal photocoagulation versus panretinal photocoagulation alone in the treatment of neovascular glaucoma. *Retina*. 2008;28:696–702.
55. Packer S, Lynch J. Ethics of comanagement. *Arch Ophthalmol*. 2002;120:71–76.
56. Digital Healthcare Wins FDA Approval for Retasure. 6-20-2009. http://www.bio-medicine.org/medicine-news-1/Digital-Healthcare-Wins-FDA-Approval-for-Retasure-1779-1/
57. Berlin J, Bruinooge SS, Tannock IF. Ethics in oncology: consulting for the investment industry. *J Clin Oncol*. 2007;25:444–446.
58. Topol EJ, Blumenthal D. Physicians and the investment industry. *JAMA*. 2005;293:2654–2657.

Chapter 16
Clinical Examples in Managing Diabetic Retinopathy

David J. Browning, Scott E. Pautler, David G. Telander, Keye Wong, Michael W. Stewart, and Abdhish R. Bhavsar

In previous chapters, the emphasis has been on a detailed understanding of a particular aspect of diabetic retinopathy. In this chapter the approach will be more topical and practical and the principles presented previously will be exemplified in characteristic situations. Actual cases will be presented with discussions regarding management. These cases were circulated among the co-authors and comments on management independently solicited and then compiled. The discussants for the cases used the comments as a springboard to review the literature and provide a synthesis that reflects both the diverse clinical judgments of the reviewers and the published evidence pertinent to the case.

16.1 Case 1: Proliferative Diabetic Retinopathy with Dense Premacular Hemorrhage in a Patient on Coumadin

A 52-year-old man with diabetes and hypertension of 24 years duration was taking warfarin for atrial fibrillation and congestive heart failure when he developed sudden painless loss of vision in the left eye. He had previously had multiple focal/grid and panretinal photocoagulation laser treatments to both eyes for diabetic macular edema and proliferative diabetic retinopathy. His visual acuity was R – 20/25, L – hand motions. The fundus of the left eye is shown in Fig. 16.1. The international normalized ratio (INR) was 2.2. How would you manage him?

D.J. Browning (✉)
Charlotte Eye Ear Nose & Throat Associates, Charlotte, NC 28210, USA
e-mail: dbrowning@ceenta.com

16.1.1 Discussion

It has been estimated that cases of dense premacular hemorrhage such as this comprise 6% of vitrectomy surgeries for complications of diabetic retinopathy, and it has been stated that this is an indication for prompt vitrectomy.[1] The rationale for skipping a period of observation and hoping for spontaneous clearing is that dense premacular hemorrhage under a bridging scaffold of posterior hyaloid results in early proliferation of fibrous membranes with traction retinal detachment.[1] It is not known whether a period of observation is detrimental in such cases. A few weeks of observation may not be risky, and would have the advantage of demonstrating to the patient that spontaneous improvement was unlikely. Patient understanding and full agreement with a surgical treatment plan is an important aspect to weigh.

Certain cases such as this one feature liquefied blood in the premacular, subhyaloid space. In these cases, rupture of the posterior hyaloid face with the neodymium YAG laser may lead to dependent movement of the blood and clearing without the need for vitrectomy.[2] The experience of others, however, is that these hemorrhages in patients with diabetes are often clotted, and if this is the case, the YAG laser approach to treatment will fail.[1] Two other approaches reported in this situation are an intravitreal injection of tissue plasminogen activator, 50 μg, or bevacizumab, 1.25 mg, together with an intravitreal injection of 0.3 ml of sulfur hexafluoride.[3,4]

D.J. Browning (ed.), *Diabetic Retinopathy*, DOI 10.1007/978-0-387-85900-2_16,

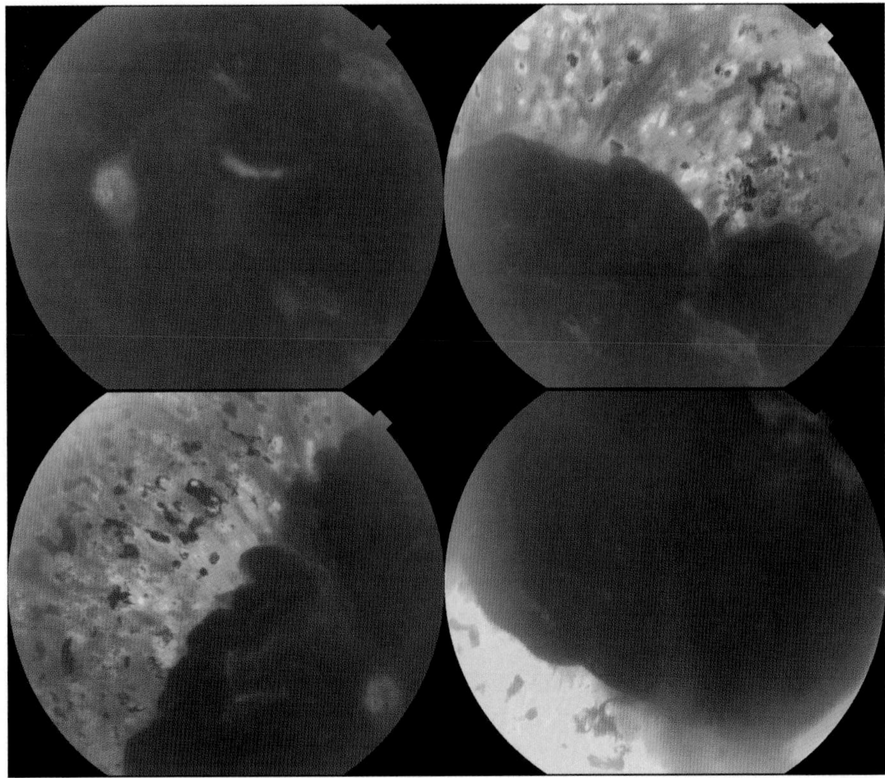

Fig. 16.1 Fundus photographs of case 1 at presentation. A dense premacular and subhyaloid clot is present in the left eye. Panretinal laser scars are present peripherally

Reports of all treatment approaches emphasize the need for complete panretinal photocoagulation to cause regression of any active neovasculariazation.[1–4]

A separate issue exemplified by this case is the management of warfarin therapy in a patient being considered for vitrectomy surgery. The growing consensus is that the warfarin need not be discontinued if there are valid medical indications for its use.[5–7] More complicated regimens of switching from warfarin to heparin, discontinuing heparin shortly before vitrectomy, reinstituting heparin after surgery, and finally converting from heparin back to warfarin appear to be unnecessary. There are no randomized controlled trials, however, to address the issue definitively and the specific details of each case together with the treating physician's experience and input from the patient's internist may be the most important determinants in management decisions.

Three technical issues arise in such a case if the ophthalmologist recommends vitrectomy surgery. First, is this a case in which 25 gauge or 20 gauge technique is preferable, or does it matter? Twenty-five gauge surgery is associated with a faster postoperative recovery, but there is concern that the 25 gauge cutter cannot resect dense fibrinous clots as efficiently as the 20 gauge cutter. Second, should a preoperative injection of bevacizumab be given to render less active any underlying neovascularization, as has been reported, especially given the anticoagulated status of the patient?[8,9] Finally, if intraoperative oozing of blood in an anticoagulated patient is a problem, what are useful approaches at surgery?

In this case, the surgeon chose 20 gauge technique and was convinced that the 25 gauge cutter would have failed to successfully resect the thick subhyaloid clot. No preoperative bevacizumab was given. Intraoperative oozing of blood was a problem and was not controllable by raising the infusion pressure or with the use of intravitreal cautery. The technique used to manage the oozing was silicone oil tamponade as has been described previously.[10–12] It is conjectural whether preoperative bevacizumab injection would have circumvented this difficulty.

The appearance of the fundus 2 days after surgery is shown in Fig. 16.2. Unrecognized preoperatively, but apparent intraoperatively, there was

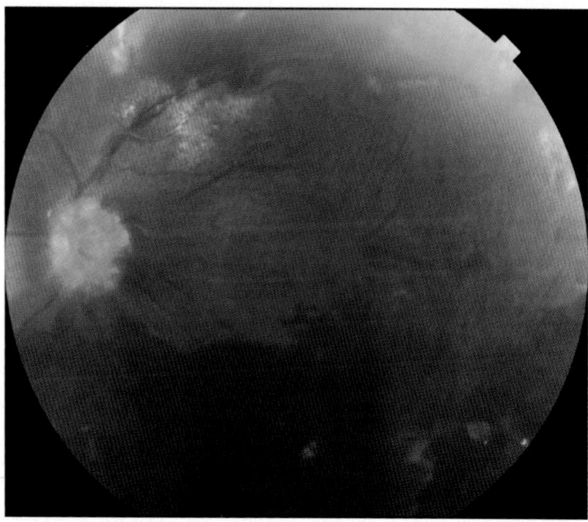

Fig. 16.2 Postoperative fundus photograph of the left eye of case 1. Silicone oil is present in the vitreous cavity. Thin subretinal hemorrhage is present in the macula

subretinal hemorrhage in addition to the premacular hemorrhage in this case, and this is clearly shown in Fig. 16.2. Subsequently the subretinal blood resolved, the silicone oil was removed from the eye, and the final visual acuity was 20/200 (Fig. 16.3).[a]

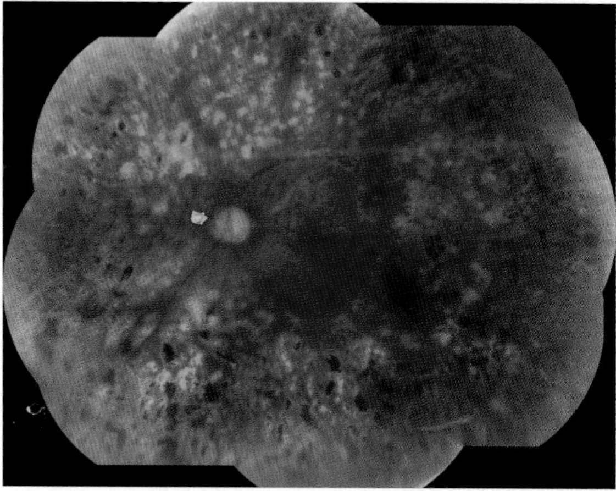

Fig. 16.3 Postoperative fundus photograph of case 1, 4 months after the fundus photograph shown in Fig. 16.2. The subretinal hemorrhage in the macula has resolved leaving pigmentary mottling. The oil was uneventfully removed and the final visual acuity was 20/200

[a] Discussed by David J. Browning MD, PhD

16.2 Case 2: Bilateral Proliferative Diabetic Retinopathy with Acute Vitreous Hemorrhage in One Eye and a Chronic Traction Retinal Detachment in the Other Eye

A 48-year-old man with type 1 diabetes for 35 years and hypertension for 15 years presented with chronic poor vision in left eye and new acute loss of vision in right eye. He reported being able to read and drive with the right eye before the sudden visual loss. The left eye visual acuity was light perception and by history had been this way for 6 months. This was the first time he had been examined by an ophthalmologist and there were no other details from the past, but there had been no previous laser treatment. The left eye had an intraocular pressure of 15 mmHg, was phakic, and had no iris neovascularization. Fundus photographs of the left disk and midperipheral fundus are shown (Figs. 16.4 and 16.5). Figure 16.4 shows a thick, florid neovascular plaque overlying the disk that has contracted and has raised the peripapillary retina into a funnel. The far peripheral retina was attached (not shown). Figure 16.6 portrays the anatomic situation. The right eye had a visual acuity of counting fingers with disk neovascularization much less severe than that present in the left eye and a new dispersed vitreous hemorrhage without traction retinal detachment.

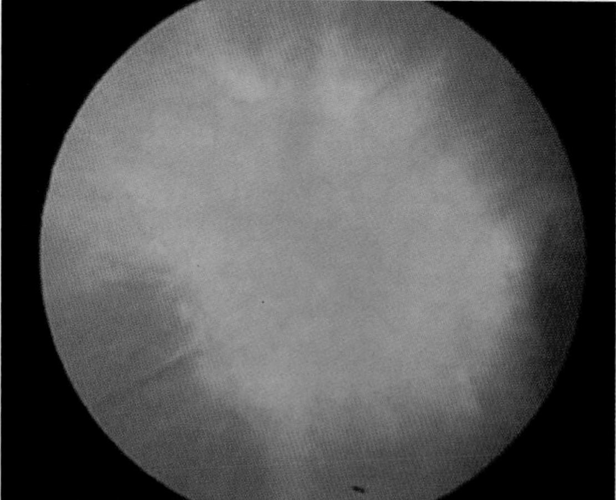

Fig. 16.4 Appearance of the left eye of case 2 at presentation. A thick neovascular plaque overlies the disk and has pulled the peripapillary retina into a tight funnel

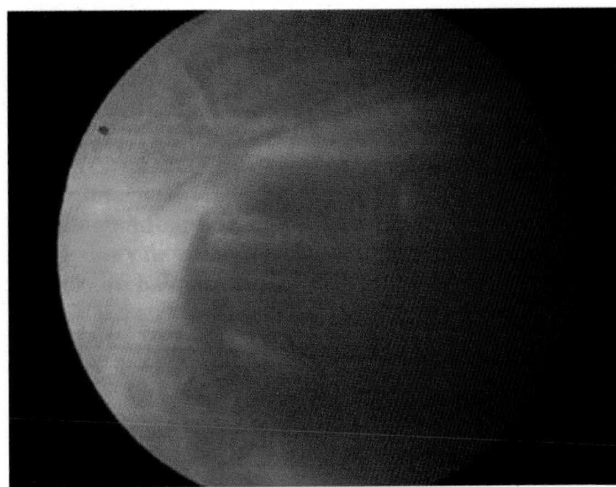

Fig. 16.5 A fundus photograph of more peripheral retina in case 2 at presentation. The far peripheral retina is attached. The midperipheral retina is detached, as shown, and no previous panretinal photocoagulation has been administered

Question: How would you manage this patient? If part of your response involves surgery of the left eye, please be detailed in the technical aspects of your approach.

16.2.1 Discussion

The four ophthalmologists who reviewed this case agreed that the management priority was to rehabilitate the right eye known to have reading vision in the recent past. This would involve a pars plana vitrectomy with panretinal laser photocoagulation. In addition, efforts should be spent to educate the patient about the importance of regular ophthalmic monitoring and care in the future, a factor missing in his past history.

The controversy in this case revolves around what to do about the left eye. One reviewer commented, "The left eye has a very poor prognosis based on poor acuity, type 1 diabetes, and long duration of traction retinal detachment, as well as the absence of panretinal photocoagulation. It is comfortable and I would like to keep it that way, so I would not operate this eye." There is ample support in the literature for this perspective. Macular traction retinal detachments present for more than 1 month have been shown to have poorer prognosis when repaired, and when the macula has been detached for greater than 6 months, older publications conclude that the risks of surgery outweigh the possible benefits.[13–16]

Counterbalancing this reasoning, it is certain that the left eye cannot improve without intervention, and it may advance to neovascular glaucoma and phthisis if observed. Unfortunately, the natural history of such eyes is not well studied, and one does not know what the spontaneous rate of progression

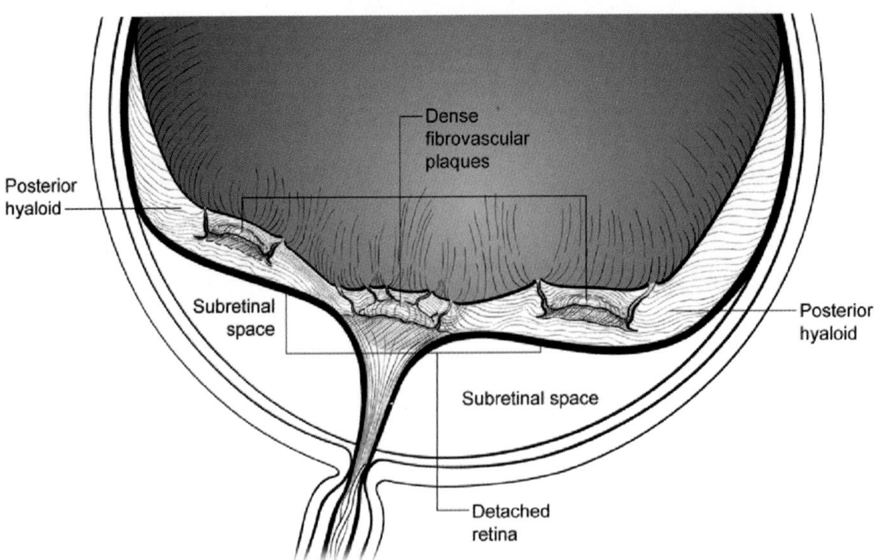

Fig. 16.6 A sketch of the anatomic configuration of the retina of the left eye in case 2

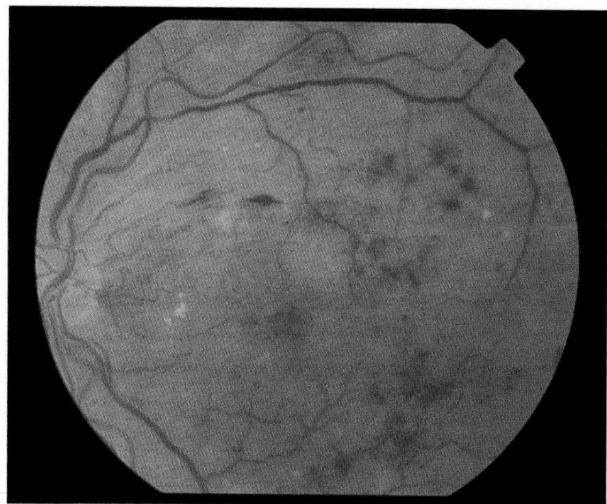

Fig. 16.7 Fundus photograph of the left eye of case 3. Neovascularization is present on the temporal disk margin. The macula is edematous with many intraretinal hemorrhages, a few lipid exudates, and a patch of neovascularization inferotemporally

to no light perception, neovascular glaucoma, and phthisis bulbi is in such eyes, but the consensus opinion of the authors is that it is relatively common. Reliable operative outcome statistics in such a case are also in short supply, and would depend on the individual surgeon's expertise. Rates of 8.7–18.6% of similar eyes progressing to no light perception after vitreous surgery and 24–67% achieving ambulatory vision have been published.[17–20] In more recent case series, it appears that vitreoretinal surgeons are more willing to operate on chronic traction macular detachments documented to be present for as long or longer than 1 year.[13,21] In view of the patient's young age, the unstable status of the right eye (better eye), and the patient's demonstrated failure to access the health care system previously, three of the four co-authors reviewing this case considered that the natural history of the left eye would probably be worse than the outcome with surgical intervention. Therefore, surgical intervention for the left eye was recommended by these co-authors after educating the patient thoroughly regarding the significant risks of surgery and possible progression to neovascular glaucoma and/or phthisis bulbi even if surgery is attempted. There were some differences in their technical approaches, however, as manifest from the following comments.

16.2.2 Opinion 1

1. Use 25 gauge instruments first and convert to 20 gauge if the membranes cannot be adequately cut with the 25 gauge instrument.
2. Use intravitreal triamcinolone to assist in visualizing the posterior hyaloid and facilitate its complete removal.

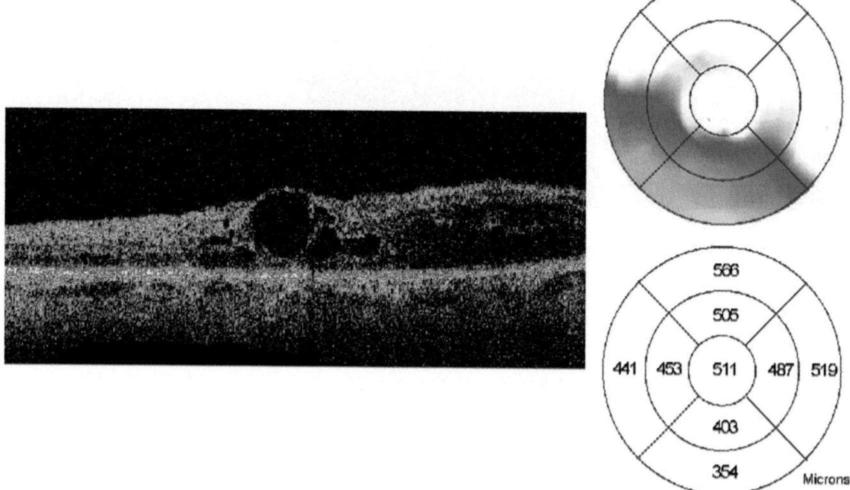

Fig. 16.8 OCT of the left eye of case 3. Marked macular thickening is present with a large foveal cyst

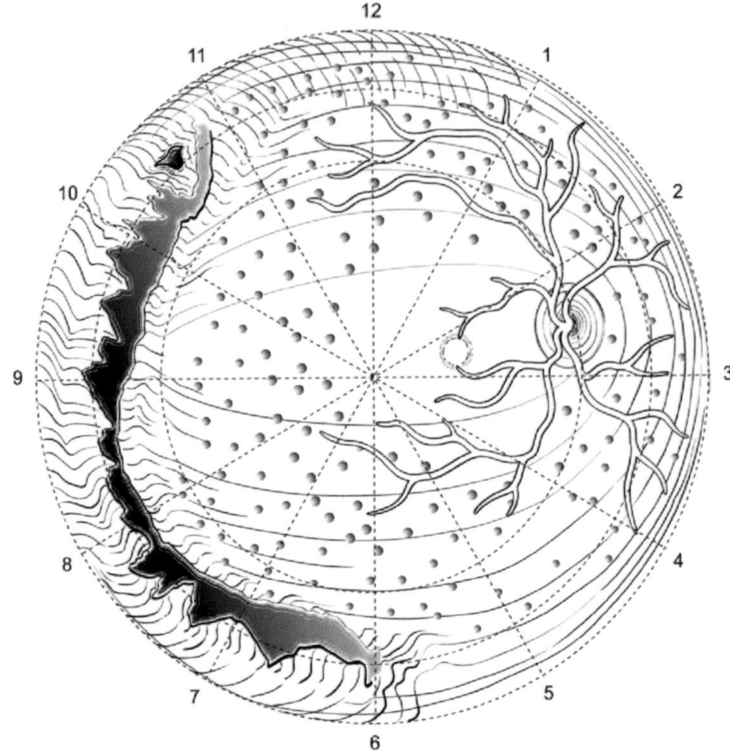

Fig. 16.9 Fundus drawing of the right eye of case 4 indicating a superotemporal horseshoe tear and a peripheral retinal detachment delimited by scarring from previously placed panretinal photocoagulation

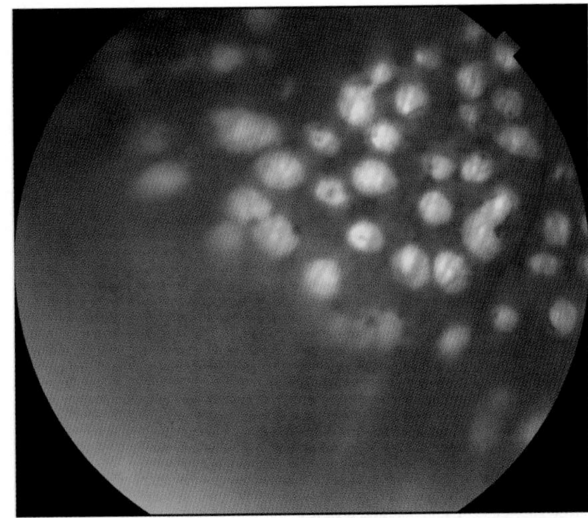

Fig. 16.10 Fundus photograph from case 4 showing 2 clock hours of a peripheral retinal detachment delimited by previously placed panretinal photocoagulation for proliferative diabetic retinopathy

3. Make no intentional retinotomies and if no intraoperative break occurs, use perfluoron to move the subretinal fluid peripherally and allow panretinal photocoagulation. If iatrogenic, unintended breaks occur intraoperatively, flatten the retina with subretinal fluid drainage through one of them, apply panretinal laser photocoagulation, and use silicone oil as a tamponade.

16.2.3 Opinion 2

1. Do not inject intravitreal bevacizumab before vitrectomy.
2. Apply panretinal photocoagulation to the attached peripheral retina in the office a few weeks before the vitrectomy.
3. Use 20 gauge instrumentation and horizontal curved scissors for membrane delamination.
4. Create a drainage retinotomy, and flatten the retina before applying panretinal photocoagulation.
5. Finish with a gas/fluid exchange using 28% sulfur hexafluoride.

16.2.4 Opinion 3

1. Inject intravitreal bevacizumab 1.25 mg 1–4 days before surgery.

2. Use 20 gauge instrumentation and vertical automated scissors.
3. Use a lighted infusion cannula to allow bimanual technique with one hand grasping and the fellow hand operating the vitrector or the scissors.
4. Apply intraoperative panretinal laser photocoagulation only to the attached peripheral retina.
5. Make no intentional retinotomies, but if an iatrogenic break occurs, aggressively resect all fibrovascular membranes, apply panretinal laser photocoagulation after flattening the retina with an air–fluid exchange, and finish the case with a silicone oil–air exchange.
6. Aim to relieve all traction on the retina, create no iatrogenic breaks, and leave the eye with its subretinal fluid to be pumped out by the retinal pigment epithelium.
7. In the office postoperatively, apply panretinal photocoagulation posteriorly (where the subretinal fluid is) after the retina flattens, which might take several weeks to occur.

In considering these various opinions, it is not possible to say which technique would offer the patient the best chance of a good outcome, as they reflect the individual aspects of different surgeons' training and experience. Furthermore, there are no randomized trials comparing specific techniques that are applicable to just such a case as this. It is worthwhile, however, to emphasize the differences of opinion and where consensus is present. The use of preoperative bevacizumab is contentious. Opinion 1 omits reference to it, opinion 2 explicitly argues against its use, and opinion 3 recommends using it. Case series have reported that use of preoperative bevacizumab reduces vascularity and intraoperative bleeding, but can cause contraction of fibrovascular membranes in approximately 5% of cases.[9,22,23] One case report has been published of a patient losing vision from hand motions to no light perception shortly after an intravitreal bevacizumab injection, but the discussants of the case were doubtful that cause and effect could be established.[24] If bevacizumab is used in such a case, the consensus of opinion seems to be that the surgery should follow within 4 days to reduce the chances of fibrovascular membrane contracture.[9] We think it is valuable to expose the reader to the spectrum of thinking about the problems raised by such a case.[b]

16.3 Case 3: Sight Threatening Diabetic Retinopathy in a Patient with Concomitant Medical and Socioeconomic Problems

A 61-year-old male was referred by an emergency room doctor. The patient was on no diabetic therapy and complained of 6 months of painless, fluctuating, blurred vision OU. He stated, "I am a borderline diabetic." He had no primary care doctor, no insurance, no Medicaid, no Medicare, no job, no money, and took no medication. The state blind commission had exceeded its yearly budget and was authorizing no more treatments until the next fiscal year.

The examination showed the following:

- Blood pressure was 165/95
- Fingerstick blood glucose in office was 283
- Best corrected visual acuity was 20/63 OU
- Phakic with early nuclear sclerosis OU
- Fundus appearance OS as shown (Fig. 16.7)
- OCT OS as shown (Fig. 16.8)
- The situation OD was similar

How would you manage this case (tests, treatment, follow-up intervals, primary care arrangements)?

16.3.1 Discussion

The patient has untreated diabetes mellitus, hypertension, diabetic macular edema (DME), and proliferative diabetic retinopathy (PDR) based on the presence of a twig of neovascularization at the temporal disk margin. The medical issues in this case are straightforward. The patient needs medical care and education about diabetes and hypertension, needs appropriate treatment to tightly control his blood sugar and blood pressure, and once this systemic treatment plan has been put in place, needs ophthalmic intervention to reduce the DME first and the PDR second (see Chapters 4, 7, and 9).[25–27]

[b]Discussed by David J. Browning MD, PhD

The treatment for the DME should be focal/grid laser photocoagulation.[28] The treatment for the PDR should be panretinal laser photocoagulation.[29] It would be preferable to have resolution of the DME before addressing the PDR, thus focal/grid laser should be applied and after 4 months, if DME persists, reapplied until either the DME has resolved or maximal treatment has been placed with refractory DME remaining.[30] In the Early Treatment Diabetic Retinopathy Study, the average number of focal/grid laser treatments required for an eye with clinically significant macular edema was 3.8, so the ophthalmologist should expect to treat this eye multiple times. In many cases, one cannot wait until DME has resolved before addressing the PDR. One may proceed with PRP together with treatment of the DME in such cases. Based on clinical experience rather than evidence from randomized clinical trials, an adjunctive agent such as intravitreal triamcinolone or bevacizumab may be useful in such a situation.[31]

The difficult issues in this case are not the medical ones, but rather the social ones. It is challenging to arrange care by an internist in the United States for such a patient. If the ophthalmologist lives in an area with a medical school, there may be provision for care of the indigent there. Some communities have clinics for the indigent, but the care may be haphazard and they are frequently understaffed. Few ophthalmologists feel qualified to treat diabetes and hypertension themselves, or some feel that they would incur unacceptable follow-up obligations and legal liability were they to begin medical therapy themselves. Thus, the systemic foundation in such a case will frequently be lacking. In such cases, the ophthalmologist can verbally encourage the preferred care at each ophthalmic visit and facilitate obtaining it as far as possible. Often the ophthalmic aspects of treatment will need to be applied regardless of optimization of the systemic factors.

The issue arises – should ancillary studies be obtained in such a situation, and is standard care to be followed? One of the panel reading this case commented that he does not change his practice based on the patient's economic circumstances (opinion#1). He would obtain a fluorescein angiogram (FA) and optical coherence tomogram (OCT), treat the patient in the preferred manner, follow-up and monitor with OCT as for anyone else, and set up a payment plan "even for $5 per month." Another reading the case would treat based on the clinical appearance only, omit both the FA and OCT, and would alter the treatment plan. This physician would begin with an intravitreal injection of triamcinolone and follow with a combined focal/grid and a full panretinal laser photocoagulation treatment 1 week later (opinion#2). Follow-up OCTs would be omitted, but visits would continue at 4-month intervals. In the discussant's experience, the ophthalmologist's approach to such cases depends on what proportion they represent of his practice. If such cases comprise <5% of the ophthalmologist's cases, the approach is often that of opinion#1. If such cases comprise 10%, 20%, or more of the practice, the approach begins to approach that of opinion#2. Ophthalmologists who practice in countries with nationalized health care seem to face fewer issues of this nature.[c]

16.4 Case 4: Asymptomatic Retinal Detachment Following Vitrectomy in a Patient Who Has Had Panretinal Laser Photocoagulation

A 62-year-old man with type 1 diabetes for 35 years and hypertension for 25 years had panretinal photocoagulation for proliferative diabetic retinopathy and focal/grid laser photocoagulation for diabetic macular edema of the right eye 3 years before. He subsequently developed a macular epiretinal membrane with persistent macular edema of this eye for which he underwent vitrectomy with membrane peeling. At routine follow-up 2 months after surgery, a peripheral rhegmatogenous retinal detachment was noted with a post-sclerotomy horseshoe tear in the superotemporal quadrant (Figs. 16.9 and 16.10). At this visit he was asymptomatic and his best corrected visual acuity was 20/40 right and 20/60 left. How would you manage this case?

[c] Discussed by David J. Browning MD, PhD

16.4.1 Discussion

Of the four retina specialists who reviewed this case and commented, all had seen a few similar cases, but they seem to be uncommon. The relevant literature is scant, reflecting this fact.[32] Two of the four reviewers responded that they would treat such an asymptomatic case, considering it to be intrinsically unstable and likely to progress. Both of these reviewers preferred to address the case with a pneumatic retinopexy. As one put it, "In spite of panretinal photocoagulation (PRP), the retinal detachment will likely progress over time. There is a small chance that it could remain stable. However, given the horseshoe tear located superotemporally, I would recommend cryoretinopexy to surround the tear followed by either a pneumatic retinopexy with 0.3–0.5 cc 100% sulfur hexafluoride (SF_6) or simply a fluid–gas exchange with 25% SF_6. This can be done in the office with subconjunctival lidocaine for anesthetic and is typically quite successful."

The other two reviewers would have managed the situation differently. One physician would simply bolster the PRP but also monitor closely for neovascularization of the iris that could be stimulated by the ischemic detached peripheral retinal detachment in a patient with diabetic retinopathy. The last physician recommended rather close observation initially, with plans to do nothing if there was no progression and to intervene with a pneumatic retinopexy or a scleral buckle operation if there were signs of progression.

The only case series published supports the notion that the previously placed panretinal photocoagulation can barricade the peripheral retinal detachment and keep it from spreading.[d]

16.5 Case 5: Management of Progressive Vitreous Hemorrhage Following Scatter Photocoagulation for Proliferative Diabetic Retinopathy

A 63-year-old female with non-insulin dependent diabetes mellitus of 10 years duration was seen on 5/28/08 with blurred vision OS for 4 days. She had a premacular and peripapillary vitreous hemorrhage without apparent disk neovascularization. A composite fluorescein angiogram demonstrating the pattern of preretinal hemorrhage in the left eye is shown in Fig. 16.11.

She underwent an initial "moderate" scatter photocoagulation on 6/4/08 (846 spots via laser indirect ophthalmoscopic delivery). She returned on 6/16/08 complaining of increasingly blurred vision in her left eye. She had an increased amount of vitreous hemorrhage in a boat-shaped configuration as shown in Fig. 16.12, with a possible focus of

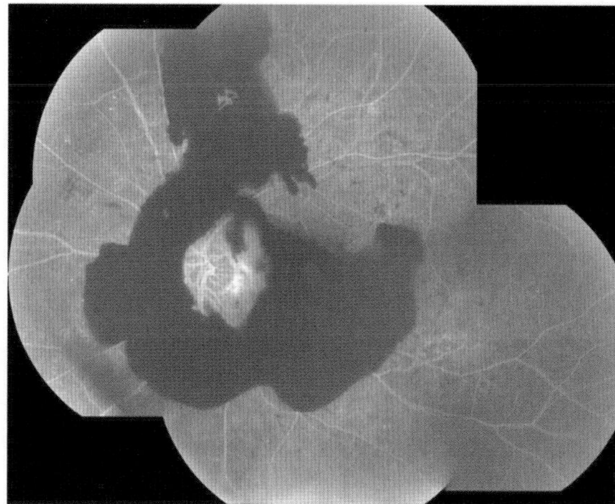

Fig. 16.11 Mosaic fluorescein angiogram of case 5 at presentation. A preretinal hemorrhage obscures the papillomacular bundle and peripapillary retina but spares the fovea

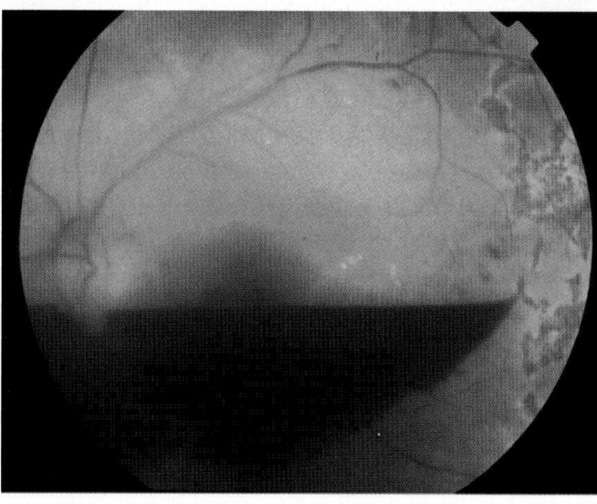

Fig. 16.12 Fundus photograph of case 5, 2 weeks after mild scatter photocoagulation

[d] Discussed by David J. Browning MD, PhD

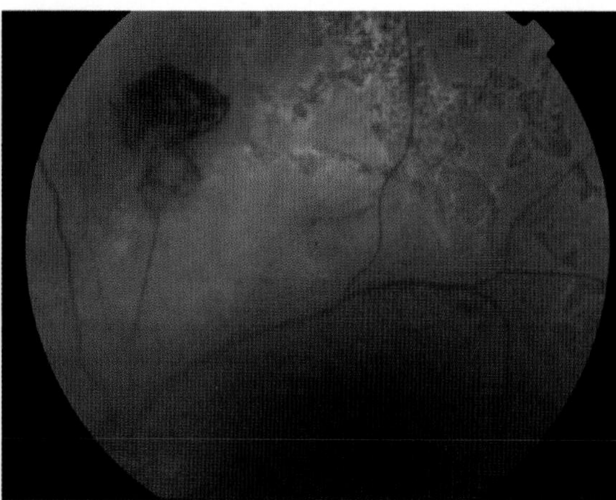

Fig. 16.13 Regressing neovascularization elsewhere, 2 weeks after mild scatter photocoagulation

regressing neovascularization elsewhere superior to the optic nerve (see Fig. 16.13).

She has NVE in the right eye nasal to the optic nerve (see Fig. 16.14) but is resistant to agreeing to panretinal photocoagulation in that eye because of the occurrence of increased hemorrhage in her left eye following panretinal photocoagulation.

Her visual acuity on 7/2/08 is 20/70 OD improving with pinhole to 20/40 and 20/400 OS. She has mild nuclear sclerotic cataracts in both eyes. How would you manage both eyes?

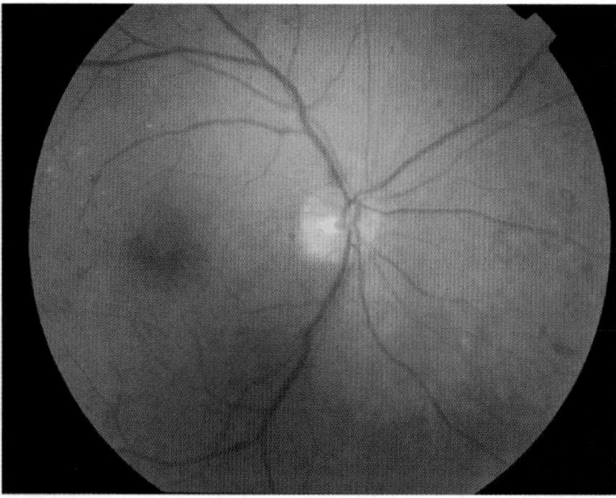

Fig. 16.14 Fundus photograph of the right eye of case 5. Neovascularization elsewhere is seen two disc diameters nasal to the optic nerve

16.5.1 Discussion

How much initial laser treatment is enough is open to interpretation. Some physicians believe that a pattern with 800 spots is not a moderate pattern of scatter laser but an incomplete pattern of scatter laser. The Diabetic Retinopathy Study (DRS) from the mid-1970s and the Early Treatment Diabetic Retinopathy Study (ETDRS) from 1980 to 1985 tested strategies of scatter photocoagulation which may need to be reinterpreted in the current era of better systemic blood sugar control, better vitrectomy techniques, and the current availability of anti-VEGF medications.

In the DRS the specified laser technique included 800–1600 argon laser burns of 500 μm spot size.[33] Scatter photocoagulation was shown to be beneficial in reducing the rate of progression to severe visual loss as compared to a strategy of observation for 2 years. This wide range of allowable laser spots were further evaluated in the ETDRS where a strategy of full scatter photocoagulation was compared to a strategy of mild scatter photocoagulation.[34] Full scatter photocoagulation comprised of 1200–1600 spots of 500 μm size. The burns were placed ½ burn width apart in comparison to the mild scatter photocoagulation pattern in which 400–650 spots of 500 μm size were placed ≥ 1 burn apart. However, unlike the DRS the ETDRS tested a strategy of allowing additional laser to be applied if NVE progressed or high-risk characteristics developed.

The study populations of the DRS differed from the patients evaluated in the ETDRS in that the ETDRS enrolled patients who had less than high-risk PDR. The 5-year rate of development of high-risk PDR in the ETDRS was 18.8% in the full scatter group vs. 26.9% in the mild scatter group vs. 38.5% in the deferral group. Therefore, an initial full scatter laser pattern is more effective in reducing the risk of progression to high-risk PDR. However, when compared to a strategy of observation every 4 months with application of laser if high-risk PDR developed there was no statistical downside to the deferral strategy. The 5-year rate of developing severe visual loss was 2.7% in the initial full scatter group vs. 2.6% in the initial mild scatter group vs. 2.2% in the deferral group. The conclusion therefore was that scatter photocoagulation prior to the development of high-risk characteristics does not reduce the risk of progressing to severe visual loss. Although the ETDRS did not evaluate patients with high-risk PDR (as in the DRS) this ETDRS data demonstrates that the lower range of laser spots studied in the DRS (800) was as effective as the upper range of laser spots allowed (1,600) in preventing severe visual loss (when given the option of adding laser at 4-month intervals). The ETDRS also demonstrated a visual cost to full scatter laser in that there was a statistically greater chance of decreased visual field and color vision deficits of full scatter laser vs. mild scatter laser and mild scatter laser vs. deferral.

Therefore it seems reasonable that even for patients with high-risk characteristics if one can provide follow-up at 4-month intervals or less, an initial mild scatter laser pattern may be as effective as full scatter in reducing the progression to severe visual loss and will also have a decreased cost of affecting visual field and color vision.

Additional data to suggest that a mild scatter laser pattern may be appropriate arise from the data from the Diabetes Control and Complications Trial. In that trial it was demonstrated that a reduction in baseline hemoglobin A1c of 10% reduced by 45% the subsequent risk of progression of diabetic retinopathy.[35] Baseline demographic data from the ETDRS revealed that 42% of the study population in 1980 had a hemoglobin A1c $\geq$ 10.[36] In a diabetic retinopathy study population from 2003 the mean hemoglobin A1c was 8.2 ± 2.2.[37] Assuming a Gaussian distribution this would translate to about 16% of patients with a hemoglobin A1c > 10. The better systemic blood sugar control currently exhibited by diabetic patients therefore translates into their natural history having a decreased risk of diabetic retinopathy progression and provides further evidence that an initial mild scatter laser pattern is not detrimental.

An additional issue exemplified by this case is the need for appropriate education of the patient regarding the natural history of untreated diabetic retinopathy. In the setting of her visual symptoms worsening after laser intervention the natural tendency is to blame the treatment. Pretreatment education would be helpful but patients may still expect that laser therapy will help them see better rather than decrease their risk of progressing to severe visual loss. In the setting that the patient questions the value of laser treatment it may be helpful to re-establish patient confidence by re-reviewing goals of therapy or to offer a second opinion. Establishing patient cooperation is critical if other therapies to include anti-VEGF injections or vitrectomy are to be considered.[e]

16.6 Case 6: Post-surgical, Inflammatory Macular Edema, or Diabetic Macular Edema?

A 77-year-old man who had previously undergone uneventful bilateral cataract surgery with intraocular lens implantation was seen with blurred vision of the left eye of several months duration. The right and left eye cataract surgeries had been done 12 and 9 months previously, respectively. His best corrected visual acuity was 20/20 right eye and 20/200 left eye. The slit lamp examination showed bilateral posterior chamber intraocular lenses in the capsular bag with clear posterior capsules and no uveitis. His fundus examination showed bilateral mild nonproliferative diabetic retinopathy. On the left, vitreomacular traction was evident (Fig. 16.15). He underwent vitrectomy with membrane peeling of the left eye with resolution of the traction and return of visual acuity to 20/50. One month later his vision dropped to 20/80. The slit lamp examination of the left eye showed no anterior chamber or vitreous cells. The post-vitrectomy optical coherence tomogram, fundus photograph, and fluorescein angiogram are shown in Figs. 16.16, 16.17, and 16.18.

- Questions: Is this post-surgical, inflammatory macular edema, or is this diabetic macular edema? If you think they can be distinguished, what clues are reliable in order to tell the two apart? Based on your interpretation of the situation, how would you manage this patient?

[e] Discussed by Keye Wong MD

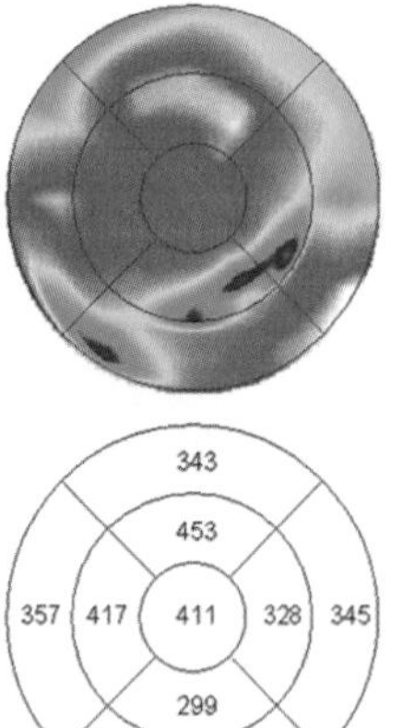

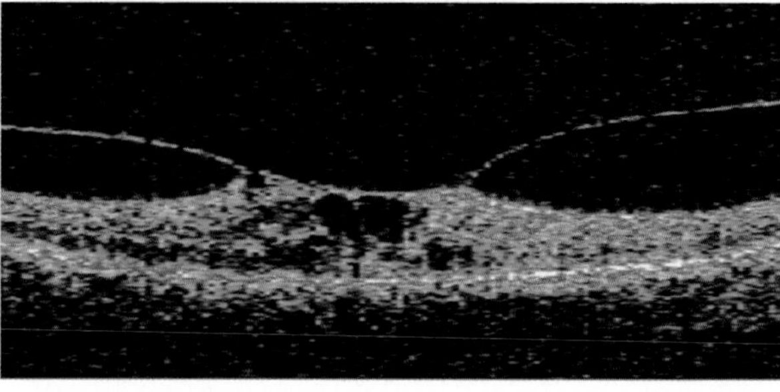

Fig. 16.15 Optical coherence tomography of the left eye of case 6 showing vitreomacular traction

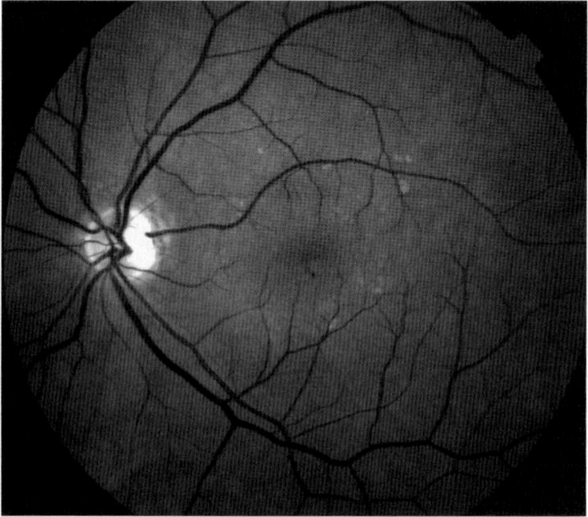

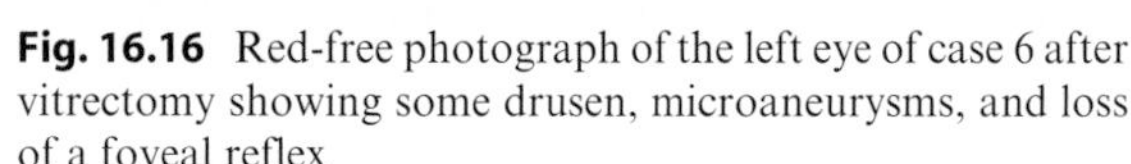

Fig. 16.16 Red-free photograph of the left eye of case 6 after vitrectomy showing some drusen, microaneurysms, and loss of a foveal reflex

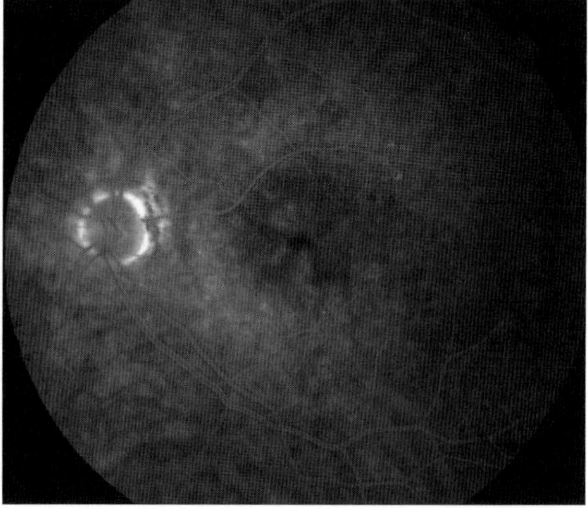

Fig. 16.17 Late frame of the fluorescein angiogram of the left eye of case 6 after vitrectomy showing late fluorescein leakage in the macula and no optic nerve head hyperfluorescence

16.6.1 Discussion

The three reviewers who commented on this case echoed each other. They all commented that this patient has three possible sources of macular edema: the improved but chronic residual macular edema that is commonly seen after surgery for macular epiretinal membranes, post-surgical inflammatory macular edema (sometimes called Irvine-Gass syndrome after cataract surgery, but potentially seen after any intraocular surgery), and diabetic macular edema (DME).[38,39]

For years ophthalmologists thought that they could distinguish the second from the third types of edema. It was commonly written that a petalloid pattern of hyperfluorescence in the macula and a hyperfluorescent optic disk in later frames of the fluorescein angiogram were signs of post-surgical inflammatory macular edema rather than DME.[40,41] However, when this impression was examined in prospective, masked studies, it did not appear that these signs were reliable in distinguishing the two types of edema.[42,43] That is, diabetic eyes that do not develop post-surgical macular edema can

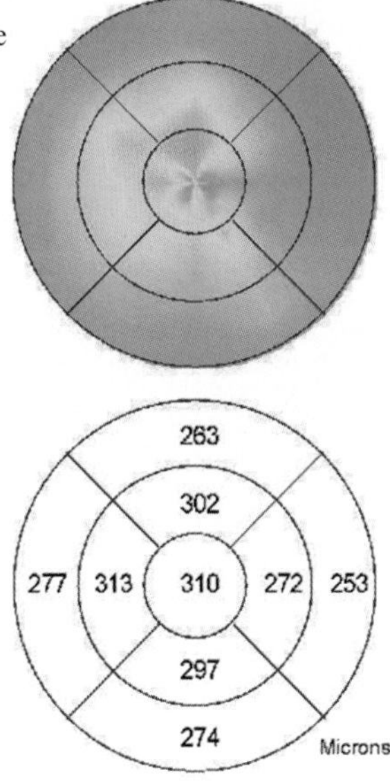

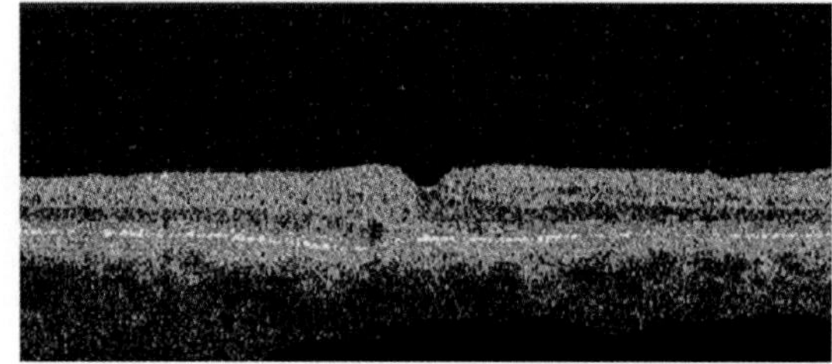

Fig. 16.18 Optical coherence tomogram of the left eye of case 6 after vitrectomy showing macular thickening but no vitreomacular traction

develop disk hyperfluorescence after surgery and petalloid macular hyperfluorescence can be seen in diabetic eyes with macular edema that have never undergone surgery.[43,44] Thus, the relative contributions of DME versus PCME in post-surgical macular thickening can be difficult to assess in mixed clinical pictures.[41,45] In the past, when it was thought that the treatments differed for the two conditions, discriminating the components had greater importance. With the discovery that anti-inflammatory drugs can improve DME and that anti-VEGF drugs can improve post-surgical macular edema, the importance of the distinction has diminished.[46–53]

With this background, there are two practical approaches that seem reasonable. If the patient is reasonably content and willing to proceed in a stepwise fashion, one could begin with the least invasive option and try topical prednisolone acetate and ketorolac for a month. If there is no improvement, then one could proceed to use periocular triamcinolone, and then if it resolves but recurs 3–4 months later, one could deduce by the process of elimination that the visible microaneurysms were of importance and selectively ablate them. If the patient is distressed and pushing the ophthalmologist for expedient relief, then a multi-pronged approach addressing all potential contributing sources at the same time would be rational – for example, simultaneous combined periocular triamcinolone plus focal photocoagulation.[f]

16.7 Case 7: Proliferative Diabetic Retinopathy with Macular Traction and Ischemia

A 43-year-old female with diabetes and hypertension known for 5 years but present probably for many years longer has had blurred vision OS>OD for several months. The best corrected visual acuity is R – 20/25, L – 20/100. The intraocular pressure is 15 OU. Neither eye has iris neovascularization. Each eye has had one session of panretinal photocoagulation with ~1,500 burns. Both fundi are shown as are the OCTs and sample frames from the fluorescein angiogram (Figs. 16.19, 16.20, 16.21, 16.22, 16.23, and 16.24). How would you manage these two eyes?

16.7.1 Discussion

The management of the right eye was controversial among the five reviewers of the case. Two reviewers thought that the neovascularization in the right eye was relatively inactive and that no further treatment

---

[f]Discussed by David G. Telander MD, PhD

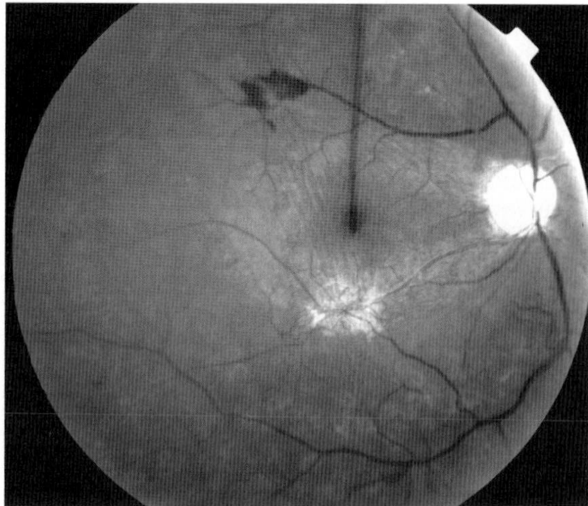

Fig. 16.19 Red-free photograph of the right eye of case 7 showing retinal neovascularization, some preretinal hemorrhage, and a macular epiretinal membrane

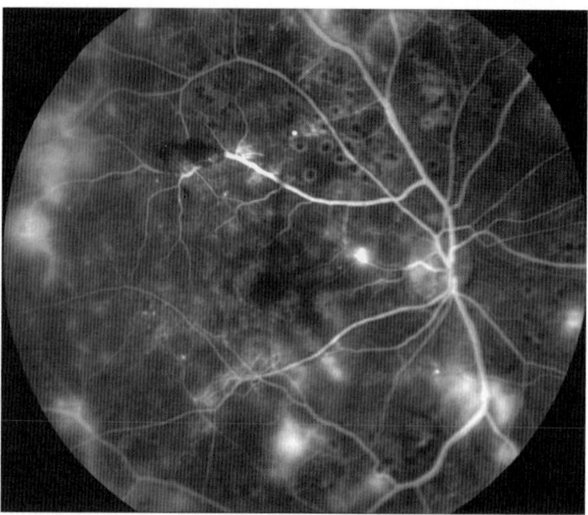

Fig. 16.21 Mid-phase frame of the fluorescein angiogram of the right eye of case 7 showing leakage from neovascularization, areas of capillary nonperfusion, and parafoveal intraretinal fluorescein leakage

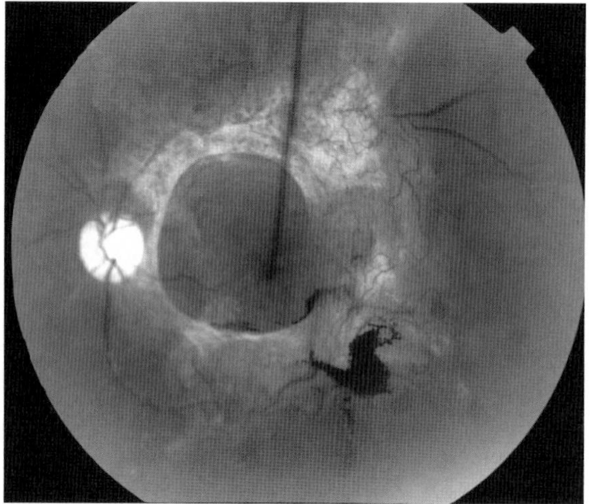

Fig. 16.20 Red-free photograph of the left eye of case 7 showing retinal neovascularization, some preretinal hemorrhage, and a ring of preretinal membranes exerting traction on the macula

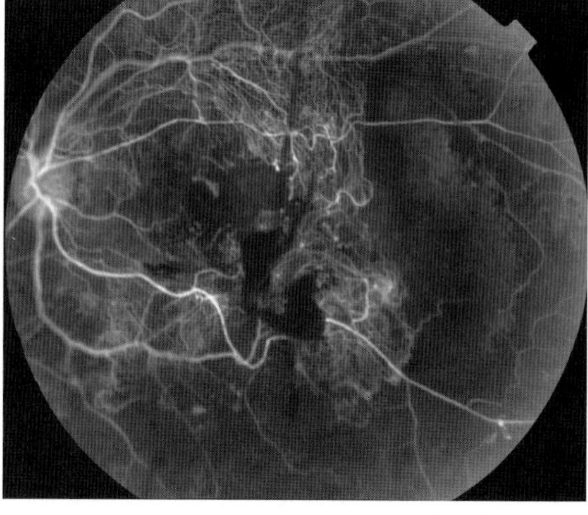

Fig. 16.22 Mid-phase frame of the fluorescein angiogram of the left eye of case 7 showing extensive areas of capillary nonperfusion in the midperiphery and an enlarged and irregularly bordered foveal avascular zone

was indicated given the good level of vision. Three reviewers thought that the neovascularization showed continued activity and that further panretinal photocoagulation (PRP) was needed, but there was considerable disagreement about how to do this. One reviewer thought that focal/grid laser should be given first for a component of diabetic macular edema, and then later that the PRP should be completed. Two reviewers thought that all of the macular thickening in the right eye was based on the epiretinal membrane (ERM). These reviewers did not think that the ERM was bad enough to recommend vitrectomy and membrane peeling. Two reviewers thought that PRP should be given alone,

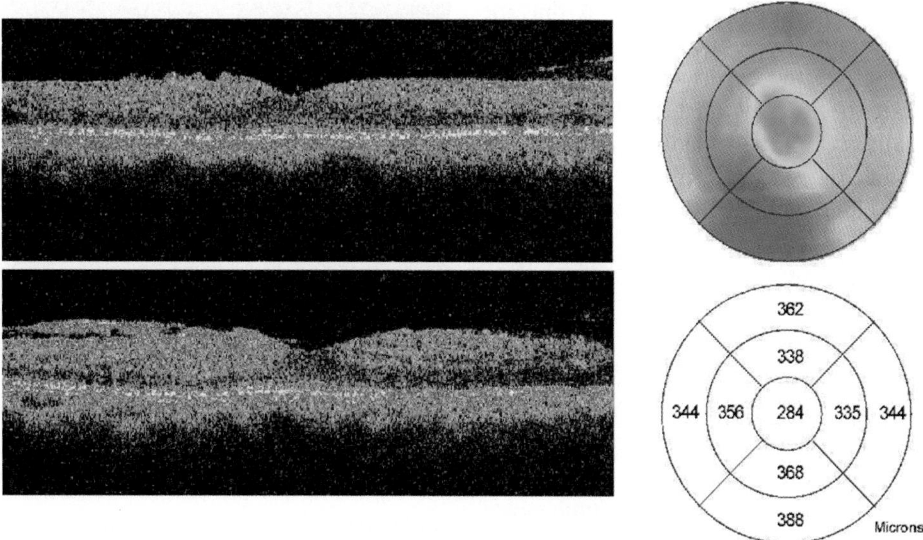

Fig. 16.23 Optical coherence tomography of the right eye of case 7 showing a macular epiretinal membrane and associated macular thickening

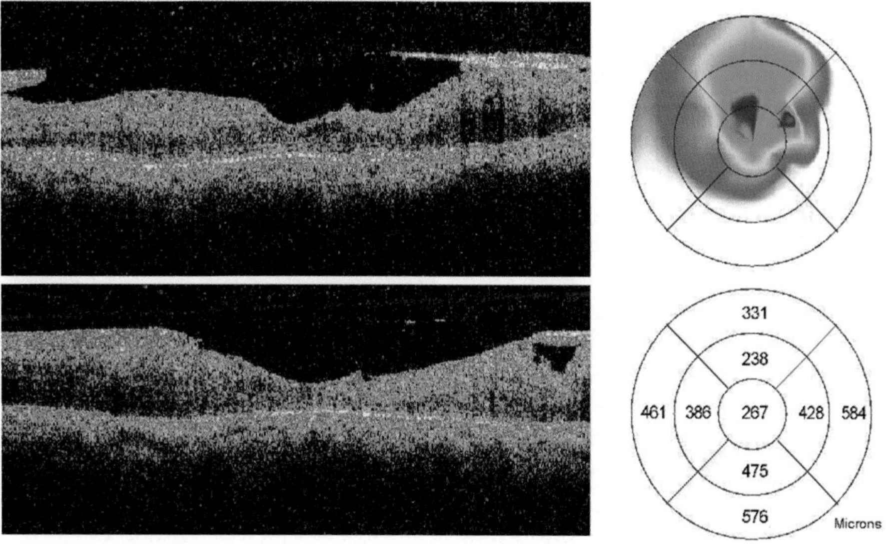

Fig. 16.24 Optical coherence tomography of the left eye of case 7 showing thick preretinal membranes and associated retinal cystic changes in the parafovea

but one favored use of pre-PRP intravitreal bevacizumab to reduce the neovascular activity rapidly. This level of disagreement in interpretation of clinical data and management is common in complicated cases of diabetic retinopathy. The point is exemplified that cases in actual practice can be ambiguous in many respects. The discussant would argue that neovascular activity in the right eye seems evident, based on the fluorescein angiogram frame, and that the need for further PRP therefore would seem to outweigh the risk that the ERM may contract and reduce vision when it is applied. Should the latter occur, prompt vitrectomy with membrane peeling should be able to remedy that eventuality. Although neovascular activity appears evident, it does not seem to be so severe as to threaten problems with hemorrhaging, thus there seems to be little reason to preface the supplemental PRP with an intravitreal bevacizumab injection, which carries a higher risk of ERM contracture than supplemental PRP alone.

For the left eye, two reviewers thought that vitrectomy was indicated to relieve the tractional component contributing to the visual loss. One of these two would preface the surgery with intravitreal bevacizumab and one would not. Neither of these two recommended further PRP before proceeding to surgery, but both would supplement the PRP at the time of surgery. Two reviewers thought that ischemia was the main cause for loss of vision in the left eye and that surgery should be deferred unless further progression to macula involving traction detachment occurred; neither of these reviewers thought that supplemental PRP to the left eye was needed. One reviewer thought that the left eye should have an intravitreal bevacizumab injection followed by completion of the PRP, but no surgery as long as the macula remained attached. Again, the diversity of opinions among experienced retina specialists is striking.

The fact that the patient presented with advanced disease suggests that follow-up is going to be a continuing concern, hence the discussant would favor completion of the PRP bilaterally to reduce the risk of subsequent vitreous hemorrhage, progressive fibrovascular proliferation with traction, and iris neovascularization. He favored no surgery of the right eye, but expected that it might be necessary if the ERM worsened later. He also favored vitrectomy surgery on the left despite the severe ischemia in hopes of removing the component of visual decline due to macular traction even though the center of the macula is not detached. Because this case was the discussant's patient that is what was done. Six months later, the visual acuities of the right and left eyes were 20/70 and 20/40, respectively. Figures 16.25 and 16.26 show the appearance of the fundi at this point.

Because of the progressive decline in vision of the right eye, vitrectomy, membrane peeling was recommended and performed. At follow-up 1 month later the visual acuity of the right eye had improved to 20/30 and the vision in the left eye had further improved to 20/30. Figure 16.27 shows the postoperative appearance of the right fundus.

Several points are illustrated. First, the assessment of visual potential based on capillary nonperfusion is fraught with error (see Chapter 8). No reviewer of this case considered that a 20/30 outcome for the left eye was possible at

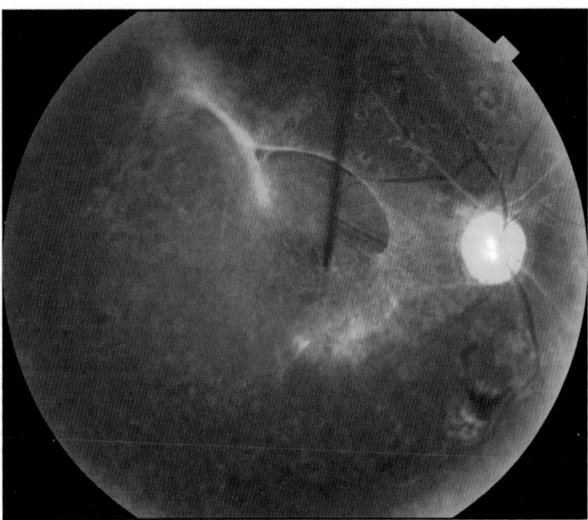

Fig. 16.25 Progressive thickening of the macular epiretinal membrane of the right eye of case 7

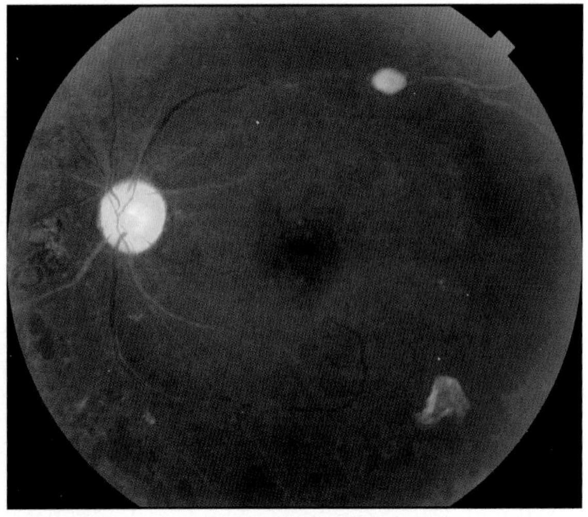

Fig. 16.26 Post-vitrectomy fundus photograph of the left eye of case 7. Release of macular traction is apparent but residual vertical retinal striae are seen

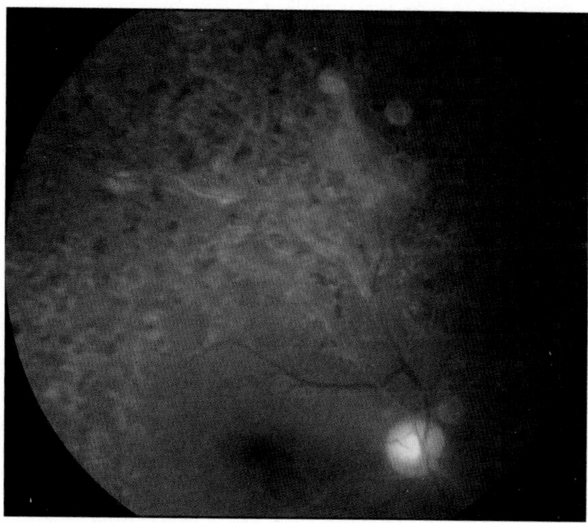

Fig. 16.27 Appearance of the right macula of case 7 after vitrectomy surgery

presentation. Second, the perception that PRP worsens contracture of fibrovascular membranes is prevalent among retina specialists, but has scant basis in peer reviewed literature.[54–56] The right eye shows worsening of an ERM temporally associated with supplemental PRP, but it cannot be said that the PRP caused the worsening. It may have occurred had PRP been withheld. It is unlikely that a clinical trial would ever be performed to determine an evidential basis for this perception. Third, the assessment of the effect of traction on visual function is also fraught with uncertainty. The center of the macula of the left eye was not detached, and several of the reviewers therefore did not consider vitrectomy surgery to be indicated, yet the case demonstrates that improvement can occur in such cases by relief of traction. Fourth, the clinical ability to judge "activity" of PDR is questionable; our reviewers were divergent in their assessments.[57] In such cases, humility and careful longitudinal follow-up to detect change may be prudent. Finally, the use of intravitreal bevacizumab as an adjunct to surgery and laser is far from standardized in 2009 as illustrated by the diversity of responses by the reviewers.[9,34,58] Greater consensus regarding proper use of this drug may evolve with continued study and especially through well-designed prospective randomized clinical trials regarding its many potential uses.[g]

16.8 Case 8: What Is Maximal Focal/Grid Laser Photocoagulation for Diabetic Macular Edema?

16.8.1 Definition of the Problem

Although it is the rule in treating diabetic macular edema (DME) that multiple treatments will be necessary over time, eventually there is no more room for focal/grid laser treatment if DME persists. In Diabetic Retinopathy Clinical Research (DRCR) Network protocols and other studies, subjective definitions of maximal focal/grid laser are used. For example, here is the definition from the ISIS-DME study: "Maximal laser treatment was defined as a point at which the investigator felt that additional laser treatment would be of no benefit based on clinical judgement and the fluorescein angiogram."[59] In DRCR Network studies, a fluorescein angiogram is not required to treat DME or to make a decision about whether maximal focal/grid laser treatment has been given. In the following cases (Figs. 16.28, 16.29, 16.30, 16.31, 16.32, 16.33, 16.34, 16.35, 16.36,

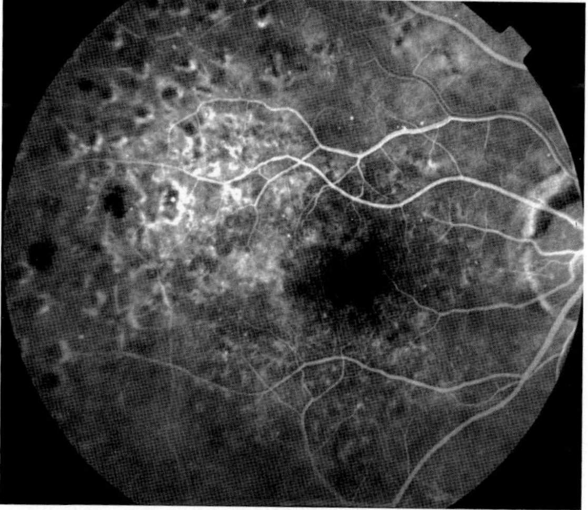

Fig. 16.28 Case 1 of 11 in a series addressing "What is maximal focal/grid laser photocoagulation?"

[g] Discussed by David J. Browning MD, PhD

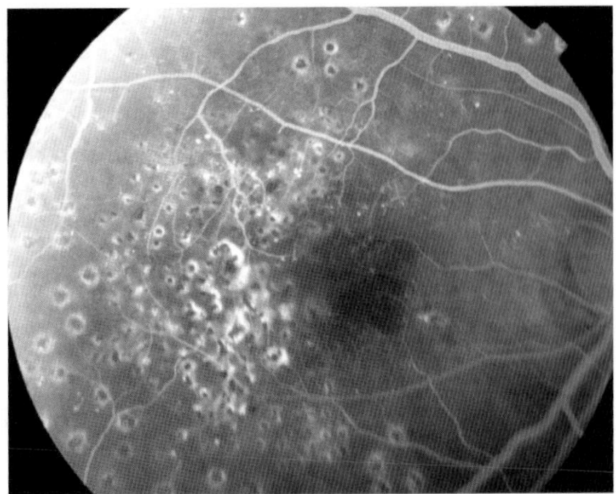

Fig. 16.29 Case 2 of 11 in a series addressing "What is maximal focal/grid laser photocoagulation?"

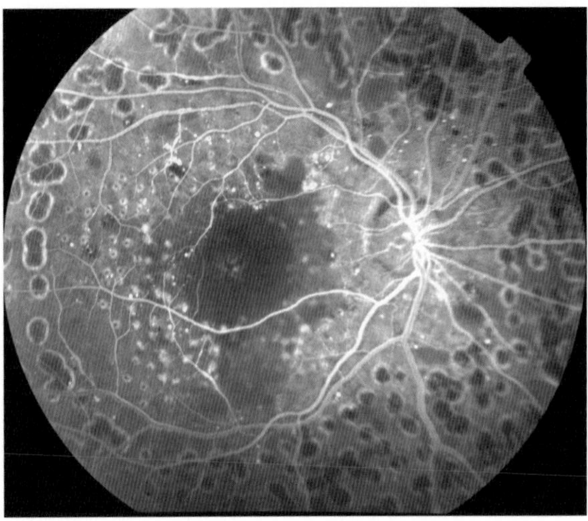

Fig. 16.31 Case 4 of 11 in a series addressing "What is maximal focal/grid laser photocoagulation?"

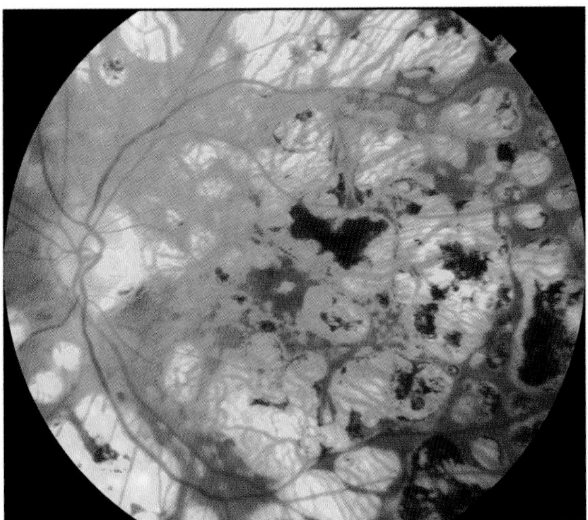

Fig. 16.30 Case 3 of 11 in a series addressing "What is maximal focal/grid laser photocoagulation?"

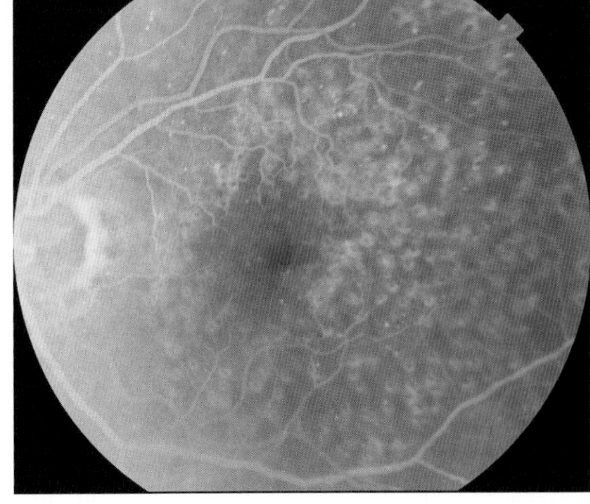

Fig. 16.32 Case 5 of 11 in a series addressing "What is maximal focal/grid laser photocoagulation?"

16.37, and 16.38), patterns of focal laser used for center-involved clinically significant macular edema (CSME) are illustrated. All cases have persistent center-involved macular edema with central subfield mean thicknesses >250 μm on OCT despite previous treatment. Which case(s) have had maximal laser treatment and, in your hands, would not be offered any further focal/grid laser photocoagulation, but instead, would be declared treatment failures to that approach and either observed or treated with alternative therapies such as intravitreal or peribulbar pharmacologic therapy or vitrectomy surgery?

16.8.2 Discussion

A better designed exercise would be to have a sample of ophthalmologists examine the same set of patients together with their customarily acquired ancillary testing, but such is not possible within the constraints of a textbook. Acknowledging the limitations of the exercise and the data presented, we think the results are interesting to consider, if only to raise the seldom discussed issue "When does

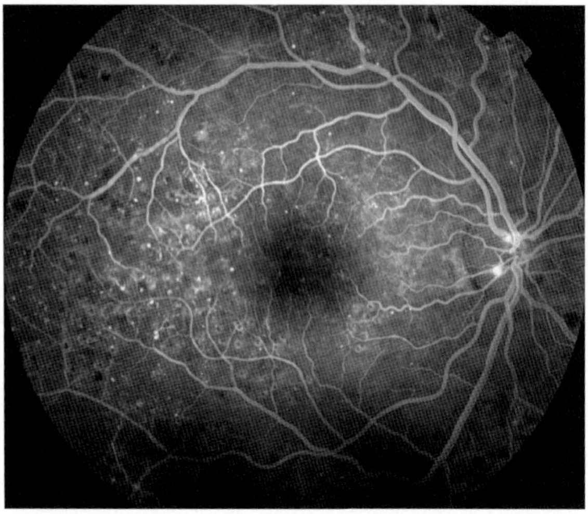

Fig. 16.33 Case 6 of 11 in a series addressing "What is maximal focal/grid laser photocoagulation?"

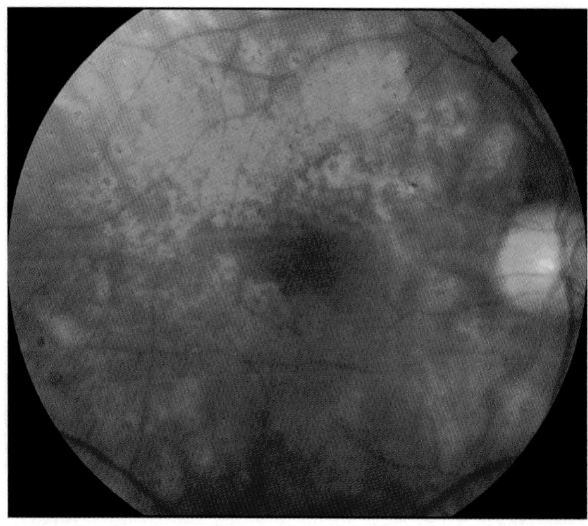

Fig. 16.35 Case 8 of 11 in a series addressing "What is maximal focal/grid laser photocoagulation?"

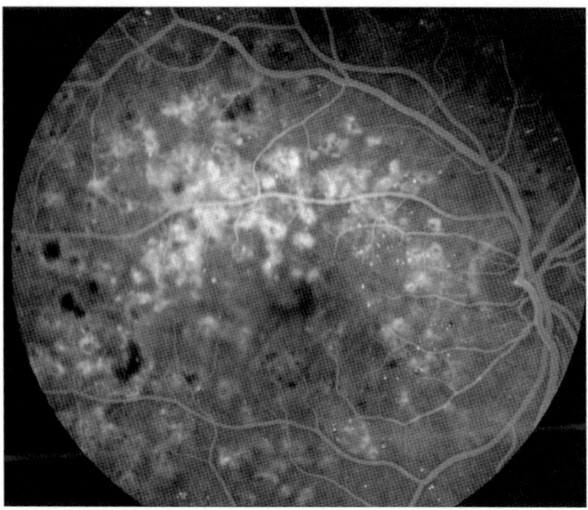

Fig. 16.34 Case 7 of 11 in a series addressing "What is maximal focal/grid laser photocoagulation?"

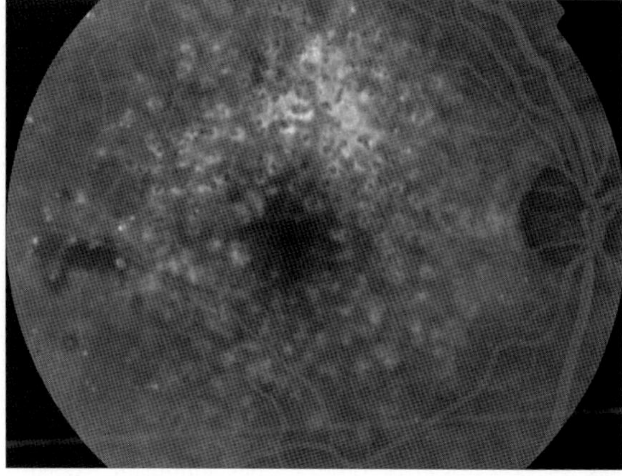

Fig. 16.36 Case 9 of 11 in a series addressing "What is maximal focal/grid laser photocoagulation?"

one stop focal/grid laser? And what is maximal treatment?" Four of the co-authors returned comments on these cases. A redaction of their responses is shown in Table 16.1. Even with the small sample size, it is apparent that clinical judgement is variable on what constitutes maximal treatment.

Doctor B was reluctant to comment on 9 of the 11 cases. He mentioned that he relies exclusively on fluorescein angiography to determine where to apply re-treatment – to focal leaking microaneurysms and ungridded areas of capillary nonperfusion – and therefore did not have as much information as he was accustomed to having to be able to respond. This was the approach outlined in the Early Treatment of Diabetic Retinopathy Study (ETDRS). In that study, "repeat fluorescein angiography was usually necessary to assess whether treatable lesions were present. All focal leaks more than 500 μm from the center of the macula were treated. Focal leaks 500 μm or less from the center of the macula were treated if the visual acuity was 20/40 or worse and if it was thought that the treatment would not destroy the remaining perifoveal capillary network. Grid

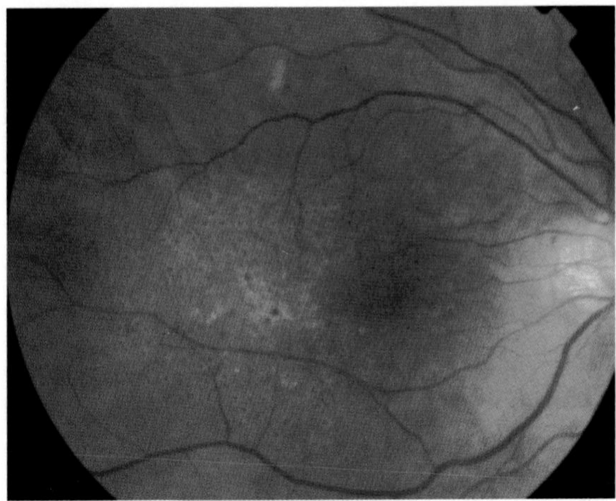

Fig. 16.37 Case 10 of 11 in a series addressing "What is maximal focal/grid laser photocoagulation?"

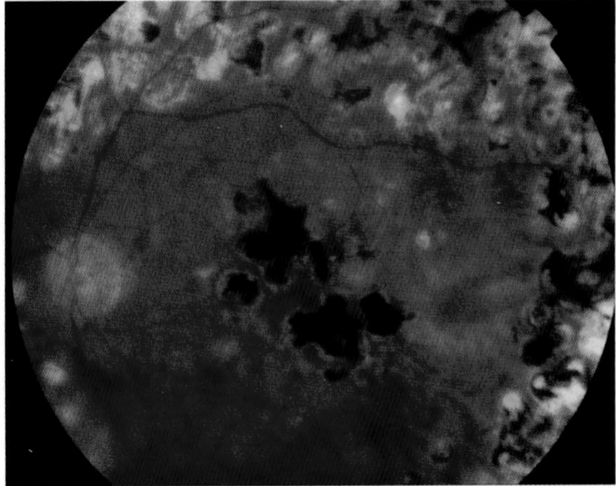

Fig. 16.38 Case 11 of 11 in a series addressing "What is maximal focal/grid laser photocoagulation?"

treatment was not usually reapplied to areas that had already been treated."[60]

Twenty years after the ETDRS, the DRCR Network reported in one of its prospective trials that 49% of cases of CSME treated with focal/grid laser underwent treatment without fluorescein angiographic guidance.[61] Internationally, the estimate is higher.[62] It is not known if outcomes are different when focal/grid laser treatment is applied with or without fluorescein angiographic guidance because a randomized clinical trial of the question has not been performed. But because previously applied laser spots may be more easily detected from fluorescein angiography than from ophthalmoscopy alone, it is possible that decisions on maximal versus submaximal treatment depend on whether the ophthalmologist obtains the angiogram to inform his judgement.[63] The point in this context is that variable use of fluorescein angiography may add to the variability among ophthalmologists in what constitutes maximal focal/grid laser.

Other pertinent comments to the question of maximal focal/grid laser were made. Three of four ophthalmologists remarked that cases 3 and 11 had received too much focal/grid laser – that is, above maximal. These cases were treated 20 years previously and demonstrate not only laser spots applied too close together and too intensely, but also the probable effects of laser scar expansion over 20 years.[64] One ophthalmologist commented that he would not treat the thickened but nonperfused area of case 4. In the ETDRS, thickened but nonperfused areas of the macula up to 2 disk diameters from the center of the macula were treated

Table 16.1 Four retina specialists' assessments of the completeness of focal/grid laser treatment in 11 exemplary cases of diabetic macular edema

Case	Doctor A	Doctor B	Doctor C	Doctor D
1	Submaximal		Submaximal	Submaximal
2	Maximal		Submaximal	Submaximal
3	Maximal		Maximal	Maximal
4	Maximal	Submaximal	Maximal	Submaximal
5	Submaximal		Submaximal	Submaximal
6	Submaximal	Submaximal	Submaximal	Submaximal
7	Submaximal		Submaximal	Submaximal
8	Submaximal		Submaximal	Submaximal
9	Submaximal		Maximal	Maximal
10	Submaximal		Maximal	Submaximal
11	Maximal		Maximal	Maximal

with the grid part of focal/grid photocoagulation, but there is a perspective that such ischemic zones need not be treated with grid laser.[60] This point of view may derive from a study on edema associated with perfused versus nonperfused branch retinal vein occlusion in which nonperfused zones of edema resolved spontaneously.[65] Although DME and macular edema in BRVO may be quite different, the extrapolation in treatment philosophy seems to exist among a subgroup of ophthalmologists.

Even if one strictly adheres to ETDRS style focal/grid treatment technique, it is apparent that considerable subjectivity creeps into the process. For example, the ETDRS protocol explicitly omits guidelines on treating microaneurysms involving the perifoveal capillary network, and there is wide variation in reading center grading of what constitutes focal versus diffuse leakage on the fluorescein angiogram (and hence where to apply focal laser).[60,66] Variation among clinician interpreters of fluorescein angiograms – and thus where they do and do not treat focally – is likely even greater than the variation of professional reading center graders.

In an era of multiple treatment approaches for DME, it is becoming less common to see examples like cases 3 and 11. Rather, futility of focal/grid is often declared after 1–2 treatments if DME persists, and a pharmacologic or surgical approach is taken instead. Nevertheless, focal/grid laser is a superior treatment to serial intravitreal triamcinolone injections, and until a randomized trial shows that some other treatment approach is better, the question of what constitutes maximal focal/grid laser treatment remains important, problematic, and topical for further study.[48,h]

16.9 Case 9: What Independent Information Does Macular Perfusion Add to Patient Management in Diabetic Retinopathy?

The AAO preferred practice pattern on Diabetic Retinopathy states that fluorescein angiography is "usually" useful to evaluate unexplained visual loss.[67] Clinicians widely embrace this perspective and look at fluorescein angiograms to assess macular ischemia. Yet the variability of these assessments is unknown. The presumption is that there is enough correlation between the clinician's interpretation of macular ischemia and levels of visual acuity that the test could be informative for patient care.

Consider the following case in this vein. The patient has had type 1 diabetes for 25 years and has previously had focal/grid laser for diabetic macular edema and panretinal photocoagulation for proliferative diabetic retinopathy. The OCT and FA are shown (CSMT = 262 μm) (Figs. 16.39 and 16.40). What are the bounds on your estimate of the visual acuity based on your interpretation of the macular perfusion?

16.9.1 Discussion

The four reviewers of this case were unanimous in stating their uncertainty in utilizing fluorescein angiography to predict current visual acuity. In spite of this uncertainty the predicted visual acuities were consistent with three reviewers predicting

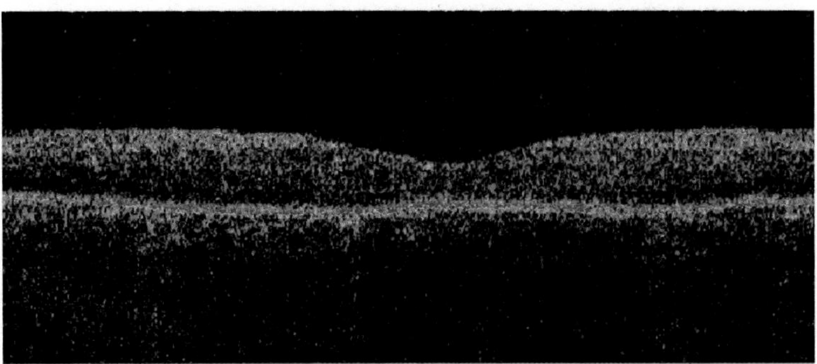

Fig. 16.39 OCT radial line scan through the fovea

[h] Discussed by David J. Browning MD, PhD

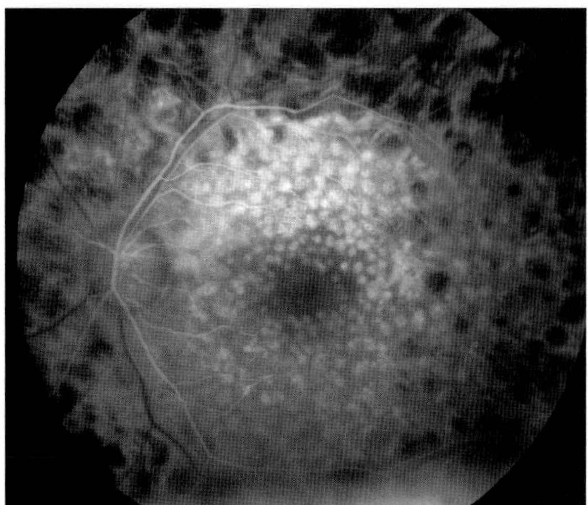

Fig. 16.40 Frame from the early venous phase of the fluorescein angiogram showing the degree of macular perfusion in an eye that has previously had both focal/grid and panretinal photocoagulation for macular edema and proliferative retinopathy, respectively

20/40 visual acuity and one reviewer predicting 20/50 visual acuity. This consistency is interesting in light of the patient's tested visual acuity of 20/200. Why were all of the reviewers so uniformly off base?

One reviewer pointed out that this case exercise reverses our traditional path of obtaining information from the patient in which a medical history (which includes duration of diabetes and history of blood sugar control) precedes an examination (which includes obtaining a visual acuity) which precedes ancillary testing (optional). The discussant believes that the consistency of the reviewers' predictions is based on the current widespread use of OCT ancillary testing in preference to fluorescein angiography. OCT technology first became available for clinical practice in 2002. Prior to availability of OCT technology the gold standard for managing diabetic macular edema was based on the Early Treatment Diabetic Retinopathy Study. Color photography and fluorescein angiography were protocol ancillary tests in the Early Treatment Diabetic Retinopathy Study and protocol administration of laser therapy was based on fluorescein angiographic guidance. In 1991 the American Academy of Ophthalmology established Diabetes 2000 as a concerted educational effort to "reduce – and possibly eliminate – preventable blindness from diabetes by the year 2000." [68] As a consequence it is not surprising that in the 1990s fluorescein angiography was utilized in clinical practice in nearly 100% of cases to manage diabetic macular edema.

In current clinical practice for management of diabetic macular edema, OCT has supplanted fluorescein angiography in its usage rate. In 2007 a DRCR.net clinical trial to investigate the effect of intravitreal bevacizumab on diabetic macular edema protocol OCTs was obtained routinely. In this setting of mandated OCT testing, the optional usage rate for obtaining fluorescein angiography was 51%.[64] In the management of diabetic macular edema this shift in usage from fluorescein angiography to OCT may be due to the reliability and reproducibility of OCT in directly measuring macular edema. In comparison, ischemia, leakage, and RPE abnormalities as assessed by fluorescein angiography have at best a variable correlation with macular edema. The reproducibility of fluorescein angiography to measure macular ischemia is variable even when angiography is performed in academic centers.[69]

Even though OCT-measured macular thickness correlates modestly with visual acuity the discussant believes that the trend for clinicians to utilize OCT preferentially over fluorescein angiography in managing diabetic macular edema leads to a bias to predict visual acuity preferentially based on OCT data.[69] The nearly normal foveal anatomy in this case probably explains the nearly normal visual acuity predicted by the four respondents.

When challenged to predict visual acuity based on macular perfusion two respondents used OCT data to help interpret the fluorescein angiogram. They suggested that the lack OCT thinning implies the lack of significant macular ischemia. These views highlight the reliance on OCT and the difficulty with subsequent lack of confidence in quantifying macular ischemia on fluorescein angiography.

The AAO preferred practice pattern in 2008 indicates that ancillary tests such as color fundus photography, optical coherence tomography, and fluorescein angiography may enhance patient care.[67] The "appropriate" role of ancillary testing in this case was touched upon by two respondents with distinctly different viewpoints. One respondent used fluorescein angiography only to guide location of laser therapy but not to prognosticate response. The ETDRS supports this approach with published guidelines to support the use of fluorescein angiography in guiding treatment but published guidelines to direct retreatment are not publicized.[70] A second respondent believed that fluorescein angiography-determined enlargement of the foveal avascular zone carries a poorer prognosis in managing diabetic macular edema and that this information is helpful in counseling patients. Although intuitively logical such subclassification of diabetic macular edema based on degree of macular ischemia has not been demonstrated to enhance patient care by allowing advice on a differential natural history or differential response to therapy.[71]

The discussant believes that the approach of the second respondent reflects a fundamental change in our current clinical expectations in managing diabetic macular edema. The Early Treatment Diabetic Retinopathy Study defined clinically significant macular edema as the indication to benefit from focal/grid laser. The demonstrated benefit of that treatment was to decrease the risk of developing moderate visual loss (defined as loss of 15 or more letters between baseline and follow-up visit). Reports with intravitreal triamcinolone, intravitreal anti-VEGF agents, and focal/grid laser photocoagulation demonstrate that visual improvement is not uncommon following treatment of diabetic macular edema.[72,73,48] When patients currently demonstrate visual loss following therapy for diabetic macular edema clinicians tend not to counsel patients that "their vision would have been even worse had treatment not been done" but instead to search for alternative therapies to reverse the decline. The discussant believes that in managing diabetic macular edema we are in a current era where loss of vision is considered a "failure" of therapy and that improvement in vision may not be an unreasonable hope.[i]

16.10 Case 10: Macular Edema Following Panretinal Photocoagulation for Proliferative Diabetic Retinopathy

A 72-year-old man with diabetes of 22 years duration had focal/grid laser photocoagulation for diabetic macular edema with regression bilaterally. His best corrected visual acuity was R – 20/63, L – 20/25. On regular follow-up he was found to have small areas of neovascularization elsewhere (NVE) without preretinal hemorrhage in each eye. He underwent panretinal photocoagulation (PRP) of the right eye and called in to report blurring 2 weeks later. He wanted to put on hold the scheduled panretinal photocoagulation of the left eye. Examination revealed vision of R – 20/63, L – 20/25. The maculas were clinically unchanged and without thickening, but the pre-PRP and post-PRP Optical Coherence Tomograms (OCT) are shown in Fig. 16.41. How would you manage this patient?

16.10.1 Discussion

This case demonstrates the importance of listening to the patient who notes vision loss even though Snellen visual acuity remains unchanged. The OCT showed recurrent macular thickening following the PRP laser, which is a known complication of this treatment.[31,74,75] OCT often detects macular edema not seen clinically, and macular edema fluctuations can cause symptoms without diminution of visual acuity.[76]

There are several reasonable management options for the right eye. One is to simply observe the eye as the edema may resolve. If the patient is sufficiently distressed that an intervention is deemed necessary, the least invasive treatment option would be a trial of topical steroidal or nonsteroidal drugs, an approach advocated by one of the five physicians who reviewed this case. There is no published evidence to support topical therapy in post-PRP recurrence of DME, but there is a biological rationale, assuming that the recurrence is based on inflammation and that the drugs can penetrate to the posterior segment. Other reasonable options would include periocular or intravitreal triamcinolone injection or intravitreal bevacizumab injection.[77,64] Periocular triamcinolone injection might be more effective than topical therapy and would be associated with a 10% risk of intraocular pressure elevation and 10% risk of ptosis.[77] Intravitreal triamcinolone would probably be more effective in

[i] Discussed by Keye Wong MD

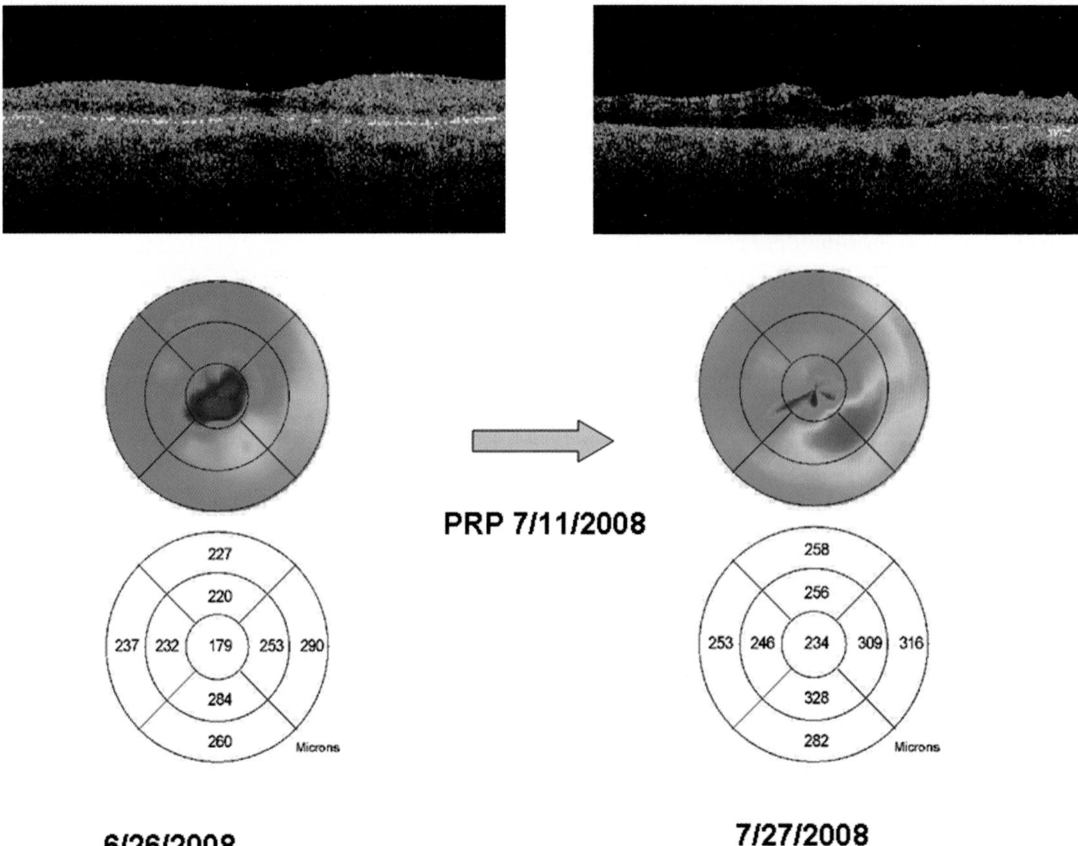

Fig. 16.41 The pre-PRP and post-PRP OCTs are shown on the *left* and *right* sides of the figure, respectively. Recurrence of diabetic macular edema after PRP is shown

reducing the edema, although with an increased risk of intraocular pressure elevation and cataract formation and the additional risk of vitreous hemorrhage, hypotony, and endophthalmitis.[72,78–81] An intravitreal injection of bevacizumab could be considered, although several reviewers thought that it is less effective than triamcinolone in such a circumstance.[82] A fluorescein angiogram might be useful; if there were angiographic evidence of worsening focal retinopathy with untreated microaneurysms then adding focal photocoagulation would be reasonable assuming maximal photocoagulation had not already been applied.

For the left eye, there is no rush to treat based on the non-high-risk characteristics of the NVE, and respect for the patient's reluctance to proceed suggests that observation for a period until the right eye stabilizes would be prudent. Ideally, the patient was told before the right eye PRP that his vision might be worse after laser, which now makes it easier to explain that this blurring will likely resolve over time with observation or with one of the treatments outlined previously. Once the right eye has improved or stabilized, then treatment of the left eye might be encouraged, but perhaps preceded by a peribulbar triamcinolone injection to reduce the chance of post-PRP DME. The PRP laser treatment might be split into small sessions to prevent reactive edema, although in an eye with no edema, there is evidence that multiple session and single session PRP are associated with similar rates of post-PRP DME.[83] An alternative acceptable plan would be continued deferral of PRP with close serial observation until high-risk characteristics were reached.[j]

[j] Discussed by David G. Telander MD, PhD

16.11 Case 11: Diabetic Macular Edema with a Subfoveal Scar

A 65-year-old woman with type 2 diabetes and hypertension for 15 years sees you with a complaint of bilateral blurred vision for 2 years. Her best corrected visual acuity bilaterally is 20/200. She is bilaterally phakic with 2+ nuclear sclerotic cataracts. She is an immigrant to the United States and has had no previous ophthalmic care. The left eye is shown (Figs. 16.42 and 16.43); the right eye is similar. How would you manage the paracentral DME in the presence of the subfoveal scar?

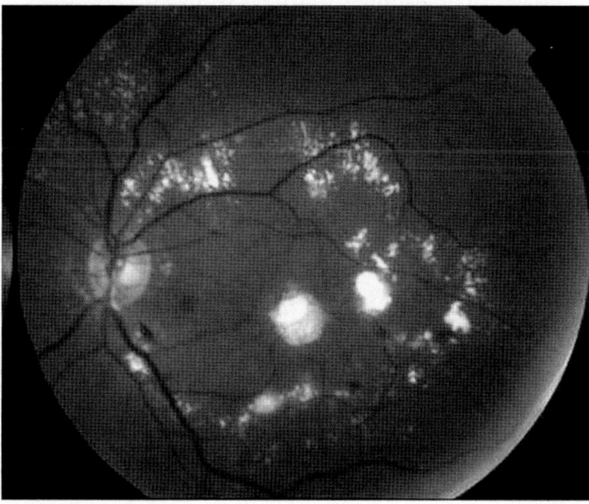

Fig. 16.42 The left eye has a subfoveal scar with surrounding macular edema

16.11.1 Discussion

The patient described has had a devastating consequence of neglected DME with dense central macular exudates evolving into subfoveal fibrosis. There is no proven treatment to prevent this complication after exudates have collected in the subfoveal space. In fact, some have proposed surgical removal of these exudates to prevent this type of scarring.[84] The patient should be educated regarding her guarded prognosis and referred for low vision counseling and services.

The goal of treatment at this point is to limit the extent of perifoveal DME and attempt to reduce the size of her central scotoma. The Early Treatment Diabetic Retinopathy Study showed that treatment of DME by focal/grid laser decreased the risk of moderate vision loss, but cases such as this were not addressed in that study. Additional macular laser may further degrade this patient's macular visual field. Recent reports from the Diabetic Retinopathy Clinical Research Network revealed that focal laser was more effective in preventing vision loss than serial injections of intravitreal triamcinolone for clinically significant macular edema, but patients such as this with subfoveal scarring were not included in the study.[47,85] This patient is phakic, making the use of intravitreal triamcinolone with its cataractogenic side effect less attractive. Anti-vascular endothelial growth factor (VEGF) therapy has demonstrated efficacy in patients with diabetic macular edema and lacks the side effect of cataract progression.[86–90] Therefore, in this case intravitreal anti-VEGF (e.g., bevacizumab) therapy may be the first step and if the edema proved to be recurrent, then combination therapy with bevacizumab plus focal/grid laser could be recommended.[k]

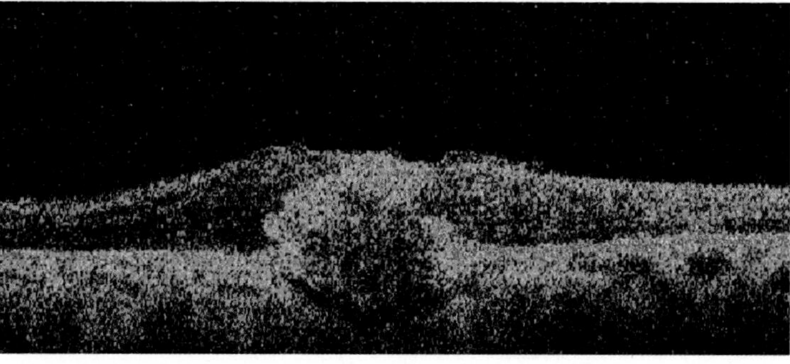

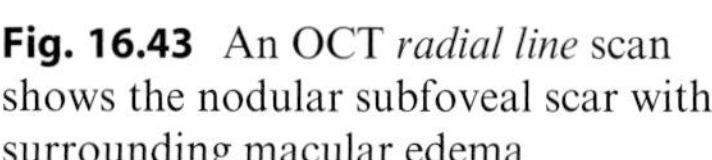

Fig. 16.43 An OCT *radial line* scan shows the nodular subfoveal scar with surrounding macular edema

[k] Discussant: David G. Telander MD, PhD

16.12 Case 12: How Does the Severity of Diabetic Macular Edema Affect the Therapeutic Approach?

16.12.1 Definition of the Problem

As a wide variety of treatment options exist for the treatment of diabetic macular edema (DME), consideration may be given to altering the therapeutic approach based on the severity of the edema. Although macular photocoagulation has withstood the test of time in the form of focal/grid laser treatment, intravitreal injection of triamcinolone acetonide (IVT) and bevacizumab (IVB) has gained popularity.[29,48,91] In the following cases (Figs. 16.44, 16.45, 16.46, 16.47, 16.48, and 16.49), a range of DME severity is presented. All examples are from patients with type 2 diabetes with ages ranging from 45 to 60 years. None have been treated previously. How should each case be managed?

Case 1:

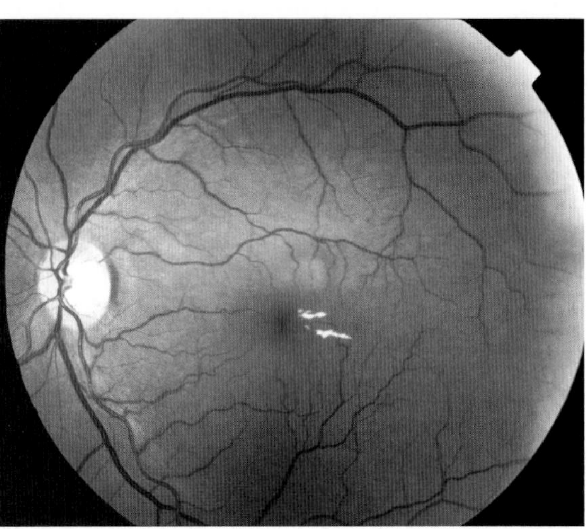

Fig. 16.44 Red-free fundus photograph of the left eye of case 1. A circinate lipid ring surrounding a few microaneurysms is present temporal to the center of the macula

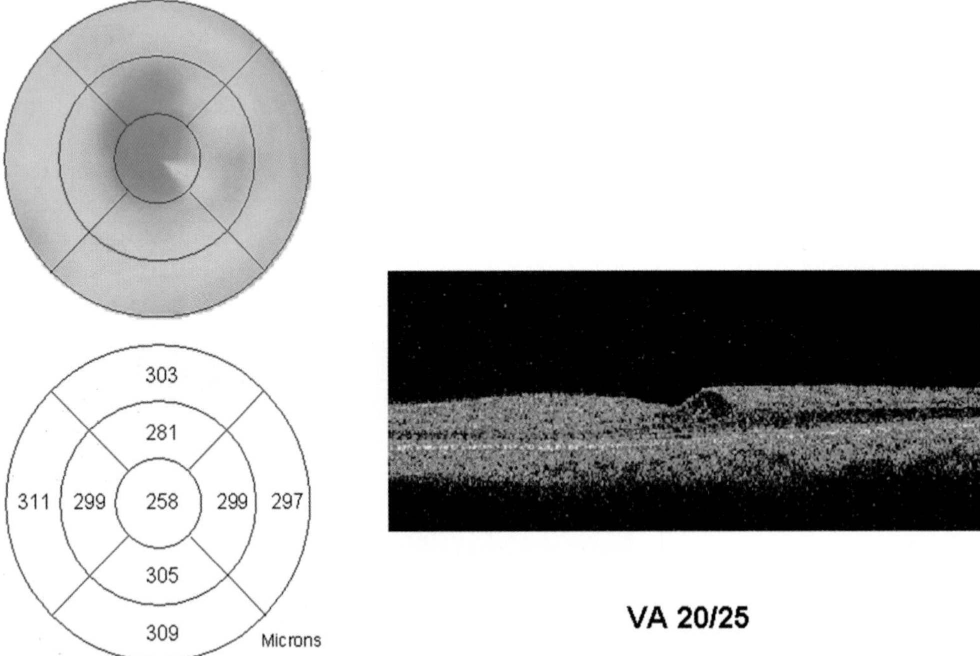

Fig. 16.45 Optical coherence tomogram of the left eye of case 1. An intraretinal cyst is present on the temporal edge of the foveal depression

Case2:

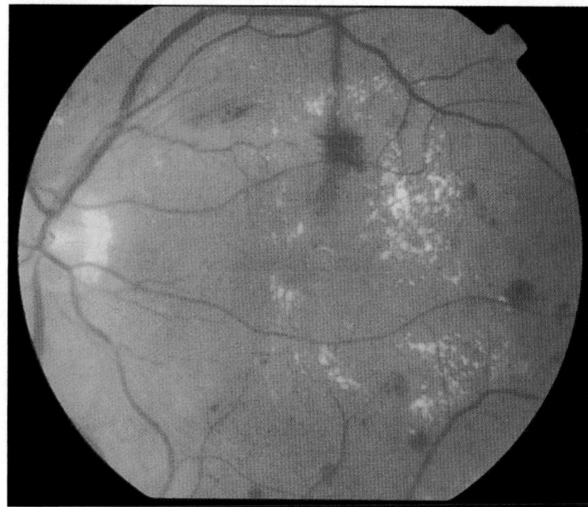

Fig. 16.46 Color fundus photograph of the left eye of case 2. Dot hemorrhages, microaneurysms, and lipid exudate rings that overlap at the center of the macula are seen

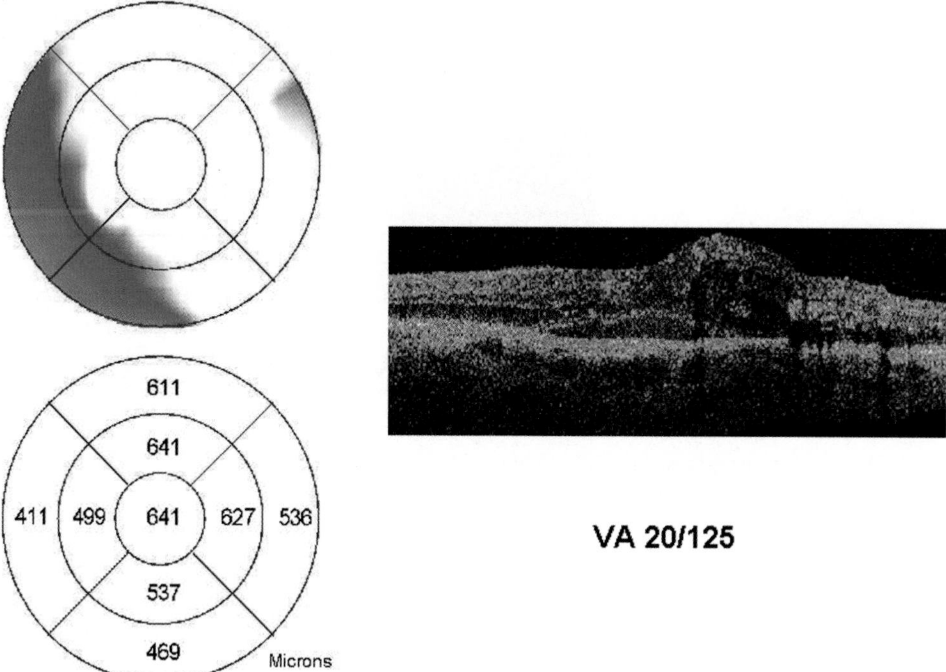

Fig. 16.47 Optical coherence tomogram of the left eye of case 2. The entire macula is thickened with the thickest point in the center of the macula

Case 3:

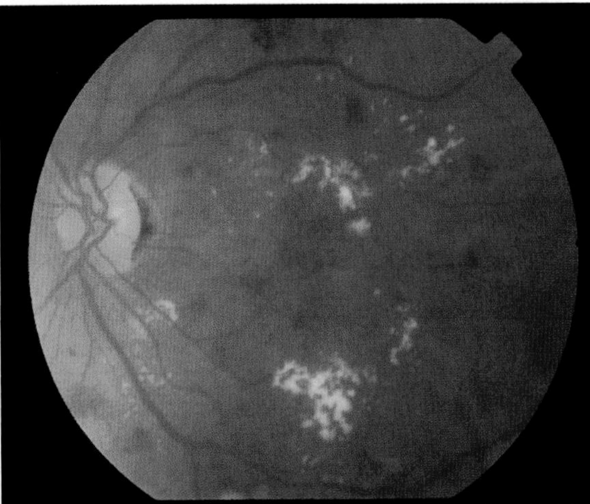

Fig. 16.48 Color fundus photograph of the left eye of case 3. Many dot hemorrhages, microaneurysms, and a lipid exudate ring that surrounds the center of the macula are seen

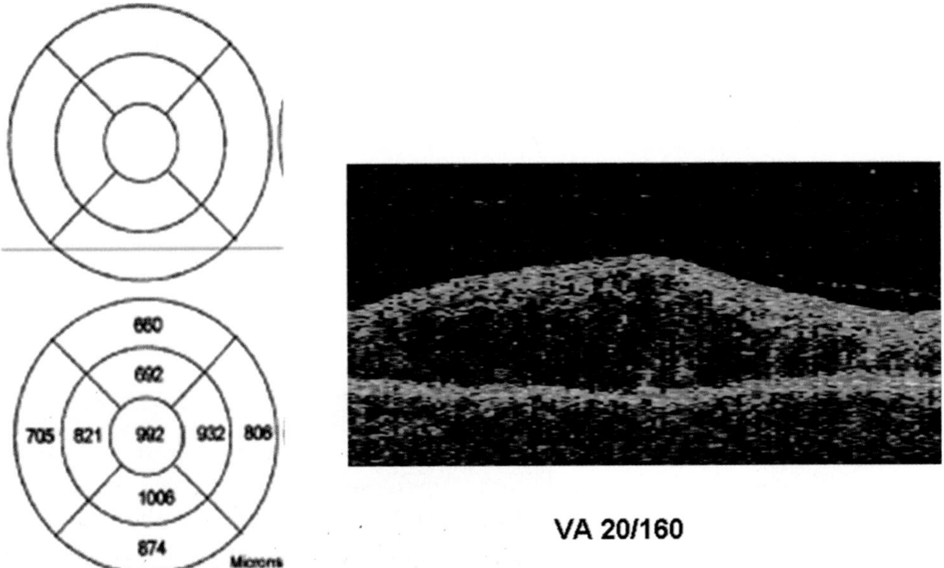

Fig. 16.49 Optical coherence tomogram of the left eye of case 3. The entire macula is massively thickened with the thickest point in the center of the macula

16.12.2 Discussion

The clinical management of diabetic macular edema requires the application of an extensive body of knowledge with the understanding that this information is incomplete. Therefore, it is not surprising that there are differences of opinion in treatment recommendations. Table 16.2 summarizes the opinions of four authors of this book. No additional clinical information was provided, which may have altered the responses. For example, several doctors indicated they obtain fluorescein angiograms to

Table 16.2 Opinions of three retina specialists on the best approach to three cases of diabetic macular edema of differing severity

Case	Doctor A	Doctor B	Doctor C	Doctor D
1	Focal	Focal	Observe vs. focal	Focal/grid
2	Grid	Focal → (4 months) add focal ± IVB/IVT	Focal/grid ± IVB/IVT	IVT and focal/grid
3	IVB → IVT (if no response to IVB)	Focal → (4 months) add focal ± IVB/IVT	Focal/grid ± IVB/IVT	IVT and focal/grid

IVB = Intravitreal bevacizumab, IVT = Intravitreal triamcinolone acetonide

detect capillary nonperfusion and to guide laser treatment. As the individual responses were elicited in a masked fashion, there was no discussion among the participants. Such discussion frequently results in less divergence of opinion, especially as assumptions regarding the clinical presentation are revealed.

CASE 1: In the case of limited macular edema and exudates within 500 μm from the foveal center with fairly good visual acuity, there was general agreement to employ macular photocoagulation. Given the lack of stereoscopic fundus photographic demonstration of retinal thickening, the doctors made the assumption that clinically significant macular edema was present in this case. However, macular edema detected by optical coherence tomography does not equate with clinically significant macular edema.[92] The central subfield macular thickness in this case was greater than 250 μm and, therefore, would have qualified for treatment in the Diabetic Retinopathy Clinical Research Network study.[48] Doctor C offered the option of initial observation with a review of the general medical status of the patient. It may have been assumed by the others that the issue of managing the metabolic syndrome had already been undertaken. Doctor C was also reluctant to risk the creation of paracentral scotomata with laser in an eye with 20/25 vision. If the patient was symptomatic from macular edema, Doctor C recommended very light treatment sparing the FAZ in an effort to avoid adverse effects. Doctor B anticipated the need for treatment close to the fovea and, therefore, recommended warning the patient of post-laser blind spots. None of the respondents recommended IVT or IVB for this case. In the literature there appears to be a similar impression that focal DME may not require adjunctive therapy.[93–95]

CASE 2: In the case of extensive macular edema with profound central macular thickening (OCT central subfield macular thickness = 641 μm) and visual acuity of 20/125, there was unanimous agreement to apply focal or grid macular photocoagulation. This agreement is consistent with the findings of the Early Treatment Diabetic Retinopathy Study (ETDRS) and the Diabetic Retinopathy Clinical Research Network (DRCR.net) reports.[29,48] The recommendations regarding the adjunctive use of intravitreal injections covered the spectrum of options. Doctor A did not recommend the use of IVB or IVT. Doctor C considered the adjunctive use of IVT/IVB at the initial treatment session in order to speed the recovery of vision, depending on patient preference and need. There is support for this approach in the literature; however, the advantages of speeding the recovery of vision need to be balanced by the well-known adverse effects of therapeutic intravitreal injection.[91,96,48] Doctor B recommended the use of IVB/IVT along with additional laser if persistent macular thickening remained four months following initial meticulous focal laser guided by fluorescein angiography. This approach suggests a step-up in therapy based on an unsatisfactory response to initial laser treatment. The results of the DRCR.net suggest that this patient likely would require more than one laser treatment in order to resolve the edema.[48] Doctor D routinely performs IVT 1–2 weeks prior to modified grid laser. Prelaser IVT may decrease short-term inflammation/edema from laser and may be of value in reducing the amount of laser energy required for macular photocoagulation via IVT-induced thinning of the macula.[97,98] Doctor C expressed concern about the possibility of permanent central visual loss from inspissation of exudates into the fovea following resolution of the macular edema. Therapy of existing foveal plaques and exudates appears to be of limited benefit.[99,100] Therefore, the possibility of prevention is appealing. Rapid resolution of exudates has been reported following IVT.[101] In addition, the anti-fibrotic effects of triamcinolone acetonide make it an interesting potential therapeutic agent in an attempt to prevent retinal pigment epithelial metaplasia in eyes threatened with foveal exudates.[102]

CASE 3: In the case of extreme macular thickening (OCT central subfield thickness = 992 μm) and 20/160 visual acuity, the management recommendations of most of the doctors mirrored their responses to case 2. However, doctor A diverged from the use of laser in this severe case of DME, preferring the use of IVB/IVT. The literature supports the notion that poor visual acuity from DME is prognostic of poor visual outcome despite intervention with laser.[103] Thus, it is not surprising that a more aggressive therapeutic stance may be taken in such cases. In the short term, IVB/IVT does appear to have a more rapid onset of effect compared with macular laser.[96,48] However, the long-term effect of persistent focal/grid macular laser was shown to be superior to IVT by the DRCR.net.[48] Randomized controlled trials are needed to better define the role of adjunctive use of IVB and IVT.[1]

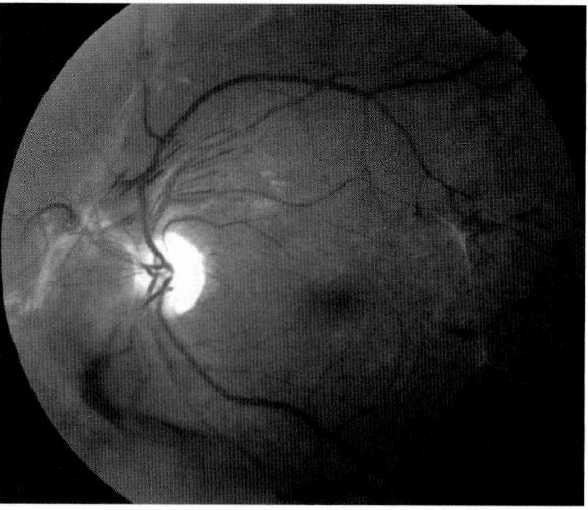

Fig. 16.50 Red-free photograph of the left eye of case 13. Disk neovascularization, vitreous hemorrhage, a macular epiretinal membrane, and traction by a membrane on the nasal disk margin are seen

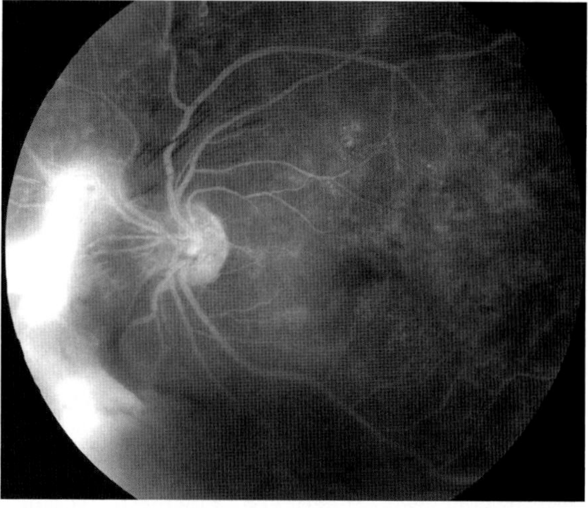

Fig. 16.51 Mid-phase frame from the fluorescein angiogram of the left eye of case 13. Hyperfluorescent leakage from the disk neovascularization, parafoveal intraretinal hyperfluorescence, and temporal midperipheral capillary nonperfusion are seen

16.13 Case 13: Management Options for a Complicated Case of Proliferative Diabetic Retinopathy with Severe Fibrovascular Proliferation, Sub-clinical Macular Edema, and Recent Vitreous Hemorrhage

16.13.1 Definition of the Problem

A 48-year-old female with type 1 diabetes mellitus of 30 years duration has previously undergone panretinal photocoagulation (PRP) with a total of 1,241 spots for proliferative diabetic retinopathy (PDR) and vitreous hemorrhage involving the left eye 6 weeks ago. Presently, she is phakic and her visual acuity is 20/20 OD and 20/30 OS. Her vitreous hemorrhage has cleared somewhat and her fundus photograph (Fig. 16.50), fluorescein angiogram (Fig. 16.51), and optical coherence tomogram (Fig. 16.52) are shown. What management recommendations would you have for this eye?

[1]Discussed by Scott E. Pautler, M.D.

16.13.2 Discussion

This patient has severe fibrovascular proliferation with vitreous hemorrhage from PDR accompanied by diabetic macular edema (DME). All of the chapter authors who reviewed this case recommended additional PRP. Although this patient has already received a PRP laser of 1,241 spots,

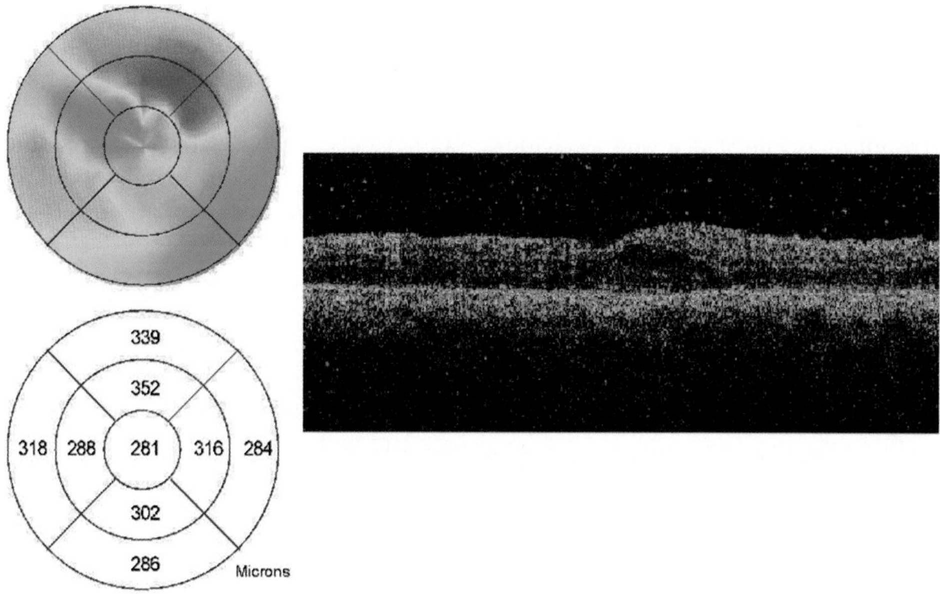

Fig. 16.52 Optical coherence tomogram of the left eye of case 13. Temporal macular thickening is seen

the details of the laser procedure were not given. If a wide-angle contact lens was used with a laser setting of 200 μm, this laser treatment does not equate to Early Treatment Diabetic Retinopathy Study (ETDRS) PRP. In the ETDRS, 1,200–1,600 laser burns were usually applied using a 500 μm laser setting with a Goldmann 3-mirror lens.[104] An equivalent PRP treatment using a 200 μm laser setting with a wide-angle lens (e.g., Volk H-R Wide Field, Volk SuperQuad 160, or Ocular Instruments Mainster PRP 165) would require approximately 3,000 laser spots (see Table 9.6). Moreover, there are proponents for the application of PRP exceeding ETDRS guidelines in cases of severe PDR.[105,106] As this case possesses high-risk features for visual loss in PDR, such as severe fibrovascular proliferation with vitreous hemorrhage and DME in a patient with type 1 diabetes, a complete 360 degree PRP extending anterior to the equator may be in order.[107–110] Finally, the literature supports the prompt completion of PRP in this case given the presence of high-risk features.[104]

This case is complicated by the presence of diabetic macular edema and preretinal membrane formation with central subfield macular thickness (CSMT) of 281 μm. The chapter authors who reviewed this case expressed concern about the potential for exacerbation of DME by additional laser and were generally inclined to offer adjunctive intravitreal pharmacotherapy.[111,102] There was divided opinion on the use of IVT vs. IVB. One group preferred IVB to avoid the risk of steroid-induced cataract and glaucoma.[102] Those who preferred IVT wished to avoid IVB-induced vitreoretinal traction retinal detachment.[112] Although there are no evidence-based guidelines at this time, there is support in the literature for the efficacy of both IVB and IVT in reducing DME in the short term.[102,112] Macular laser should be considered for long-term control of DME.[29,48]

The presence of severe fibrovascular proliferation (FVP) and preretinal membrane formation in this case places the retina at risk for traction retinal detachment. The fundus photograph (Fig. 16.51) shows early evidence of preretinal traction in the way of mild macular heterotopia with inferior macular dragging, though no history of metamorphopsia or diplopia was given. The presence of severe FVP prompted one group of doctors to avoid the use of IVB for DME. However, it appears that progressive traction retinal detachment may occur in PDR following IVB, PRP, or in the natural history of PDR.[113,114,112,110] Although there is reason to believe that the anti-fibrotic effects of triamcinolone acetonide may mitigate this risk, there is no definitive evidence to date.[102]

Given the seriousness of the retinopathy in this patient, extensive pretreatment counseling is essential. With or without treatment this eye is at risk of visual loss. The patient should understand that extensive laser treatment is anticipated and vitrectomy surgery may be needed in an effort to preserve vision. The alternatives, risks, benefits, and limitations of treatment are routinely reviewed. Finally, clear information on the benefits of optimal management of systemic disease is given to the patient.[m,115,116]

16.14 Case 14: How Is Diabetic Macular Ischemia Related to Visual Acuity?

16.14.1 Definition of the Problem

The clinician may be faced with the dilemma of attempting to predict the visual outcome in a case of diabetic retinopathy complicated by diabetic macular ischemia. For example, a patient may present with a combination of diabetic macular edema and ischemia, or combined preretinal membrane and macular ischemia. In these situations a general determination must be made regarding the visual potential in order to weigh various management options. The following exercise is designed to explore the confidence of the clinician in predicting the best corrected visual acuity based on the magnitude of macular capillary dropout (Fig. 16.53).

A 73-year-old man has had type 2 diabetes mellitus for 11 years and hypertension for 25 years. He has had multiple focal/grid macular laser and panretinal photocoagulation treatments in the past and is bilaterally pseudophakic. Presently, there is no evidence of diabetic macular edema (DME) detected by fundoscopy or optical coherence tomography (Fig. 16.53). What visual acuity would you predict based on the degree of macular capillary

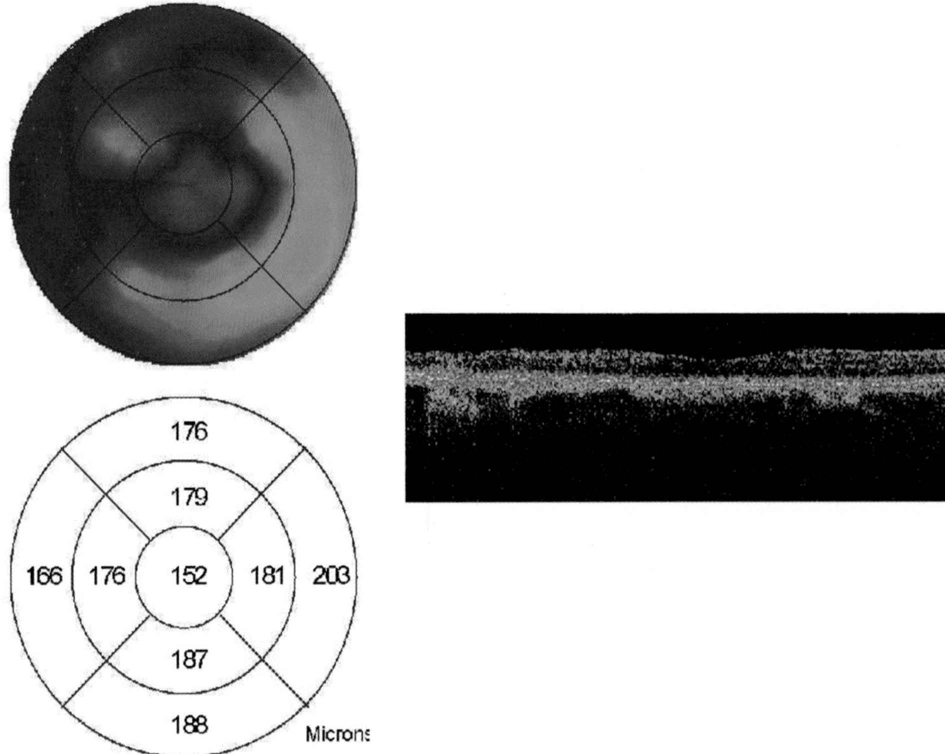

Fig. 16.53 Optical coherence tomography of the right eye of case 14

[m] Discussed by Scott E. Pautler, M.D.

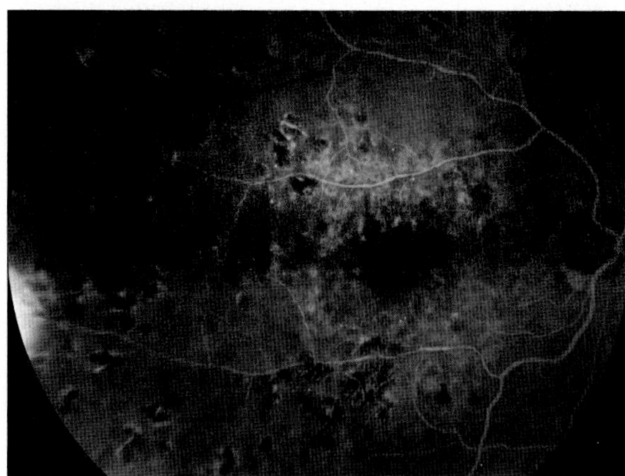

Fig. 16.54 Early-phase frame of the fluorescein angiogram from the right eye of case 14

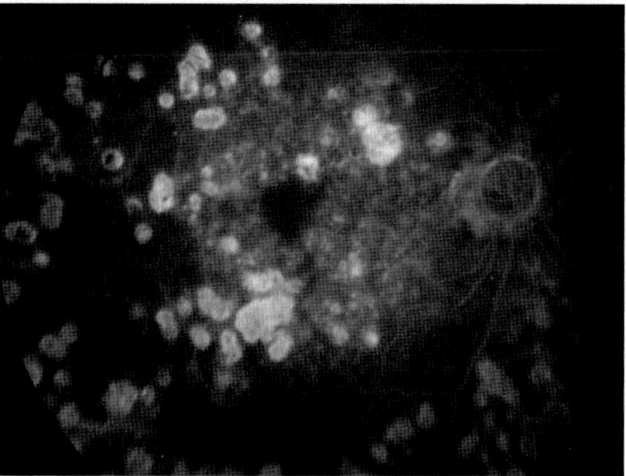

Fig. 16.55 Late-phase frame from the fluorescein angiogram of the right eye of case 14

nonperfusion shown on the fluorescein angiogram (Figs. 16.54 and 16.55)?

16.14.2 Discussion

This patient has severe diabetic macular ischemia. The optical coherence tomogram (OCT) shows loss of inner retinal structural details as shown on the line scan and generalized thinning of the macula is evident on the false color map. The central subfield macular thickness (CSMT) is remarkably reduced at 152 μm. There is no evidence of preretinal membrane or vitreomacular traction. Although we cannot rule out the possibility of permanent structural damage from past DME, there is no sign of degenerative cystic change. The early-phase fluorescein angiogram (FA) reveals no significant central macular defects in the retinal pigment epithelium. Central macular capillary nonperfusion is detected on the late phase of the FA as an area of relative hypofluorescence surrounded by low-grade diffuse leakage of fluorescein. Although the area of the foveal avascular zone is not given, it appears to be approximately equal to one disc area (1.77 mm^2). Thus, the primary vision-limiting factor for this eye is diabetic macular ischemia (DMI).

The chapter authors who independently reviewed this case were asked to comment on their ability to predict the visual acuity based on the presence of severe DMI. In general, the doctors expressed a fairly low confidence in their ability to reliably predict the visual acuity of this patient. Doctor A commented on the irregularity of the foveal avascular zone (FAZ), but interpreted the OCT as showing a "relatively physiologic foveal architecture." He predicted a range of visual acuity from 20/40 to 20/300. Doctor B estimated the diameter of the irregular FAZ to be 1,000–1,700 μm, which he interpreted to be consistent with 20/100 to 20/300 vision. Doctor C expressed a very low confidence in predicting vision by offering a range from 20/40 to count fingers. The actual best corrected visual acuity in this case was 20/100.

The literature offers limited information regarding the impact of diabetic macular ischemia on visual acuity. The most specific data correlating visual acuity with FAZ area was published by Arend et al.,[117] who studied diabetic eyes with video-fluorescein angiography using a scanning laser ophthalmoscope for high-resolution images of the foveal avascular zone. Image analysis software was used to calculate the area of the FAZ in a masked fashion without prior knowledge of the visual acuity. In their study, decreased visual acuity correlated significantly with increasing FAZ area ($R^2 = 0.51$). Visual acuity less than 20/50 was found to be consistent with an FAZ $\geq$ 0.55 mm^2. Their study was limited to 30 diabetic eyes and showed considerable latitude in visual acuity for any given FAZ area measurement (Fig. 8.16). Thus, it is not surprising that there was such a wide range on opinions among the authors who responded to this exercise.[n]

[n] Discussed by Scott E. Pautler, M.D.

References

1. O'Hanley GP, Canny CLB. Diabetic dense premacular hemorrhage. A possible indication for prompt vitrectomy. *Ophthalmology*. 1985;92:507–511.
2. Raymond LA. Neodymium. YAG laser treatment for hemorrhages under the internal limiting membrane and posterior hyaloid face of the macula. *Ophthalmology*. 1995;102:406–411.
3. Yang CM, Chen MS. Tissue plasminogen activator and gas for diabetic premacular hemorrhage. *Am J Ophthalmol*. 2000;129:393–394.
4. Shih CW, Yang CM, Chen MS, Wang TJ. Intravitreal injection of bevacizumab and gas for diabetic premacular hemorrhage and active fibrovascular proliferation. *Graefe's Arch Clin Exp Ophthalmol*. 2008;246: 1547–1551.
5. Dayani PN, Grand MG. Maintenance of warfarin anticoagulation for patients undergoing vitreoretinal surgery. *Arch Ophthalmol*. 2006;124:1558–1565.
6. Fu AD, McDonald HR, Williams DF, et al. Anticoagulation with warfarin in vitreoretinal surgery. *Retina*. 2007; 27:290–295.
7. Charles S, Rosenfeld PJ, Gayer S. Medical consequences of stopping anticoagulant therapy before intraocular surgery or intravitreal injections. *Retina*. 2007;27:813–815.
8. Mason JO III, Nixon PA, White MF. Intravitreal injection of bevacizumab (avastin) as adjunctive treatment of proliferative diabetic retinopathy. *Am J Ophthalmol*. 2006;142:685–688.
9. Arevalo JF, Maia M, Flynn HW Jr, et al. Tractional retinal detachment following intravitreal bevacizumab (Avastin) inpatients with severe proliferative diabetic retinopathy. *Br J Ophthalmol*. 2007;92:213–216.
10. Joussen AM, Joeres S. Benefits and limitations in vitreoretinal surgery for proliferative diabetic retinopathy and macular edema. *Dev Ophthalmol*. 2007;39:69–87.
11. Kroll P, Gerding H, Busse H. Retinale proliferationen als komplikation retinaler chirurgie mit silikonoltamponade. *Klin Monatsbl Augenheilkd*. 1989;195:145–149.
12. Lucke KH, Foerster MH, Laqua H. Long -term results of vitrectomy and silicone oil in 500 cases of complicated retinal detachments. *Am J Ophthalmol*. 1987;104:624–633.
13. La Heij EC, Tecim S, Kessels AGH, Liem ATA, Japing WJ, Hendrikse F. Clinical variables and their relation to visual outcome after vitrectomy in eyes with retinal traction detachment. *Graefe's Arch Clin Exp Ophthalmol*. 2004;242:210–217.
14. Flynn HW, Chew EY, Simons BD, Barton FB, Remaley NA. Pars plana vitrectomy in the early treatment diabetic retinopathy study. ETDRS report number 17. The early treatment diabetic retinopathy study research group. *Ophthalmology*. 1992;99:1351–1357.
15. The Diabetic Retinopathy Vitrectomy Study Research Group. Early vitrectomy for severe vitreous hemorrhage in diabetic retinopathy. *Arch Ophthalmol*. 1985;103: 1644–1652.
16. Ho T, Smiddy WE, Flynn HW Jr. Vitrectomy in the management of diabetic eye disease. *Surv Ophthalmol*. 1992;37:190–202.
17. Azen SP, Scott IU, Flynn HW, et al. Silicone oil in the repair of complex retinal detachments. A prospective observational multicenter study. *Ophthalmology*. 1998; 105:1587–1597.
18. Castellarin A, Grigorian R, Bhagat N, et al. Vitrectomy with silicone oil infusion in severe diabetic retinopathy. *Br J Ophthalmol*. 2003;87:318–321.
19. Michels RG, Wilkinson CP, Rice TA. Vitreous surgery. In: Klein EA ed. *Retinal Detachment*. 1st ed. St. Louis, Mo: CV Mosby Co; 1990:Chap. 13.
20. Imamura Y, Minami M, Ueki M, et al. Use of perfluorocarbon liquid during vitrectomy for severe proliferative diabetic retinopathy. *Br J Ophthalmol*. 2003;87:563–566.
21. Oshima Y, Sima C, Wakabayashi T, et al. Microincision vitrectomy surgery and intravitreal bevacizumab as a surgical adjunct to treat diabetic traction retinal detachment. *Ophthalmology*. 2009;116:927–938.
22. Avery RL. Regression of retinal and iris neovascularization after intravitreal bevacizumab (Avastin) treatment. *Retina*. 2006;26:352–356.
23. Avery RL, Pearlman J, Pieramici DJ, et al. Intravitreal bevacizumab (Avastin) in the treatment of proliferative diabetic retinopathy. *Ophthalmology*. 2006;113: 1695–1705.
24. Murakami Y, Kusaka S, Oshima Y, et al. Diagnostic and therapeutic challenges. *Retina*. 2008;28:1357–1360.
25. Diabetes Control and Complications Trial Research Group. Progression of retinopathy with intensive versus conventional treatment in the diabetes control and complications trial. *Ophthalmology*. 1995;102:647–661.
26. UK Prospective Diabetes Study (UKPDS) Group. Intensive blood-glucose control with sulphonylureas or insulin compared with conventional treatment and risk of complications in patients with type 2 diabetes (UKPDS 33). *Lancet*. 1998;352:837–853.
27. UK Prospective Diabetes Study Group. Tight blood pressure control and risk of macrovascular and microvascular complications of type 2 diabetes: UKPDS 38. *BMJ*. 1998;317:703–713.
28. Early Treatment Diabetic Retinopathy Study Research Group. Photocoagulation for diabetic macular edema-early treatment diabetic retinopathy study report number 1. *Arch Ophthalmol*. 1985;103(12):1796–1806.
29. The Diabetic Retinopathy Study Research Group. Four risk factors for severe visual loss in diabetic retinopathy. *Arch Ophthalmol*. 1979;97, 654–655.
30. McDonald HR, Schatz H. Macular edema following panretinal photocoagulation. *Retina*. 1985;5:5–10.
31. Bandello F, Polito A, Pognuz DR, Monaco P, Dimastrogiovanni A, Paissios J. Triamcinolone as adjunctive treatment to laser photocoagulation to laser panretinal photocoagulation for proliferative diabetic retinopathy. *Arch Ophthalmol*. 2006;124:643–650.
32. Hudson HL, Chong LP, Frambach DA, et al. Encircling panretinal laser photocoagulation may prevent macular detachment after vitrectomy for proliferative diabetic retinopathy. *Int Ophthalmol*. 1994;18:101–104.

33. DRS Research Group. Photocoagulation treatment of proliferative diabetic retinopathy: clinical application of Diabetic Retinopathy Study (DRS) findings. DRS Report #8. *Invest Ophthalmol Vis Sci*. 1981;88:583–600.
34. ETDRS Research Group. Early photocoagulation for diabetic retinopathy. ETDRS report #9. *Ophthalmology*. 1991;98:766–785.
35. DCCT Study Group. The relationship of glycemic exposure (Hgb A1c) to the risk of development and progression of diabetic retinopathy in the DCCT. *Diabetes*. 1995;44:968–983.
36. ETDRS Research Group. Early treatment diabetic retinopathy study design and baseline patient characteristics. ETDRS report #7. *Ophthalmology*. 1991;98:741–756.
37 Diabetic Retinopathy Clinical Research Network. Comparison of modified-ETDRS and mild macular grid laser photocoagulation strategies for diabetic macular edema. *Arch Ophthalmol*. 2007;125:469–480.
38. Massin P, Allouch C, Haouchine B, et al. Optical coherence tomography of idiopathic macular epiretinal membranes before and after surgery. *Am J Ophthalmol*. 2000; 130:732–739.
39. Massin P, Haouchine B, Gaudric A. Macular traction detachment and diabetic edema associated with posterior hyaloidal traction. *Am J Ophthalmol*. 2001;132:599.
40. Gupta A, Gupta V. Diabetic maculopathy and cataract surgery. *Ophthalmol Clin North Am*. 2001;14:625–637.
41. Browning DJ. Diabetic macular edema: a critical review of the Early Treatment Diabetic Retinopathy Study (ETDRS) series and subsequent studies. *Comp Ophthalmol Update*. 2000;1:69–83.
42. Dowler JGF, Sehmi KS, Hykin PG, Hamilton AMP. The natural history of macular edema after cataract surgery in diabetes. *Ophthalmology*. 1999;106:663–668.
43. Escaravage GK, Cohen KL, Patel SB, et al. Quantification of macular and optic disc hyperfluorescence after phacoemulsification in diabetes mellitus. *J Cataract Refract Surg*. 2006;32:803–811.
44. Otani T, Kishi S. Correlation between optical coherence tomography and fluorescein angiography findings in diabetic macular edema. *Ophthalmology*. 2007;114: 104–107.
45. Squirrell D, Bhola R, Bush J, Winder S, Talbot JF. A prospective, case controlled study of the natural history of diabetic retinopathy and maculopathy after uncomplicated phacoemulsification cataract surgery in patients with type 2 diabetes. *Br J Ophthalmol*. 2002; 86:565–571.
46. Gillies MC, Sutter FK, Simpson JM, et al. Intravitreal triamcinolone for refractory diabetic macular edema: two-year results of a double-masked, placebo-controlled, randomized clinical trial. *Ophthalmology*. 2006;113: 1533–1538.
47. Diabetic Retinopathy Clinical Research Network. A randomized trial comparing intravitreal triamcinolone acetonide and focal/grid photocoagulation for diabetic macular edema. *Ophthalmology*. 2008;115(9): 1447–1449.
48. Arevalo JF, Garcia-Amaris RA, Roca JA, et al. Primary intravitreal bevacizumab for the management of pseudophakic cystoid macular edema: pilot study of the Pan-American collaborative retina study group. *J Cataract Refract Surg*. 2007;33:2098–2105.
49. Mason JO III, Albert MA Jr, Vail R. Intravitreal bevacizumab (Avastin) for refractory pseudophakic cystoid macular edema. *Retina*. 2006;26:356–358.
50. Johnson MW. Etiology and treatment of macular edema. *Am J Ophthalmol*. 2009;147:11–21.
51. Cervera E, Diaz-Llopis M, Udaondo P, Garcia-Delpech S. Intravitreal pegaptanib sodium for refractory pseudophakic macular edema. *Eye*. 2008;22:1180–1182.
52. Cheema RA, Al-Mubarak MM, Amin YM, Cheema MA. Role of combined cataract surgery and intravitreal bevacizumab injection in preventing progression of diabetic retinopathy. A prospective randomized study. *J Cataract Refract Surg*. 2009;35:18–25.
53. Paccola L, Costa RA, Folgosa MS, et al. Intravitreal triamcinolone versus bevacizumab for treatment of refractory diabetic macular oedema (IBEME study). *Br J Ophthalmol*. 2008;92:76–80.
54. Wade EC, Blankenship GW. The effect of short versus long exposure times of argon laser panretinal photocoagulation on proliferative diabetic retinopathy. *Graefe's Arch Clin Exp Ophthalmol*. 1990; 228:226–231.
55. Ryan SJ. Traction retinal detachment. XLIX Edward Jackson Memorial Lecture. *Am J Ophthalmol*. 1993;115:1–20.
56. Larsson LI, Nuija E. Increased permeability of the blood-aqueous barrier after panretinal photocoagulation for proliferative diabetic retinopathy. *Acta Ophthalmol Scand*. 2001;79:414–416.
57. Foos RY, Kreiger AE, Nofsinger K. Pathologic study following vitrectomy for proliferative diabetic retinopathy. *Retina*. 1985;5:101–106.
58. El-Batarny AM. Intravitreal bevacizumab as an adjunctive therapy before diabetic vitrectomy. Clin Ophthalmol. 2008;2:709–716.
59. Kim JE, Pollack JS, Miller DG, Mittra RA, Spaide RF, ISIS Study Group. ISIS-DME. A prospective, randomized, dose-escalation intravitreal steroid injection study for refractory diabetic macular edema. *Retina*. 2008;28:735–740.
60. Early Treatment Diabetic Retinopathy Study Research Group. Treatment techniques and clinical guidelines for photocoagulation of diabetic macular edema-Early treatment diabetic retinopathy study report number 2. *Ophthalmology*. 1987;94:761–774.
61. Diabetic Retinopathy Clinical Research Network, Scott IU, Edwards AR, Beck RW, Bressler NM, Chan CK et al. A phase II randomized clinical trial of intravitreal bevacizumab for diabetic macular edema. *Ophthalmology*. 2007;114:1860–1867.
62. Bailey CC, Sparrow JM, Grey RHB, Cheng H. The national diabetic retinopathy laser treatment audit. I. maculopathy. *Eye*. 1998;12:69–76.
63. Akduman L, Olk RJ. Subthreshold (invisible) modified grid diode laser photocoagulation in diffuse diabetic macular edema (DDME). *Ophthalmic Surg Lasers Imaging*. 1999;30:706–714.
64. Schatz H, Madeira D, McDonald R, Johnson R. Progressive enlargement of laser scars following grid laser photocoagulation for diffuse diabetic macular edema. *Arch Ophthalmol*. 1991;109:1549–1551.

65. Finkelstein D. Ischemic macular edema recognition and favorable natural history in branch vein occlusion. *Arch Ophthalmol.* 1992;110(10):1427–1434.
66. Early Treatment Diabetic Retinopathy Study Group. Classification of diabetic retinopathy from fluorescein angiograms. ETDRS Report Number 11. *Ophthalmology.* 1991;98:807–822.
67. Chew EY, Benson WE, Blodi BA, et al. *Diabetic Retinopathy Preferred Practice Pattern.* American Academy of Ophthalmology; 2008.
68. Patz A, Smith RE. The ETDRS and diabetes 2000. *Ophthalmology.* 1991;98:739–740.
69. Browning DJ, Glassman AR, Aiello LP, et al. Relationship between optical coherence tomography-measured central retinal thickness and visual acuity in diabetic macular edema. *Ophthalmology.* 2007;114:525–536.
70. ETDRS Research Group. Treatment techniques and clinical guidelines for photocoagulation of diabetic macular edema. ETDRS Report # 2. *Ophthalmology.* 1987;94:761–774.
71. Early Treatment Diabetic Retinopathy Study Research Group. Focal photocoagulation treatment of diabetic macular edema-relationship of treatment effect to fluorescein angiographic and other retinal characteristics at baseline: ETDRS report number 19. *Arch Ophthalmol.* 1995;113:1144–1155.
72. Martidis A, Duker JS, Greenberg PB, et al. Intravitreal triamcinolone for refractory diabetic macular edema. *Ophthalmology.* 2002;109:920–927.
73. Arevalo JF, Fromow-Guerra J, Quiroz-Mercado H et al. Primary intravitreal bevacizumab (Avastin) for diabetic macular edema: results from the Pan-American Collaborative Retina Study Group at 6-month follow-up. *Ophthalmology.* 2007;114:743–750.
74. McDonald HR, Schatz H. Visual loss following panretinal photocoagulation for proliferative diabetic retinopathy. *Ophthalmology.* 1985;92:388–393.
75. Higgins KE, Meyers SM, Jaffe MJ, Roy MS, de Monasterio FM. Temporary loss of foveal contrast sensitivity associated with panretinal photocoagulation. *Arch Ophthalmol.* 1986;104:997–1003.
76. Browning DJ, McOwen MD, Bowen RM Jr, O'Marah TL. Comparison of the clinical diagnosis of diabetic macular edema with diagnosis by optical coherence tomography. *Ophthalmology.* 2004;111:712–715.
77. Diabetic Retinopathy Clinical Research Network. Randomized trial of peribulbar triamcinolone acetonide with and without focal photocoagulation for mild diabetic macular edema. A pilot study. *Ophthalmology.* 2007;114:1190–1196.
78. Jonas JB, Degenring R, Kreissig I, Akkoyun I. Safety of intravitreal high-dose reinjections of triamcinolone acetonide. *Am J Ophthalmol.* 2004;138:1054–1055.
79. Gillies MC, Kuzniarz M, Craig J, Ball M, Luo W, Simpson JM. Intravitreal triamcinolone-induced elevated intraocular pressure is associated with the development of posterior subcapsular cataract. *Ophthalmology.* 2005;112:139–143.
80. Gillies MC, Simpson JM, Billson FA, et al. Safety of an intravitreal injection of triamcinolone: results from a randomized clinical trial. *Arch Ophthalmol.* 2004;122: 336–340.
81. Moshfeghi DM, Kaiser PK, Scott IU, et al. Acute endophthalmitis following intravitreal triamcinolone acetonide injection. *Am J Ophthalmol.* 2003;136: 791–796.
82. Shimura M, Nakazawa T, Yasuda K, et al. Comparative therapy evaluation of intravitreal bevacizumab and triamcinolone acetonide on persistent diffuse diabetic macular edema. *Am J Ophthalmol.* 2008 May;145(5): 854–861. Epub 2008 Mar 6.
83. Diabetic Retinopathy Clinical Research Network. Observational study of the development of diabetic macular edema following panretinal (scatter) photocoagulation given in 1 or 4 sittings. *Arch Ophthalmol.* 2009; 127:132–140.
84. Takagi H, Otani A, Kiryu J, Ogura Y. New surgical approach for removing massive foveal hard exudates in diabetic macular edema. *Ophthalmology.* 1999;106(2): 249–256; discussion 56-7.
85. Beck RW, Edwards AR, Aiello LP, et al. Three-year follow-up of a randomized trial comparing focal/grid photocoagulation and intravitreal triamcinolone for diabetic macular edema. *Arch Ophthalmol.* 2009;127(3):245–251.
86. Ozkiris A. Intravitreal bevacizumab (Avastin) for primary treatment of diabetic macular oedema. *Eye.* 2009; 23(3):616–620.
87. Soheilian M, Ramezani A, Bijanzadeh B, et al. Intravitreal bevacizumab (avastin) injection alone or combined with triamcinolone versus macular photocoagulation as primary treatment of diabetic macular edema. *Retina.* 2007;27(9):1187–1195.
88. Kook D, Wolf A, Kreutzer T, et al. Long-term effect of intravitreal bevacizumab (avastin) in patients with chronic diffuse diabetic macular edema. *Retina.* 2008; 28(8):1053–1060.
89. Kumar A, Sinha S. Intravitreal bevacizumab (Avastin) treatment of diffuse diabetic macular edema in an Indian population. *Indian J Ophthalmol.* 2007;55(6):451–455.
90. Arevalo JF, Sanchez JG, Fromow-Guerra J, et al. Comparison of two doses of primary intravitreal bevacizumab (Avastin) for diffuse diabetic macular edema: results from the Pan-American Collaborative Retina Study Group (PACORES) at 12-month follow-up. *Graefes Arch Clin Exp Ophthalmol.* 2009;247(6):735–743.
91. Schwartz SG, Flynn HW, Jr. Pharmacotherapies for diabetic retinopathy: present and future. *Exp Diabetes Res.* 2007;2007:52487.
92. Xie XW, Xu L, Wang YX, Jonas JB. Prevalence and associated factors of diabetic retinopathy. The Beijing Eye Study 2006. *Graefes Arch Clin Exp Ophthalmol.* 2008;246(11):1519–1526.
93. Spandau UH, Derse M, Schmitz-Valckenberg P, Papoulis C, Jonas JB. Dosage dependency of intravitreal triamcinolone acetonide as treatment for diabetic macular oedema. *Br J Ophthalmol.* 2005;89(8):999–1003.
94. Chieh JJ, Roth DB, Liu M, et al. Intravitreal triamcinolone acetonide for diabetic macular edema. *Retina.* 2005;25(7):828–834.
95. Martidis A, Duker JS, Greenberg PB, et al. Intravitreal triamcinolone for refractory diabetic macular edema. *Ophthalmology.* 2002;109(5):920–927.
96. Soheilian M, Ramezani A, Obudi A, et al. Randomized trial of intravitreal bevacizumab alone or combined with

triamcinolone versus macular photocoagulation in diabetic macular edema. *Ophthalmology*. 2009;116(6):1142–1150.

97. Kang SW, Sa HS, Cho HY, Kim JI. Macular grid photocoagulation after intravitreal triamcinolone acetonide for diffuse diabetic macular edema. *Arch Ophthalmol*. 2006;124(5):653–658.
98. Iida T. Combined triamcinolone acetonide injection and grid laser photocoagulation: a promising treatment for diffuse diabetic macular oedema? *Br J Ophthalmol*. 2007;91(4):407–408.
99. Takaya K, Suzuki Y, Mizutani H, Sakuraba T, Nakazawa M. Long -term results of vitrectomy for removal of submacular hard exudates in patients with diabetic maculopathy. *Retina*. 2004;24(1):23–29.
100. Avci R, Inan UU, Kaderli B. Long -term results of excision of plaque-like foveal hard exudates in patients with chronic diabetic macular oedema. *Eye*. 2008;22(9): 1099–1104.
101. Larsson J, Kifley A, Zhu M, et al. Rapid reduction of hard exudates in eyes with diabetic retinopathy after intravitreal triamcinolone: data from a randomized, placebo-controlled, clinical trial. *Acta Ophthalmol*. 2009;87(3):275–280.
102. Cunningham MA, Edelman JL, Kaushal S. Intravitreal steroids for macular edema: the past, the present, and the future. *Surv Ophthalmol*. 2008;53(2):139–149.
103. Early Treatment Diabetic Retinopathy Study Research Group. Early photocoagulation for diabetic retinopathy. ETDRS report number 9. Early Treatment Diabetic Retinopathy Study Research Group. *Ophthalmology*. 1991;98(5 Suppl):766–785.
104. The Early Treatment Diabetic Retinopathy Study Research Group. Techniques for scatter and local photocoagulation treatment of diabetic retinopathy: Early Treatment Diabetic Retinopathy Study Report no. 3. The Early Treatment Diabetic Retinopathy Study Research Group. *Int Ophthalmol Clin*. 1987;27(4): 254–264.
105. Aylward GW, Pearson RV, Jagger JD, Hamilton AM. Extensive argon laser photocoagulation in the treatment of proliferative diabetic retinopathy. *Br J Ophthalmol*. 1989;73(3):197–201.
106. Vine AK. The efficacy of additional argon laser photocoagulation for persistent, severe proliferative diabetic retinopathy. *Ophthalmology*. 1985;92(11): 1532–1537.
107. Yeh PT, Yang CM, Yang CH, Huang JS. Cryotherapy of the anterior retina and sclerotomy sites in diabetic vitrectomy to prevent recurrent vitreous hemorrhage: an ultrasound biomicroscopy study. *Ophthalmology*. 2005;112(12):2095–2102.
108. Mosier MA, Del PE, Gheewala SM. Anterior retinal cryotherapy in diabetic vitreous hemorrhage. *Am J Ophthalmol*. 1985;100(3):440–444.
109. Neely KA, Scroggs MW, McCuen BW. Peripheral retinal cryotherapy for postvitrectomy diabetic vitreous hemorrhage in phakic eyes. *Am J Ophthalmol*. 1998; 126(1):82–90.
110. McLeod D. A chronic grey matter penumbra, lateral microvascular intussusception and venous peduncular avulsion underlie diabetic vitreous haemorrhage. *Br J Ophthalmol*. 2007;91(5):677–689.
111. Mason JO, III, Yunker JJ, Vail R, McGwin G, Jr. Intravitreal bevacizumab (Avastin) prevention of panretinal photocoagulation-induced complications in patients with severe proliferative diabetic retinopathy. *Retina*. 2008;28(9):1319–1324.
112. Arevalo JF, Maia M, Flynn HW Jr, et al. Tractional retinal detachment following intravitreal bevacizumab (Avastin) in patients with severe proliferative diabetic retinopathy. *Br J Ophthalmol*. 2008;92(2):213–216.
113. Early Treatment Diabetic Retinopathy Study Research Group. Early photocoagulation for diabetic retinopathy. ETDRS report number 9. Early Treatment Diabetic Retinopathy Study Research Group. *Ophthalmology*. 1991;98(5 Suppl):766–785.
114. Yang CM, Su PY, Yeh PT, Chen MS. Combined rhegmatogenous and traction retinal detachment in proliferative diabetic retinopathy: clinical manifestations and surgical outcome. *Can J Ophthalmol*. 2008;43(2): 192–198.
115. The Diabetes Control and Complications Trial Research Group. The effect of intensive treatment of diabetes on the development and progression of long-term complications in insulin-dependent diabetes mellitus. The Diabetes Control and Complications Trial Research Group. *N Engl J Med*. 1993;329(14): 977–986.
116. Matthews DR, Stratton IM, Aldington SJ, Holman RR, Kohner EM. Risks of progression of retinopathy and vision loss related to tight blood pressure control in type 2 diabetes mellitus: UKPDS 69. *Arch Ophthalmol*. 2004;122(11):1631–1640.
117. Arend O, Wolf S, Harris A, Reim M. The relationship of macular microcirculation to visual acuity in diabetic patients. *Arch Ophthalmol*. 1995;113:610–614.

Subject Index

D.J. Browning (ed.), *Diabetic Retinopathy*, DOI 10.1007/978-0-387-85900-2,

D

E

Printed in the United States of America